Dental Materials

Clinical Applications for Dental Assistants and Dental Hygienists

FOURTH EDITION

Dental Materials

Clinical Applications for Dental Assistants and Dental Hygienists

W. STEPHAN EAKLE, DDS, FADM

Professor of Clinical Dentistry Emeritus,
Department of Preventive and Restorative Dental Sciences,
School of Dentistry, University of California,
San Francisco, California

KIMBERLY G. BASTIN, CDA, EFDA, CRDH, MS

Assistant Professor and Director of Dental Hygiene,
State College of Florida Manatee-Sarasota,
Bradenton, Florida

ELSEVIER

3251 Riverport Lane
St. Louis, Missouri 63043

DENTAL MATERIALS: CLINICAL APPLICATIONS FOR DENTAL ASSISTANTS
AND DENTAL HYGIENISTS, FOURTH EDITION

ISBN: 978-0-323-59658-9

Previous editions copyrighted 2016, 2011, 2003.

Library of Congress Control Number: 2020900776

Content Strategist: Joslyn Dumas
Senior Content Development Manager: Luke Held
Senior Content Development Specialist: Kelly Skelton
Publishing Services Manager: Deepthi Unni
Senior Project Manager: Manchu Mohan
Design Direction: Renee Duenow

Printed in India

Last digit is the print number: 9 8 7 6 5

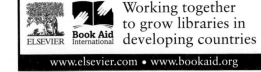

Reviewers

Jennifer Cooper, RRDH, BSc, MSc
Coordinator, Dental Assisting
Fanshawe College
London, Ontario, Canada

Stephanie Meredith, RDH, BS, MSDH
Program Director, Sarah Whitaker Glass School of Dental
    Hygiene
West Liberty University
West Liberty, West Virginia

Kathy Ann Pierce, CDA, RDA, EFDA, BS
Faculty, Health Sciences
Western Iowa Tech Community College
Sioux City, Iowa

Amanda R. Reddington, LDH, MHA, CDA, EFDA
Clinical Assistant Professor Dental Assisting and Dental
    Hygiene
University of Southern Indiana
Evansville, Indiana

Preface

LIFELONG LEARNING

The subject of dental materials is rapidly changing as researchers and manufacturers develop new materials and improve those currently in use. Consequently, dental hygienists and dental assistants are challenged to keep up with the new materials, their physical properties, their handling characteristics, and their clinical applications. As important members of the dental team, they must be adept at placing or assisting in the placement of dental materials, and they play a valuable role in the maintenance of dental materials once they are in the mouth. Dental hygienists and dental assistants also are instrumental in educating patients in the home maintenance of restorations and prostheses and what to expect with a new prosthesis. As allied oral health providers, dental hygienists and dental assistants play major roles in preventive education and therapy in most practices. To stay current, they must be lifelong learners who know how to use available resources to update their knowledge. *Dental Materials: Clinical Applications for Dental Assistants and Dental Hygienists* provides the foundation for that lifelong learning for the new student and serves as an important update on new materials and improvements in materials for the practicing assistant or hygienist. In addition, it provides them with sound criteria for evaluating steps in the restorative process in which they will play a role, such as making accurate alginate and elastomeric impressions, cord retraction and selection and application of a matrix for composite and amalgam.

KEY GOALS

The goal of *Dental Materials: Clinical Applications for Dental Assistants and Dental Hygienists* is to provide students with the following:
- The principles of dental materials so they can understand the rationale for the use of these materials
- The opportunity to apply newly gained knowledge through clinical and laboratory procedures
- The ability to evaluate their work using accepted criteria
- The opportunity to test their knowledge and prepare for board examinations
- The opportunity to apply critical thinking through the use of case-based discussion questions

FEATURES

The chapters have the following components:
- **Learning and performance objectives** to guide students in learning.
- **Key terms** listed and defined in the order of their presentation in the chapters and highlighted in the chapters in colored print.
- **Basic principles and applications, physical properties, and handling characteristics** of the dental materials presented in each chapter.
- **Generous use of color illustrations and photography throughout to aid learning.**
- **Helpful clinical tips or precautions** regarding the use of the materials, highlighted in boxes set apart from the main text for emphasis.
- **Illustrated clinical and laboratory procedures** presented in step-by-step instructions so that students can practice common applications of the materials. Notes at the top of the procedure sheets guide the clinician as to precautions for patients or clinicians and alert the clinician when procedures may not be allowed by all state dental boards.
- **Competency assessment forms** for each procedure to test skills attainment located on the Evolve website.
- **Review questions** to enable students to test their comprehension of the subject matter and prepare for examinations; answers are provided at the end of the book.
- **Case-based discussion topics** that encourage students to relate what they have learned to the actual application in the dental office. Instructors may want to use them as topics for group discussions.
- **Reference lists** at the end of each chapter to help students find additional information about the principles, procedures and properties of the dental materials discussed.
- **Links to instructional videos are available on the EVOLVE website** to enhance and reinforce materials presented.

NEW TO THIS EDITION

- New illustrations and clinical photographs throughout
- Additional instructional videos with links found on the Evolve website to supplement learning from the text
- New Clinical tips and Cautions
- Bioactive dental materials are presented

- Expanded information on staining and glazing ceramic restorations
- Additional information on mercury safety practices
- Enhanced information on amalgam matrix and wedge placement
- Illustrated information on the crystalline structure of metals
- CAD/CAM technology applied to implant planning, placement and restoration including digital impressions
- Air polishing for implant cleaning: indications and contraindications
- Suture materials
- New illustrated procedures: removal of sutures; fabrication of custom impression trays with Triad material; making a wax bite registration; fluoride varnish application; and silver diamine fluoride application
- Luting cements have been reorganized according to their composition and the section on resin cements has been expanded to include more on self-adhesive resin cements
- The section on surgical dressings has been expanded and illustrated steps for placement and removal have been added
- A section on digital dentures explaining the use of CAD/CAM technology for denture construction.
- New information on detection and management of denture sores to aid home care
- Use of CAD/CAM Provisional Materials
- Introduction to 3-D printing
- Introduction to probiotics
- Expansion of information on whitening products
- Expansion of information on fluoride varnish, and new material on silver diamine fluoride
- Expanded information on powders utilized in air polishing to include glycine and erythritol
- Expansion of information on thumb sucking devices, palatal expanders, and crossbite correctors.

EVOLVE

An expanded Evolve website is key to this edition. The Evolve website provides a variety of resources for both instructors and students.

FOR INSTRUCTORS

- TEACH Instructor's Resource Manual (includes answer keys, lesson plans, PowerPoints, and student handouts)
- Test Bank
- Image Collection

FOR STUDENTS

- Practice Quizzes
- Competency forms
- Instructional video links

A NOTE TO EDUCATORS

Dental Materials: Clinical Applications for Dental Assistants and Dental Hygienists is written to be easily comprehended by students with varying amounts of science in their educational backgrounds. Learning and performance **objectives** draw the students' attention to the important concepts and features of the materials. **Key terms** are not only listed but also defined at the start of each chapter. Helpful **clinical tips** are used throughout the chapters to call attention to clinical points to which the student may not have been exposed, and **cautions** are noted where appropriate for the safety of both the patient and the clinician. The book is generously illustrated to help with the comprehension of clinical and **laboratory procedures**, especially for our visual learners. The procedures help the students to see how the materials are actually used, and when students apply their newly gained knowledge, the procedures reinforce learning. **Review questions** help reinforce what the students have learned and help prepare them for board examinations. **Case-based discussion** topics can be used for group discussions and bring the flavor of real-life dentistry to the application of dental materials.

Additional material is included on the Evolve website. **Chapter quizzes** (270 total questions) help students prepare for classroom and board exams. **Competencies** are included for each procedure so that students can evaluate their own efforts and also receive feedback from their instructors.

YOUR COMMENTS, PLEASE

The authors would appreciate suggestions or comments regarding this book because it is written with your needs in mind. We hope instructors and students will enjoy this book and gain as much from it as we have intended.

W. Stephan Eakle, Stephan.
Stephan.Eakle@ucsf.edu
Kimberly G. Bastin
bastink@scf.edu

Acknowledgments

The authors express their appreciation to the many people whose contributions to this edition were invaluable. We thank the dental researchers and clinicians upon whose work this book is based. We thank them for clinical illustrations that enhance the quality of this edition and help the learner to visualize what cannot be defined solely by the written word. We thank our colleagues for their expertise and suggestions. We thank the dental manufacturers who provided technical information on dental materials and relevant illustrated procedures. Without your assistance this edition would not have been complete.

The authors thank the editorial team at Elsevier, in particular Joslyn Dumas, Luke Held, Kelly Skelton and Manchu Mohan for their commitment, encouragement, and tireless efforts in bringing this fourth edition to fruition.

A special thanks to our family members Sheila Eakle, Rachel, Olivia, Sam and Emi for your energy and inspiration; to Jimmy Bastin who continually provided encouragement, feedback, guidance, and support; to Toni McLeroy a friend and colleague who is always a positive influence and cheerleader; and our friends, and colleagues for their patience when we were not available to them and for their enthusiastic and endless support throughout this endeavor.

We also owe a debt of gratitude to previous authors, Bill Bird and Carol Hatrick, who provided the initial impetus to write this book and devoted countless hours to conceiving and writing previous editions. We thank you for your dedication and superb efforts on behalf of students and educators.

To all of you we remain most grateful.

Contents

Introduction to Dental Materials

Chapter Objectives

Upon completion of this chapter, the student should be able to:

1. Discuss the importance of the study of dental materials for the allied oral health practitioner.
2. Discuss why it is necessary that the allied oral health practitioner have an understanding of dental materials in the delivery of dental care.
3. Discuss evidence-based decision-making (EBDM) as it relates to dental materials; what questions might you ask yourself or your practice to ensure you are increasing the potential for successful patient care outcomes?
4. Review the historical development of dental materials.
5. List and compare the agencies responsible for setting standards and specifications of dental materials.
6. Discuss the requirements necessary for a consumer product to qualify for the ADA Seal of Acceptance.

The study of dental materials (biomaterials) is the science covering the evolution, development, properties, manipulation, care, and evaluation of materials used in the treatment and prevention of dental diseases and the interactions of these materials with the tissues of the face and mouth. Specifically, it includes principles of engineering, chemistry, physics, and biology. Dental biomaterials science is continually evolving as dentistry keeps up with the requirements for delivering optimal health care while delivering minimally invasive dentistry.

The tooth and the tooth's supporting structure, esthetics, and function are important considerations for the patient's overall well being. The dentist, dental assistant, and dental hygienist should have a working knowledge of why materials behave as they do and how we can help to maximize their performance. Through the understanding of how the basic principles of biomaterials affect the choice, manipulation, patient education, and care of all materials used to assist in rendering dental services, the dental team can help to ensure the ultimate success of a patient's dental work and contribute to their quality of life.

THE ROLE OF THE DENTAL AUXILIARY IN THE USE OF DENTAL MATERIALS

Since 1970 efforts have been made to employ allied oral health practitioners (also referred to in text as dental auxiliaries), dental assistants, and dental hygienists, in the performance of intraoral tasks to efficiently deliver health care and to enhance the productivity of the dentist. Until 1970 only the dental hygienist was permitted to perform intraoral functions in all states. Although laws vary from state to state virtually every state has modified, updated, and made changes to its state restrictions to allow for the performance of intraoral procedures by all allied oral health practitioners.

At present, several states allow for the placement as well as care of restorative and other therapeutic agents in the patient's mouth by dental auxiliaries which includes the new category of advance practice dental therapist.

In the traditional role, the dental assistant is most directly responsible for the delivery of dental materials within specific guidelines outlined by the dental manufacturer while the dental hygienist's responsibilities more frequently include the care of the restorative material once it has been placed and the application of some therapeutic and preventive agents. Expanded function auxiliaries provide restorative services after the dentist has prepared the tooth for restoration. These services may include placement and carving or finishing of the restorative material, placement of retraction cord, and taking the preliminary impression for crown and bridge restorations and/or endodontic procedures. The dental therapist may provide basic preventive and restorative treatment to children and adults in affiliation with or under the general supervision of a dentist. Typically these dental therapists work primarily in settings that serve low socioeconomic populations or in a dental health professional shortage area. State regulations determine the training and scope of practice for the expanded function auxiliary and the dental therapist.

All oral health practitioners must have a complete understanding of the potential hazards in the manipulation and disposal of materials and be educated to handle them safely. Background knowledge of the basic principles of dental materials is also essential to appreciate the selection of a particular restoration or treatment procedure for individual patient application. It becomes, in many circumstances, the auxiliary's role to educate the patient in the reasons that the dentist has recommended a particular restorative or therapeutic material or the choices the patient may have for a particular circumstance.

Dental materials are classified as preventive, restorative, or therapeutic materials. The search for the perfect material, designed to prevent disease, treat disease, or restore tooth structures, continues to elude the profession. There have been many important improvements in dental materials in recent years; however, despite these improvements, the ideal material does not yet exist. The perfect material would be biocompatible, esthetic, bond permanently to the tooth structures, and be useful in repairing or regenerating missing tissues.

This may seem an overwhelming task given the ever-growing variety and changes of materials available; recommendations for their use or disuse; and rapidly developing techniques in their manipulation, placement, and care. Professional journals, weblinks, dental materials manufacturers or manufacturer's representatives, and other resources can provide invaluable information. The knowledgeable dental auxiliary reviews products recommended and used by their office to provide a reliable resource for their patients and the dentist.

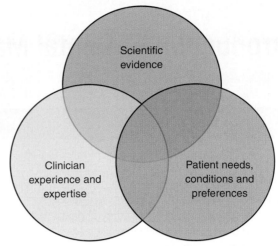

FIG. 1.1 The elements of evidence-based dentistry. (From Sakaguchi RL, Powers JM: *Craig's Restorative Dental Materials*, (ed 13). St. Louis, 2012, Mosby.)

EBDM into your practice: How does your practice make decisions regarding the techniques, technology, and products used? How do you analyze the published scientific literature to make sure a product provides a clinical benefit to the patient? Do you try product samples before giving them to your patients? How does your office stay informed about the newest advances in dentistry? How do you incorporate the patient's needs and choices into your decision-making process?

Evidence alone does not replace clinical expertise or input from the patient. EBDM requires an understanding of new concepts and the development of new skills. The clinician must be able to incorporate the best research evidence along with clinical expertise and patient preferences. Developing an evidence-based approach to addressing patient problems will greatly increase the potential for successful patient care outcomes by understanding the cause-and-effect relationship between biomaterials selected and the success of the treatment rendered. The ADA offers a website (http://ebd.ada.org/) for dentists and their patients to access the most current, clinically relevant information. This approach is based on scientific research and clinician expertise and is tailored to the patient's needs (Fig. 1.1).

Why Study Dental Materials?

To enhance safety: Appropriate handling and disposal of dental materials

To promote awareness: Awareness of the overall success of a particular material's properties in dental applications

To maintain materials properly: Recognition of dental materials present in oral cavity; effective cleaning, polishing, and instrumentation

To deliver correctly: Accurate knowledge of the behavior of a dental material on application, correct manipulation of material, effective delivery or assistance in delivery of material

To educate patients: Ability to present options concerning dental material choices, maintenance of materials present

---

EVIDENCED-BASED DENTISTRY

The American Dental Association (ADA) defines evidence-based dentistry as an approach to oral health care that requires the judicious integration of systematic assessments of clinically relevant scientific evidence, relating to the patient's oral medical history, with the dentist's clinical expertise and the patient's treatment needs and preferences. Searches through the scientific literature identify thousands of citations for materials and techniques in restoring and treating oral structures. With this wealth of scientific information, evidence-based decision-making (EBDM) helps the clinician make decisions about what is relevant to incorporate into practice. The following questions should be asked in order to appropriately incorporate

THE HISTORICAL DEVELOPMENT OF DENTAL MATERIALS

The concept of using materials for restoration, replacement, or beautification to alter the appearance and/or function of the natural dentition predates Christianity. Just as today, the diet of our caveman ancestors was a chief contributor to dental disease. Although they were rarely afflicted with dental caries because of the lack of refined sugars, excessive wear from a diet containing sand, dirt, and grit produced occlusal surfaces of teeth

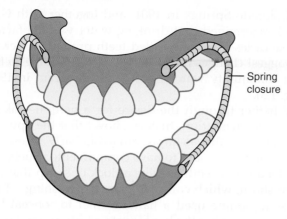

Spring closure

Spring closed denture

FIG. 1.2 A denture with spring closure, much like those worn by George Washington.

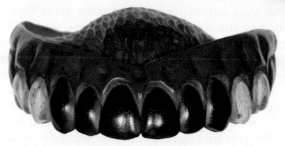

FIG. 1.3 A denture of carved black and white ivory teeth.

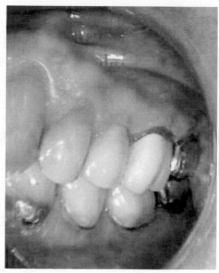

FIG. 1.4 Class V gold foil restoration on the facial surface of the mandibular first premolar.

often worn to the pulp with resultant abscess formation. Examination has revealed mummies that show loss of teeth due to abscess and periodontal disease as early as 2500 B.C.E. Research published in the *Proceedings of the National Academy of Sciences* has revealed the presence of toothpicks among the oldest known human fossils, dating 1.77 million years ago. Much is found in the literature about treatment options, including remedies based on potions and prayer, but no evidence of restorative dentistry exists until around 600 to 300 B.C.E. The Etruscans, who once lived in the area of present-day Tuscany, created bridges of gold rings and natural, as well as, cadaver teeth. By the Christian Era the Romans, who quite valued their teeth, had become skilled at restoring teeth with gold shells, fixed bridges, and partial and full dentures; although through the Middle Ages and into the mid-1800s most dental treatment consisted of extraction and artificial replacements.

Casts constructed of plaster from wax impressions were developed in Prussia in the mid-eighteenth century. Hippopotamus ivory bases with human and animal teeth replacements were popular. However, because it was so difficult to carve ivory and the denture bases did not fit well, retention of dentures was accomplished by joining the maxillary and mandibular dentures with springs forcing the two parts against the arches. Pierre Fauchard, considered the father of modern dentistry, devotes a portion of his book, The Surgeon-Dentist, published in 1728, to this technique. George Washington had several sets of such dentures, losing one tooth after another until, at the time of his inauguration in 1789, he had only one tooth left (Fig. 1.2). In France in the late 1700s, work was being done to improve denture teeth by firing them from porcelain. In 1788 King Louis XVI bestowed on a Parisian dentist an inventor's patent for porcelain teeth. For denture bases the Goodyear brothers gained a patent for rubber called vulcanite in 1844, and this remained

the primary denture base material until World War II. Dentures were made from many materials; depicted in (Fig. 1.3) is a denture base elaborately carved in wood with carved black and ivory teeth.

Silver paste is first mentioned by the Chinese in 659 C.E.; more than 1000 years later, in 1800, it was produced in France from "shavings from silver cut from coins mixed with enough mercury to form a sloppy paste." Health problems arising from the high mercury content of this early amalgam prompted the American Society of Dental Surgeons in 1846 to pass a resolution not to use amalgam under any circumstances. The disagreement over the value and safety of amalgam came to be called the "Amalgam War," and it did not end until 1895 when G.V. Black developed an acceptable amalgam formula.

Gold remained popular for the restoration and decoration of teeth and gained in popularity in 1855 when cohesive gold foil, which could be condensed directly into the cavity preparation, was introduced (Fig. 1.4). At the same time dental cements were introduced. Patterned after a technique for cementing tiles to floors, the first mixtures of cements, using zinc oxide with a weak phosphoric acid, were developed. In 1907, William Taggart demonstrated a casting method to produce gold inlays. In 1932 synthetic resins were introduced; these resins soon replaced rubber as the denture base of choice. At this time synthetic resins also became a popular tooth-colored alternative and, together with the introduction of the acid-etch technique in 1955, evolved into one of the most popular of the restorative materials, composite resins.

Preventive dentistry had an early beginning as well, with fluoride first mentioned in 1874 and dispensed in England at this time for the prevention of caries. Frederick McKay is credited with noting dental fluorosis

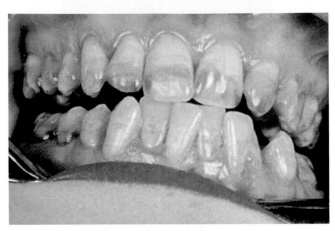

FIG. 1.5 Severe dental fluorosis.

in Colorado Springs in 1901, and together with G.V. Black determined that drinking water was the factor. These caries-free but mottled teeth prompted McKay to suggest changes in the water supply, leading to the first community water fluoridation program in 1945 (Fig. 1.5).

Whether through the desire for a natural look or more ornamentation, history shows that the appearance of the teeth was important to our early ancestors. King Solomon is said to have complimented Sheba on her teeth: "thy teeth are like a flock of sheep that are even shorn, which come up from the washing." Empress Josephine used a handkerchief to conceal her bad teeth, turning the hankie into a fashion accessory. In 1295 Marco Polo wrote of the people of southern China covering their teeth with thin plates of gold. This use of gold may have suggested the socioeconomic status of the individual as well as serving a protective purpose. In the mid-1800s, California railroad king Charles Crocker had a gold crown, embedded with diamonds to form the cusps, placed on one of his molars.

The history of dental materials and techniques in the restoration, replacement, and beautification of our teeth is full of ingenuity (Table 1.1). Even early man knew the importance of maintaining these important structures and more often than not suffered the pain

TABLE 1.1   Historical Development of Dental Materials

ERA	DEVELOPMENTS
Ancient times	600-300 B.C.E.—Etruscans practice dentistry with artificial teeth and gold work
Middle Ages	700—Chinese medical text mentions "silver paste" for replacement of tooth structure
Sixteenth century	1530—*The Little Medicinal Book for All Kinds of Diseases and Infirmities of the Teeth*, the first book devoted entirely to dentistry, is published in Germany. Written for barbers and surgeons who treated the mouth, it covers practical topics such as oral hygiene, tooth extraction, drilling teeth, and placement of gold fillings
Eighteenth century	Casts constructed of plaster and wax for the construction of dentures with finely carved ivory teeth, animal and cadaver teeth Pierre Fauchard introduces the technique of joining maxillary and mandibular dentures with springs and hinges. This was done to compensate for the weight of the dentures, which made retention of the maxillary denture virtually impossible Denture teeth fired from porcelain in France First dental assistant employed by C. Edmund Kells of New Orleans
Nineteenth century	Denture bases made of rubber by the Goodyear brothers Silver coins mixed with mercury as the first dental amalgam "Amalgam War"—American Society of Dental Surgeons passes a resolution not to use amalgam G.V. Black develops an acceptable amalgam formula Silicate cements developed for esthetic restorations Cohesive gold foil introduced
Twentieth century	Dr. William Taggart develops the method to cast gold inlays Dr. Alfred Fones opens the first school for dental hygienists Development of acrylic resin for fillings and dentures Fluoride placed in community drinking water Development of the acid-etch technique for bonding Composites replace silicate cements for esthetic restorations Light-activated composites Modern ceramics are developed for esthetic restorative alternatives First commercial home tooth-whitening product marketed

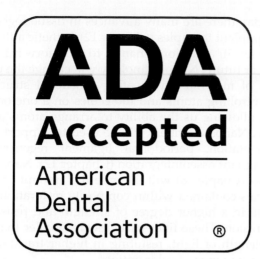

FIG. 1.6 The American Dental Association (ADA) Seal of Acceptance.

associated with their neglect. Through centuries of dental practice dental professionals have been challenged with the restoration of tooth and oral structures lost to disease and trauma.

THE AGENCIES RESPONSIBLE FOR STANDARDS

Most of the triumphs and atrocities of dentistry were discovered by trial and error, mainly at the expense of the patient. It is only in more recent times that the study of dental materials includes standards set forth to evaluate a material or technique before it is tried in the patient's mouth. In 1839 the first such attempt was made when the American Society of Dental Surgeons was formed to fight against the use of amalgam by forbidding its members to use silver amalgam for restoring lost tooth structure. In 1930 the first of the American Dental Association Specifications was for amalgam alloy.

AMERICAN DENTAL ASSOCIATION

Dentistry continued to try to elevate and regulate the practice of the profession with the establishment of the American Dental Association (ADA) in 1859. In 1866 an ADA committee prepared a statement on a toothpaste, claiming "it cut teeth like so much acid." By 1930, the ADA had established guidelines for testing products and awarded the first Seal of Acceptance in 1931 (Fig. 1.6). Members of the ADA's Council on Scientific Affairs and ADA staff scientists reviewed dental drugs, materials, instruments, and equipment for safety and effectiveness before awarding the ADA seal. The ADA seal has evolved since its inception; in 2005 the ADA decided to phase out the seal for professional products and to award it only to consumer products. Although the ADA review process is strictly a voluntary program, more than 300 consumer dental products carry the ADA Seal of Acceptance. Most common among these are toothpaste, toothbrushes, mouth rinses, floss and other interdental cleaners, sugar-free chewing gum, and denture adherents and cleansers.

The consumer and dentist alike recognize this important symbol of a dental product's safety and effectiveness. The ADA Seal of Acceptance is designed to help consumers make informed decisions about the safety and efficacy of products. Consumers can be confident in products bearing the ADA seal as these products have undergone voluntary and strict testing. The ADA review process outlines a broad spectrum of requirements that must be met to qualify for the ADA seal. A list of products and guidelines for qualification for the ADA Seal of Acceptance are available online at http://www.ada.org.

In July 2006, the ADA began a new program to evaluate professional dental products: the "ADA Professional Product Review." The *ADA Professional Product Review* is a newsletter which is mailed to ADA members quarterly with the *Journal of the American Dental Association*. This resource is a publication of the ADA's Council on Scientific Affairs and includes extensive laboratory performance data and clinician feedback.

The American National Standards Institute (ANIS) was founded in 1918. The mission of this not-for-profit organization is to enhance the global competitiveness of U.S. businesses while helping to ensure the safety and health of consumers and protection of the environment. The development of ANSI/ADA Specification Number 41, Recommended Standard Practices for Biological Evaluation of Dental Materials, represents the establishment of biological tests for dental materials.

U.S. FOOD AND DRUG ADMINISTRATION

The U.S. Food and Drug Administration (FDA) is one of the oldest consumer protection agencies and is charged with protecting the public by ensuring that products meet certain standards of safety and efficacy. The original Pure Food and Drug Act of 1906 did not include provisions to ensure medical and dental device safety or claims. In 1976 the Medical Device Amendments were signed to give the FDA regulatory authority over medical and dental devices that are now classified and regulated according to their degree of risk to the public. Dental materials, considered devices by the FDA, as well as over-the-counter products sold to the public, are subject to control and regulation by the FDA Center for Devices and Radiological Health. There are three classifications of medical (including dental) devices, grouped according to the amount of control needed to ensure their safety and efficacy:

Class I: Lowest risk, good manufacturing standards and record-keeping practices, materials such as examination gloves and prophylaxis (prophy) paste, and some over-the-counter products.

Class II: Products required to meet performance standards set by the FDA or ADA, products such as amalgam and composite materials.

Class III: The most regulated devices, which support or sustain human life; include such products as endosseous implants and bone-grafting materials. These require premarket approval of the FDA, involving scientific review to ensure their safety and effectiveness.

INTERNATIONAL AGENCIES

Two international agencies, the FDI World Dental Federation and the International Organization for Standardization (ISO), represent the standards used to develop specifications and testing at the international level. These standards are developed through the ISO's technical committee for dentistry (ISO/TC 106). In Canada's Medical Devices Regulations, dentistry manufacturers that apply for a license to distribute materials used in dentistry within Canada must provide a valid certificate showing that their quality management system complies with the ISO standard for quality systems (ISO 13485:2003). To receive such a certificate, manufacturing companies are audited to ensure their procedures are in line with requirements set out in the standard. These international standards are invaluable in supplying today's high demand for dental materials and devices.

There have been many advances in the quality and efficacy of dental materials; the challenge to dental professionals is to use evidence-based practice to critically review the claims, performance, and long-term end-product results of the materials and devices chosen. The input of the allied oral health practitioner is imperative in the successful choice of these materials to deliver quality service to the patient.

FUTURE DEVELOPMENTS IN DENTAL BIOMATERIALS

The dental materials used today are much better than those used in the past, but they are still far from being ideal. Materials continue to be developed and techniques in their manipulation improved. Despite much more effort in health promotion and disease prevention, dental caries is a major global public health problem. Dental restorations are still needed. The World Health Organization (WHO) and the United Nations Environment Programme (UNEP) meeting in 2010 has strengthened the work to reduce risks to human health and the environment from the use and release of mercury by recommending alternatives to amalgam containing restorations (Chapter 10). Periodontal disease continues to be a leading cause of tooth loss despite technologies to improve homecare and patient education. Advances in periodontal surgery, restorative dentistry, and implant therapies have enabled people to retain their teeth (Chapter 12). The demand for esthetics has driven the increase in whitening systems (Chapter 8), esthetic restorations (Chapters 6 and 9), and orthodontic procedures (Chapters 5 and 19).

Today there are many advances in tissue regeneration; implant therapies (Chapter 12); esthetic adhesion (Chapter 5); and biomechanics to look forward to in the near future. Nanotechnology will change the properties of materials by creating functional structures by controlling atoms and molecules on a one-on-one basis, allowing us the ability to arrange atoms as we desire. Nanoscale fibers will be used to support bone augmentation, periodontal ligament regeneration, and implant osseointegration (Chapter 12). Nanocomposites (Chapter 6) will increase the amount of filler particles contained within composite restorations, resulting in a higher degree of strength and resistance to abrasion. These filler particles are smaller than the wavelength of light, resulting in higher translucence and a vast range of color options.

The ADA, FDA, and ISO are committed to continuing to evaluate, test, monitor, and assess risks and review claims and labels of all materials used in dentistry (Chapter 4). Current research is concentrating on bringing technology to the dental office, making dental appointments faster, minimally invasive, and more comfortable for the patient and resulting in optimum patient-centered care. The allied oral health practitioner will continue to play an important role in the successful delivery, manipulation, and maintenance of these and other materials and technologies. Embrace the study of dental materials, for it is the advancement of this science that will ultimately change the way we look at the replacement of oral structures. We look forward to the future.

Case-Based Discussion Questions

1. Compile a list of 5 to 10 dental products that display the ADA Seal of Acceptance and are found in your local drug store or supermarket.
   How is the seal displayed on these items? Ask family and friends if the seal is important in their selection of a dental product. How does the presence of the seal affect your recommendation of a particular product?
2. Research a dental product by using the Internet or by contacting a manufacturer's representative.
   What information is available? What type of research has been done? How is the product marketed? What assistance is available to the consumer or dental office?

BIBLIOGRAPHY

American Dental Association (ADA). Home page. Available at http://www.ada.org.

ADA:ADA Dental Product Guide. Available at http://www.ada.org/en/publications/ada-dental-product-guide/.

ADA:History of Dentistry Timeline. Available at http://www.ada.org/en/about-the-ada/ada-history-and-presidents-of-the-ada/ada-history-of-dentistry-timeline.

ADA:ADA Policy on Evidence-Based Dentistry. Available at http://www.ada.org/en/about-the-ada/ada-positions-policies-and-statements/policy-on-evidence-based-dentistry.

ADA: ADA Seal Products. Available at http://www.ada.org/en/science-research/ada-seal-of-acceptance/ada-seal-products.

Forrest JL, Miller SA, Overman PR, et al: *Evidence-Based Decision Making: A Translational Guide for Dental Professionals*, Philadelphia, 2009, Lippincott Williams & Wilkins.

International Standards Organization (ISO)/TC 106: Dentistry. Available at http://www.iso.org/iso/iso_catalogue/catalogue_tc/catalogue_tc_browse.htm?commid=51218.

Ring ME: *Dentistry: An Illustrated History*, New York, 1993, Harry N. Abrams.

U.S. Food and Drug Administration: Home page. Available at http://www.fda.gov.

Wynbrandt J: *The Excruciating History of Dentistry*. New York, 1998, St. Martin's Press.

Oral Environment and Patient Considerations

Chapter Objectives

Upon completion of this chapter, the student should be able to:

1. Discuss the qualities of the oral environment that make it challenging for long-term clinical performance of dental materials.
2. Describe the long-term clinical requirements of therapeutic and restorative materials.
3. List and give examples of four types of biting forces and the tooth structures most ideally suited to them.
4. Define stress, strain, and ultimate strength and compare the ultimate strength of restorative materials during each type of stress to tooth structures.
5. Explain how moisture and acidity in the mouth can affect dental materials.
6. Explain how galvanism can occur in the mouth and how it can be prevented.
7. Discuss thermal conductivity and thermal expansion and contraction, and compare the values of thermal expansion and conductivity of restorative materials with those of tooth structures.
8. Explain how mechanical and chemical adhesion, or bonding, work to retain restorations.
9. Describe the factors that determine successful adhesion, including wettability, viscosity, film thickness, and surface characteristics.
10. Describe microleakage and how it can lead to recurrent decay and postoperative sensitivity.
11. Define biocompatibility and discuss why requirements for biocompatibility may fluctuate.
12. Describe tooth color in terms of hue, value, and chroma.
13. Discuss the characteristics of oral biofilm and its role in the etiology of dental caries and periodontal disease.
14. Explain the importance of detection of restorations and methods for detection.

Key Terms

Adhesion the act of sticking two things together. In dentistry, it is used to describe the bonding or cementation process. Chemical adhesion occurs when atoms or molecules of dissimilar substances bond together and differs from cohesion in which attraction among atoms and molecules of like (similar) materials holds them together

Adverse Response an unintended, unexpected, and harmful or unwelcomed response of an individual to dental treatment or biomaterial

Auxiliary Materials materials used to fabricate and maintain restorations, directly or indirectly

Biocompatible the property of a material that allows it not to impede or adversely affect living tissue

Biofilm a complex community of oral microorganisms living on surfaces within the mouth. When these colonies are found on teeth or restorations, they are commonly called dental plaque

Bonding to connect or fasten; to bind

Chroma the intensity or strength of a color (e.g., a bold yellow has more chroma than a pastel yellow)

Coefficient of Thermal Expansion the measurement of change in volume or length in relationship to change in temperature

Compressive Force force applied to compress an object

Corrosion deterioration of a metal caused by a chemical attack or electrochemical reaction with dissimilar metals in the presence of a solution containing electrolytes (such as saliva)

Dimensional Change a change in the size of matter. For dental materials, this usually manifests as expansion caused by heating and contraction caused by cooling

Exothermic Reaction the production of heat resulting from the reaction of the components of some materials when they are mixed

Fatigue Failure a fracture resulting from repeated stresses that produce microscopic flaws that grow

Film Thickness the minimal obtainable thickness of a layer of a material. It is particularly important in the context of dental cements

Flexural Stress bending caused by a combination of tension and compression

Fracture Toughness a measure of the energy needed to fracture a material

Galvanism an electrical current transmitted between two dissimilar metals in a solution of electrolytes

Hue the color of a tooth or restoration. It may include a mixture of colors, such as yellow-brown

Insulators materials having low thermal conductivity

Interface the surface between the walls of the preparation and the restoration or between two dental materials

Microleakage leakage of fluid and bacteria caused by microscopic gaps that occur at the interface of the tooth and the restoration margins

Opaque optical property in which light is completely absorbed by an object

Percolation movement of fluid in the microscopic gap of a restoration margin as a result of differences in the expansion and contraction rates of the tooth and the restoration with temperature changes associated with ingestion of cold or hot fluids or foods

Resilience a measure of the energy needed to permanently deform a material

Restorative Materials materials used to reconstruct tooth structure

Retention a material's ability to maintain its position without displacement under stress

Shearing Force force applied when two surfaces slide against each other

Solubility susceptible to being dissolved

Strain distortion or deformation that occurs when an object cannot resist a force

Stress the internal force, which resists the applied force

Surface Energy the electrical charge that attracts atoms to a surface

Tarnish discoloration resulting from oxidation of a thin layer of a metal at its surface. It is not as destructive as corrosion

Tensile Force force applied in opposite directions to stretch an object

Therapeutic Materials materials used to treat disease

Thermal Conductivity the rate at which heat flows through a material

Torsion *or* Torque a twisting force that combines tensile and compressive forces

Translucency optical property in which varying degrees of light pass through or are absorbed by an object

Transparent optical property in which light passes directly through an object

Ultimate Strength the maximum amount of stress a material can withstand without breaking

Value how light or dark a color is. A low value indicates a darker color and a high value indicates a brighter color

Viscosity the ability of a liquid material to resist flow, e.g. ketchup is more viscous than water

Vitality a life-like quality

Water Sorption the ability to absorb moisture

Wetting the ability of a liquid to wet or intimately contact a solid surface. Water beading on a waxed car is an example of poor wetting

---

To become effective in the selection, manipulation, and handling of dental materials it is important that the auxiliary have an appreciation for the complexity and challenges of the oral environment. Dental biomaterials placed and used within the oral cavity must be biocompatible, durable, nonreactive under acid or alkaline conditions, compatible with other materials, and esthetically acceptable. Eating by itself introduces hot and cold extremes, acidic or alkaline foods and beverages, hard or sticky foods, and heavy biting pressure. These factors may degrade the materials over time, affect marginal integrity, roughen the surfaces, or fracture the restorative materials. Materials must be selected that have physical and mechanical properties that can hold up in these conditions. The severity of the conditions in the oral environment may vary somewhat from patient to patient and in specific circumstances.

The degree of compatibility may depend on how and/ or how long the material is expected to survive in the oral environment. Therapeutic materials, those used to treat disease, are generally used for short periods of time whereas restorative materials, those used to reconstruct tooth structure, are expected to remain in contact with tissues for indefinite lengths of time. Consider the following cases. If a therapeutic agent were to be used to treat a specific condition, such as a denture sore, it would need to be biocompatible with the tissues but would not need to last long. If the material were being used as a permanent restoration, such as a gold crown, biocompatibility and longevity would both be required.

Patient concerns, questions, and demands must also play a part in the decision process. The patient should be brought into the decision process very early. Tooth-colored materials are frequently requested by the patient, but may present limitations in their use under certain circumstances. Patients are frequently looking for the best esthetic choice and may not be aware of the limitation of that choice. The patient may desire porcelain or composite veneers to cover discolored anterior teeth or to close spacing (FIG. 2.1). If the patient has parafunctional habits such as clenching or grinding, the choice of porcelain may result in the chipping or wearing of the opposing teeth or of the restorations themselves. On the other hand, composite veneers may wear down excessively under the same conditions. The patient(s) needs to be educated as to the limitations imposed by their particular oral condition(s) and the appropriate restorative choices in order to produce long-lasting results. The auxiliary is frequently involved in this education and must have a good understanding of how materials function in the oral environment.

CLASSIFICATION OF DENTAL MATERIALS

Dental materials may be classified by their use: preventive/therapeutic materials, restorative materials, and auxiliary materials.

PREVENTIVE/THERAPEUTIC MATERIALS

Preventive/therapeutic materials are used to prevent disease or trauma or for their therapeutic action on the teeth or oral tissues. Included in this category are materials such as pit and fissure sealants to help prevent

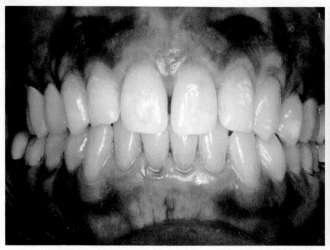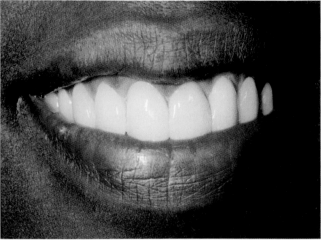

FIG. 2.1 Closing a diastema (i.e., a space) between teeth #8 and #9 with composite restorative material. (Courtesy of Dr. Stephan Eakle.)

caries, mouth guards to mitigate the effects of parafunctional habits and injury due to athletic activities, and materials used for their antibacterial effects such as those found in some restorative and base materials. Also included in this category are fluoride and fluoride-containing materials to prevent or reduce the progression of caries.

RESTORATIVE MATERIALS

Restorative materials include those materials used to repair or replace tooth structure lost to oral disease or trauma or to change the appearance of the teeth. Restorations are classified as direct and indirect. Direct restorations are placed immediately and directly into a prepared tooth in a pliable state that then sets to harden. This procedure can be done in a single office visit. Indirect restorations involve customized tooth replacements that require fabrication outside the mouth usually in a lab. These restorations usually require a second appointment to fit and cement the restoration.

AUXILIARY MATERIALS

Auxiliary materials include those materials used to fabricate and maintain restorations, directly or indirectly. Materials such as impression materials, gypsum, dental waxes, and finishing and polishing materials are also included in this category.

BIOCOMPATIBILITY

Materials must be **biocompatible**; that is, they must not impede or adversely affect living tissue and should interact to the benefit of the patient. The study of dental biomaterials must include a thorough understanding of each material's biological properties; all materials contain potentially irritating ingredients. Responses may include postoperative sensitivity, toxicity, and hypersensitivity. A material may be acceptable for use or

fabrication on hard tissues (tooth structure), whereas it may not be acceptable for use on soft tissues. Some materials may be therapeutic in small quantities or if in contact with tissues for short periods of time, but also may be irritating or toxic with longer contact or in larger quantities or higher concentrations. Topical fluoride is of great benefit when used according to the manufacturer's directions, but can be irritating to soft tissues and even excessively etch enamel if an acidulated version is used. Dentistry is not alone in its attention to the development of biocompatible materials; orthopedics must consider biocompatibility in the placement of joint prostheses, as does cardiology in the placement of catheters and prosthetic heart valves. All must consider the short-term and long-term functional and biocompatible responses of any material.

Postoperative sensitivity is often associated with dental operative procedures. This may be due to the toxicity of the restorative, preventive, or therapeutic material or bacterial invasion into or near the pulpal tissues.

ADVERSE RESPONSE

A patient may have an **adverse response** to a dental material. The response may be due to the material itself or may be due to breakdown products of its components in the oral environment. An example of an adverse response is seen with patients allergic to some metals, particularly nickel. There is evidence of nickel allergies in 10% to 20% of the population, particularly in women. It is thought that they become sensitized to nickel by wearing jewelry containing it. Some nickel-containing alloys are used in dentistry for fabrication of crowns, bridges, partial denture frameworks, or in orthodontic wires. Evidence of allergic reactions to nickel may be seen at crown margins of metal-based crowns (FIG. 2.2), on a patient's lips when wearing some orthodontic appliances, and on a patient's attached gingiva in contact with the metal framework of a removable prosthesis.

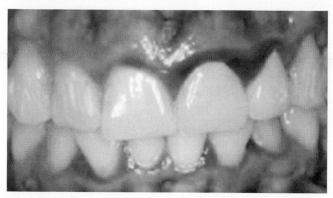

FIG. 2.2 Allergic reaction to nickel. Porcelain-fused-to-metal crowns have been placed on teeth #9 and 10. The tissue is red and inflamed and bleeds easily because of chronic inflammation from allergy to the metal in the crown.

A complete health history, questioning of the patient, and a thorough examination of oral tissues can help to identify hypersensitive individuals. Frequently, several different materials are used in combination to produce a restoration, such as a porcelain-fused-to-metal crown cemented with glass ionomer cement. The use of multiple materials makes it more difficult to determine which material is responsible for the adverse response. In general, materials intended for permanent replacement of tooth structures should exhibit no adverse biologic responses as well as be of benefit to the patient.

In subsequent chapters the limitations as well as precautions for the use of each material will be clearly outlined.

ORAL FACTORS AFFECTING DENTAL MATERIALS

A number of factors in the oral environment will have an effect on the functioning and durability of the dental materials used in the oral cavity and thus will have an influence on which material the clinician will select.

BIOMECHANICS

The function of a material depends on the physical and mechanical properties (see Chapter 3 Physical and Mechanical Properties of Dental Materials) of that material as well as on how the material is being asked to perform. Designs for restorations require an understanding of the biomechanical properties of the material. Much like an engineer, the dentist must design a dental bridge by taking into consideration the load that will be placed on the bridge, the length of the span, and the stability of the supporting structures. For example, a material may be used successfully to restore anterior teeth, where biting forces are not as strong, whereas this same material may be undesirable to restore the occlusal surfaces of posterior teeth, where biting forces are heavier. Excessive wear of a material may occur when a stronger material applies force against a weaker material such as porcelain against composite resin

and may be intensified by surface roughness on the porcelain and by parafunctional habits such as clenching or grinding. Dentists must consider the performance of a material based on a thorough knowledge of the material's properties, the intended application of the material, and the impacting factors in each patient's oral environment.

FORCE, STRESS AND STRAIN

FORCE

A force is a push, pull or twist (or combination of these) applied to a material. When a weight is placed on an object, the weight applies force to that object. The force applied at the surface creates **stress** within the object that tries to resist the weight. If there was no resistance to the weight, then the material would be flattened or displaced.

Materials used to restore teeth must withstand varying degrees of force, or *load*, applied through muscular action resulting in the pushing or pulling of a restoration by the teeth or food bolus during mastication. For some patients the forces come from parafunctional habits such as clenching or grinding (called *bruxism*). Normal biting force varies among individuals and from one area of the mouth to another. Biting force is largely a measurement of the strength of the muscles of mastication and the surface area over which the force is applied during the normal chewing of foods. When clenching or grinding, this force is increased due to the lack of a food cushion and the resultant direct contact of tooth surfaces. Normal masticatory forces on the occlusal surface of molar teeth average 90 to 200 pounds per square inch and can increase to as much as 28,000 pounds per square inch on a cusp tip. Masticatory forces are greatest in the molar region and gradually decrease moving toward the anterior part of the mouth from premolars to incisors. Denture wearers apply 40% less force than patients with intact dentitions, but denture wearers whose dentures are supported by implants or roots regain much of the biting force.

A study of the anatomy of teeth reveals that each kind of tooth shape (i.e., incisor, premolar, molar) is designed to apply specific types of force. The three basic types of force are as follows:
- *Compressive Force*, force applied to compress or squeeze an object; crushing biting forces. Posterior teeth are ideally suited for this type of force. Their large occlusal surface and multi-rooted base are well suited to resist a crushing force.
- *Tensile Force*, force applied at each end of a material in opposite directions to stretch an object or pull it apart. When tensile force is applied to a rubber band it is stretched.
- *Shearing Force*, force applied when two surfaces slide against each other in opposite directions. When the maxillary and mandibular incisors are used for cutting, shearing forces are applied. When we use the anterior teeth to bite into food, we slide

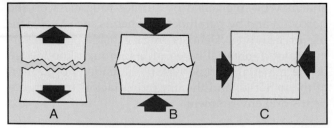

FIG. 2.3 Types of stress and strain. **A,** Tensile stress pulls and stretches a material. **B,** Compressive stress pushes it together. **C,** Shearing stress tries to slice it apart. (From Bird DL, Robinson DS: *Torres and Ehrlich Modern Dental Assisting* (ed 11). Philadelphia, 2015, Saunders.)

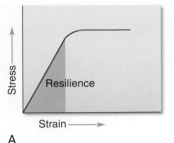

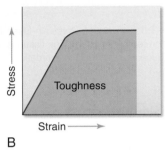

FIG. 2.4 Stress-strain curves for a material. **A,** Dark blue area under the curve shows resilience (resistance to permanent deformation) **B,** Large area under the curve shows toughness (energy needed to cause fracture) (From Sakaguchi RL, Powers JM: *Craig's Restorative Dental Materials* (ed 13). St. Louis, 2012, Mosby.)

the mandibular teeth forward or to the side across the the maxillary teeth to shear it off.

Torsion

Another type of force is **torsion or torque.** It is a twisting force that has tensile and compressive forces. This force is more descriptive of normal masticatory events. When we chew we combine compressive, tensile, and shear forces resulting in torsion. When a patient wears full dentures, he or she may complain that the dentures become dislodged when they chew certain foods. This is because of torque on the dentures, which are not well suited to withstand the combination of compressive, tensile, and shear forces while eating (FIG. 2.3).

> **Clinical Tip**
>
> Dislodging of dentures is often due to tipping forces and possibly torque that breaks the peripheral seal causing the loss of suction and results in the movement of the denture away from the ridge.

The forces used in chewing a sticky caramel candy are different from those used in chewing a peanut. The caramel is compressed as the person bites down and it sticks to the teeth. Then, it is torn apart by tensile forces as the jaws separate. The peanut is crushed by compressive forces and ground with shearing forces as the upper and lower posterior teeth slide across each other in the chewing cycle.

Flexure

Flexure or bending force is a combination of compressive, tensile, and shear forces. When a long plastic rod is flexed into an arch-shape, compression occurs on the inside surface of the arch and tension occurs on the outside of the arch while shear occurs inside of the rod itself.

Stress and Strain

When a force is exerted on a tooth or restorative material, the tooth or material creates stress to resist the force. Stress is expressed as pounds per square inch (psi) or megapascals (MPa) in the metric system. If an object is

fixed in position, it may be deformed by the force if the magnitude is great enough, and the object is considered strained. Stress, then, is the amount of force exerted from within an object to resist an external force and **strain** is the amount of change that the force has produced in the object. When the strain is caused by a compressive force the object is shortened while a tensile force causes the object to lengthen. If the object does not return to its original shape after the stress is removed, it has undergone permanent deformation. If the object returns to its original shape, the change is called elastic deformation. The effect on the object is determined by the size of the force, the point or area of contact, and the direction in which the force is applied. If a force is applied over a large surface area, the stress generated is less than if the same force is applied to a small area. The large surface area helps to dissipate the impact of the force.

Stress-Strain Curve

Each material has its unique relationship between the stresses placed on it and the strains that develop in reaction to those stresses. This relationship is known as the stress-strain curve. The curve is determined by plotting the amount of deformation that occurs at each magnitude of applied stress (compressive or tensile loading). It is useful in comparing how materials can withstand loading. Thus, it can help in selecting an appropriate dental material, for example, to use in restoring the biting surfaces of a lower molar. It can show which material is strong enough and stable enough for that application (FIG. 2.4).

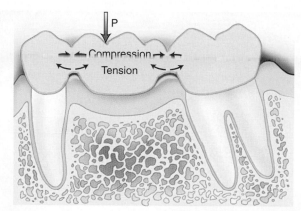

FIG. 2.5 Stresses on a bridge. (From Anusavice KJ, Shen C, Rawls H: *Phillips' Science of Dental Materials* (ed 12). St. Louis, 2013, Saunders.)

TABLE 2.1	Ultimate Compressive and Tensile Strengths of Tooth and Restorative Structures	
STRUCTURE	ULTIMATE COMPRESSIVE STRENGTH (lb/in²)	ULTIMATE TENSILE STRENGTH (lb/in²)
Enamel	56,000	1,500
Dentin	43,000	4,500
Amalgam	45,000-64,000	7,000-9,000
Porcelain	21,000	5,400
Composite resin	30,000-60,000	6,000-9,000
Acrylic	11,000	8,000

The normal process of chewing rarely involves only one type of stress; complex stress combinations are more common. For example, dental bridges are subject to flexural stress when compressive forces placed on the occlusal surface of the bridge bend the bridge downward and tensile forces on the tissue side of the bridge stretch upward in response (FIG. 2.5).

Materials may be suited to one type of stress but fail during another. If the force is exerted over a large area, the tooth structures can more adequately handle the stress. When the force is exerted over a small area the increase in pressure may result in fracture. Consider the force exerted on the floor by a woman wearing flat shoes and then changing into high spike heels. The woman's weight supported by both types of shoes is the same, so there is no difference in force. However, because there is a difference in area, the pressure on the surface contacted is drastically different. This is the reason that teeth or restorations may fracture when subjected to stresses by small, very hard objects, such as a popcorn kernel or cherry pit.

Fracture Toughness Strength

Fracture toughness is a mechanical property of materials that measures the energy needed to fracture a material. When increasingly higher forces are applied to a material it will eventually fracture and the point of fracture is called the **ultimate strength.**

Resilience

Resilience indicates the energy needed to permanently deform a material. Brittle materials such as composites, amalgam, or ceramics are not resilient and do not deform readily and will fracture if loaded too much. Any flaws in the materials will cause stress to concentrate in those areas and ultimately reduce the strength of the material leading to fracture. Values of compressive and tensile forces applied to tooth structure and restorative materials are expressed in Table 2.1. Use the table to compare the ultimate compressive and tensile strengths of tooth structure types to the various restorative materials to understand why a certain material

may function better in one application than another. As you can see, amalgam and composite resins more closely replicate enamel in compressive strength, whereas porcelain falls short. Porcelain is brittle and more likely to fracture under compressive stresses, especially those that are directed onto a small area. (Note: Porcelain is one type of ceramic material described in Chapter 9. It is one of the weaker ceramic materials but is very esthetic.)

Fatigue Failure

During mastication, stresses occur repetitively over time. Failures rarely occur in a single-force application; rather, they occur when stress is frequently repeated. These repeated stresses may produce microscopic flaws that grow over time, resulting in fracture: this is known as **fatigue failure**. A metal wire bent repeatedly will eventually break; this is another example of fatigue failure. Teeth and restorative materials under function or bruxism are subjected to repeated stresses by a mixture of forces applied in a variety of directions and intensities. As a result they may crack or fracture. Additionally, conditions of the oral cavity such as moisture, temperature, and pH fluctuations may also contribute to fatigue failure.

MOISTURE AND ACID LEVELS

The oral cavity is always in contact with moisture in the form of foods, saliva, and blood. This moisture can vary from acid to alkaline depending on foods, beverages, medications, and the amount of acid-producing bacteria present (biofilm).

EFFECT OF pH

The normal resting pH of saliva ranges from 6.2 to 7.0 (neutral), but can fluctuate higher or lower by several points during the course of a day Many materials that would be compatible in a neutral environment will not be compatible in an acidic one. Some beverages are slightly or very acidic. Citrus fruits and sports drinks contain citric acid and can attack enamel and some restorative materials. Acidulated topical fluorides can

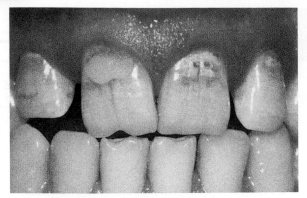

FIG. 2.6 "Washed out" glass ionomer restoration on tooth #8 is stained owing to porosities and the solubility of this restorative material.

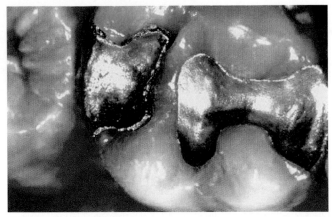

FIG. 2.7 Two amalgam restorations. *Left:* A low-copper amalgam with severe marginal breakdown. *Right:* A high-copper amalgam restoration with minimal marginal discrepancy. Both restorations were placed at the same time. (From Anusavice KJ: *Quality Evaluation of Dental Restorations: Criteria for Placement and Replacement.* Chicago, 1989, Quintessence Publishing.)

also attack some materials such as glass ionomer cements, composite resins, and ceramics.

Most materials are adversely affected by moisture either during placement or in the long-term clinical behavior of the material. The breakdown of many restorative materials is directly related to the effects of moisture, acid, and stress. Materials designed for long-term retention in the mouth must not rapidly deteriorate under these conditions.

Solubility

Desirable materials should have low **solubility,** that is, not susceptible to being dissolved in a solvent, and in the case of the oral environment saliva is the main solvent. Gold and porcelain are retained in the oral environment for many years because of their insoluble nature. Glass ionomer cement materials, frequently used as tooth-colored restorations, are much more soluble. They tend to "wash out" or change in mass over time, requiring replacement (FIG. 2.6).

Water Sorption

Some materials also have the undesirable characteristic of **water sorption** or the ability to absorb moisture; this may result in staining or a slight swelling of the material. Staining of resins and acrylics from repeated exposure to coffee, tea, and other dyed beverages is due to water sorption. Dentures placed in a glass of water will take up the liquid and become slightly larger. Some acrylics will absorb both odors and tastes from foods due to microscopic porosity in the material. Directions on routine home care can help alleviate this problem for the patient. (See Chapter 17 Polymers for Prosthetic Dentistry.)

Corrosion

Metals suffer from the effects of moisture and acidity, with the exception of noble metals such as gold and platinum. The deterioration or dissolution of the metal in response to a chemical attack (acid), or in an electrochemical reaction with other metals because of the moisture and acid present in the oral environment, is called **corrosion**. Metals such as steel cannot be used in the oral cavity because the metal breaks down in the wet environment, becoming iron oxide (commonly known as *rust*). When steel is coated first with a barrier to corrosive components, the barrier gives steel its stainless quality. Dental amalgams are particularly susceptible to corrosion, causing marginal breakdown and discoloration of tooth structures. (See Chapter 10 Dental Amalgam.) The result of corrosion is also seen on dental instruments that are processed in autoclaves due to oxidation of the metal's surface. Corrosion begins at the surface of the metal and migrates deeper into the metal than **tarnish,** that is limited to the surface and can be seen as discoloration. Corrosion can accelerate in crevices between tooth and restoration and on rough surfaces. Polishing of amalgams to produce a smooth surface has been recommended to help delay this process. In high-copper amalgams this may not be as critical to their longevity since they are more corrosion resistant than low-copper amalgams (FIG. 2.7).

GALVANISM

An environment containing moisture, electrolytes, and dissimilar metals makes the generation of an electric current possible. The ions in the saliva facilitate the movement of electrical current from one type of metal to another. The phenomenon of electric current being transmitted between two dissimilar metals is called **galvanism**. The current may result in stimulation to the pulp, called *galvanic shock*. The classic example of a metal fork touching a metal restoration or the biting on aluminum foil will be familiar to anyone with metal restorations, and unfamiliar to those who have no metal restorations. Some patients may even feel a galvanic shock or report a metal taste when instruments are used against the surface of a restoration. When it becomes necessary

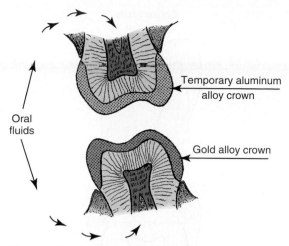

FIG. 2.8 Galvanism illustration of how dissimilar metals in opposing teeth can create a galvanic current with saliva providing a solution of electrolytes.

TABLE **2.2**	Thermal Properties of Tooth and Restorative Structures	
STRUCTURE	**COEFFICIENT OF THERMAL EXPANSION ($\times 10^{-6}$/°C)**	**THERMAL CONDUCTIVITY (K [mcal cm]/ cm²sec°C)**
Enamel	11	2.0
Dentin	8	1.30
Amalgam	20–28	54
Gold	15	350
Porcelain	15	2.50
Composite resin	26–40	2.60

to place differing types of metal restorations such as a gold crown in contact with an amalgam restoration, insulation under the restorations in the form of bases or liners can help to lessen the stimulation. Provisional (temporary) aluminum crowns placed opposite or adjacent to amalgam or metal crowns can also cause this phenomenon (FIG. 2.8). In this situation the selection of a polycarbonate or acrylic provisional crown would be a better choice. In time the galvanic stimulation will fade as oxides form on the surface of the metal, acting as an insulator against the galvanic current.

TEMPERATURE

EXPANSION AND CONTRACTION

The ingestion of hot and cold foods and beverages and smoking may alter the temperature of the oral environment. With few exceptions, all forms of matter expand when they are heated and contract when cooled, resulting in **dimensional change**. Atoms or molecules in a material vibrate over a greater range when the material is heated causing it to expand. Acceptable materials used as restorations and replacement of tooth structure should have characteristics of expansion and contraction similar to tooth structures. Excessive expansion of a restoration within a tooth may result in the fracture of cusps; excessive contraction may result in leakage of fluids and bacteria into the open gaps, resulting in sensitivity. Expansion and contraction are measured as the **coefficient of thermal expansion (CTE)**, the measurement of change in volume or length in relationship to change in temperature. (Refer to Table 2.2 to review the values of thermal expansion.)

Amalgam readily heats up and expands or cools and contracts with a small temperature change, whereas composite resin is not a good conductor of temperature and requires a greater temperature change to expand or contract. Both of these materials have rates of expansion and contraction that differ significantly enough from enamel and dentin that the marginal integrity of the restoration may be compromised. The difference in CTE value of unfilled acrylic and sealants with tooth structure is the highest, and the value of gold is the closest to human teeth.

Repeated shrinkage and expansion of a restoration during ingestion of cold and hot fluids and foods produces the opening and closing of a gap with movement of oral fluids between the restoration and the tooth surface; a phenomenon called **percolation**. Percolation allows the ingress of bacteria and oral fluids and may lead to recurrent caries, staining, and pulpal irritation.

THERMAL CONDUCTIVITY

Thermal conductivity is the rate at which heat flows through a material over time. Enamel and dentin are poor thermal conductors, whereas metals are excellent conductors. Gold is one of the best thermal conductors, even better than amalgam. Nonmetals such as ceramics, composites, acrylics, and cements are very poor conductors. Poor conductors can be used as restorations or as insulators. For instance, a patient wearing a denture may not sense the temperature of a liquid because of the insulation produced by the acrylic denture base.

When a metal restoration conducts temperature changes into the tooth from foods and beverages taken into the oral cavity, the pulp of the tooth may feel the resultant stimulation as sensitivity, particularly if the overlying dentin is thin. Dentin acts as a natural insulator, but when it is too thin, temperature changes may be felt by the pulp. Amalgam and gold have much higher values of thermal conductivity than dentin and enamel; a hot cup of coffee may transmit heat readily through these metals, resulting in pulpal stimulation. A piece of ice placed on an amalgam restoration may conduct stimulation to the pulp in as little as 2 to 3 seconds. When metal restorations are placed close to the pulp of the tooth, material such as a cement is often placed between the tooth structure and the restoration to act as an insulating base to delay and absorb the transfer of temperature. Metals placed against tissue such as a partial denture framework and some orthodontic appliances can also conduct temperature to the soft tissues.

Table 2.2 gives values of thermal expansion and thermal conductivity. Compare values for restorative materials with those for tooth structures to determine the potential for marginal leakage through percolation and/or the need for insulation. When there is a large difference between the CTE for the restorative material, such as amalgam, and that for the tooth structure the percolation will be greater. Note that whereas composite has a higher CTE compared with tooth structure, bonding it to the tooth structure helps to prevent percolation.

In addition to temperature considerations for materials already present in the mouth, it is important to consider the temperature of materials as they are placed into the mouth. Icy cold water used when mixing alginate may cause the patient pain when the very cold alginate contacts metal restorations. The components of some materials when mixed may result in a chemical reaction that produces heat. For example, when the powder and liquid of a chairside denture reline material are mixed, the reaction produces heat (an **exothermic reaction**). If the material is left in the mouth while this reaction is occurring, it is possible that the tissues could receive a thermal burn.

 Clinical Tip

An exothermic reaction must be minimized by proper mixing and handling to prevent excess heat from coming into contact with a susceptible tooth surface. Acrylic used to make temporary crowns and bridges in the mouth will release heat as it polymerizes and sets. If left in the mouth too long, the heat can damage the pulp or burn any soft tissues it contacts.

RETENTION

An important factor in the selection of a material is how it will be retained within or on the tooth. The **retention** of a material is its ability to maintain its position without displacement under stress. Retention may be secured through mechanical, chemical **adhesion,** or **bonding** mechanisms between materials.

MECHANICAL AND CHEMICAL RETENTION

Mechanical retention involves the use of undercuts or other projections into which the material is locked in place. The undercuts used in a typical amalgam preparation are an illustration of mechanical retention (FIG. 2.9). Note that the opening of the cavity preparation is smaller than the internal floor of the preparation. Once the material is hardened in place, it is retained through this design.

When a significant amount of tooth structure has been removed, undercuts can no longer be successfully used, because the cusps or other parts of the tooth will be undermined and weakened. At this time the clinician may wish to place a restoration covering

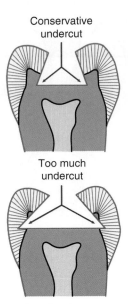

FIG. 2.9 The retentive undercuts of a conservative preparation *(top)* and an excessively undercut reparation that compromises the remaining tooth structure *(bottom)*.

the remaining tooth structure (a crown) and hold it in place with a dental cement. Dental cement retains the restoration by chemically and/or mechanically connecting the two surfaces. Glass ionomer cement will chemically bond to the mineral component of tooth structure and can also mechanically retain a crown.

BONDING

Bonding is a term commonly used when describing the retention of materials. Bonding of materials occurs when the tooth surface is prepared with an acid-etch technique to create microscopic roughness and pores in enamel and dentin. A fluid bonding material is then allowed to flow into the roughened surfaces and pores and when hardened it mechanically locks into the tooth structure. See Chapter 5 Principles of Bonding, Figure 5.9 and 5.10. Restorative materials that adhere chemically to the bonding material are then placed. This technique offers several advantages in producing retention. It requires less removal of healthy tooth structure because no undercuts are necessary, it produces a stronger retentive force between tooth and restoration, and it can seal the margin of the restoration to prevent the seepage of bacteria and fluids through percolation. (See Chapter 5 Principles of Bonding.)

Many of today's restorative materials use a combination of mechanical and chemical or bonding adhesion for optimal retention. Retention by mechanical undercuts alone will not adequately seal the margins of a restoration and will frequently place tooth structure in jeopardy of fracture when undercuts leave vulnerable areas of tooth structure unsupported. Bonding requires the intimate contact of surfaces to produce the best bond strength. The strength of the bond is measured by applying shearing and tensile stresses.

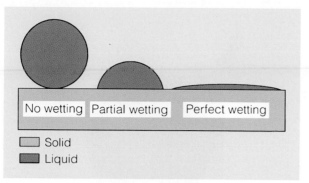

FIG. 2.10 Wetting characteristics of a liquid on a solid surface. (From Van Noort R: *Introduction to Dental Materials* (ed 14). London, 2013, Mosby, p. 53.)

Factors Affecting Bond Strength

Several factors can affect this bond strength and the success of a material as an adhesive. These include wetting, viscosity, film thickness, and surface characteristics of the tooth, restoration, and adhesive.

Wetting. **Wetting** is the degree to which a liquid adhesive is able to spread over the surface of a tooth and restorative material. This wettability is based on the contact angle between the liquid and the tooth surface. The lower the contact angle the better the liquid adhesive spreads onto the surface of the tooth (FIG. 2.10). (See also Chapter 5 Principles of Bonding.) The Teflon surface of cooking equipment exhibits poor wettability, that is, the liquids bead up on the surface rather than spreading out. The better the adhesive is able to spread on the surface of the tooth and restoration, the more retentive it is. Microscopic surface roughness such as that created by etching enamel will increase the wetting of the surface by the liquid.

Viscosity. **Viscosity**, that is, the resistance of a liquid material to flow, can hinder the ability of a liquid to wet a material. Materials with high viscosity are thicker and do not flow well, and therefore may not be effective in wetting an area. Viscosity also can affect the film thickness of an adhesive or cement.

Film thickness. **Film thickness** is the minimal thickness obtainable by a layer of a liquid material after it sets under pressure and is particularly important in working with dental cements. When cementing a crown, if the film thickness of the cement is too great, it may keep the crown from seating completely. A thin film of cement is desirable to allow the cement to completely wet the surfaces and for excess material to flow from under the crown when it is seated under pressure during cementation.

Surface characteristic. Surface characteristics are other factors that affect the adhesive retention of a material. They include the cleanliness of a surface, moisture contamination, surface texture, and surface energy of the restoration and tooth. As mentioned previously, adhesion depends on intimate contact of surfaces. Even slight contamination can prevent contact. Debris from the tooth preparation, microorganisms in biofilm, and products of saliva are often impossible to completely eliminate. Surface irregularities may prevent complete wetting of the surfaces. Microscopic surface irregularities can trap air as the adhesive flows over them, resulting in incomplete wetting of the surface.

Surface energy. The surface energy of liquids is also called surface tension. The molecules at the surface of a liquid or solid are aligned differently than in the center. In the center the molecules are in balance with the molecules that surround them. At the surface, however, there is an imbalance in the attraction between molecules causing them to be attracted to the larger mass of molecules in the center. This attraction or force directed inward causes an energy level at the surface. With liquids, if the surface energy is high, the liquid can flow readily over a solid substrate. When liquids bead up on a surface, such as on wax or many plastics, the surface has low surface energy.

Solids also develop surface energy. When enamel is etched, a high surface energy is created that can attract liquids across the surface. If newly etched enamel comes in contact with just a little saliva, a molecular film of saliva is drawn across the surface by the high energy causing contamination. Liquids generally wet or spread over high surface energy surfaces better. Metals, ceramics, and enamel have high surface energies.

Many situations present conditions that are not favorable for retention of materials. The dentist is responsible for the mechanical design of the preparation, but is not solely responsible for other factors. In many states, allied oral health practitioners routinely place therapeutic and restorative materials. In addition, the dental assistant plays an essential role in delivering materials and controlling the conditions of the oral environment during their delivery. An understanding of the factors that influence retention is essential to achieving a successful restoration.

MICROLEAKAGE

The need for replacement of restorative materials can be significantly influenced by microleakage. The surface between the walls of the tooth structure (preparation) and the restoration is called the **interface**. If this tooth/restoration interface is not sealed there may be a space into which fluids and microorganisms can penetrate. This seepage of harmful materials is called **microleakage** and is responsible in part for recurrent decay, marginal staining, and postoperative sensitivity. Microleakage may be due to the deterioration of the dental material, percolation due to differences in CTE, or lack of adhesion of the material to the tooth. It is easy

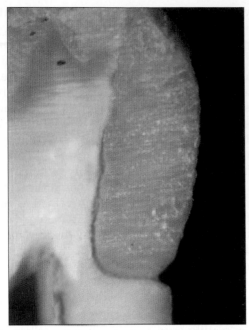

FIG. 2.11 Microleakage allows the seepage of fluids and microorganisms into the restoration–tooth structure interface. Microleakage can be seen as a pink dye penetrating along the internal surface of the Class II composite restoration. (From Sakri MR, Kippal P, Patil BC, Haralur SB: Evaluation of microleakage in hybrid composite restoration with different intermediate layers and curing cycles. *J Dent Allied Sci* 5(1):14–20, 2016.)

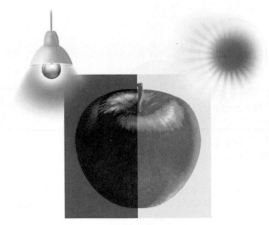

FIG. 2.12 Example of metamerism: the apple changes color depending on the light source used to illuminate it. (From Sakaguchi RL, Powers JM: *Craig's Restorative Dental Materials* (ed 13). Philadelphia, 2012, Saunders, p. 58.)

to understand why the seepage of bacteria and other fluids between preparation and restoration sets up an environment for recurrent decay and staining. Postoperative sensitivity may be due to microleakage as well (FIG. 2.11). (Please also refer to Figs. 5.21 and 6.3 for pictures of microleakage.) Tubules found within the hard material of the dentin are filled with fluids under pressure from the pulp. When the enamel of the tooth is removed fluids can flow out of the much larger dentinal tubules and outside chemicals and bacteria can flow in causing irritation of the pulp and sensitivity. Procedures for ensuring the proper seal of the dentinal tubules are described in Chapter 5 (Principles of Bonding).

ESTHETICS AND COLOR

Esthetic dentistry is a rapidly growing elective procedure which is in high demand and may be of equal if not greater concern to the patient than function. Our eyes sense light through the cone cells in the retina in three different ranges of wavelength: red, green, and blue. Having three types of color-sensing cells doesn't limit us to just three colors. The stimulation of two or more types of cone cells, the amount of light they detect, and the interpretation of that light by our brain determine the overall response to a particular color. Mixtures of red, green, and blue light allow you to see many colors. The television mixes these primary colors of light to produce full color pictures. Three components—hue, chroma, and value—describe the resultant color:

Hue is the dominant color of the wavelength detected. Tooth colors are predominantly seen in the yellow and brown range.

Chroma refers to the intensity or strength of the color; teeth are rather pale in color.

Value describes how light or dark the color is. Teeth have value ranges at the light end of the value scale. As we age the tooth value gets darker.

The color of teeth and ceramic and composite resin restorations is influenced by their optical properties. Light that reaches the surface of the tooth or restoration can be transmitted through it, absorbed by it, and scattered or reflected by it. If light passes directly through an object (like window glass) it is **transparent.** If light is completely absorbed, scattered, and/or reflected by the object it is **opaque**. Light is reflected off the surface (called reflectance) depending on the surface texture and amount of polish. Usually teeth and esthetic restorations will reflect light and transmit light to various degrees giving the tooth or restoration a life-like quality called **vitality**. Manufacturers over time have adjusted the components of composite resins so that they can absorb, transmit, scatter and reflect light to mimic natural tooth structure. The same can be said for modern ceramics.

Individuals see these many colors, components, and reflections of color somewhat differently in different situations. This phenomenon, known as **metamerism** means that colors look different under different light sources (FIG. 2.12). It is important that we have a standardized measure of color such as a shade guide to give us an objective measure (FIG. 2.13). It is also important that we produce an environment that reduces the possibility of extraneous color reflection producing an inaccurate color match for the restoration. A detailed discussion on shade selection is presented in Chapter 9 (Dental Ceramics).

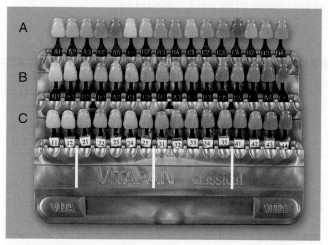

FIG. 2.13 Tab arrangements of the Vitapan classical shade guide. Manufacturer's arrangement according to **A,** hue, **B,** value scale, and **C,** lightest to darkest. (From Paravina RD, Powers JM: *Esthetic Color Training in Dentistry*. St. Louis, 2004, Mosby.)

ORAL BIOFILM AND DENTAL MATERIALS

It is important to have a basic understanding of **oral biofilm**, what it is, how it functions in health and disease, and how to manage it to maintain a healthy mouth. The oral biofilm is a three dimensional, complex, structured community of microorganisms that can be found on mucous membranes, teeth, intracoronal (fillings) and extracoronal (crowns) restorations, dental implants, and removable prostheses. Over 700 species of microorganisms can colonize the mouth. These microorganisms include bacteria, viruses, and fungi. In any one individual approximately 200 of these species may exist as part of the normal oral microbiota. Of these, bacteria are found in the greatest numbers and species.

The oral biofilm exists in a dynamic symbiotic (beneficial to host and microorganisms) relationship with the host. The biofilm provides some level of protection for the structured community of microorganisms from invading bacteria, fungi and viruses, and toxic substances such as antibiotics or chemicals. The biofilm also provides a type of circulatory system for the uptake of nutrients (derived from adjacent tissues, from salivary secretions, from other microorganisms, and from the host diet) and for elimination of metabolic by-products through water-filled spaces between colonies.

FORMATION OF ORAL BIOFILM

Biofilm (or dental plaque) forms on teeth soon after they erupt. Likewise, it quickly re-forms after a professional cleaning and forms on newly placed restorations. The initial layer on the surfaces of the teeth or restorations comes from salivary and gingival crevicular fluid components such as proteins, glycoproteins, lipids, albumin, and mucin and is called the acquired pellicle. That layer acts as a base to which bacteria can attach. The majority of the first colonizers is from the *Streptococcus*

genus (e.g., *S. mutans, S. salivarius*) and occupies up to 90% of the surface while other early colonizers occupy the remainder. The early colonizers are mostly gram positive bacteria (they have a thick cell wall that retains a stain used in the laboratory). Within a couple weeks gram negative bacteria (they have a thin cell wall that does not retain the stain) begin to proliferate. Later colonizers are mostly anaerobes (they thrive where there is little or no oxygen) that can contribute to periodontal disease, and they attach to the growing plaque. As the bacterial community grows, the adherent bacteria form a protective matrix from extracellular polysaccharides they secrete. The matrix can help in protecting them from competing microorganisms, antibiotics, and antibacterial mouth rinses. A state of microbial homeostasis (a stable state of equilibrium) forms until it is thrown out of balance by factors affecting the oral environment, such as change in the host immune system, dietary changes, or other systemic changes. Oral factors such as the temperature of the oral cavity, the pH of the saliva, and available nutrients affect the rate of growth of the bacterial plaque. The temperature can change rapidly with the introduction of hot or cold foods and beverages. The pH can vary from its normal range of 6.5 to 7.5 by the introduction of sugars that are metabolized by certain bacteria with resultant acid production. Acidic and alkaline foods can also alter the pH, but the saliva dilutes and buffers the foods so that gradually the saliva returns to its normal range. This pH balancing may not happen in patients with dry mouth or saliva with low buffering capacity.

BIOFILM AND ORAL DISEASE

Most of the bacteria in the biofilm are harmless, but pathogens are present in small numbers. If systemic or oral conditions change, the potential exists for certain pathogens for both tooth decay and/or periodontal disease to proliferate and cause disease.

Changes in the diet to consumption of foods high in sugars and fermentable carbohydrates can cause a proliferation of acid-producing and acid-tolerant bacteria such as mutans-type streptococci and lactobacilli. These bacteria can cause dental caries. Changes in other oral factors can cause the growth of periodontal pathogens leading to gingivitis, periodontitis, and peri-implantitis.

PROBIOTICS

Prescribed antibiotics can kill beneficial bacteria as well as pathogens. It can, then, be a challenge to maintain a healthy level of beneficial bacteria in the mouth and gut. Numerous studies have shown that the introduction of beneficial bacteria called probiotics can help. Probiotics are live microorganisms that are consumed by an individual to promote health. The bacteria are added to milk, yogurt, or sour cream or are available as tablets, capsules, or drops. Probiotics are becoming more popular as a way to increase the numbers of helpful bacteria to the G.I. tract and even the mouth. By increasing the numbers of beneficial bacteria, they can help suppress the harmful bacteria. They help promote a healthy digestive tract and immune system.

Studies conducted over the past 15 years have shown beneficial oral effects in managing dental caries risk by reducing mutans streptococci in plaque and saliva; in managing periodontal disease risk by reducing periodontal pathogens and thereby, reducing bleeding on probing and gingival bleeding; by managing peri-implantitis risks; and by reducing the numbers of Candida (a common fungus in the mouth that causes thrush) by inhibiting its growth. As more evidence is made available and guidelines are established on dosage and types of bacterial species to use for specific oral diseases, it is anticipated that general dentists and specialists will begin to use probiotics on a routine basis for management of these diseases.

BIOFILM AND SYSTEMIC DISEASES

More and more research studies are showing a correlation between periodontal disease and certain systemic diseases such as heart disease, diabetes, some respiratory ailments, and certain complications with pregnancy. It is believed that the ulceration of the gingival sulcus caused by the bacteria in subgingival plaque allows pathogenic bacteria to enter the bloodstream and affect distant organ systems (FIG. 2.14).

BIOFILM ON DENTAL MATERIALS

Biofilm (dental plaque) on oral structures is well documented as having a primary role in the formation of dental caries and periodontal diseases. The role of biofilm adhesion on dental material is less well known. Surface roughness has a direct correlation with biofilm accumulation. Roughness from abrasion, coronal polishing agents, hand and ultrasonic scaling, and lack of finishing (smoothing and shaping) and polishing after fabrication or initial placement of a restoration are all associated with increased biofilm accumulation. Biofilm accumulation at the margins of rough or faulty restorations may, in part, contribute to the development of recurrent caries. Biofilms do not accumulate as readily on polished cast alloys and ceramic restorations, possibly because of their smooth surfaces. Amalgam tends to have a biofilm that is less active likely because of the affect of mercury on the bacterial population. Control of biofilm accumulation on dental implants has been shown to play a significant role in the ultimate success of the implant. Fluoride-releasing materials found in some restorations can counteract the acids produced by biofilms. Dentures tend to develop a biofilm that is high in Candida (a yeast) and is associated with chronic irritation of the underlying oral mucosa known as denture stomatitis. Occasionally, the denture stomatitis requires treatment with antifungal medication to clear it up. So, prevention is the best treatment.

MANAGING THE ORAL BIOFILM

Currently, we do not have a means of totally eliminating pathogens in the oral biofilm, but we can manage the biofilm so that a healthy mouth can be maintained. The American Dental Association recommends twice daily brushing and daily flossing as a basic minimum oral hygiene routine. Tooth brushing with a fluoride-containing paste can be accomplished with manual or power brushing. Interdental cleaning is commonly done with dental floss, but a variety of other aids are available such as toothpicks, balsa sticks (Stimu-Dents®), interproximal plastic cleaners (GUM Soft-picks®) and oral irrigators (WaterPik®). Additional oral hygiene measures may include tongue brushing or scraping. ADA accepted antimicrobial mouth rinses, especially those with a combination of essential oils (e.g. Listerine®) or chlorhexidine (e.g. Peridex®), can be helpful in managing gingivitis and supragingival plaque.

It is important for denture wearers to clean their dentures daily with a denture brush and non-abrasive paste and use a denture soak to remove the adherent biofilm.

 Caution

It is important that the oral health practitioner carefully identify the locations and types of restorations present in the patient's mouth and take precautions to avoid altering their surfaces while instrumenting teeth or adjacent restorations.

DETECTION OF RESTORATIVE MATERIALS

Oral health care professionals must be able to identify restorative materials within the oral environment to treat them appropriately. Heavy pressure during scaling, the use of sonic and ultrasonic scaling (uses high frequency vibrations) or air polishing (air-driven stream of fine abrasive particles to smooth the surface), and inappropriate use of polishing agents may gouge or scratch the surface of a restoration (FIG. 2.15). The placement of therapeutic agents such as acidulated fluoride may etch the surface of the restoration.

Identification of restorative materials, which may be obvious with amalgam materials, may also be difficult when identifying tooth-colored materials such as composite resin or ceramics. In addition, restorations may be composed of different materials, such as a ceramic inlay cemented with resin-based cement. Identification of restorative materials may be by appearance, location, tactile sensitivity, and radiography. A well-matched tooth-colored restoration may be difficult to distinguish from natural tooth structures. Well-developed tactile sensitivity skills with a dental explorer, adequate illumination, liberal use of air to dry the teeth and restorations, and even magnification may be needed to detect some esthetic restoration. The location of margins, especially

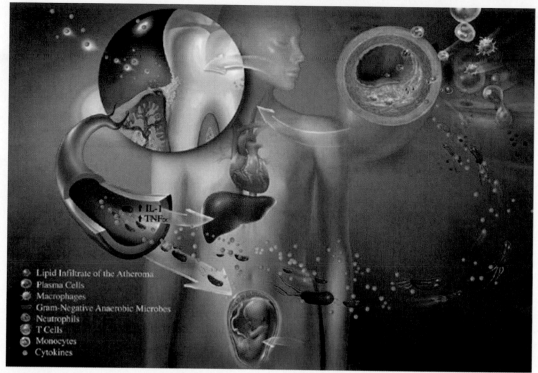

FIG. 2.14 Subgingival plaque bacteria and/or their by-products may gain access to distant sites in the body through the circulatory system and may potentially contribute to systemic inflammation. In this way, a dental biofilm infection may contribute to various systemic diseases and conditions. (From McNeil J Dent Hygiene vol 81, No 5, Oct 2007 Fig 4)

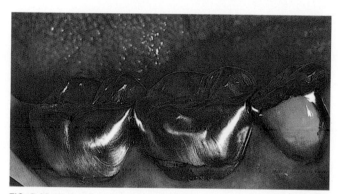

FIG. 2.15 The scratched surface of these gold crowns is due to inappropriate use of polishing agents.

those placed subgingivally, make visual inspection of many materials impossible. Drying the teeth well often makes detection of composites easier. Saliva tends to hide the distinction between the tooth surface and the margins of the restoration as well as the differences in the texture and luster (shininess) of the restoration surfaces.

Tactile evaluation of the tooth surface can be a helpful means of clinical assessment. The surface of some composite and glass ionomer restorations may feel rougher than enamel. Tracing the enamel surface onto the restoration with the sharp tip of an explorer is the best way to distinguish this difference. The clinician may detect a smooth surface on the enamel and a "scratchy" surface on the restoration. This difference may be noticed at the cavosurface margin (the margin of the cavity preparation that meets the tooth surface).

Once the presence of a restoration is identified, the entire cavosurface margin should be evaluated. The cavosurface margin should be almost undetectable as the tip of the explorer passes from the restoration to the tooth. Sealants have a smooth glassy surface covering the anatomical pits and fissures of the tooth surfaces; the explorer feels like it is skating on ice. Porcelain has a very smooth glassy surface, and the explorer glides easily over the surface (FIG. 2.16). Note the tip of the explorer as it glides against the margin of the restoration.

Adequate direct illumination and transillumination are helpful for the detection of many anterior restorations. With transillumination light can pass through teeth to varying degrees based upon the intensity of the light and the thickness of the teeth. A mouth mirror placed lingual to the incisors can reflect the operatory light through these thin teeth. The light will not pass through the restoration as well as enamel so it will stand out. This, along with the knowledge that most anterior restorations are prepared from the lingual surface to preserve as much natural enamel on the facial surface as possible, will help in the identification of many class III and IV restorations.

Magnification and the liberal use of air will help to distinguish the glossy surface of enamel versus the more opaque surface of composite and resin restorations. (However, highly polished newer generations of composites allow them to be polished to a very smooth, lustrous surface similar to enamel.)

Radiographs are a valuable tool for the detection of restorations and the assessment of restorative components. Most modern composites are radiopaque, but

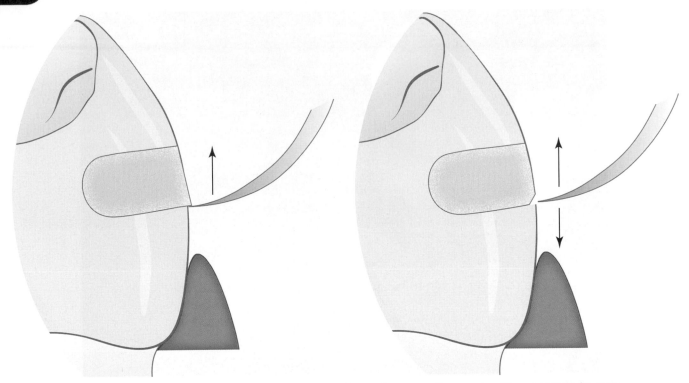

FIG. 2.16 The restoration margin in the first drawing extends over the cavosurface margin of the preparation (an overhanging margin) causing a trap for food and biofilm and if located on the proximal surface, will make flossing difficult. The restoration margin in the second drawing does not meet the cavosurface margin of the preparation (a deficient margin) causing a trap for biofilm and possibly lead to recurrent caries.

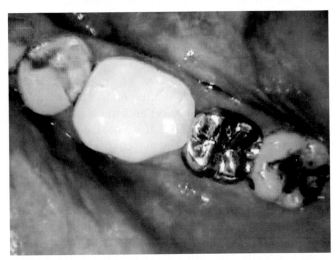

FIG. 2.17 Tooth-colored restorative materials may be difficult to detect. Tooth #17 DO amalgam; tooth #18 gold crown over an implant; tooth #19 porcelain fused to metal crown; tooth #20 DO composite restoration.

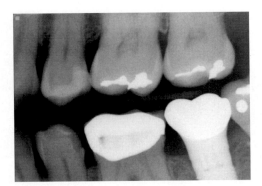

FIG. 2.18 Radiograph of the restorations in Fig. 2.17. Note the radiopacities: composite #13 DO, amalgam #14, #15, and #17, gold crown #18 implant and PBM crown #19. Radiolucency of older type composite is seen in #20 DO.

some older ones are radiolucent. Glass ionomers are radiopaque, as are many resin-based cements and ceramics (FIGS. 2.17 and 2.18 illustrate various types of restorative materials as seen intraorally as well as their corresponding radiographic appearance). Note that the restoration on tooth #20 is an older radiolucent type of composite material whereas the composite on #13 is a radiopaque type. The other radiopaque restorative materials include the amalgam restorations seen on teeth #14, #15, and #17, as well as the gold crown on an implant #18 and a porcelain fused to metal crown on #19.

For most difficult-to-detect restorations, it is necessary to use a combination of the above-described methods to determine the presence and type of material before clinical procedures are performed.

Conditions for Assessing Restoration

- Dry field
- Good lighting
- Sharp explorer
- Radiographs
- Magnification
- Good knowledge of the material

SUMMARY

The oral environment presents unique challenges to the successful use of dental materials as restorative and therapeutic agents. An understanding of the limiting factors in this environment and an appreciation for how these limitations affect the selection of materials are essential to the successful use of dental materials. Materials used must be biocompatible, exhibit long-term clinical durability, and be esthetically acceptable. No one material is superior in all of these areas. The allied oral health care practitioner must have an understanding of the limitations as well as the criteria for selection of therapeutic and restorative materials. With this knowledge he or she can educate the patient about the materials used in their mouths as well as select and properly manipulate and maintain materials to ensure their ultimate success.

INSTRUCTIONAL VIDEOS

See the Evolve Resources site for a variety of educational videos that reinforce the material covered in this chapter.

Get Ready for Exams!

Review Questions

Select the one correct response for each of the following multiple-choice questions.

1. The safe interaction of a dental material with the rest of the body is defined as the material's
   a. radioactivity
   b. carcinogenicity
   c. biocompatibility
   d. therapeutic reaction

2. The study of dental materials includes knowledge of
   a. the chemical reactions of the material
   b. the physical reactions of the material
   c. the ways to manipulate the material
   d. all of the above

3. The internal reaction to an externally applied force is called
   a. strain
   b. stress
   c. hardness
   d. elasticity

4. When increasingly higher forces are applied to a material it will eventually fracture and the point of fracture is called
   a. fatigue fracture
   b. tensile strength
   c. ultimate strength
   d. compressive fracture

5. Material subject to repeated stresses such as in mastication may be subject to fracture due to
   a. flexural stress
   b. force exerted over a large area
   c. forces stretching an object
   d. fatigue failure

6. Which of the following restorative materials is the most soluble?
   a. Amalgam
   b. Glass ionomer
   c. Porcelain
   d. Acrylic

7. Corrosion is of greatest concern for which of the following restorative materials?
   a. Gold
   b. Composite resin
   c. Amalgam
   d. Porcelain

8. Surface discoloration of a metal restoration is called
   a. corrosion
   b. tarnish
   c. crystallization
   d. metallurgy

9. Restorative materials with values of thermal conductivity similar to enamel include
   a. gold
   b. composite resin
   c. amalgam
   d. silver

10. Susan has just had an MOD amalgam placed on tooth #30. When biting, this tooth is in contact with a gold crown on tooth #3. Susan complains of electric shock sensation and metal taste. This is most likely due to
    a. galvanism
    b. corrosion
    c. tarnish
    d. metamerism

11. Microleakage may be responsible for
    a. recurrent decay
    b. marginal staining
    c. postoperative sensitivity
    d. all of the above

12. Excessive film thickness of cements may cause
    a. an increase in retention
    b. a decrease in marginal leakage
    c. improper seating of the restoration
    d. fracture of the restoration

13. The leakage of fluids and debris extending along the tooth-restoration interface is called
    a. metamerism
    b. trituration

Continued

Get Ready for Exams!—cont'd

  c. microleakage
  d. deformation
14. Colonies of bacteria growing on the teeth are called
  a. principle invaders
  b. parasites
  c. dental plaque
  d. primary intruders
15. Color shades can vary depending on the incident light or source of light. This effect is called
  a. spectrum
  b. chroma
  c. meniscus
  d. metamerism

16. The term that describes the intensity of color is
  a. hue
  b. value
  c. chroma
  d. opacity
17. Oral biofilm is
  a. a slick film of mucus that develops on surfaces within ther mouth
  b. composed of bacteria only
  c. considered normal or healthy when non-pathogens keep harmful microbes in balance
  d. is a complex organization of microorganisms on oral surfaces and restorations

For answers to Review Questions, see the Appendix.

Case-Based Discussion Topics

1. A 45-year-old businessman comes to your dental office with the chief complaint of having to wear a maxillary removable partial denture. He wishes to have this removable prosthesis replaced with a fixed bridge. Examination reveals that the partial denture replaces teeth #6 through #11.

Discuss the stresses that would be placed on a bridge of this span.

2. A 25-year-old school teacher comes to your office with the chief complaint of losing a distal-incisal class IV composite from tooth #9. She explains that this restoration has been in place for only a few days.

Discuss the factors that might affect the bond strength of this restoration and what you can do to help prevent this from happening again.

3. Look into a mirror, or position yourself to examine someone else's mouth, and check the following:
  a. Check how tooth surfaces contact on the posterior, middle, and anterior teeth when in normal occlusion, biting edge-to-edge on anterior teeth, and moving the jaw laterally and front to back.

Which forces are being exerted by these teeth and when?
  b. Check for metal and resin restorations. Place a piece of ice on the enamel of a tooth, on the metal restoration, and on the resin restoration.

How long does it take to feel sensation to the pulp for each? What is this property called?
  c. Look at the gingival, middle, and incisal/occlusal third of anterior and posterior teeth.

How does the color of the area change; is there a change in translucency or opacity? Place something bright red close to the teeth, and direct the dental lamp or other bright light onto the teeth. How do these factors affect the color?

BIBLIOGRAPHY

Anusavice KJ: *Phillips' Science of Dental Materials* (ed 12). Philadelphia, 2013, Saunders.

Bird DL, Robinson DS: *Torres and Ehrlich Modern Dental Assisting* (ed 11). Philadelphia, 2015, Saunders.

Gurenlian JR: The role of dental plaque biofilm in oral health. *J Dent Hyg* 81(5):116, 2007.

Marsh PD: Ecological events in oral health and disease: new opportunities for prevention and disease control? *J Calif Dent Assoc* 45(10):525–537, 2017.

Twetman S, Jørgensen MR, Keller MK: Fifteen years of probiotic therapy in the dental context: what has been achieved? *J Calif Dent Assoc* 45(10):539–545, 2017.

Powers JM, Wataha JC: *Dental Materials: Foundations and Applications* (ed 11). St. Louis, 2017, Elsevier.

Sakaguchi RL, Powers JM: Fundamentals of materials science. In *Craig's Restorative Dental Materials* (ed 13). St. Louis, 2012, Mosby (Chapter 4).

Van Noort R: Principles of adhesion. In *Introduction to Dental Materials* (ed 4). London, 2013, Mosby (Chapter 1.9).

Physical and Mechanical Properties of Dental Materials

Chapter Objectives

Upon completion of this chapter, the student should be able to:

1. Define primary and secondary bonds and give an example of how each determines the properties of the material.
2. Describe the three forms of matter and give a defining characteristic of each.
3. Define density and explain the relationship of density, volume, and crystalline structure.
4. Define hardness and describe how hardness contributes to abrasion resistance.
5. Define elasticity and give an example of when elasticity is desirable in dental procedures.
6. Relate stiffness and proportional limit, and describe how these properties apply to restorative dental materials.
7. Define ductility and malleability and explain how these characteristics contribute to the edge strength of a gold crown.
8. Explain the difference between toughness and resilience.
9. Define brittleness and discuss how this property applies to restorative dental materials.
10. Define viscosity and thixotropy and describe the clinical significance of each.
11. Differentiate between therapeutic, preventive, and restorative materials.
12. List and describe the three main types of restorative dental materials.
13. Describe the reaction stages a material undergoes to acquire its final state.
14. Describe the variables in the manipulation of a material.

Key Terms

Primary Bonds strong bonds with electronic attractions; ionic bonds, covalent bonds, metallic bonds

Secondary Bonds weaker bonds than primary bonds; hydrogen bonds, van der Waals forces, London Dispersion Forces

Brittle hard materials that break easily when stress is applied. They break suddenly with little plastic deformation, e.g., glass.

Density the measure of the c weight of a material compared with its volume

Hardness the resistance of a solid to penetration

Ultimate Strength the maximum amount of stress a material can withstand without breaking

Elasticity the ability of a material to recover its shape completely after deformation from an applied force

Elastic Deformation deformation of a material that recovers its original shape and size when the force is removed

Elastic Limit the greatest stress a structure can withstand without permanent deformation

Plastic Deformation deformation of a material causing permanent changes in size or shape due to an applied force

Yield Stress the stress at which plastic deformation begins; also called yield point on a stress-strain curve

Stiffness a material's resistance to deformation

Young's Modulus or Elastic Modulus measures the resistance of a material to being deformed.

Resilience the ability of a material to absorb energy without permanent deformation

Toughness the ability of a material to resist fracture

Ductility the ability of an object to be pulled or stretched under tension without rupture

Malleability the ability to be compressed and formed into a thin sheet without rupture

Edge Strength the ability of a material to withstand fracture at a thin edge, such as at margins of a restoration

Durability the ability of a material to withstand damage due to pressure or wear

Viscosity the ability of a liquid material to resist flow

Thixotropy a characteristic of some gels and liquids that they will flow more readily under mechanical force such as mixing, stirring, or shaking.

Direct Restorative Materials restorations placed directly into a cavity preparation

Indirect Restorative Materials materials used to fabricate restorations outside the mouth that are subsequently placed into the mouth

Permanent Restorations restorations expected to be long-lasting

Temporary Restorations restorations expected to last several days or weeks

Intermediate Restorations restorations expected to last several weeks to months

Mixing Time the amount of time allotted to bring the components of a material together into a homogeneous mix

Working Time the lapse of time from the start of mixing the material until it begins to harden and is no longer workable because it has reached its initial set

Initial Set Time coincides with the end of working time and is the time at which the material can no longer be manipulated in the mouth

Final Set Time the time needed for the reaction that begins when the material is mixed to go to completion, and the material hardens to its permanent state

Chemical Set Materials materials that set through a timed chemical reaction with the combination of a catalyst and base

Light-Activated Materials materials that require light in the blue wave range to initiate a reaction

Dual Set Materials materials that polymerize either from exposure to light in the blue wave range or from a chemical reaction

Shelf Life the useful life of a material before it deteriorates or changes in quality

---

To predict how a material will react under oral conditions, it is necessary to have an understanding of its physical properties. Chapter 2 (Oral Environment and Patient Considerations) discussed how the oral environment could affect and challenge the properties of dental materials. This chapter discusses how those properties are achieved, how they influence the clinician's choice of a material, and how and when properties can be manipulated. Both physical and mechanical properties must be considered when choosing the best restorative dental material. Physical properties are those properties of materials that can be measured and observed without having to change the composition of the material and they help describe it. Physical properties include properties such as color, thermal conductivity, and solubility. Mechanical properties are properties that define the material's ability to perform in the oral environment and resist stresses and strains. Mechanical properties are considered a subset of physical properties and include properties such as elasticity, ductility, durability, and ultimate strength.

Electrochemical properties are seen in the reactions of materials as they set or their reactions to corrosive elements in the oral environment and their chemical stability and durability in the mouth.

To begin a discussion of the properties of dental materials, it is important to begin with a review of the physical structure of matter.

PHYSICAL STRUCTURE

ATOMS

Atoms are the basic building blocks of matter. They are composed of particles called neutrons, protons, and electrons (Fig. 3.1). Protons have positive electrical charges; electrons have negative charges and neutrons have no electrical charges. Neutrons and protons being heavier than electrons form the nucleus in the center of the atom. Electrons are found in orbits (also called shells) around the nucleus. It is the outermost orbit in which electrons (called valence electrons) will interact with other atoms. The numbers and configuration of electrons in their orbits affect how reactive they are with other atoms. Some atoms have space within their outer orbits while other atoms have extra electrons in

their outer orbits. Atoms attempt to form the most stable configurations possible by filling their outermost orbits with electrons when bonding with other atoms. To do this, they will transfer or share electrons.

TYPES OF BONDS

Two categories of bonds are formed between two atoms; strong bonds are called **primary bonds** and weaker bonds are called **secondary bonds**.

Primary Bonds

Primary bonds are the strongest bonds that hold atoms together because they involve the transferring or sharing of electrons. The three types of primary bonds (Fig. 3.2) are:

- Covalent bonds
- Ionic bonds
- Metallic bonds

Covalent Bonds

Covalent bonds represent a type of bond that occurs when two nonmetal atoms share electrons in their outer shells, creating full shells for both (Fig. 3.2B). Many covalent bonds form gasses (hydrogen molecule, H_2) or materials with low melting points. Covalent bonds occurring in a network configuration are very strong.

Structure of atom

FIG. 3.1 The atomic structure. Heavy neutrons and protons form the nucleus of the atom and electrons circle around the nucleus in shells or orbits.

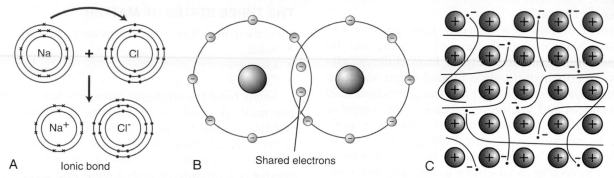

FIG. 3.2 Primary Bonds. **A**. Ionic bond, characterized by electron transfer from one element (Na) to another (Cl). **B**. Covalent bond, characterized by electron sharing and very precise bond orientations. **C**. Metallic bond, characterized by electron sharing and formation of a "cloud" of electrons that bonds to the positively charged nucleus in a lattice. (From Anusavice KJ, Shen C, Rawls H: *Phillips' Science of Dental Materials* (ed 12). St. Louis, 2013, Saunders.)

Diamond is a good example of a strong network covalent bond; it is hard and has a high melting point. Some materials are made up of chains of covalent bonds; polymers used in plastic and rubber are good examples of long chains of covalently bonded atoms.

Ionic Bonds

When atoms gain or lose electrons they become electrically charged and are called ions. Positively charged (+) ions are called cations and negatively charged (-) ions are called anions. Ions that have opposite charges have electrostatic attractions for each other. When they combine, one atom gives up electrons from its outer shell and the other atom gains electrons. The energy that holds these atoms together to form a molecule is called ionic bonding. Salt or sodium chloride is an example of ionic bonding (Fig. 3.2A).

Materials bonded in this way, such as ceramics, are usually brittle when they are pulled or bent and are poor electrical conductors. Ionic bonding can also be seen in gypsum products and phosphate-based cements.

Metallic Bonds

When atoms join to form metals, they bond in an entirely different manner than with covalent or ionic bonding, but they still attempt to form stable outer orbits. Multiple atoms in a lattice arrangement share a large pool of valence electrons that move throughout the material. This sea of electrons passing among the atoms produces what is called metallic bonding (Fig. 3.2C). Imagine filling a bucket with marbles and then adding water. The marbles are arranged in a structured manner and the water fills the spaces between them. The water is like the sea of electrons that is shared by the metal atoms represented here as marbles.

It is this type of bonding with freely flowing electrons that is responsible for many of the physical properties seen with metals such as their strength or ability to conduct heat and electricity, to be formed into shapes such as coins or jewelry (malleable), or stretched into wires (ductile) like those used in orthodontics.

Combinations of Primary Bonds

Many materials contain more than one type of primary bond.

SECONDARY BONDS

Secondary bonds, broadly called **van der Waals forces**, are very different than primary bonds. Unlike primary bonds, no transfer or sharing of electrons occurs. Secondary bonds are forces found between molecules in the same material (i.e., attractions between water molecules) rather than forces that bond atoms (together into a molecule) such as covalent bonding of hydrogen and oxygen atoms to form a water molecule. The secondary bonds are created by various types of electric dipoles. A dipole is created when electrons are unequally shared between atoms within a molecule forming positive and negative charge centers at each end of the molecule causing an electrical imbalance. Secondary bonds are much weaker than primary bonds.

Three examples of secondary bonds include
- Hydrogen bonds (dipole-dipole forces)
- Permanent dipoles
- Temporary dipoles

Hydrogen Bonds

Hydrogen bonds are dipole-dipole inactions. They exist in molecules where electrons are not shared equally and thus have electrical poles. In the case of water, hydrogen is attracted to the larger oxygen atom. Although electrons are shared between the hydrogen and oxygen atoms, these electrons are unbalanced, spending more time around the oxygen atom. This causes a partial negative charge on the oxygen side of the molecule, and a partial positive charge on the hydrogen side setting up two opposite electromagnetic poles called a dipole. They act like a magnet attracting opposite charges. These bonds are responsible for many of the properties of water such as solvent properties, cohesion (sticks to itself), adhesion (sticks to other materials), and density. Hydrogen bonds are the strongest of the secondary bonds but still much weaker than primary bonds.

Permanent Dipoles

Permanent dipoles in a molecule have positive and negative charge centers that do not fluctuate and the molecule must consist of atoms from different elements. A permanent dipole is formed when one atom in a molecule has a stronger electron attraction than another atom and, therefore, becomes more negative in its charge. Then, the other atom becomes more positive in its charge. This electrical imbalance creates an electric dipole. When the attraction between dipoles in adjacent molecules causes them to interact, they form weak bonds between the molecules. Hydrochloric acid (HCl) is an example of a polar molecule where the molecules are held together by permanent dipole-dipole forces.

Temporary (Induced) Dipoles

All atoms and molecules have electron clouds. Within a bond the electrons are in constant motion and can oscillate. For brief nanoseconds electrons may be clustered more to one side creating a charge that quickly disappears. The temporary negative charge will attract a temporary positive charge from a nearby molecule, a process called the London dispersion force of attraction. For example, the interaction between iodine molecules is a temporary dipole bond. The London dispersion force is the weakest of the secondary bonds. It is responsible for the condensation of nonpolar atoms or molecules into liquids or solids with a drop in temperature.

Types of Bonds

PRIMARY BONDS
Strong bonds that bind atoms of a molecule
1. Ionic bonds—one atom gives up electrons and another atom gains electrons in the outer shell
2. Covalent bonds—two nonmetal atoms share electrons in their outer shell
3. Metallic bonds—multiple atoms in a lattice configuration share a sea of electrons that move throughout the lattice.

SECONDARY BONDS
Weak bonds that are adhesive forces acting between molecules (broadly called van der Waals forces)
1. Permanent dipole interactions—negatively charged pole in one atom attracts positively charged pole in an adjacent atom to form weak bonds
2. Temporary dipole interaction—constantly circulating electrons in one molecule cluster briefly causing a negative charge that attracts a positive charge form a nearby molecule; called London dispersion force. The weakest of the secondary bonds.
3. Hydrogen bonds—dipole-dipole interaction involving hydrogen atoms where a positive electromagnetically charged atom (commonly hydrogen) attracts a strongly negatively charged atom (adjacent dipole) to bind hydrogen to a larger atom (i.e., oxygen). These are the strongest of the secondary bonds.

THE THREE STATES OF MATTER

Matter exists in three states or phases:
- Solid
- Liquid
- Gas

Solids have the strongest attraction between atoms and molecules and have both shape and volume; a liquid has volume but no definite shape; and a gas has neither definite shape nor volume. Most materials are mixtures of more than one state of matter. For example, plaster is a mixture of both a solid and a liquid, and fluoride foams are a mixture of a liquid and a gas (air) under pressure. Gases are used mostly as propellants in dispensing or mixing dental materials. Therefore, this chapter will limit the discussion to the general properties common to solids and liquids.

Solids

In solids the atoms are packed tightly together and this restricts their movement providing them with a fixed shape. Primary bonds hold the atoms of solids together, giving them strength and stability. Solids maintain their shape and resist forces that try to deform them. Solids are found in two main forms: crystalline or amorphous. Crystalline solids have an ordered three-dimensional symmetrical pattern or lattice network that repeats throughout the crystal (Fig. 3.3). There are 14 different types of lattice structures. Many minerals such as table salt are crystalline solids. Because of their structure crystalline solids cannot be compressed into smaller shapes. Within the lattice structure all bonds between particles are equal so that when heat is applied all the bonds are broken at the same time producing a definite melting point. Ice transforms from a solid state to a liquid state at its melting point of 0° C at standard atmospheric pressure.

Noncrystalline solids called **amorphous** solids have atoms in nonrepeating arrangements similar to liquids. They do not have a definite melting point but soften gradually as heat is applied. Examples of amorphous solids include many dental waxes and glass-type ceramics.

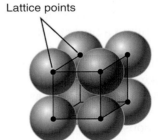

Lattice points

Simple cubic lattice cell

FIG. 3.3 Lattice network in a crystalline solid. Depicted is a simple cubic lattice cell. (From Lattice Structures in Crystalline Solids by Rice University.)

Liquids

Unlike the molecules of a solid, molecules in a liquid state are not confined to patterns; therefore, liquids can easily change shape and can flow. The study of this flow is the science of rheology. Fluid flow can be steady or unsteady, and flow has a major influence on the handling or delivery of dental materials. For example, impression materials that are placed around the prepared tooth must flow readily to capture the fine details of the preparation while impression materials that are placed in the impression tray should exhibit less flow. The movement of a liquid will depend on the characteristics of the liquid and the surface on which it is placed. Chapter 2 defines these characteristics and their relationships in the discussion of bonding.

Viscosity is the resistance of a liquid to flow. Values of viscosity depend on the nature of the fluid; thin liquids have low viscosity and thicker liquids have high viscosity. Water flows readily, and therefore has very low viscosity, whereas higher viscosity liquids (tree sap, for example) have greater ability to resist flow. The viscosity of liquids usually decreases as the temperature increases. Some viscous liquids will flow more readily under stress (a property called **thixotrophy**), for example, when they are mixed, shaken, stirred, or manipulated. Fluoride gels are often advertised as thixotropic. This gives the operator control of the gel while it is in the delivery tray, so that it does not drip out when inserted into the patient's mouth. Once the material is in the mouth, the patient is instructed to chew on the tray, decreasing the material's viscosity and allowing it to flow into pits and fissures and interproximally to improve penetration into all surfaces.

Gypsum products when mixed with water are a slurry (a watery mixture) that can be poured into an impression to create a solid cast when it hardens. Some materials like waxes appear solid but are really supercooled liquids. They can be caused to flow under loading forces or can deform under light stresses.

Liquids when heated eventually vaporize or boil. Water transforms from a liquid state to a gas state (steam) at its boiling point of 100 °C at standard atmospheric pressure. The lower the atmospheric pressure, the lower will be the boiling point.

PROPERTIES OF DENTAL MATERIALS

Properties of dental materials are of three basic types: physical, mechanical, and chemical (or electrochemical).

PHYSICAL PROPERTIES

Physical properties are those properties that can be observed and measured without changing the composition of the material. Physical properties include such things as melting and boiling points, density, viscosity, thermal conductivity, and thermal expansion (see Chapter 2 Oral Environment and Patient Considerations, section on Temperature), and optical properties such as color

(see Chapter 2 Oral Environment and Patient Considerations, section on Esthetics and Chapter 9 Ceramics, section Optical Properties and section Shade Taking).

Density is a measure of the weight a material has compared with its volume. It is a measure of the compactness of matter, or how much mass is squeezed into a given space. A brick and a sponge of the same dimensions have the same volume but the brick is much denser (Fig. 3.4). The sponge has many large air spaces throughout. If you squeeze the sponge, the volume and the air spaces are reduced and the sponge becomes denser (less spacing is seen between atoms). The close spacing of the crystalline structure gives the greatest density. Enamel is the densest of the tooth structures, and gold is a dense restorative material.

MECHANICAL PROPERTIES

Mechanical properties are a subset of physical properties. They are physical properties that are seen when a load or force is applied to a material. They include such properties as hardness, stress, strain, fatigue, strength, elasticity, stiffness, resilience, toughness, ductility, malleability, and durability.

Hardness is the resistance of a solid to penetration. Hardness is also used to define a material's resistance to wear and abrasion. The hardness of a dental structure or material determines the extent to which it is scratched by an abrasive material. Enamel and porcelain, two of the hardest materials, are more resistant to being scratched than are cementum and dentin, or composite resins and gold crowns. For this reason it is very important that the type of restorative material or tooth surface be determined first, before beginning procedures with abrasive agents.

Hardness tests. There are several tests designed to measure the hardness of materials, and they all measure the material's resistance to being indented. Knoop hardness is the value usually given for dental materials. The testing head is shaped like a pyramid for the Knoop and Vickers tests, a cone for the Rockwell test, and a ball for the Brinell test. The Knoop test uses lower pressures for pressing the diamond head into the material than the Vickers test, so it can be used to test a variety of materials including thin or brittle materials

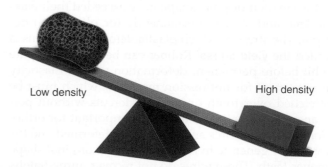

FIG. 3.4 The sponge on the left is porous and low in density while the brick on the right lacks porosity and is very dense. So, the brick weighs more even though the two are about the same in volume.

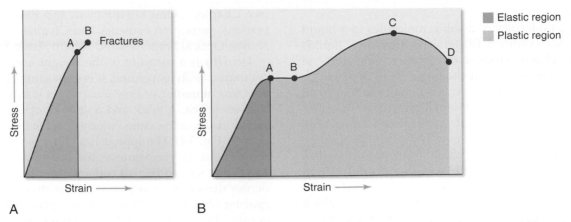

FIG. 3.5 Stress-strain curve **A,** Curve for brittle materials. Brittle material reaches its elastic limit (A) and then quickly fractures (B) with added stress. **B,** Curve for ductile materials. Ductile material reaches its elastic limit (A) and begin to distort (B). This plastic deformation continues until the material reaches its breaking stress (C). Unlike brittle materials, it fails slowly until it reaches its fracture point (D).

such as ceramics. The size of the indentation is measured and the hardness is calculated based upon this size. The smaller the indentation, the harder is the material. The Vickers test is used mostly for testing metals.

Stress develops within a material when a force is applied (see Chapter 2 Oral Environment and Patient Considerations, section on Force, Stress and Strain). The larger the area over which the force is distributed, the less will be the stress. Stress can occur singularly or in various combinations depending on the directions of the applied forces.

When a solid is subjected to an external force of sufficient magnitude, it undergoes change in size and shape and is considered strained. The amount of stress placed on a material at the time it breaks is known as its **ultimate strength**. A material does not necessarily have to break when subjected to an external compressive, shearing, or tensile force; it may deform. If this deformation is not permanent and the material recovers from the force completely, it has good **elasticity** and has undergone **elastic deformation**. A rubber band is an example of a material with elasticity. Plastic deformation, on the other hand, occurs when a force or stress produces an irreversible change in a solid material's shape or size.

Not all materials return to their original shape when the deforming force is removed. Materials that do not return to their original shape have exceeded their **elastic limit** and start to permanently (or plastically) deform. The stress at which **plastic deformation** begins is called the **yield stress**. Rubber can be deformed quite a bit before permanent deformation occurs. Elasticity is important for impression materials, which must be stretched over tooth or bony undercuts without permanent deformation. Elasticity is important for orthodontics, where wires and springs are deformed and the force they generate in returning to their original shape moves teeth. These wires do not recover immediately; rather, they recover over a period of time and with some degree of permanent deformation. This slow progressive recovery is important in the controlled movement of teeth.

The relationship between stress and strain is useful for comparing properties of materials so the best material can be selected for a given application. The relationship can be plotted on a graph with values of stress on the vertical axis and values of strain on the horizontal axis. The resultant curve plotted on the graph represents a behavior of a material when subjected to a load. It provides useful information about the strength and ductility of materials and can compare the response of different materials to the same load. The stress-strain curve for each material is unique, but it is possible to find some characteristics in common among various groups of materials. For example, stress-strain curves for brittle materials or ductile materials have similar characteristics (Fig. 3.5). The stress-strain curve for brittle materials such as porcelain has only an elastic region followed by fracture of the material. There is no yield point and the ultimate strength and the fracture strength are the same. **Young's modulus** measures the resistance of a material to being deformed. The **stiffness** of a material, i.e., the lack of elasticity, means that it resists being deformed and it is measured by Young's modulus (also called elastic modulus). Stiffer materials have a higher modulus; enamel has a high modulus. Restorative materials should have a modulus that is compatible with tooth structure. We usually do not want dental restorations to bend or compress when a force is applied, so materials such as amalgam, composite resin, and ceramics should be stiff.

Resilience is the amount of energy a material can absorb without permanent deformation. Impression materials and orthodontic wire must be resilient to be successful. When an impression is removed from the patient's mouth it needs to deform to be slipped over the contours of the oral structures. To be an accurate impression it is equally important that the material returns completely to the original shape of the oral structures impressed.

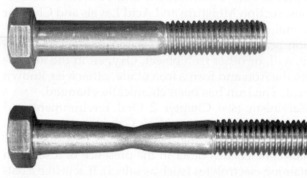

FIG. 3.6 Ductility. Stainless steel is an example of a very ductile metal. When placed under enough stress, it will elongate significantly before it fractures. (Courtesy Fastenal Company, Winona, MN.)

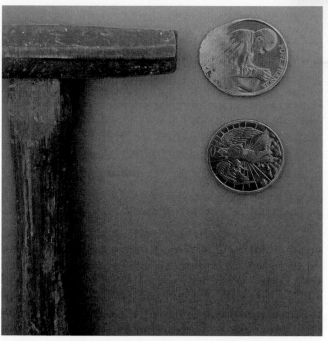

FIG. 3.7 Malleability. The two coins are made from a malleable metal and were originally the same size. The left side of the top coin has been pounded with a hammer to a thin edge without breaking. This property is is an indication of malleability. (Courtesy Dr. Steve Eakle.)

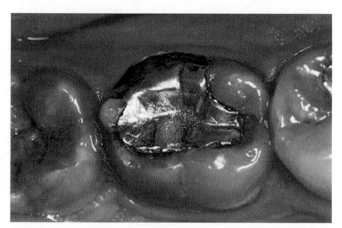

FIG. 3.8 An amalgam restoration with severe breakdown of the margins creating a space or ditch between the amalgam and the cavity preparation. (Courtesy of S. Geraldeli. From Anusavice KJ, Shen C, Rawls H: *Phillips' Science of Dental Materials* (ed 12). St. Louis, 2013, Saunders, p. 357.)

Toughness is the ability of a material to absorb energy without fracture; restorative materials must exhibit toughness. Brittle materials have limited toughness because small amounts of deformation will cause fracture. Traditional porcelain restorations are much more likely to fail on the occlusal surfaces of posterior teeth than are gold restorations. Newer ceramic materials such as zirconia are very tough.

Pulling or stretching of orthodontic wire under tensile stress is a measure of its **ductility** (Fig. 3.6), that is, the amount of dimensional change it can withstand without breaking. Gold is very ductile since it can be elongated close to 20%. Materials with poor ductility are classified as **brittle**. These materials are much weaker when subjected to tensile forces than to compressive forces. Porcelain is brittle and cannot undergo much tensile stress without fracture; its ultimate strength is about equal to its elastic limit. Gold is not only ductile, but it is malleable too (Fig. 3.7). **Malleability** means that it responds easily to compressive stress and can be hammered into a thin sheet without fracture. The combination of malleability and ductility gives this metal the ability to resist fracture even at fine margins, giving gold **edge strength**. These characteristics allow for the superior edge strength of gold crowns. Amalgam does not have good edge strength. If an insufficient amount of amalgam is present at the edge of a restoration, the forces of mastication will likely cause fracture of the material at the margin (Figures 3.8 and 3.9). In most cases noble metals tend to be ductile and malleable, but ceramics are brittle. Ceramics and composites are described as brittle, because they will sustain little strain before they fracture.

Fatigue occurs within a material when it is subjected to repeated stresses and can result in a sudden failure or fracture of the material. Microscopic flaws or cracks develop within the material that progress with repeated loading. This can be seen when a strip of metal is bent back and forth repeatedly until it breaks. Likewise, weak cusps of a tooth may fracture over time from repeated chewing forces placed on them (Fig. 3.10).

Durability refers to the ability of a material to withstand damage due to pressure or wear. Both porcelain and metal are very durable, resilient, and tough and can absorb stress without breaking. Porcelain is brittle, however, and cannot withstand shearing stresses as well as metals. Metals are very durable but not as esthetic as porcelain. All-ceramic crowns have replaced porcelain in many applications, and provide excellent mechanical properties as well as esthetics. Amalgam is durable and provides longevity and a cost-effective alternative. Amalgam restorations lack esthetics and contain mercury, which some offices have chosen to eliminate from their environment. Composites provide a durable option in areas where esthetics are important, but can they stain and do not resist abrasion as well as the other restorative choices. The new nanocomposite materials have improved this restorative choice. To adequately evaluate the best restorative choice, durability and esthetics are both important.

CHEMICAL PROPERTIES

Chemical properties are those that involve a chemical reaction that changes the material into one or more different materials. Atoms have been rearranged and a new material is formed. Some of the chemical reactions in the mouth involve an electrical current and these are called electrochemical reactions. **Corrosion** is the most common electrochemical property seen in the oral cavity and is seen most often with metals (see

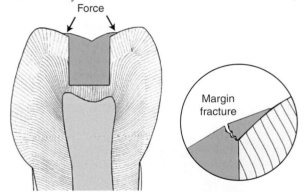

FIG. 3.9 Chipping of the margins of an amalgam restoration. Amalgam is a brittle material. If a thin edge of amalgam is left overlapping the enamel at the margin after carving, this excess amalgam may fracture away under chewing forces creating ragged margins or a gap that collects plaque. (From Anusavice KJ, Shen C, Rawls H: *Phillips' Science of Dental Materials* (ed 12). St. Louis, 2013, Saunders, p. 357.)

Chapter 2 Oral Environment and Patient Considerations, section Moisture and Acid Levels and Chapter 10 Amalgam, Fig. 10.3). A very common form of corrosion seen in your neighborhood is a rusting iron gate, nail, or other iron object. Oxygen in the air oxidizes the iron and forms iron oxide, otherwise known as rust. The iron has been chemically changed.

Galvinism (see Chapter 2 Oral Environment and Patient Considerations, section Galvinism) is an electrochemical reaction that occurs when two dissimilar metals contact each other in the presence of a solution containing electrolytes (such as saliva). It acts like a battery and produces an electric current causing the patient to experience electric shocks and/or a metallic taste.

CLASSIFICATION OF MATERIALS

Restorative dental materials can be classified by their composition and divided into the categories of metals and their alloys, ceramics, and polymers.

Metals have properties such as strength, ability to conduct electricity and heat, malleability, ductility, and luster. Metals and their alloys are used for amalgam restorations, implants, partial denture frameworks, and crowns and bridges.

Ceramics are strong but generally are rigid and brittle and melt at high temperatures. They are poor conductors of heat and electricity. Ceramics are popular for esthetic crowns and veneers.

Polymers can occur in long chains that give certain properties depending on how the chains are linked to each other. Some polymers can be flexible, easily shaped, and rubbery, while others can be hard, rigid, and difficult to mold into shapes. They can be used for denture bases and denture teeth, for example.

Composite resins are combinations of polymers and ceramics. The polymer component allows the material

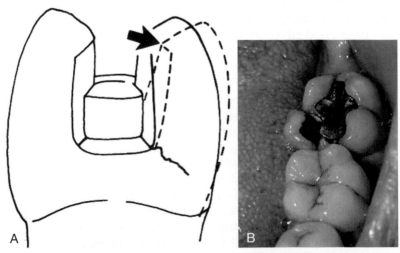

FIG. 3.10 Material fatigue. **A,** Crack develops and propagates under cusp as it flexes under repeated chewing pressure. **B,** Fatigue fracture of ML cusp of lower 2nd molar. (Courtesy Dr. Steve Eakle.)

to adapt to the walls of the cavity preparation and be shaped, while the ceramic component adds wear resistance and provides color and other optical properties for esthetics.

Materials also can be classified by their application, how they will be used and fabricated, and their expected longevity. As stated in Chapter 2, they may be preventive, therapeutic, or restorative:

Preventive materials: Preventive materials are directed toward preventing the occurrence of oral disease, trauma to teeth and jaws, and promoting oral health. Fluorides, pit and fissure sealants, and polyethylene materials for sports guards are preventive materials.

Therapeutic materials: Therapeutic materials are used in the treatment of disease and include materials such as medicated bases or topical treatments for periodontal disease.

Restorative materials: Restorative materials represent the largest classification. This classification applies to any filling, inlay, crown, bridge, implant, or partial or complete denture that restores or replaces lost tooth structure, teeth, or oral tissue. Restorative materials may be used for short-term (temporary crowns, cements) or for long-term use (permanent restorations, prosthetic, implant, and orthodontic appliances).

Restorations may be further classified as **direct restorative materials** or **indirect restorative materials**. Direct restorative materials are fabricated directly in the mouth, whereas indirect restorative materials are fabricated outside the mouth (often in dental laboratories, using replicas of the patient's dentition) and then placed in the patient's mouth.

Some materials such as amalgams and composites may be fabricated directly in the mouth. Other materials, because of convenience or toxicity or other physically harmful characteristics, need to be fabricated indirectly, outside the mouth, and then placed into the oral environment. Porcelain, for instance, needs to be fired to temperatures higher than 1000 °F, making indirect fabrication necessary.

Materials are classified by longevity, that is, how long they are expected to hold up in the oral cavity. Although all materials will degrade, wear, or fracture over time, **permanent restorations** are expected to be a long-lasting replacement for missing, damaged, or discolored teeth. **Temporary restorations**, also called *provisional restorations*, are used for short periods of time, several days to weeks. They function in the place of the permanent restoration to protect the teeth, prevent sensitivity and unwanted tooth movement, maintain the health and contours of the periodontal tissues, enable the patient to function normally, and provide temporary esthetics in the prepared area. **Intermediate restorations**, like provisional restorations, are placed for a limited time; however, the time may extend from several weeks to months. These restorations are not expected to replace tooth structure permanently and are

generally used when there is other ongoing treatment such as orthodontics or implant therapy that is needed before a permanent restoration is required.

COMPOSITION

Materials may be classified by their composition. Components and the reactions of those components may aid classification of materials. Many types of dental materials require the combination of two components to form the resulting final material. These initial two components may begin as water and powder, liquid and powder, paste and liquid, paste and paste, or paste and initiator (blue light). Dental plaster begins with water and powder components. Composite restorations may require a paste, with blue light as an initiator. Many of these components are classified as catalyst and base; the catalyst is responsible for the speed at which the reaction occurs and is often the liquid component. Components may be measured and dispensed as catalyst and base or packaged in predosed amounts.

 Clinical Tip

Standardization of measurements in predose packages eliminates the errors produced in measuring.

REACTION ACTIVATED BY MIXING

When components are mixed together, a reaction occurs. This reaction may be physical, involving the evaporation or cooling of liquid, or it may be chemical, creating new primary bonds. Most reactions of the two components result in a solid structure. Before the material reaches its ultimate solid state, the process goes through stages: the manipulation stage and the reaction stage. Both stages are defined in units of time. The manipulation stage includes the mixing time and working time, and the reaction stage includes the initial set and final set times. **Mixing time** is the length of time the dental auxiliary has to bring the components together into a homogeneous mix. To allow the clinician the full working time, mixing times must be strictly observed. The **working time** is the time from mixing the material until it begins to harden and is no longer workable because it has reached its initial set. The **initial set time** coincides with the end of working time and it occurs when the material no longer can be manipulated in the mouth. The **final set time** is that time needed for the reaction that begins when the material is mixed to go to completion, and the material hardens in its permanent state (Fig. 3.11).

Mixing and working times often offer some control variables. Mixing slowly and cooling the components may increase the working time; the addition of more catalyst may decrease the working time. Control of these variables is important for some situations. For instance, when working with pediatric patients, or

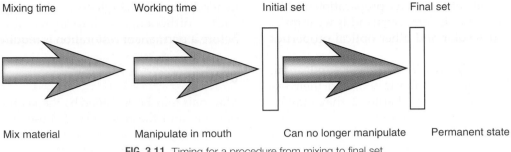

Mixing time   Working time   Initial set   Final set

Mix material   Manipulate in mouth   Can no longer manipulate   Permanent state

FIG. 3.11 Timing for a procedure from mixing to final set.

patients who have a limited opening, decreasing the working time would be desirable. When one is working with a large amount of restorative material, an increase in the working time may be required, so that the material can be manipulated for a longer time. The amount of working time also may be controlled by how the reaction stage is initiated. **Chemical set materials** are those that set through the timed chemical reaction of a catalyst and base. Once the two components come in contact with each other, the chemical reaction begins and continues through the reaction stage. The clinician has little or no control of the time, except cooling the material before mixing. For this reason many clinicians have selected light-activated systems for their materials. **Light-activated materials** use a light source in the blue light range to initiate the reaction stage (Fig. 3 12, and see Chapter 6, section on Light Curing for a detailed discussion). Both components are present in the material but do not react until the material comes in contact with the blue light source, thus giving the clinician unlimited working time. **Dual set materials** have a slow chemical set that is activated when components are mixed but the set can be accelerated by light curing. This gives the clinician much more control of the working time and gives assurance of complete setting in deeper or more difficult-to-access areas of the mouth or preparation.

The setting times, initial and final, are important to the auxiliary as well as the clinician. The material must not be disturbed after the initial set has occurred. Moisture and pressure controls are frequently important during the initial set. Moisture contamination, from saliva and blood, during the initial set time may have an adverse effect on many dental materials, causing them to fail. Continued firm pressure from biting force or from holding the material firmly in the mouth is essential for materials needing intimate contact with the tooth, such as dental cements. The final set of the material may occur while the patient is still in the office or several hours later. Many amalgam restorations reach their final set 8 hours or more after placement. Appropriate patient postoperative instructions on when and what to eat, what to avoid, or how to place pressure on the restoration are essential to avoid fracture of these materials. The accompanying box gives an example of

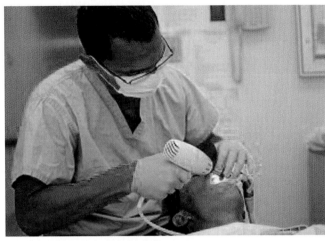

FIG. 3.12 Light curing unit that emits light in the blue wave range is used to cure light-activated material in the mouth.

manipulation instructions for dental cement, including units of time.

Variables in the manipulation of the material begin with the ratios of the components.

Manipulation of Dental Cement for Cementation of a Crown, Expressed in Units of Time

MANIPULATION STAGE
Powder-to-liquid ratio: 2 scoops of powder to 4 drops of liquid
  Mixing time: Mix all of the powder aggressively into the liquid for about 30 seconds
  Working time: Spread the cement over all the internal surfaces of the crown; the working time is 2.5 minutes

REACTION STAGE
Initial set time: Wait 2 minutes after placement; remove the excess cement with an appropriate instrument. Knotted floss can be used in the interproximal areas
  Final set time: Oral set time is approximately 6 minutes.

MANIPULATION OF MATERIALS

Manipulation of a material's components is an important consideration for the dental auxiliary. It is through this manipulation that the final characteristics of the material are achieved. Some materials offer some variation in their manipulation; others are very technique sensitive and even the slightest variation will have a detrimental effect on the final product. Variables in the manipulation of the material begin with the ratios of the components.

RATIOS OF COMPONENTS

The manufacturer, using the weight or volume of the components, recommends specific ratios. Many materials are produced as separate components that need to be measured and dispensed according to manufacturers' recommendations. Manufacturers also produce materials in pre-measured units, eliminating the need to measure and dispense the components, thus standardizing the ratios. Changing the ratios of the materials by adding more catalyst may result in a faster reaction; increasing the amount of water or liquid component may also result in a less dense, weaker material. These ratio changes are variables that permit the clinician to alter manipulation and reaction times for some materials but are contraindicated with other materials because of adverse effects. Manufacturers give directions as to when variation is needed and how much variation in ratio the material can withstand without adverse results. The auxiliary is most often responsible for measuring and dispensing the components; strict adherence of ratios is required for some materials whereas others allow some flexibility.

EFFECT OF TEMPERATURE AND HUMIDITY

External variables such as the temperature of the material and the room temperature and humidity can also play an important part in the manipulation of materials. In general, high temperatures and humidity will accelerate the reaction of a material's components, and low temperatures and humidity will retard the reaction.

MIXING OF COMPONENTS

How the components of a material are mixed, that is, quickly or slowly, on a paper pad or a glass slab, or by hand-mixing or using automix dispensers, will affect the final material and its consistency (Fig. 3.13). Materials mixed slowly on cool glass will usually produce a slower reaction. Automixed materials will give a more consistent result because the materials are mixed by equipment in a standardized manner with controlled proportions, eliminating the variables of human error.

SHELF LIFE

The **shelf life** of a material refers to the length of time a material can be stored before it becomes unsuitable for use. The shelf life varies from material to material and will be impacted by how it is stored. Temperature extremes and high humidity should be avoided. Plaster and other gypsum products will begin to deteriorate if exposed to high humidity. Material should be stored

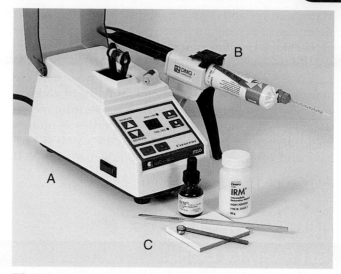

FIG. 3.13 Types of material mixing. **A,** Device called a triturator is used to mix encapsulated, pre-measured materials. **B,** A gun-type automixing dispenser mixes materials contained in a two-barrel cartridge (one barrel with base and one with catalyst) by expressing them through a mixing tip. **C,** Powder and liquid hand-mixed material that will be mixed on a paper pad (or a slab) with a metal spatula. A scoop for the powder is seen on the pad.

in sealed containers. Some materials require refrigeration to prolong their useful life, and others need to be protected from direct light and may be packaged in light-blocking containers. Always refer to manufacturers' directions to determine conditions of storage and expiration. Check with the dental supplier to see that materials are shipped under conditions that will not adversely affect the shelf life such as seasonal temperature variations. The expiration date for all materials stored in the office should be monitored carefully. Materials should be organized such that older materials are used before new shipments to prevent them from expiring. Many materials will lose their potency or fail to set properly if they have passed their expiration date. While some materials may be able to be used a few months beyond their expiration date, it is risky to use them, because they may lack their optimum performance and the treatments they were used with may fail. The American Dental Association requires materials that meet its specifications to stamp a date of production on the packaging of the material.

SUMMARY

The physical structure of a material helps to define the characteristics expected from that material. The success of dental materials is directly related to the choices the dental auxiliary makes in selecting and manipulating the components while keeping in mind those variables that cannot be altered. Controlling variables of manipulation and reaction stages has become increasingly important with more sophisticated materials and more challenging clinical situations. Hand-mixing of materials allows for some control of manipulation and reaction stages. However, inconsistencies in mixing and time demands have become problematic in many clinical situations. Manufacturers are producing materials in a variety of forms to address these concerns. Pre-measured materials are manufactured to standardize the amount of catalyst and base included in the mix, thus preventing inconsistencies in resultant physical properties. Automix materials standardize the amount of catalyst and base and produce a consistent homogeneous mix. It is important to refer to manufacturers' directions for instruction on storage, proportioning, and mixing, and on variables that may be altered to produce the best final results for a given clinical scenario.

INSTRUCTIONAL VIDEOS

See the Evolve Resources site for a variety of educational videos that reinforce the material covered in this chapter.

Get Ready for Exams!

Review Questions

Select the one correct response for each of the following multiple-choice questions.

1. A defining characteristic of a solid is that it has
   a. shape and volume
   b. shape only
   c. neither shape nor volume
   d. volume but no shape

2. The type of primary bond where atoms share electrons in their outer shells is called
   a. atomic bond
   b. covalent bond
   c. ionic bond
   d. metallic bond

3. The correct term for describing the maximal amount of stress a material can withstand without breaking is
   a. toughness
   b. elasticity
   c. ultimate strength
   d. ductility

4. When the weight of a material increases in relationship to its volume, this is described as
   a. elastic
   b. resilient
   c. dense
   d. hard

5. Hardness determines the material's ability to
   a. deform an object
   b. break an object
   c. be easily compressed
   d. resist scratching

6. When deformation is not permanent and a material recovers, it has good
   a. toughness
   b. elasticity
   c. malleability
   d. ductility

7. Resistance to flow is known as
   a. viscosity
   b. film thickness
   c. density
   d. curing

8. Thixotropic materials are those that
   a. have poor viscosity
   b. flow under mechanical forces
   c. flow at higher temperatures
   d. flow at lower temperatures

9. Mixing time is the length of time from
   a. the beginning of mixing to the end of setting time
   b. the beginning of mixing to the initial set time
   c. the beginning of mixing to the beginning of working time
   d. the beginning of mixing to the end of working time

10. A material mixed slowly on a cooled glass surface will
    a. have a shorter working and setting time
    b. have a shorter working and longer setting time
    c. have a longer working and setting time
    d. have a longer working and shorter setting time

For answers to Review Questions, see the Appendix.

Case-Based Discussion Topics

1. Mary Smith has come to your office for a crown preparation on tooth #18. The dentist has recommended a porcelain-fused-to-metal crown for this area. The tooth is prepared with a tapered margin and a final impression taken.

   How would the stiffness of the impression material affect the accuracy of the final impression? If Mary grinds or clenches her teeth, how will this affect the new restoration and resto-

Get Ready for Exams!—cont'd

rations on the opposing teeth? Why is metal's edge strength an important characteristic for this preparation?

2. Bill Miller is scheduled for an orthodontic appointment; he has been in full orthodontic treatment for several months, resulting in the alignment of his teeth.

Give two important properties of the orthodontic wire used in this movement. How do these properties contribute to this movement?

3. You have been asked to prepare cement for a final cementation appointment.

What cement control variables would be desirable if this was a multiunit bridge? How might these variables be manipulated?

4. While attending your state dental convention, you find a great deal on dental plaster. To take advantage of this offer, you must buy five 25-pound containers. When the plaster is delivered to the office, you find that there is not enough space to store the material, so it is decided to store it in the dentist's garage. Although the material in the first container has normal setting reactions, material in containers opened later are inconsistent in their working and setting times.

What may account for these inconsistencies?

BIBLIOGRAPHY

Anusavice KJ, Shen C, Rawls H: *Phillips' Science of Dental Materials* (ed 12). Philadelphia, 2013, Saunders.

Bird DL, Robinson DS: *Modern Dental Assisting* (ed 12). St. Louis, 2018, Elsevier.

Darby ML, Walsh MM: *Dental Hygiene: Theory and Practice* (ed 4). St. Louis, 2015, Saunders.

Powers JM, Wataha JC: *Dental Materials: Foundations and Applications* (ed 11). St. Louis, 2013, Elsevier.

Sakaguchi RL, Powers JM: *Craig's Restorative Dental Materials* (ed 13). St. Louis, 2012, Mosby.

Van Noort R: *Introduction to Dental Materials* (ed 4). St. Louis, 2013, Mosby.

4 General Handling and Safety of Dental Materials in the Dental Office

Chapter Objectives

Upon completion of this chapter, the student should be able to:

1. Identify five job-related health and safety hazards for employees in dental offices, and explain the methods of prevention for each one.
2. Explain the components of the Occupational Safety and Health Administration Hazard Communication Standard.
3. Describe the ways that chemicals can enter the body.
4. Describe the employee and employer responsibility for safety training.
5. Describe the basic infection control methods for the handling of dental materials in the treatment area.
6. Identify the concepts and benefits of *going green* in the dental practice.
7. Discuss how the ADA Top Ten Initiatives of sustainability can be incorporated into a general dental practice.

Key Terms

Particulate Matter extremely small particles (e.g., dust from dental plaster or stone)

Personal Protective Equipment (PPE) gloves, masks, gowns, eyewear, and other protective equipment for the employee

Bio-Aerosol a cloudlike mist containing droplets, tooth dust, dental material dust, and bacteria of a particle size less than 5 microns (μm) in diameter

Splatter small particles that may contain blood, saliva, oral particulate matter, water, and microbes

Hazardous Chemical a chemical that can cause burns to the skin, eyes, lungs, etc., is poisonous, or can cause fire

Toxicity the degree to which a product or a chemical can cause damage to the body

Flash Point the lowest temperature at which the vapor of a volatile substance will ignite with a flash; a low flash point means that a substance can catch fire easily

Ignitable a material or chemical that can erupt into fire easily

Corrosive usually an acid or strong base that can cause damage to metals and equipment, a gradual chemical destruction of metallic materials, as the rusting of metal instruments

Reactive the reaction of opposing chemical substances that creates a different end product

Safety Data Sheet (SDS) printed product reports from the manufacturer containing important information about the chemicals, hazards, handling, cleanup, and special PPE related to a product

---

Dental health care personnel use a wide variety of chemical-containing dental materials for patient treatment and laboratory procedures. All chemicals are capable of causing harmful effects if they are absorbed into the human body. The safety of the patient and the dental professional handling dental materials is of paramount concern. Safety for the work environment is a shared commitment of the dental team and the patient. Clinicians should be very familiar with the regulations for safe practice in the prevention of transmission of potentially pathogenic microbes to both patients and dental personnel. This chapter concentrates on how to prevent exposure to potentially hazardous materials. All dental personnel must understand the safe use, cleanup, and disposal methods for all the materials used in the dental office. This chapter also discusses compliance with governmental regulations and explains health and safety procedures.

MATERIAL HAZARDS IN THE DENTAL ENVIRONMENT

EXPOSURE TO PARTICULATE MATTER

During the manipulation of many dental materials, **particulate matter** can be generated. Items such as gypsum products, alginate, microblasting (sandblasting with very fine particles) materials, and pumice may generate dust during handling. Gypsum models, processed acrylic, porcelain, and various restorative materials may generate dust during the grinding and polishing processes. Pneumoconiosis is a fibrotic lung disease that can be caused by chronic exposure to these dusts. Black Lung Disease is the diagnosis for coal miners who got this disease from inhaling coal dust. It is important for each person handling and manipulating these materials to have and use the proper **personal protective equipment (PPE)** such as dust or surgical masks, eyewear, gowns, and (when appropriate) hair covering or tieback. Appropriate exhaust ventilation in dental laboratories where grinding or trimming of materials is performed is equally important.

Material Hazards in the Dental Office

- Exposure to particulate matter
- Exposure to biological contaminants
- Exposure to airborne contaminants
- Exposure to toxic effects of chemicals
- Exposure to mercury

EXPOSURE TO BIOLOGICAL CONTAMINANTS

Dental personnel come in contact with a variety of microorganisms via exposure to blood, body fluids, or oral and respiratory secretions. These microorganisms may include hepatitis B virus (HBV), hepatitis C virus (HCV), human immunodeficiency virus (HIV), herpes simplex virus (HSV), or other viruses and bacteria. Dental personnel can be protected from the occupational transmission of infectious diseases through strict adherence to the requirements of the Occupational Safety and Health Administration (OSHA) and the Canadian Centre for Occupational Health (CCOH) Bloodborne Pathogens Standard, and to the infection control guidelines issued by the Centers for Disease Control and Prevention (CDC). A further excellent resource for the dental team is the Organization for Safety, Asepsis, and Prevention (OSAP). Most U.S. states have regulations specific to infection control for dentistry. It is imperative the dental auxiliary is familiar with both state and federal regulations and guidelines. Dental personnel must consider the possibility that equipment, storage containers, and dental materials may become contaminated during handling. Therefore it is important to use proper barrier protection such as overgloves or plastic covers when handling bottles, cans, or tubes that contain many of the dental materials used in a modern dental practice (Fig. 4.1).

Areas and equipment in each operatory must be clearly marked so that dental personnel know which area or item is potentially contaminated thus allowing the necessary precautions be taken in handling that item. If you are unsure, use a protective covering or disinfect the item with the appropriate germicide.

BIO-AEROSOLS IN THE DENTAL SETTING

A **bio-aerosol** (*bio,* living; *aerosol,* mist) is a cloudlike mist containing microbes such as bacteria, viruses, molds, fungi, and yeast. Airborne microorganisms can be found in any building. Air conditioning systems, humidifiers, carpets, wall coverings, and plants can easily become microbial breeding grounds.

DENTAL BIO-AEROSOLS

In addition to the usual sources of airborne microorganisms, bio-aerosols and **splatter** in the dental office are even more complex. This is because the aerosols and splatter created during many dental procedures contain

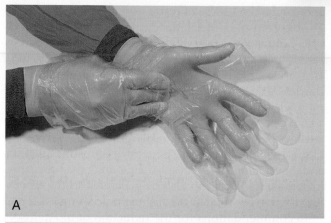

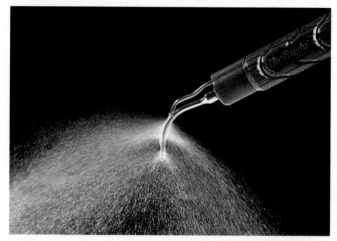

FIG. 4.1 A, Overgloves are used to prevent cross-contamination when multiple-use dental material containers and dispensers are handled. **B,** Syringe is barrier protected with a disposable plastic cover.

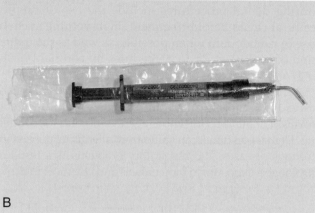

FIG. 4.2 Aerosol and droplets generated by ultrasonic scaler procedures. (Photo © Hu-Friedy Mfg. Co., Inc. [Chicago, IL]; used with permission.)

oral fluids, blood, dental materials, powder, latex particles, and dust from metal, composites, and hygiene procedures (Fig. 4.2). Particles that exit the patient's mouth during dental procedures can be separated into two categories. Those particulates that are greater in diameter than 50 microns (μm) can be considered splatter. The larger splatter particulates can land on the provider's eyewear, skin, and PPE; or on other spaces and equipment and on the floor in the treatment area as far away as 3 feet. The smaller particulates (less than 50 μm) are the aerosols. These remain airborne from minutes to hours and can be the source of respiratory infection if inhaled. The bio-aerosols and splatter created by the dental handpiece, ultrasonic scaler, and by air abrasion procedures can contain particles of human teeth, oral fluids, bacteria and viruses, old restorations, lubricating oil, and abrasive powder. The use of a slurry of certain air-water powder products during hygiene procedures (use of the ultrasonic scaler and air polishing) has been implicated in the creation of bio-aerosols. Aerosols are generated from soft tissue treatments with lasers and electrosurgical units and may contain gases, tissue debris, and other infectious materials. Aerosols can also be generated in the laboratory during grinding and polishing procedures.

Recommendations for the reduction of bio-aerosols during dental procedures include the use of preprocedural rinses before treatment, high-volume suction, use of rubber dam when possible, as well as the reduction of biofilm prior to procedures by coronal polishing, or by brushing and flossing.

When the amount of bio-aerosol in the environment exceeds the capacity of the air filtration system, allergens, toxins, irritants, and infectious agents will continue to build up. Dental personnel can suffer from allergic responses, infectious diseases, and respiratory problems as a result of prolonged exposure to bio-aerosols and chemical irritants.

 Clinical Tip

Make sure the clinical or laboratory environment where aerosols are generated is well ventilated and the air is not recycled in the system. Use PPE appropriate for the type of aerosol exposure, i.e., special high-filtration masks may be needed.

Management of Bio-Aerosols in the Dental Environment

The effects of bio-aerosols can be minimized in dental offices through the following procedures:
- Monitor HVAC (heating, ventilation, and air-conditioning) systems to ensure optimal performance for the removal of particulates and to eliminate excess moisture.
- Clean the air filtration system frequently.
- Use proper oral and laboratory evacuation and ventilation techniques during bio-aerosol–producing procedures.
- Use a vacuum dust collection system during dust-producing laboratory procedures.
- Use high-volume suction during all intraoral procedures that produce aerosol.
- Use rubber dams (to minimize exposure to oral fluids).
- Use preprocedural mouth rinses.
- Conduct preprocedural removal of biofilm through coronal polishing, brushing, and flossing.
- Wear appropriate PPE:
  - Masks
  - Protective clothing such as an overgown or lab jacket
  - Proper eyewear and face shields
  - Gloves; minimize the use of latex products and use powder-free gloves
- Keep all containers tightly covered.
- Pour chemicals rather than spraying.
- Use lids on ultrasonic cleaners and other chemical containers.

CHEMICAL SAFETY IN THE DENTAL OFFICE

HAZARDOUS CHEMICALS

A **hazardous chemical** is defined as any chemical that has been shown to cause a physical or health hazard. It can be any substance which can catch fire, react, or explode when mixed with other substances, or is corrosive or toxic. It is the chemical manufacturers' and importers' responsibility to assess the hazards of their products and pass this information on to consumers through the **Safety Data Sheet (SDS)**. Many dental materials contain more than one chemical (Fig. 4.3).

How Chemicals Enter the Body

- Inhalation
- Direct contact with the skin or eyes
- Absorption through the skin
- Ingestion (eating or drinking)
- Invasion directly through a break in the skin

SKIN AND EYES

The skin is an effective barrier for many chemicals; however, some chemicals are absorbed through the skin. In general, the skin must be in direct contact with the chemical for this to happen. Absorption also may occur directly through a break in the skin such as cuts, open sores, or chapped hands. After repeated contact with some chemicals, a skin disease called *dermatitis* may occur. Adverse occupational reactions in the form of hand or facial dermatitis are not uncommon in dental personnel. These reactions seem to be most often associated with exposure to acrylates, formaldehyde, latex, and rubber additives which can be the result of exposure to dental materials or the components that make up PPE.

Other chemicals, such as acids, can break down the outer layer of the skin, causing burns, and are extremely harmful to the eyes. In the bonding technique for all ceramic crowns, hydrofluoric acid is used to etch the prosthesis to enhance the bond to the tooth. Hydrofluoric acid (HF) is extremely dangerous; anyone handling this acid must be well informed about the risks and safety requirements in handling the material and how to handle potential accidental exposure. Eye exposure may result in permanent damage or even blindness. Flushing the eyes at the eyewash station for at least 15 minutes and immediate medical attention are recommended. Exposure to HF is not limited to contact with the skin and eyes; inhalation of this potent acid is of equal concern. Adequate ventilation must be used.

INHALATION

Inhalation of materials via gases, vapors, or dusts is a common route of chemical exposure for dental personnel. Some chemicals can cause damage directly to the lungs in the form of pneumoconiosis. Among dental personnel, prolonged exposure to

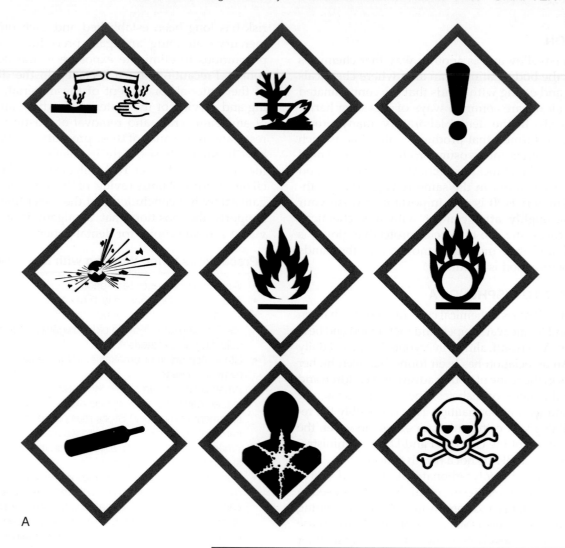

A

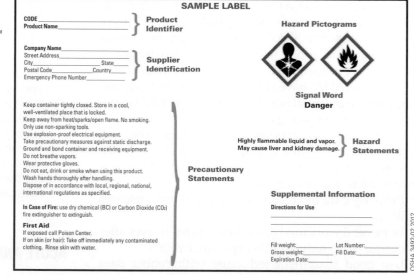

OSHA® QUICK CARD™

Hazard Communication Standard Labels

OSHA has updated the requirements for labeling of hazardous chemicals under its Hazard Communication Standard (HCS). As of June 1, 2015, all labels will be required to have pictograms, a signal word, hazard and precautionary statements, the product identifier, and supplier identification. A sample revised HCS label, identifying the required label elements, is shown on the right. Supplemental information can also be provided on the label as needed.

For more information:

OSHA® Occupational Safety and Health Administration   (800) 321-OSHA (6742)   www.osha.gov

www.osha.gov

SAMPLE LABEL

CODE _____ } Product Identifier
Product Name _____

Company Name _____
Street Address _____ } Supplier Identification
City _____ State ____
Postal Code _____ Country ____
Emergency Phone Number _____

Keep container tightly closed. Store in a cool, well-ventilated place that is locked.
Keep away from heat/sparks/open flame. No smoking.
Only use non-sparking tools.
Use explosion-proof electrical equipment.
Take precautionary measures against static discharge.
Ground and bond container and receiving equipment.
Do not breathe vapors.
Wear protective gloves.
Do not eat, drink or smoke when using this product.
Wash hands thoroughly after handling.
Dispose of in accordance with local, regional, national, international regulations as specified.

In Case of Fire: use dry chemical (BC) or Carbon Dioxide (CO_2) fire extinguisher to extinguish.

First Aid
If exposed call Poison Center.
If on skin (or hair): Take off immediately any contaminated clothing. Rinse skin with water.

Hazard Pictograms

Signal Word
Danger

Highly flammable liquid and vapor. } **Hazard**
May cause liver and kidney damage. **Statements**

Precautionary Statements

Supplemental Information

Directions for Use
_____
_____
_____

Fill weight: _____ Lot Number: _____
Gross weight: _____ Fill Date: _____
Expiration Date: _____

OSHA 3492-02 2012

B

FIG. 4.3 Modern Dental Assisting: **A,** Hazard Communication Standard pictograms. **B,** Sample label. (From Occupational Safety and Health Administration. Available at http://www.osha.gov/dsg/hazcom/index.html.)

dusts containing metal or silica has led to pneumoconiosis. Other chemicals may not directly affect the lungs but are absorbed by the lungs and sent via the bloodstream to other organs such as the brain, liver, or kidneys, where they may cause damage. PPE such as masks or a proper respirator and adequate ventilation must be considered and used as appropriate for each procedure.

INGESTION

Ingestion (swallowing) is another way that chemicals can enter the body. Eating in an area where chemicals are used, and eating with hands that are contaminated with chemicals, are common ways of ingesting harmful chemicals. In the dental laboratory, many procedures are performed that produce contaminants such as metal grindings and gypsum products. It is essential to not eat in the clinical or laboratory area and food should not be stored in the same refrigerator as other dental materials. It is also important to wash your hands thoroughly after contact with any chemical. In many cases, the use of special protective gloves is indicated, and they must be removed and the hands washed before food is handled.

EXPOSURE TO BISPHENOL A

Bisphenol A (BPA) is a chemical currently used to harden plastics, and to line water pipes, and metal food and beverage cans. As a result, almost everyone is exposed daily to BPA. An association has been found between higher BPA levels in the urine of young adults and children and increased diagnosis of diabetes, obesity, cardiovascular disease, and liver abnormalities. This is possibly the result of BPA's weak estrogenic properties; however, the current position of the U.S. Food and Drug Administration (FDA) is that BPA is not a health concern.

BPA is found in polycarbonate plastics and epoxy resins. A form of epoxy resin containing BPA is used in some dental sealants and composites. Resins containing the BPA derivative bis-DMA are more likely to release some BPA at low levels over those containing another BPA derivative, bis-GMA. Glass ionomer sealants do not produce BPA residue. Dental products are less likely to cause exposure to BPA than consumer products made with plastic and epoxy resin. The U.S. Department of Health and Human Services and the American Dental Association (ADA) have called for more research to understand the potential human health effect of BPA exposure, especially in young children.

There are recommended steps to reduce the incidence of BPA exposure during sealant and composite placement. Each of these steps is also important for a successful restorative result:

1. Properly cure the resin—under-cured resin releases BPA.
2. Wipe off the uncured (air-inhibited) resin layer after curing—this reduces BPA exposure by 95%.
3. Use good placement technique with rubber dam isolation or four-handed dentistry with high-volume suction.
4. Use high-volume suction when adjusting sealants, composites, or orthodontic brackets.

EXPOSURE TO MERCURY

There is a known health risk to dental health care personnel from exposure to elemental mercury. This risk has long been established and each office using mercury-containing amalgam procedures must take precautions to eliminate exposure to the dental personnel. Precautions must be taken in the dispensing of the material, placement of the material, condensing and carving of the material, handling and storage of amalgam scrap, and removal of existing amalgam restorations. Because of these precautions many offices have begun to phase out the use of mercury-containing materials (see Chapter 10 Amalgam). The ADA Council on Scientific Affairs review of the literature on amalgam safety has concluded that the "scientific evidence supports the position that amalgam is a valuable, viable and safe choice for dental patients."

Precautions When Working with Mercury

- Work in a well-ventilated space.
- Avoid direct skin contact with mercury.
- Avoid inhaling mercury vapor; use high-volume evacuation whenever removing old amalgam restorations or adjusting new materials.
- Store mercury in unbreakable, tightly sealed containers away from heat.
- When preparing amalgam for restorations, use preloaded capsules. (This avoids exposure during measurement of mercury.) Stock multiple sizes of amalgam capsules to minimize amalgam waste.
- When mixing amalgam, always close the cover before starting the amalgamator.
- Reassemble amalgam capsules immediately after dispensing the amalgam mass. (The used amalgam capsule is highly contaminated with mercury and is a significant source of mercury vapor if left open.) Place empty amalgam capsule in a airtight container marked "Amalgam Capsule Waste for Recycling."
- Store leftover scrap amalgam (i.e., unused amalgam) in a tightly closed container.
- Disinfect scrap amalgam (amalgam that has been retrieved from dental unit traps) in a solution of bleach and water. Then place the amalgam in the container with other scrap alloy.
- Clean spills, using appropriate procedures and equipment; do *not* use a household vacuum cleaner or high-velocity evacuation (HVE). (Dangerous fumes from the mercury can be released into the air.)
- Place contaminated disposable materials into polyethylene bags, seal them, and dispose of them according to state/province and local regulations.

ACUTE AND CHRONIC CHEMICAL TOXICITY

The **toxicity** of a chemical, and thus its harmfulness, depends directly on the dose, length of exposure, and frequency of exposure.

ACUTE CHEMICAL TOXICITY

Acute chemical toxicity results from high levels of exposure over a short period of time. This frequently is caused by a large chemical spill in which the exposure is sudden and unexpected. The effects of this type of toxicity are felt right away. The symptoms of acute overexposure to chemicals may include dizziness, fainting (syncope), headache, nausea, and vomiting.

CHRONIC CHEMICAL TOXICITY

Chronic chemical toxicity results from repeated exposures, usually to lower doses, over a much longer period of time such as months or years. The effects of chronic toxicity can include cancer, neurologic deficits, and infertility.

For example, a single exposure to a high concentration of benzene may cause dizziness, headache, and unconsciousness; long-term daily exposure to low levels of benzene may eventually cause leukemia. Another example is that of beryllium, a metal used in partial denture frameworks. When grinding beryllium frameworks for adjustment, one must avoid inhaling the dust because it is a toxic hazard which can lead to lung disease. A proper mask or respirator must be worn.

PERSONAL AND CHEMICAL PROTECTION

HAND PROTECTION

Appropriate hand hygiene is the most important step that the health care personnel can take to prevent the transmission of infectious diseases in the dental setting. When routine dental treatment is being performed hand washing with plain soap, hand antisepsis with antimicrobial soap, or cleansing with an alcohol hand rub should be utilized. Alcohol handrubs may be effective; however, soap and water is necessary to clean the hands when they are visibly soiled with dirt, blood, or bodily fluids.

Fingernail integrity is an integral part of hand hygiene. Nails should be short with smooth edges not extending beyond fingertips. Artificial nails, tips, and extenders are not recommended as they may harbor bacteria. If nail polish is worn, it should be maintained with a smooth appearance. Once fingernail polish has become chipped or nails grow out showing margins of the polish at the cuticle, bacterial growth is encouraged.

Procedure gloves (patient treatment gloves) worn during patient care do not provide adequate protection when chemicals are handled. When exposed to chemical disinfectants, antiseptics, resins, and bonding agents the patient treatment gloves may degrade. When degradation of gloves occur, contaminates and chemicals can be pulled through the glove like a wick and onto the hands. Chemical-resistant gloves such as nitrile utility gloves are recommended for wear during chemical handling (Fig. 4.4). With the many materials on the market, the manufacturer's SDS instructions should be consulted to determine the compatibility of the glove material with various chemicals. Some individuals develop sensitivity to latex; however, a proper dermatologic diagnosis is required

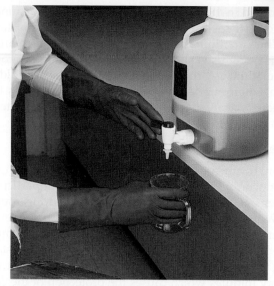

FIG. 4.4 Nitrile utility gloves, because they are resistant to chemicals, are used to handle disinfectants, acids, and hazardous chemicals. (Courtesy Lab Safety Supply, Janesville, WI.)

before a latex reaction can be distinguished from sensitivity to some other chemical. To ensure patient treatment gloves maintain their integrity and protective features, they should be worn no longer than 60 minutes and be changed when moisture on the internal surface is visible, become tacky on the exterior surface, or become ripped or torn.

EYE PROTECTION

Serious damage to the eyes, including blindness, may result from chemical accidents. It is necessary to protect the eyes from exposure to all dental materials including fumes and splashes while chemicals such as alcohol or methyl methacrylate monomer, acid, or other solvents are poured. The acids used for bonding procedures can be splashed into the eyes during rinsing from the etched teeth. Protective eyewear with side shields and splash shields are available from many manufacturers and must be worn when handling materials and in patient care settings.

PROTECTIVE CLOTHING

Protective clothing such as disposable overgowns or laboratory jackets should be worn over uniforms and personal clothing to protect the clinician from blood-borne pathogens and dental materials. The most effective overgowns and laboratory jackets button up to the neck, cover the legs to the top of the knee when in both a seated or standing position, and have elastic at the wrist. Water-resistant overgowns are more effective in protecting the clinician than laboratory jackets as the lab jackets are not impervious to liquids. Overgowns and lab jackets are not to leave the facility once worn and potentially contaminated by blood-borne pathogens. Overgowns should be disposed of or sterilized as indicated by the manufacturer. Lab jackets should be laundered in the dental office or processed by a laundry service that specializes in handling biohazardous items.

When manipulating chemicals, the type of chemical that is being used should guide the selection of protective clothing. A rubber or neoprene apron should be worn when one is mixing or pouring chemicals that are caustic; can stain; or would saturate, penetrate, or damage regular fabric.

INHALATION PROTECTION

Patient treatment masks are necessary to protect the clinician not only from the spread of infection but particulate matter described earlier in the chapter. During routine dental treatment the mask should be changed after every patient, every sixty minutes, or when it becomes damp or wet. The necessity to change the mask frequently stems from the mesh in the mask beginning to break down after twenty minutes which causes the protection of the clinician to decrease the longer the mask is worn.

The masks worn during patient care may or may not provide adequate protection when one is working with chemicals, depending on the quality of mask. The facemask should be fluid repelling and provide respiratory protection. If the job requires frequent pouring or mixing of chemicals, sensitive or allergic individuals might need a National Institute of Occupational Safety and Health (NIOSH)–approved dust and mist respirator facemask. Several masks are on the market for personnel with sensitive skin; these masks are free of dyes and chemicals and have a lint-free cellulose inner layer.

CONTROL OF CHEMICAL SPILLS

MERCURY SPILL

Mercury spill kits should be available in all dental offices that use amalgam for restorations (Fig. 4.5). Exposure to even small amounts of mercury is very hazardous to workers' health. Mercury can be absorbed through the skin or by the inhalation of mercury vapors.

The spill kit for small amounts of mercury should contain mercury-absorbing powder, mercury sponges, and a disposal bag. A mask and utility-type gloves should be worn when cleaning a mercury spill.

FLAMMABLE LIQUIDS

Many solvents used with dental materials have a very low **flash point** and can easily ignite when used near open flame such as a Bunsen burner or an alcohol torch. Take extreme caution when using flammable products (e.g., the liquid monomer for acrylic or acetone). The SDS for each product describes the flammability of that product.

ACIDS

As mentioned previously, phosphoric, hydrofluoric, and hydrochloric acids are used during manipulation of various dental materials. Splashing any of these acids on the skin, eyes, or clothing can cause severe

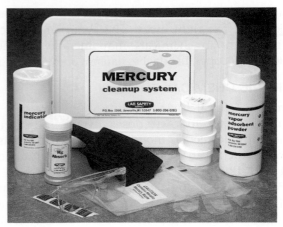

FIG. 4.5 Mercury spill kit. Note its compact size for convenient storage. (Courtesy of Lab Safety Supply Inc. [Janesville, WI].)

burns or damage. Flushing with water immediately is essential to prevent severe injury.

EYEWASH

OSHA regulations require an eyewash unit to be installed in every place of employment where chemicals are used. A wide variety of styles are available. The standard eyewash unit attaches directly to existing faucets for emergencies yet still allows normal faucet use. When turned on, the eyewash unit will irrigate the eyes with a soft, wide flow of water as necessary to bathe away contaminants without causing additional damage. As an employee, you must be trained in proper use of the eyewash station. It is recommended that eyewash stations be inspected frequently to ensure water flow. Some manufacturers suggest running them for several minutes periodically to discharge any potential built-up biofilms or infectious agents. A posting of suggested times for eyewashing after an exposure (Table 4.1) and directions for the proper use of the particular type of eyewash unit should be placed nearby the eyewash station (Fig. 4.6).

VENTILATION

Good ventilation is a necessity when dealing with any type of chemical. Dental offices should be equipped with special exhaust systems for fumes and dust in the laboratory and in radiographic processing areas. For example, vapors from chemicals used in radiographic processing can cause contact dermatitis and irritation of eyes, nose, throat, and respiratory tract. Other laboratory areas may be laden with fine dust particles from grinding or chemical vapors such as from acrylic monomer or pickling acid (used to remove oxides from cast metals).

GENERAL PRECAUTIONS FOR STORING CHEMICALS

All dental materials contain chemical components, and some are more hazardous than others. Careful

Table 4.1   OSHA Recommendations for Eyewashing

CHEMICAL EXPOSURE TO THE EYE	TIME PERIOD FOR EYEWASHING
Non-irritants or mild irritant	5 minutes
Moderate to severe irritant	15 to 20 minutes
Nature of contaminate unknown	20 minutes
Corrosives	30 minutes
Strong alkalis (sodium, potassium, or calcium hydroxide)	60 minutes

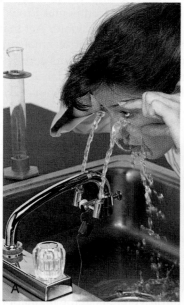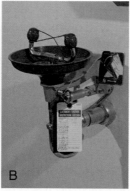

FIG. 4.6 **A,** Faucet-mount eyewash and eye/face-wash station. **B,** Wall-mounted eyewash station showing inspection record. (**A,** Courtesy of Lab Safety Supply Inc. [Janesville, WI]. **B,** Courtesy of Dr. Mark Dellinges.)

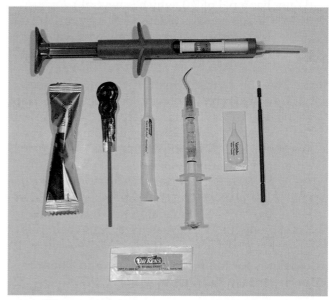

FIG. 4.7 Examples of single-use items (dental floss, fluoride varnish, temporary restorative materials, cement cartridge, and etching solution).

use and storage of dental materials is essential to ensure these products retain their therapeutic activity and identity. Changes in the chemical composition of materials can occur for many reasons. When changes take place, the product may no longer retain its effectiveness. Expiration dates must be reviewed and out-of-date material should be disposed of properly. A basic "safe" policy for the storage of dental medications and chemicals is to keep them in original containers when possible and a dry, cool, dark place where they are not exposed to direct sunlight. Many single-dose products have been developed to eliminate cross-contamination and reduced effectiveness of the product due to evaporation or contamination (Fig. 4.7).

DISPOSAL OF CHEMICALS

EMPTY CONTAINERS

Even empty containers can be hazardous because they often hold residues that can burn or explode. Never fill an empty container with another substance because a

dangerous chemical reaction could occur. Follow the label and the SDS on how to dispose of empty containers. (Safety Data Sheets are discussed later in this chapter.)

Tips to Aid in the Safe Use and Effectiveness of Dental Materials

Follow instructions: The manufacturer has already determined the best methods of protective packaging and storage. Therefore the manufacturer's instructions for storage, manipulation, and protection should be followed.

Light, heat, and air: Exposures to light, heat, and air are the prime factors in the deterioration of many bonding solutions. Changes in color, viscosity, or curing time are the most common signs of deterioration.

Expiration date: The substance's expiration date should always be noted. To maintain the proper chemical reactions, materials should be replaced when the expiration date is reached. Also, new supplies should always be stocked behind the current inventory so that the oldest product is used first.

HAZARDOUS WASTE DISPOSAL

A waste is considered hazardous if it has certain properties or chemicals that could pose dangers to human health and the environment after being discarded. In general, waste is classified as hazardous if it has any of the following characteristics:

Ignitable: The substance is **ignitable** if it is flammable or combustible.

Corrosive: The substance is **corrosive** if it is highly acidic (pH less than 2.0) or basic (pH greater than 12.5). (Water has a pH of 7.0, which is neutral.)

Reactive: The substance is **reactive** if it is chemically unstable or explosive, reacts violently with water, or is capable of giving off toxic fumes when mixed with water.

Toxic: The substance is toxic if it contains arsenic, barium, chromium, mercury, lead, silver, or certain pesticides. (*Note:* Dental amalgam, asbestos, lead foil, and radiographic processing solutions are examples of hazardous waste that may be regulated differently by individual states and provinces.)

Listed by the U.S. Environmental Protection Administration (EPA) and the Canadian Environmental Protection Agency (CEPA): Several hundred chemicals are listed by the EPA/CEPA as hazardous chemicals.

Guidelines for Minimizing Exposure to Chemical Hazards in the Dental Office

- Keep a minimum amount of hazardous chemicals in the office.
- Read the labels and use only as directed.
- Store according to the manufacturer's directions.
- Keep containers tightly covered.
- Avoid mixing chemicals unless consequences are known.
- Wear appropriate personal protective equipment (PPE) when handling hazardous substances.
- Wash hands immediately after removing gloves.
- Avoid skin contact with chemicals; immediately wash skin that has come in contact with chemicals.
- Maintain good ventilation.
- Do not eat, drink, smoke, apply lip balm, or insert contact lenses in areas where chemicals are used.
- Keep vaporizing chemicals away from open flames and heat sources.
- Always have an operational fire extinguisher handy.
- Know and use proper cleanup procedures.
- Keep neutralizing agents available for strong acid and alkaline solutions.
- Dispose of all hazardous chemicals according to SDS instructions.

Regulations for hazardous waste disposal vary among states and provinces, and heavy fines may be imposed for those individuals who knowingly violate regulations. More important than the legal penalties are the environmental damage and the pollution of surface and groundwater that can result from improper handling, transportation, and disposal of hazardous wastes. The solutions from the wet processing of dental radiographs are not permitted in the public sewer systems, and if they are disposed of in private septic systems, they can cause those systems to fail. The disposal limits, either down the drain or in landfill, of x-ray film, lead foil, disinfectants, and acid etch are also regulated by either county or state regulatory agencies and can vary widely throughout the United States.

An example of a regulation that can improve wastewater and groundwater is the regulation requiring use of the amalgam separator. The Environmental Protection Agency mandated under the Clean Water Act that in July 2017 dental practices must control amalgam waste through the use of amalgam separators certified by the International Organization for Standardization (ISO, standard 11143). These separators can remove 95% of the amalgam "fine" waste and prevent it from going into the sewer system. Mercury from dental amalgam can end up in the soil, atmosphere, and groundwater through several routes including wastewater discharges from dental practices as well as throwing out amalgam scrap in the office waste. Mercury from dental amalgams may also be released through the burial and cremation of individuals with amalgam restorations. The amount of mercury released from dental amalgam and the result of the conversion into the ecosystem is highly variable. The aquatic and soil contribution of mercury from dental amalgams is considered to be very low and there have been several improvements to the regulation in the disposal of scrap amalgam in many states. The ADA has provided a "best practices management" for handling amalgam with the intent of reducing amalgam release into the environment (Table 4.2).

DENTAL LABORATORY INFECTION CONTROL

OSHA mandates that the dental laboratory have the same infection control protocols as the dental office. Dental laboratories may be a part of the dental office or may be off-site and owned and operated by dental laboratory technicians not employed by the office. Effective communication must be established with facilities within the office or off-site to prevent disease transmission from contaminated items entering the dental laboratory. In addition, dental laboratories are obligated to make sure that the products delivered back to the dental operatory are free of contaminants. Dental laboratory technicians must adhere to the same standard precautions for the prevention of health-related diseases from the materials they handle.

For example, impressions, casts, and dental prostheses are often moved back and forth between laboratories and dental operatories. These items may be contaminated with blood and saliva which allows microorganisms to be transferred to the laboratory environment and back to the dental operatory. Microbes have been cultured from set gypsum dental casts for up to 7 days.

Table 4.2	American Dental Association (ADA) Best Management Practices for Amalgam Waste
DO	**DON'T**
Use pre-capsulated alloys and stock a variety of capsule sizes	Use bulk mercury
Recycle used disposable amalgam capsules	Put used disposable amalgam capsules in regular trash, bio-hazard, or infectious waste containers
Salvage non-contact amalgam, store, and recycle	Put non-contact amalgam waste in regular trash, biohazard, or infectious waste containers
Salvage contact amalgam pieces from restorations after removal for recycle	Put contact amalgam waste in regular trash, biohazard, or infectious waste containers
Use chair-side traps, vacuum pump filters, and amalgam separators to capture amalgam and recycle their contents	Rinse devices containing amalgam over drains and sinks as amalgam waste may be lost and travel into the city water system
Recycle teeth that contain amalgam restorations (ensure the amalgam recycler will accept the extracted teeth and verify if the teeth require disinfection)	Dispose of extracted teeth that contain amalgam restorations in regular trash, biohazard, or infectious waste containers
Manage amalgam waste through recycling	Flush amalgam waste down the drain or toilet
Use wastewater line cleaners that minimize dissolution of amalgam	Use bleach or chlorine containing cleaners to flush wastewater lines

Good communication and standardized protocols are essential for effective infection control. If there is ever a doubt as to the status of an incoming or outgoing case, the appropriate disinfection process must be completed before the item may be handled or placed in the patient's mouth.

Infections Control Communication between Laboratory and Dental Office

- Disinfection status of incoming and outgoing cases
- Utilization of appropriate shipping and receiving containers
- Designated receiving and shipping areas and protocols
- Designated production areas

All equipment used in the dental laboratory must be single-use items or handled with standard precautions for prevention of cross-contamination. Even though cases are appropriately disinfected before entering the production area, dental lathes, handpieces, burs, brushes, rag wheels, and other laboratory equipment should be disinfected or sterilized daily. The dental lathe should be protected with a functional shield surrounding the lathe to prevent spatter, aerosols, and the possibility of flying debris (Fig. 4.8).

Appropriate PPE must be worn in the dental laboratory to protect individuals from biological contaminants, bio-aerosols, and chemical contact and inhalation. Appropriate ventilation and/or air-suction motors are important for these areas.

The dental office and dental laboratory must follow the same infection control guidelines to protect health care personnel and patients from bloodborne pathogens. Standard precautions, appropriate personal protective equipment, and good communication between the laboratory and the office are all components of successful infection control protocols.

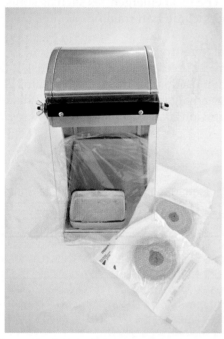

FIG. 4.8 Picture of a lathe splash hood lined with a disposable bag, a removable dish for a new mix of pumice, and sterilized rag wheels attached.

OCCUPATIONAL SAFETY AND HEALTH ADMINISTRATION HAZARD COMMUNICATION STANDARD

OSHA has created standards to protect the safety of workers. Dental office personnel should be very familiar with the Bloodborne Pathogens Standard. This section addresses the standard that protects workers who are at risk of chemical exposure: the Hazard Communication Standard.

OSHA issued the Hazard Communication Standard because employees have "the right and the need to know" the identity and hazards of chemicals that they use in the workplace. The Hazard Communication Standard, also known as the Employee Right to Know Law, requires employers to implement a hazard communication program.

HAZARD COMMUNICATION PROGRAM

OSHA has been enforcing a Hazard Communication Standard (HCS) since 1983. A chemical hazard communication program has five parts: the written program, the chemical inventory, the Safety Data Sheet (SDS), labeling of containers, and employee training.

Written Hazard Communication Program

The written program must identify by name all employees who are exposed to hazardous chemicals and identify the person responsible for the program. In addition, it must describe how chemicals are handled in the workplace, must include a description of all safety measures and an explanation of how one should respond to chemical emergencies such as spills or exposures, and include staff training.

Chemical Inventory

The chemical inventory is a comprehensive list of every product used in the office that contains chemicals, including amalgam, bonding agents, disinfectants, and impression materials. Each time a new product is added to the office, it must be added to the chemical list and the SDS for that product must be placed in the SDS file.

The office will frequently appoint a staff member to be the hazard program coordinator. This person will be responsible for maintaining the chemical inventory and updating the SDS file.

Safety Data Sheets

The basic elements of the safety sheet uses a combination of signal words and standardized pictograms to communicate hazards associated with a specific chemical (Fig. 4.3). Safety Data Sheets (SDSs) contain health and safety information about each chemical in the office. SDSs provide comprehensive technical information and are a resource for employees/providers who work with chemicals. They describe the physical and chemical properties of a material; health and environmental health hazards; protective measures; precautions for safe handling, use, and storage; emergency and first aid procedures; and spill-control measures. The manufacturers of products must provide SDSs, and an SDS must be obtained for every chemical used in the office. Manufacturer's typically enclose the SDS in the box with delivery of the product. SDSs should be organized in binders so that employees/providers have ready access to them and can easily locate a particular SDS (Box 4.1).

Box **4.1**	Explanation of the Safety Data Sheet

HAZARD COMMUNICATION SAFETY DATA SHEETS

   The Hazard Communication Standard (HCS) requires chemical manufacturers, distributors, or importers to provide Safety Data Sheets (SDSs) (formerly known as Material Safety Data Sheets or MSDSs) to communicate the hazards of hazardous chemical products. As of June 1, 2015, the HCS will require new SDSs to be in a uniform format, and include the section numbers, the headings, and associated information under the headings below:

   Section 1, Identification includes product identifier; manufacturer or distributor name, address, phone number; emergency phone number; recommended use; restrictions on use.

   Section 2, Hazard(s) identification includes all hazards regarding the chemical; required label elements.

   Section 3, Composition/information on ingredients includes information on chemical ingredients; trade secret claims.

   Section 4, First-aid measures includes important symptoms/effects, acute, delayed; required treatment.

   Section 5, Fire-fighting measures lists suitable extinguishing techniques, equipment; chemical hazards from fire.

   Section 6, Accidental release measures lists emergency procedures; protective equipment; proper methods of containment and cleanup.

   Section 7, Handling and storage lists precautions for safe handling and storage, including incompatibilities.

   Section 8, Exposure controls/personal protection lists OSHA's Permissible Exposure Limits (PELs); ACGIH Threshold Limit Values (TLVs); and any other exposure limit used or recommended by the chemical manufacturer, importer or employer preparing the SDS where available as well as appropriate engineering controls; personal protective equipment (PPE).

   Section 9, Physical and chemical properties lists the chemical's characteristics.

   Section 10, Stability and reactivity lists chemical stability and possibility of hazardous reactions.

   Section 11, Toxicological information includes routes of exposure; related symptoms, acute and chronic effects; numerical measures of toxicity.

   Section 12, Ecological information[1]

   Section 13, Disposal considerations

   Section 14, Transport information

   Section 15, Regulatory information

   Section 16, Other information, includes the date of preparation or last revision.

NOTE: Since other Agencies regulate this information, OSHA will not be enforcing Sections 12 through 15(29 CFR 1910.1200(g)(2)).
Employers must ensure that SDSs are readily accessible to employees.
See Appendix D of 1910.1200 for a detailed description of SDS contents.
From OSHA.gov.

LABELING OF CHEMICAL CONTAINERS AND SAFETY DATA SHEETS

The responsibility for labeling of chemicals is with the manufacturer or distributor. Containers must be labeled to indicate manufacturer's name, address, and telephone number; product name or identifier; signal words for warning or hazards; hazard statements; and precautionary statements and pictograms (Fig. 4.9).

All chemicals in the dental office must be labeled. In many cases, the manufacturer's label is suitable. However, when the chemical is transferred to a different container, the new container must also be labeled. For example, when a concentrated chemical such as acrylic monomer is transferred to a small bottle for use in the treatment area or laboratory, the bottle must be labeled. No official labeling

system is required, and a variety of styles are available on the market (Fig. 4.10) (Procedure 4.1). Even affixing to the new container a photocopy of the label from the original container is acceptable. The most important considerations are that the labeling system should be easy to use, in legible condition, and provide all the information from the original label including words, pictures, and symbols. All employees must be properly trained to understand and read the labels.

LABELING EXEMPTIONS

Some products, such as pharmaceuticals directly dispensed to the patient by the pharmacy and drugs intended for personal consumption by the employee for use in the workplace (such as aspirin), are exempt. Other examples of exempted products are food, alcoholic beverages, and cosmetics packaged for consumer use.

National Fire Protection Association Labels

The National Fire Protection Association (NFPA) has a labeling system that is frequently used to label containers of hazardous chemicals. This system consists of blue, red, yellow, and white diamonds filled with numerical ratings from 0 to 4. Categories are identified as follows: health (blue); flammability (red); reactivity (yellow); and special hazard symbols, such as "OXY" for oxidizers (white).

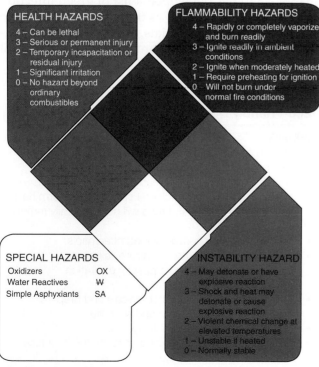

HAZARDOUS MATERIALS CLASSIFICATION

HEALTH HAZARDS
4 – Can be lethal
3 – Serious or permanent injury
2 – Temporary incapacitation or residual injury
1 – Significant irritation
0 – No hazard beyond ordinary combustibles

FLAMMABILITY HAZARDS
4 – Rapidly or completely vaporize and burn readily
3 – Ignite readily in ambient conditions
2 – Ignite when moderately heated
1 – Require preheating for ignition
0 – Will not burn under normal fire conditions

SPECIAL HAZARDS
Oxidizers   OX
Water Reactives W
Simple Asphyxiants SA

INSTABILITY HAZARD
4 – May detonate or have explosive reaction
3 – Shock and heat may detonate or cause explosive reaction
2 – Violent chemical change at elevated temperatures
1 – Unstable if heated
0 – Normally stable

FIG. 4.9 Hazard Communication Standard pictograms. Secondary chemical container labeling. (From Bird DL, Robinson DS: *Modern Dental Assisting* (ed 11). St. Louis, 2015, Elsevier.)

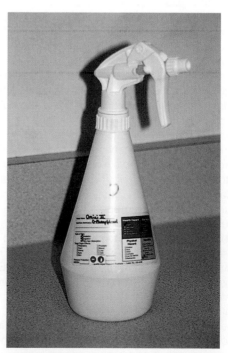

FIG. 4.10 Labeling of chemical transferred to a secondary container. (From Bird, D, Robinson D: *Modern Dental Assisting* (ed 12). St. Louis, 2018, Elsevier)

Guidelines for Chemical Labeling

The label must contain the following information:
- Name, address, and phone number of the manufacturer or responsible party
- Product name or identifier
- Signal word for warning or hazard
- Hazard statement
- Precautionary statement
- Pictogram(s)

Employee Training

Employee training is essential for a successful hazard communication program. Staff training is required (1) when a new employee is hired, (2) when a new chemical product is added to the office, and (3) once a year for all continuing employees. Records of each training session must be kept on file and retained for at least 5 years. Although the dentist is responsible for providing the training, the hazard program coordinator is responsible for routinely following these safety precautions.

The chemical training program for employees must include the following:
- Use of hazardous chemicals
- All safety practices, including all warnings
- Required personal protective devices
- Safe handling and disposal methods

Outline for a Hazard Communication Training Program

1. Discuss requirements of the Hazard Communication Standard.
2. Prepare a written communication plan for the office (location, use, etc.).
3. Explain the hazards of the chemicals.
4. Ensure that employees can interpret warning labels and the Safety Data Sheet (SDS).
   a. Product identifier, chemical name, code number or batch number
   b. Signal work—indicates the severity of the hazard
   c. Pictogram—OSHA has designated eight pictograms (Box 4.2 provides examples of two of the eight pictograms)
   d. Hazard statement—nature of the hazard
   e. Precautionary statements—how to minimize or prevent adverse effects resulting from exposure, storage, or handling of a hazardous chemical
   f. Name, address, and phone number of the manufacturer, distributor, or importer.
5. Discuss how to obtain more information.
6. Discuss taking measures to protect oneself and others:
   a. Office safety procedures
   b. Available personal protective equipment (PPE)
   c. Instructions for reporting accidents and emergencies
   d. Information about first aid
   e. Information regarding proper storage
7. Present methods and observations that can be used to detect the presence or release of a hazardous chemical.
8. Provide a question-and-answer opportunity.
9. On completion, ask employees to sign a training record that will remain in their personnel file.

Responsibilities of the Hazard Program Coordinator

- Read and understand the Hazard Communication Standard.
- Implement the written hazard communication program.
- Compile a list (chemical inventory) of products in the office that contain hazardous chemicals.
- Obtain Safety Data Sheets (SDSs).
- Update the SDS file as new products are added to the office inventory.
Inform other employees of the location of the SDS file.
- Label containers appropriately.
- Provide training to other employees.

ECO-CONSCIENCE GREEN PRACTICES

What about protecting your office and the environment? The process of preventing the transmission of disease and performing dental procedures involves equipment and products that produce waste, consume excess energy, and use toxic chemicals. To accomplish this there are traditional and environmentally friendly products, supplies, and procedures available. The average dental practice disposes of hundreds of pounds of paper and plastic waste each year. There must be effective compromises to maintain an eco-friendly practice while not compromising the safety of the patient. Chris H. Miller (Indiana University School of Dentistry, Indianapolis, IN) has developed a list of green infection control "do's and don'ts" as they relate to recyclable and biodegradable materials, energy and water conservation, waste management, and infection control standards.

Eco-Friendly Do's and Don'ts

THE DO'S
- Choose reusables instead of disposables when possible.
- Use alcohol hand rubs instead of hand washing. If hands are visibly soiled, clinical staff must perform hand washing as alcohol hand rubs will not physically remove debris.
- Use trigger/pump sprays instead of aerosols.
- Establish better inventory control to eliminate discarding excess product past its expiration date.
- Ensure accurate mixing of chemicals and prepare amounts based on use-life and shelf-life.
- Switch to digital instead of film x-ray.
- Ensure sterilizers and cleaning units are full to reduce number of cycles per day.
- Use products made from recycled materials.
- Use products that are recyclable.

BOX 4.2   OSHA Pictograms

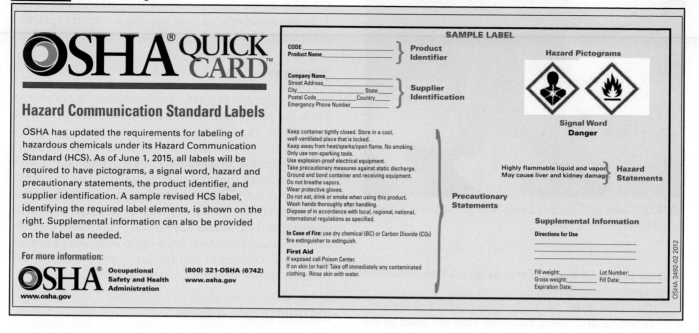

THE DONT'S

- Don't use paper (i.e., biodegradable) instead of plastic surface barriers, because paper will allow penetration of moisture and microbes.
- Don't reuse standard sterilization wraps and pouches, because they were not designed to maintain sterility after more than one use.
- Don't use woven cloth (e.g., denim) as sterilization wraps and then reuse it, because it is not a good microbial barrier.
- Don't use a disinfectant that has a reduced concentration of an active ingredient unless there is evidence of its efficacy.
- Don't shorten cleaner or sterilization cycles just to save energy.
- Don't reuse items that are sold as disposable.

Dental facilities can do their part to sustain the environment while continuing to prevent disease transmission. We are all encouraged to "reduce, reuse, recycle, and rethink."

American Dental Association Council on Dental Practice "Go Green" Subcommittee Recommendations

Top Ten Initiatives
- Install an amalgam separator.
- Turn off equipment when not in use.
- Reuse paper scraps.
- Use recycle bins and create a "Green Team" to bring items to recycle centers.
- Recycle shredded confidential patient information.
- Convert to digital technology.
- Install solar or tinted shades.
- Install locked or programmable thermostats.
- Install high-efficiency light bulbs.
- Use nontoxic cleaners and don't use too much disinfectant.

The dental auxiliary is most frequently responsible for ordering supplies. Choosing cost-effective greener options to address environmental contamination and waste may begin with small steps and gradually build to an office that is environmentally responsible.

PATIENT SAFETY

It is extremely important for the health care provider to consider the safety of the patient while care is given and various materials and chemicals are used. First consideration should be given to protection of the patient's eyes. It is recommended that protective eyewear be supplied to the patient if he or she does not wear glasses. The same type of general protective eyewear as used by the practitioner will do. Patient protective eyewear should be washed and disinfected between patients. Although some patients prefer dark glasses to shield their eyes from the dental unit light, most providers prefer to use clear lenses so they can observe the patient's eyes and facial expressions during treatment as a clue to the patient's level of comfort (Fig. 4.11).

 Caution

Be certain that protective eyewear has been dried thoroughly after treatment with disinfectant, to avoid inadvertent contamination of the patient's skin or eyes.

Another vital safety consideration is the patient's airway. The use of high-velocity evacuation (HVE) and a rubber dam whenever possible is excellent practice. During rinsing of chemicals such as acid for etching, the patient may experience an unpleasant, bitter taste and may have a gagging reaction. The patient should be

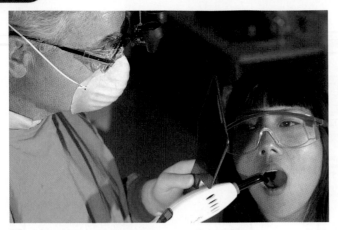

FIG. 4.11 Patient and clinician wearing protective eyewear; a protective light shield is being used.

warned of this taste, and the rinse should be controlled to minimize discomfort.

Patients are more aware than ever before of the various chemicals and filling materials that are used in the dental practice. It is essential that the dental auxiliary be as familiar as possible with hazards and reactions that can occur when these materials and chemicals are used. The SDS is the best source of this information along with the directions for use supplied with the product manufacturer.

SUMMARY

The management of a safe environment in the dental office is the responsibility of the employer and of all who work there. The safe use of any chemical or material is the responsibility of the user at the time. The safety of the patient is the responsibility of the dental team. Familiarity with each material or chemical used by the dental team is a must. This text provides general and technical information, but specific hazards are best determined by referring to the manufacturer's instructions and the SDS. Keep yourself informed, keep up to date with the standards, and continue to inquire "how can I protect myself, patients, fellow workers, and the environment,"?

INSTRUCTIONAL VIDEOS

See the Evolve Resources site for a variety of educational videos that reinforce the material covered in this chapter.

Procedure 4.1 Safety Data Sheet and Label Exercise

See Evolve site for Competency Sheet.

Consider the following with this procedure: safety glasses are recommended for the patient, PPE is required for the operator, ensure appropriate safety protocols are followed, and check your local state guidelines before performing this procedure.

Use the information found on the Safety Data Sheet (SDS) for acid etchant (conditioner) for pit and fissure sealant.

EQUIPMENT/SUPPLIES

SDS for product and labeled product
Pen
Secondary label (Refer to FIG. 4.3)

PROCEDURE STEPS

1. What is the product name and identifier? (This information is found in the product identification section of the SDS.)

2. What is the manufacturer's name, address, and emergency phone number? (This information is found in the product identification section of the SDS.)

3. What precautionary statements should be included on the label? (This information is found in the exposure controls/personal protection section of the SDS.)

4. What hazard pictograms and signal word should be included? (This information is found in the hazards identification section of the SDS.)

5. What is the hazard statement(s) associated with this product? (This information is found in the hazard identification section of the SDS.)
   What supplemental information should be included?

Get Ready for Exams!

Review Questions

Select the one correct response for each of the following multiple-choice questions.

1. When one is working with dental materials, the most common work-related health and safety hazards are:
   a. exposure to mercury, exposure to particulate matter, exposure to perfume, and exposure to airborne contaminants
   b. exposure to particulate matter, exposure to biological contaminants, exposure to noise, exposure to perfume, and exposure to airborne contaminants
   c. exposure to particulate matter, exposure to biological contaminants, exposure to perfume, and exposure to airborne contaminants
   d. exposure to mercury, exposure to particulate matter, exposure to biological contaminants, and exposure to toxic effects of chemicals

2. The proper PPE to be worn during handling of dental materials that can generate particulate matter consists of:
   a. safety glasses, surgical or special dust mask, heavy-duty utility gloves, and overgloves
   b. lab coat or overgown, surgical or special dust mask, heavy-duty utility gloves, and vinyl examination gloves
   c. safety glasses, lab coat or overgown, surgical or special dust mask, and heavy-duty utility gloves
   d. safety glasses, lab coat or overgown, and surgical or special dust mask

3. There are multiple hazards associated with the use of the dental lathe in the laboratory, which is NOT a hazards associated with the use of the dental lathe?
   a. Flying debris
   b. Aerosols
   c. Spatter
   d. Mercury vapor

4. Ways in which chemicals can enter the body include:
   a. inhaling, through cuts in the skin, and by touching the product of a reaction
   b. swallowing, inhaling, and by touching the product of a reaction
   c. swallowing, inhaling, and through cuts in the skin
   d. swallowing, through cuts in the skin, and by touching the product of a reaction

5. What is the most important step the dental auxiliary can take to prevent the transmission of infectious disease?
   a. Wear a dust and mist respirator face mask
   b. Utilize nitrile utility gloves
   c. Practice appropriate hand hygiene

6. Eyewash stations are:
   a. never to be tested because they create a mess
   b. best used at the end of the day for tired eyes
   c. required to have a posted set of instructions
   d. best used in an emergency only if the employee has had training in their use

7. What are the best ways to minimize exposure to chemical hazards in the dental office?
   a. Read the label and place in a secondary container to keep the original fresher
   b. Place in a secondary container to keep the original fresher, and keep a log of all chemicals ever purchased
   c. Read the label, and store according to the manufacturer's directions
   d. Place in a secondary container to keep the original fresher, and store according to the manufacturer's directions

For answers to Review Questions, see the Appendix.

Case-Based Discussion Topics

1. Discuss the various items in an SDS. Take out an SDS for a sealant kit and identify all of the precautions required for handling the various components and identify the pictograms used.
   What if it is light-cured versus chemical-cured?

2. Regarding secondary labeling:
   Discuss the requirements and exceptions to the use of secondary labels.

3. Discuss some of the aerosols and bio-aerosols used in the dental office.
   Give examples of procedures that are most likely to generate these aerosols, and describe how they can be eliminated or reduced. (Hint: Don't forget about disinfecting and sterilizing procedures and the treatment performed on patients.)

4. Patient safety:
   Discuss the various procedures that must be in place to ensure patient safety.

5. Cross-contamination:
   Describe the procedures used to control cross-contamination and health care personnel exposure to the various materials that may be passed from a dental office to a dental laboratory. For example, what can you do to prevent cross-contamination and bacterial exposure of the dental office and laboratory personnel and patient from a dental impression?

BIBLIOGRAPHY

American Dental Association (ADA) Best Management Practices for Amalgam Waste. Available at http://www.ada.org/~/media/ADA/Member%20Center/Files/topics_amalgamwaste_brochure.

Association (ADA) Council on DentalAmerican Dental Association (ADA) Council on Dental Practice, American Dental Assistants Association (ADAA): Go green: It's the right thing to do. *The Dental Assistant* March/April 2012.

Bird DL, Robinson DS: *Modern Dental Assisting* (ed 12). Philadelphia, 2018, Elsevier/Saunders.

Bird DL, Robinson DS: *Modern Dental Assisting* (ed 11). Philadelphia, 2014, Elsevier/Saunders.

Cuny E: Changes to the OSHA hazard communication standard: are you ready? *Inside Dental Assisting*, November/December 2013.

Donaldson K: Is your office environmentally responsible? *RDA Magazine*, 2011.

Jacks M: Protecting Yourself. *Dimensions of Dental Hygiene* 9(8), August 2011, 26–29.

MacDonald G: Chemical hazards: regulations, identification and resources. *J Calif Dent Assoc* 17(12), 1989.

Miller C, Long T, Molinari J: Protect against oral aerosols and splatter, *Dental Products Report*, 2009.

Miller CH: *Infection Control and Management of Hazardous Materials for the Dental Team* (ed 6). St. Louis, 2009, Mosby.

Mount GJ, Hume WR: Appendix 1. In: *Preservation and Restoration of Tooth Structure*. St. Louis, 1998, Mosby.

Powers JM, Wataha JC: *Dental Materials: Properties and Manipulation* (ed 10). St. Louis, 2013, Mosby.

Terézhalmy GT, Huber MA: Environmental infection control and in oral healthcare settings. A Continuing Education Course offered at dentalcare.com. Available at http://www.dentalcare.com/en-US/dental-education/ce-courses/ce363

Terézhalmy GT: Clinical Practice Guideline for an Infection Control/Exposure Control Program in the Oral Healthcare Setting. A Continuing Education Course offered at dentalcare.com. Available at http://www.dentalcare.com/en-US/dental-education/ce-courses/ce342

U.S. Department of Labor: *Hazard Communication Standard: Labels and Pictograms*. 2013. [OSHA Brief] DSG BR 3636.

Wallace S, St. Cyr W: *Sustainability challenge*, Dimensions of Dental Hygiene, March 2014;12(3):23–24,26.

RESOURCES

Canadian-Wide Standard (CWS) on Mercury for Dental Amalgam Waste. Available at http://www.ccme.ca/ourwork/water.html?category_id=118

International Organization for Standardization (ISO). Dentistry—Amalgam Separators (ISO 11143). Available at http://www.iso.org/iso/catalogue_detail.htm?csnumber=42288 (2008).

Organization for Safety, Asepsis, and Prevention (OSAP): Home page. Available at http://www.osap.org/

Principles of Bonding

Chapter Objectives

Upon completion of this chapter, the student should be able to:

1. Discuss the effects of acid etching on enamel and dentin.
2. Describe the basic steps of bonding.
3. Explain the differences between bonding to enamel and bonding to dentin.
4. Discuss the significance of the smear layer.
5. Describe "wet" dentin bonding.
6. Compare etch-and-rinse and self-etch bonding techniques.
7. Explain how the hybrid layer is formed and its importance in bonding to dentin.
8. Explain how universal adhesives differ from etch-and rinse and self-etch adhesives.
9. Discuss the factors that interfere with good bonding.
10. Discuss the adverse effects of microleakage at restoration margins.
11. Describe how to bond ceramic veneers.
12. Describe the bonding of orthodontic brackets.
13. Explain the differences in bonding to enamel, dentin, metal, and ceramic.
14. List the factors that contribute to tooth sensitivity after bonding.
15. Etch enamel and dentin with phosphoric acid as permitted by state law.
16. Apply a bonding system to etched enamel and dentin as permitted by state law.

Key Terms

Bond *or* Bonding to connect or fasten; to bind. Items are jointed together at their surfaces in three main ways: by mechanical adhesion (physical interlocking), by chemical adhesion, or by a combination of the two

Adhesion the act of sticking two things together. In dentistry the term is used frequently to describe the bonding or cementation process. Chemical adhesion occurs when atoms or molecules of dissimilar substances bond together. Adhesion differs from cohesion, in which attraction among atoms and molecules of like (similar) materials holds them together

Etching *or* Conditioning terms used interchangeably to describe the process of preparing the surface of a tooth or restoration for bonding. The most common etching material (etchant) is phosphoric acid

Primer a low-viscosity resin applied as the first layer to penetrate etched surfaces to enhance bonding

Cure *or* Polymerize a reaction that links low molecular weight resin molecules (monomers) together into high molecular weight chains (polymers) that harden or set. The reaction can be initiated by strictly a chemical reaction (self-cure), by light in the blue wave spectrum (light-cure), by a combination of the two (dual-cure), or by heat

Wetting ability of a liquid to wet or intimately contact a solid surface. Water beading on a waxed car is an example of poor wetting

Wet Dentin Bonding bonding to dentin that is kept moist after acid etching to facilitate penetration of bonding resins into the etched dentin

Smear Layer a tenacious surface layer of debris resulting from cutting the tooth during cavity preparation. It is composed mostly of fine particles of cut tooth structure

Bonding Agent a low-viscosity resin that penetrates porosities and irregularities in the surface of the tooth or restoration created by acid etching for the purpose of facilitating bonding

Hydrophilic an attribute that allows a material to tolerate the presence of moisture

Hydrophobic an attribute that does not allow a material to tolerate or perform well in the presence of moisture

Etch-and-Rinse (also called Total-Etch) Technique a clinical technique that includes etching of both enamel and dentin as a separate step from the application of bonding agents. Products that use this technique are called Etch-and-Rinse Bonding Systems.

Self-Etch Bonding System a bonding system that does not use a separate etching procedure with phosphoric acid. The acid is contained in the resin primer and no rinsing is needed

Selective etching technique where enamel is etched first with phosphoric acid prior to the application of self-etch acidic primers that lack sufficient acidity to produce a good etch of the enamel

Universal Bonding System a bonding system capable of bonding to tooth structure as well as most restorative dental materials.

Hybrid Layer a resin-dentin layer formed by intermixing of the dentin bonding agent with collagen fibrils exposed by acid etching and the etched dentin surface. It serves as an excellent resin-rich layer onto which the restorative material, such as composite resin, can be bonded

Oxygen-Inhibited Layer (also called *air-inhibited layer*) a layer of unset resin on the surface of a polymerized resin that is prevented from curing by contact with oxygen in the air

Microleakage leakage of fluid and bacteria that occurs at the interface of the tooth and the restoration margins and is caused by microscopic gaps

Percolation movement of fluid into and out of the microscopic gap of the restoration margin as a result of differences in expansion and contraction rates of the tooth and the restoration with temperature changes

Contamination contact with a substance that interferes with bonding or lessens the chemical or mechanical properties (e.g., contamination of the etched surface of the tooth with saliva before bonding)

Hydrodynamic Theory of Tooth Sensitivity theory that explains how pain is caused by movement of pulpal fluid in open (unsealed) dentinal tubules. Actions that cause a change in the pressure on the fluid within the dentinal tubules stimulate a pain response from nerve fibers in the odontoblastic processes that extend into the dentinal tubules from the pulp

---

Adhesive materials are used on a daily basis in the modern dental practice. Adhesive materials are beneficial for many restorative and preventive procedures. They provide a seal between the tooth and the restoration and seal the dentinal tubules to reduce postoperative sensitivity. They enhance retention of the restoration so that more conservative preparations can be made, and they may increase the strength of the prepared tooth to resist fracture. Materials bonded to tooth structure may themselves be more resistant to fracture than materials that are not bonded. For example, porcelain veneers are thin, brittle and fragile until they are bonded to the tooth, and then they are very fracture resistant.

Adhesives are used for a wide variety of dental procedures. The dental auxiliary must be familiar with the terms and processes used in bonding of various restorative and preventive materials, to be knowledgeable, effective members of the dental team. The dental assistant will be involved in helping the dentist perform bonding procedures many times each day. In some states trained hygienists and assistants may etch tooth structure and apply bonding agents and place sealants and composite resins. Additionally,the dental hygienist may perform periodontal treatments that might affect bonded restorations. Therefore it is important that the dental auxiliary understands the properties and handling characteristics of the bonding materials and the processes involved in their use.

BASIC PRINCIPLES OF BONDING

In dentistry, the term **bond, or bonding,** is used in several ways. It is used to describe the process of attaching restorative materials, such as a composite resin, to a tooth by **adhesion** (the attraction of atoms or molecules of two different contacting surfaces). When describing cosmetic restorations such as porcelain or composite veneers, patients often use the term "bonding," for example, "The dentist is bonding my front teeth." Bonding also is the basis for several other dental procedures, such as the placement of orthodontic brackets and fixed retainers. It is used to describe some of the materials used in the process of placing restorations. For example, bonding resin is placed on the etched tooth surface before light-curing. Manufacturers often use the word "bond" in the trade names of their bonding resins, such as Prime & Bond *NT* (Dentsply Sirona) and OptiBond Solo Plus (Kerr Corporation).

PREPARATION FOR BONDING RESTORATIONS

The first step in the bonding process involves preparation of the surface of the tooth or the restoration (or both) to receive the material that will be bonded to it. Preparing the tooth surface usually includes removing plaque and debris first. This is best done with a slurry of pumice and water applied with a bristle brush or rubber cup (Fig. 5.1). Avoid prophy paste since it may contain flavoring oils that interfere with etching. Then, **etching** or **conditioning** the enamel or dentin (or both) with an acid is done next. The most commonly used acid is phosphoric acid in concentrations ranging from 10% to 38%. Acid removes mineral from the surface to create roughness or microscopic porosity.

BONDING TO THE ETCHED SURFACE

When a resin bonding agent or **primer** is flowed over the etched surface, it penetrates into the microscopic pores. When it hardens (**cures** or **polymerizes**), it creates projections called *resin tags* that lock into the tooth, creating a mechanical bond called *micromechanical retention*. The resin bonding agent will then chemically bond to other resins placed over it, such as composite resin. The chemical bond, called a *primary bond*, is a true adhesion between atoms or molecules of the composite resin and the bonding resin. (See Chapter 3 Physical and Mechanical Properties of Dental Materials for a discussion on types of bonds.) The chemical bond is stronger than a physical bond, called a *secondary bond,* which is a weak physical attraction between two surfaces such as the adhesion of paint to a metal surface. Roughening the metal surface by sandblasting increases the adhesion of the paint by mechanical retention, much in the way that acid etching roughens the surface of the enamel to achieve mechanical retention.

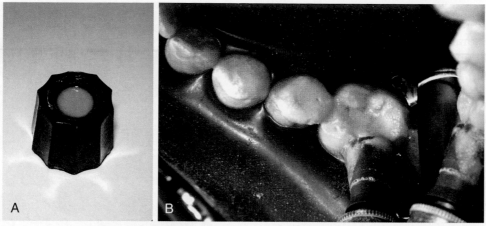

FIG. 5.1 Cleaning the tooth before bonding. **A,** Slurry of pumice and water used to remove plaque, pellicle and debris prior to acid etching. **B,** Rubber cup with slurry of pumice used at low speed to clean the enamel surface before bonding procedures.

SURFACE WETTING

Acid etching also increases the ability of liquids to wet the surface of the tooth by creating high surface energy. High surface energy helps to attract the resin to the etched surface. The adhesive must have a surface tension that is lower than the surface energy of the etched enamel. High surface energy can also attract contaminants (such as saliva), so good isolation is important. If saliva contamination occurs, drying the surface will leave residues that will interfere with the bond. The surface must be re-etched.

Good **wetting** increases the intimate contact of the bonding resin with the etched tooth structure, improving the penetration of resin to form tags and thereby improving the bond. Surfaces that are poorly wetted will cause beading of the liquid, similar to water on a newly waxed car. Each bead of water stands up on the surface of the car with a high angle of contact. On an unwaxed car, the water easily spreads out and has a low angle of contact (Fig. 5.2). Bonding agents are usually not very viscous (thick), so they will flow readily and wet the etched surface.

BOND STRENGTH

The strength of the bond obtained is usually measured by determining the force needed to separate the two joined materials. The force needed to break the bond is divided by the cross-sectional area of the bonded surfaces to arrive at the value for the bond strength. Most bond tests pull the bonded materials apart (tensile bond strength) or apply forces at approximately 90 degrees to the bonded interface of the materials until the bond fails (shear bond strength). The value for the bond strength is reported as megapascals (MPa). One megapascal equals 150 pounds per square inch (psi). Choosing materials with good bond strengths to tooth structure can enhance the longevity of the restoration and potentially allow for more conservative preparations, because cutting into healthy tooth structure to create mechanical locks can be minimized.

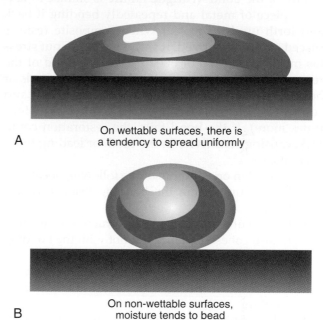

A On wettable surfaces, there is a tendency to spread uniformly

B On non-wettable surfaces, moisture tends to bead

FIG. 5.2 Acid etching of enamel increases its ability to be wetted by a resin bonding agent, resulting in a stronger bond. **A,** A low contact angle indicates good wetting as the liquid spreads over the surface. **B,** A high contact angle indicates poor wetting as the liquid beads on the surface like water on a waxed car.

Bonding to enamel usually achieves consistently high bond strengths of around 30 MPa (4500 psi). The bond strength to dentin is usually less than to enamel and varies according to how mineralized the dentin is and how deep into the dentin the cavity preparation extends. The dentin near the dentinoenamel junction (DEJ) has fewer dentinal tubules (about 15,000 to 20,000/mm^2), occupying 14% of the dentin surface, and they are smaller in diameter than in the dentin closer to the pulp. Deeper dentin contains more tubules (about 45,000 tubules/mm^2) and they are larger in diameter, occupying 20% to 30% of the dentin surface. Fluid flows from the pulp into the tubules on a constant basis. Therefore deeper dentin will be wetter from the flow of pulpal fluid through the tubules. Wetter dentin with more and larger holes (tubules) is more difficult to bond to consistently than is shallower dentin. Water will cause a deterioration of the dentin adhesives over-time. The restoration may stay in place but the dentin adhesive layer may have become porous.

Durability of the Bond

How long the bond lasts is more important than how high the initial bond strength is. Over time, exposure of the bonding agents to moisture may cause them to degrade (hydrolyze). In addition, repeated stresses on the bond caused by chewing pressures and temperature changes that cause different amounts of expansion and contraction between the restoration and the tooth structure (measured by the coefficient of thermal expansion) will gradually cause fatigue failure of the bond. (Fatigue failure is similar to taking a piece of metal and repeatedly bending it back and forth until it breaks.) When composite resin is placed and polymerized, it shrinks and can put stress (as much as 20 MPa or 3000 psi) on the bond of the resins to the tooth. In addition, hot and cold foods or beverages can cause composite resin to expand and contract much more so than the tooth (about four times more). If the bond fails, the restoration could leak, causing sensitivity in the tooth or leading to recurrent caries.

Bonds fail in one or more of the following locations:
1. failure occurs within the bonding resin (cohesive failure)
2. failure occurs within the tooth structure or restoration (also cohesive failure but not with the bonding resin)
3. failure occurs at the interface between the bonding resin and the tooth structure or restoration (adhesive failure).

It is thought that proteolytic enzymes called *matrix metalloproteinases* can cause breakdown of the resin bond to dentin. To stop the effect of these proteolytic enzymes, chemicals that inhibit them are being tested. One of these inhibitors is chlorhexidine. The durability of the bond may be enhanced by scrubbing the dentin with chlorhexidine before bonding. Further testing and a protocol on how to use it appropriately are needed.

ETCHING ENAMEL AND DENTIN

ENAMEL ETCHING

Michael Buonocore introduced acid etching of enamel into dentistry in the 1950s after observing industrial applications of 85% phosphoric acid on metal to enhance adhesion of paints and resins. Enamel is composed of thousands of rods (prisms) that extend from the dentin to the tooth surface in a radial fashion. Each rod has many millions of crystals composed of hydroxyapatite with about 20% carbonate inclusions. These carbonate imperfections add to the solubility of the crystals in

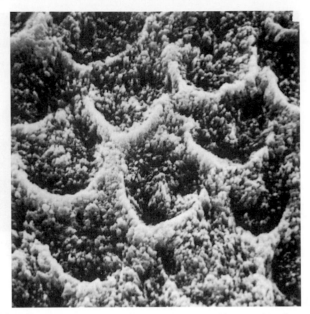

FIG. 5.3 An etched enamel surface as seen in this scanning electron micrograph has numerous peaks and valleys and surface roughness that provide retention and greatly increase the surface area for bonding. (From Phillips RW, Moore BK: Synthetic resins. In: *Elements of Dental Materials for Dental Hygienists and Dental Assistants*, Philadelphia, 1994, Saunders.)

acid. Proteins, lipids, and water in small quantities are found in microscopic spaces between the crystals.

Etching of enamel removes a small portion of the surface, reduces the ends of the enamel rods, and opens microscopic porosities between adjacent rods (Fig. 5.3). Etching creates a highly roughened surface with many tiny spaces and micropores into which the bonding resin can lock. The durability and strength of the bond to the enamel depends on how well the etch pattern is developed. Among the many different acids tested, phosphoric acid provides the best etch pattern. Bond strengths to enamel from phosphoric acid etching range from 20 to 50 MPa, depending on which test of bond strength is used.

 Caution

Do not rub or scrub the enamel surface with a hard instrument after etching. The portions of the enamel rods exposed by etching are very fragile and will break with light pressure. If this occurs, the available sites for resin tag formation will be greatly reduced and thus will affect the strength of the bond.

Etching Times

The enamel of permanent teeth is usually etched for 20 to 30 seconds with 37% phosphoric acid. Although etching times as short as 10 seconds appear to give good clinical results in some teeth, research results suggest that 20 to 30 seconds is optimal. Highly mineralized teeth may be more resistant to etching and may require up to 60 seconds of etching. Primary teeth should be etched for longer periods (60 seconds or more), because the surface of the enamel has a prism pattern

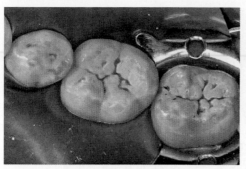

FIG. 5.4 Acid-etched enamel surfaces for bonding appear frosty white.

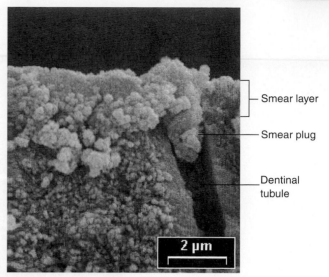

FIG. 5.6 Cutting of tooth structure with a rotary instrument forms a layer of cutting debris called the *smear layer*, as seen in this scanning electron micrograph. It is removed by acid etching so that it does not interfere with the formation of a bond. (Courtesy of Grayson Marshall, University of California School of Dentistry [San Francisco, CA].)

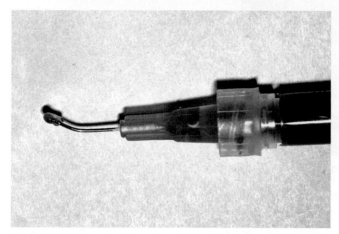

FIG. 5.5 Gel acid etchant in a syringe with a dull needle delivery tip. The gel has been dyed blue as a visual aid for its placement and removal.

that is not as well structured, is considered aprismatic (without a regular prism pattern), and is more resistant to deep resin tag formation. The etched surface should have a frosty appearance when dried (Fig. 5.4). However, when a cavity preparation involves the etching of both enamel and dentin, and the preparation is left slightly moist for **wet dentin bonding**, it cannot be determined whether the enamel has a frosty appearance.

Etchant Liquid or Gel

The acid etchant comes as a liquid or a gel. Often, coloring agents are added so the practitioner can see where the etchant is on the tooth. Liquid etchants are usually applied with a brush, a small cotton pellet, or a small sponge. Gels are more popular because they stay in place, whereas liquids tend to run without control. Gels contain silica as a thickener. They are usually applied by brush or dispensed from a syringe through a fine needle or brush tip (Fig. 5.5). The recommended rinsing time for acid gels is approximately 10 seconds or longer. Rinsing times shorter than 5 seconds may not remove residual silica. Rinsing times for liquid etchants can be shorter—5 to 10 seconds.

DENTIN ETCHING

The dentin has higher water and organic content (about 50% by volume) than does enamel (only about 12% by volume) and lower mineral content (about 50% by volume) compared to 88% for enamel. It contains a collagen matrix woven throughout the mineral component (hydroxyapatite) and a system of dentinal tubules through which fluids from the pulp flow.

Smear Layer

When a cavity preparation is cut with rotary or hand instruments, a layer of cutting debris forms on the surface of the cut dentin and enamel. This layer, called the **smear layer**, is composed mostly of cut tooth structure (hydroxyapatite and collagen) and may also contain plaque, bacteria, saliva, and even blood (Fig. 5.6). The smear layer sticks tenaciously to the dentin surface, plugs the openings of dentinal tubules greatly reducing the permeability of the dentin, and cannot be washed off with use of an air-water spray. The smear layer is about 2 microns (μm) thick and interferes with the formation of a bond to dentin. (A coarse diamond bur will produce a thicker smear layer than a fine diamond or carbide bur.)

Bonding systems that use phosphoric acid to etch the enamel and dentin dissolve the smear layer and rinse it away. Bonding systems that use acidic primers to etch the enamel and dentin penetrate the smear layer and incorporate it into the bonding agent, since there is no rinsing used with these systems. Regardless of the etching method, the smear layer is removed or modified so the bonding agents can penetrate the etched surfaces. Early bonding systems that did not etch the dentin had low bond strengths to dentin because the smear layer was in the way.

Phosphoric Acid Etching of Dentin

Etching dentin with phosphoric acid dissolves the smear layer and smear plugs in the tubules first, and then dissolves portions of the hydroxyapatite crystals

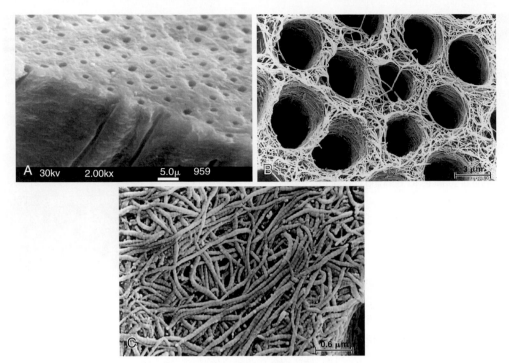

FIG. 5.7 A, Normal dentin with dentinal tubules. **B,** Acid etching of the dentin removes some of the mineral exposing the collagen fibers of the matrix, as seen in this scanning electron micrograph. C. Higher magnification of collagen fibrils. (**A,** from Sakaguchi R, Powers J: *Craig's Restorative Dental Materials*, ed 13, St. Louis, Elsevier. **B and C,** From Heymann H, Swift E, Ritter A: *Sturdevant's Art & Science of Operative Dentistry*, ed 6, St. Louis, 2013, Elsevier.)

from the surface of the dentin, creating a porous surface and exposing the meshwork of collagen fibrils that are part of the dentin matrix (Fig. 5.7, B, C). Because dentin is not as highly mineralized as enamel, it should be etched for shorter periods, typically for 10 seconds. With a 10-second etch, mineral is removed up to 5 μm in depth from the area between the tubules (intertubular dentin) and from around the periphery of the tubules (peritubular dentin) as well as in the opening of the tubules. Acid that goes into the tubules is neutralized by the fluids that flow from the pulp. When hydroxyapatite is removed from the dentin surface, it leaves a roughened, porous surface (but not the same as with enamel, because there are no rods or prisms) and exposes collagen fibrils.

When etching both enamel and dentin as in a coronal cavity preparation, it is best to apply the acid to the enamel first for 10 seconds, and then to the dentin for 10 seconds. That way enamel will be etched for a total of 20 seconds and dentin only 10 seconds. Etching dentin for 20 seconds or longer opens the tubules too wide and removes hydroxyapatite mineral to too great a depth. Over-etching will expose too much collagen matrix, causing it to act as a thick barrier and making it more difficult to coat the dentin and seal the tubules with the resin **bonding agent**. Over-etching dentin can result in a weaker bond and in post-treatment sensitivity.

Etching sclerotic dentin. Sclerotic dentin is dentin in which the dentinal tubules have become highly calcified by way of minerals deposits. This can occur as a

result of bacterial invasion from dental caries causing irritation of the odontoblasts (cells in the pulp that produce dentin) which have extensions into the tubules. The irritated odontoblasts try to protect themselves from the irritant and lay down a protective mineral wall. Also as part of the caries process, some of the mineral that is removed from the dentin as it is demineralized gets deposited into the tubules. Sclerotic dentin can also occur from injury to odontoblasts during cavity preparation for deeper restorations.

Studies have also shown that dentin of people over 55 is more mineralized than that of younger people. Sclerotic dentin being more mineralized is harder than normal dentin and has a glassy appearance. These factors make it more difficult to etch. To add some surface roughness for bonding, some clinicians use a diamond bur to abrade it before etching. Some studies suggest pre-etching the sclerotic dentin with phosphoric acid for 10 to 15 seconds before using self-etching bonding systems.

Moist dentin for bonding. After etching acid is removed by rinsing for at least 10 seconds. A gentle stream of air is used to remove excess water. However, the dentin is left slightly moist so that it glistens but without any puddles of water (Fig. 5.8). It is critical at this stage not to over-dry the dentin. The dentin surface must be moist to keep the collagen fibrils fluffed up. If the dentin is dried too much, the collagen fibrils collapse and form a dense surface that occludes the tubules and blocks adequate penetration by the dentin bonding resin. On the other hand, too much water remaining on the etched

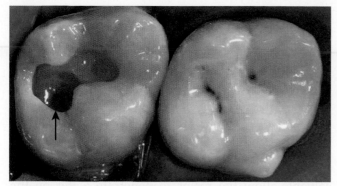

FIG. 5.8 Moist dentin for bonding after rinsing off acid. It should glisten with moisture but not have any puddles of water. (From Heymann H, Swift E, Ritter A: *Sturdevant's Art & Science of Operative Dentistry*, ed 6, St. Louis, 2013, Elsevier.)

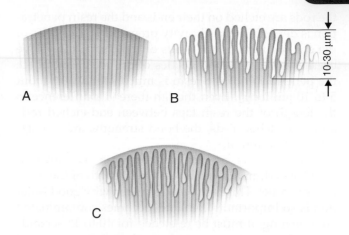

FIG. 5.9 Bonding to enamel. **A,** Unetched enamel rods **B,** Etched enamel rods C. Bonding resin mechanically bonding to etched enamel rods. (© Elsevier Collection.)

dentin dilutes the resin primer, makes it difficult for the resin to displace the water trapped in the collagen fibrils and produces a potential pathway for leakage. Both over-drying and under-drying can produce an incomplete sealing of the dentinal tubules and a much weaker bond, because the dentin-resin interface will separate more easily. A good dentinal seal helps eliminate bacterial leakage and postoperative sensitivity.

Etching Enamel and Dentin (Etch-and-Rinse Technique with 37% phosphoric acid)

	Enamel	Dentin
Etching Time	20 seconds	10 seconds
Rinsing Time	10 seconds	10 seconds
Moisture Content for Bonding	Very dry	Slightly moist (but no puddles)
Clinical Appearance	Frosty white (Fig. 5.4)	Glistening (Fig. 5.8)

 Clinical Tip

To restore moisture to overdried dentin, soak a cotton pellet in water and place it on the dentin for 10 to 20 seconds. Rewetting the dry dentin will allow the collapsed collagen fibrils to re-expand. If you wet it by squirting water on the dentin, then you will have to blow the excess water off and may overdry it again.

Enamel and Dentin Bonding

Enamel bonding resins. Bonding agents are low-viscosity resins that flow well into the microscopic porosities and irregularities of the etched surfaces. When bonding to enamel alone, the process is much simpler than bonding to dentin and the enamel can be dried completely. Etching of enamel creates a high-energy, low-tension surface that makes the surface easier to wet. A high-energy surface attracts the molecules in the resin bonding agent to improve penetration into the porous, etched enamel. Bonding to enamel alone requires only a low-viscosity liquid resin monomer that will penetrate into the spaces on and between enamel rods

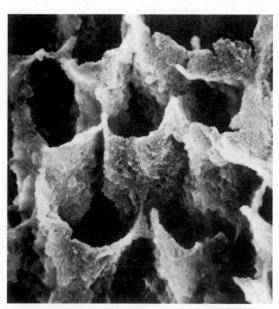

FIG. 5.10 A bonding resin placed on etched enamel penetrates the porous surface and forms resin extensions or tags that lock into the enamel and form a mechanical bond. This scanning electron micrograph shows the resin tags left after the enamel was dissolved away. (From Phillips RW, Moore BK: Synthetic resins. In: *Elements of Dental Materials for Dental Hygienists and Dental Assistants*, Philadelphia, 1994, Saunders.)

created by acid etching (Fig. 5.9). The liquid may simply be an unfilled resin or may include small amounts of very tiny filler particles to enhance the strength of the resin.

Resin tags. When the resin is cured by a chemical process or by light activation, it locks into the microscopic spaces and irregularities, producing resin tags that are 10 to 20 μm long and 5 to 6 μm in diameter (Fig. 5.10). The resin tags secure the resin to the enamel and create a very strong bond (shear bond strength of more than 20 MPa). The length of the resin tags is determined in part by the orientation of the etched enamel rods. If the enamel on the surface of the tooth is etched (as with bonding orthodontic brackets), then the rods are etched on their ends and the resin penetration is deep. In a class I cavity preparation, the sides of the enamel rods on the walls of the preparation have been exposed. When the sides of the rods are etched, the penetration of the resin is much shallower (about 5 to 10 μm long). Even though there is a difference in the length of the resin tags between end-etched rods and side-etched rods, the bond strengths are not significantly different.

Contaminants on the surface, such as saliva or blood, can dramatically lower the strength of the bond to the enamel. This is one major reason why good isolation is so important. If enamel becomes contaminated after etching, it must be re-etched for 10 to 15 seconds before the bonding process is continued. Because most restorative procedures involve etching both enamel and dentin, a dentin primer and a bonding resin that can be used on both the etched enamel and dentin are preferred.

 Clinical Tip

Good isolation is critical for good bonding. A major cause of bond failure leading to microleakage, recurrent caries and loss of retention of the restoration is contamination of the etched tooth surface. If the etched tooth surface is contaminated by saliva or blood, rinse thoroughly, re-isolate and re-etch for 10 to 15 seconds.

Dentin Bonding Resins

Resin components. Dentin bonding resins can be viewed as two components. The first is a resin primer that penetrates etched dentin and enamel and lays down a resin layer. The primer is composed of **hydrophilic** (water-tolerating) monomers and molecules that allow it to penetrate water. HEMA (2-hydroxyethyl methacrylate) is commonly used as a primer monomer. The second component is an adhesive resin that is applied over the primer. The adhesive resins commonly used are bis-GMA (bisphenol-A-glycidyl dimethacrylate), TEGDMA (triethylene glycol dimethacrylate), and urethane dimethacrylate (see Chapter 6 Composites, Glass Ionomers, Compomers).

The two resins chemically bond to each other, that is, the initial resin bonding material prepares (or primes) the tooth surface, much in the way that a primer is applied to wood before painting so that the paint will adhere better. The second resin then chemically bonds to the primer. In an effort to simplify the bonding technique, many manufacturers have combined the primer and bonding resin into one bottle to eliminate one step in the process.

"Wet" dentin bonding. Bonding to moist dentin ("wet"dentin bonding) was the first technique to achieve good bond strengths to dentin. As mineral is removed from the surface of the dentin by acid etching, the fibrils of the collagen matrix are exposed. By keeping the dentin moist, the fibrils stay spread out.

However, if the dentin is dried, the fibrils collapse into a thick mass that prevents the bonding resin from penetrating the etched dentin. A primer is more important on dentin than enamel because the primer contains hydrophilic groups that penetrate wet, etched dentin and keep the meshwork of collagen fibrils expanded so that the adhesive resin can penetrate.

Solvents. For the resin to penetrate through the water on moist dentin, it must be dissolved in a solvent that can penetrate water and carry the resin with it. The solvents allow the resins to penetrate water on the dentin and in the dentinal tubules, and to penetrate around collagen fibrils and into porosities in the tooth surfaces created by etching. The solvents are primarily acetone, ethanol (ethyl alcohol), or a combination of ethanol and water. In general, the solvent is the largest portion of the bonding agent, making up 60% or more of the material. Acetone is a highly volatile solvent. Its rapid evaporation may require that two or more coats of the bonding resin be applied to ensure adequate sealing of the dentin. An example of a bonding resin with acetone is Prime & Bond *NT* (Dentsply Sirona). Ethanol evaporates more slowly, so it may need a longer drying time. An example of a bonding agent with ethanol is OptiBond Solo Plus (Kerr Corporation). All bottles of bonding agents should be recapped immediately after the material is dispensed, to prevent evaporation of the solvent, which leads to gradual thickening of the resin left in the bottle with less ability to penetrate etched dentin. Unit-dose (single-use) packaging of bonding resins avoids some of these problems associated with bonding resins in bottles, as well as infection control issues.

After the primer is placed, it is dried before it is cured to remove the solvent and the remaining water. The resin adhesive bonds to the resin primer and provides a resin-rich layer that will chemically bond to **hydrophobic** (water-repelling) resin restorative materials such as composite resin that are placed over it. See Procedure 5.1 for bonding to enamel and dentin.

Self-etching technique. Bonding systems that do not use phosphoric acid etching instead use an acidic primer that etches and primes in the same step. Acidic primers (being hydrophilic) use water as a solvent. The water allows the acid component to ionize and become active for etching tooth structure. Water can also rewet the collagen fibrils if they have collapsed from drying to allow penetration by the primer. No rinsing and drying are needed after the acidic primer is applied.

 Clinical Tip

Bonding resins should not be dispensed before the operator is ready to place them. Otherwise, the solvent (such as acetone or ethanol) will evaporate prematurely, leaving a bonding resin with reduced ability to penetrate moist dentin.

Benefits of Bonding Restorations

- Enhances retention of the restoration
- Allows more conservative cavity preparations
- Regains some of the strength of the tooth lost by cavity preparation
- Strengthens brittle restorative materials such as porcelain veneers
- Seals the dentinal tubules
- Reduces microleakage and the associated sensitivity or recurrent caries

BONDING SYSTEMS

History of the Development of Bonding Systems

Bonding systems for enamel and dentin have undergone rapid changes over the past four decades (Box 5.1). The composites that became commercially available in the early 1960s were placed without etching or bonding agents. By the beginning of the 1970s, dentists were beginning to etch the enamel with acid and place a self-cured, unfilled bonding resin on the enamel only. This is considered to be the first generation of bonding agents. A number of different acids were tested, but phosphoric acid gave the best results. Great concern was expressed about putting a strong acid (like phosphoric acid) on dentin for fear of damaging the pulp. The dentin was covered with a liner such as calcium hydroxide for protection.

By the late 1970s and early 1980s, both enamel and dentin bonding resins (second generation) were being used, and they were light-cured. The dentin still was not etched, so the bonding resin placed on dentin was merely bonding to the smear layer. The resulting bonds to dentin were very weak bonds (2 to 6 MPa). Later in the 1980s, it was discovered that the smear layer was interfering with the ability of the bonding resins to bond to dentin. Acidic components of the bonding systems (third generation) were used to remove the smear layer, but the dentin was not adequately etched and it was dried. So, bonding resins did not penetrate the dentin surface in a meaningful way. Therefore bond strengths were still relatively low (bond strength of 12 to 15 MPa).

By the start of the 1990s, etching both enamel and dentin with phosphoric acid was an accepted technique, first called the total-etch technique but now commonly called the *etch-and-rinse* technique. Not only was the smear layer removed, but the surface of the dentin was etched and kept moist, allowing for the penetration of hydrophilic resin primers into the etched dentin surface. The bond strength to dentin increased to about 20 to 30 MPa. John Kanca introduced the "wet" dentin bonding technique in the United States. Primer and bonding resins were applied separately (two bottles—fourth generation) or combined into one bottle (fifth generation).

By the latter part of the 1990s, primers with acidic components that could etch enamel and dentin (called **self-etching systems**) were introduced and were light-cured or dual-cured (both light and chemical cures).

Box **5.1**	Time Line of Development of Bonding Systems

Enamel Etch: 1960s and 1970s—dentin was not etched. Bonding agents attached to etched enamel, and the smear layer blocked adhesion to dentin. First and second generations of bonding systems

    Products: First generation—*Cervident* (S.S. White); second generation—*Scotchbond* (3M ESPE), *Dentin Adhesit* (Ivoclar Vivadent)

↓

Etch-and-Rinse (Enamel and Dentin Etch and Rinse):
1980s—smear layer was removed by etching dentin but bonding agents could not penetrate dried, collapsed collagen layer. Third and fourth generations of bonding systems

    Early 1990s—"wet" dentin bonding introduced. Two-bottle (fourth generation) bonding systems. Highest bond strengths (but technique sensitive)

    Products: Third generation: *Scotchbond II* (3M ESPE), *Tenure* (DenMat), *XR-Bond* (Kerr Dental)

    Fourth generation: *Scotchbond Multi-Purpose* (3M ESPE), *OptiBond FL* (Kerr Dental), *ALL-BOND 2* (BISCO)

    Mid-1990s—one-bottle systems (fifth generation). High bond strength. Unit-dose packaging available

    Products: *Prime & Bond* NT (Dentsply International), *OptiBond Solo Plus* (Kerr Dental), *ExciTE* (Ivoclar-Vivadent), *Adper Single Bond Adhesive* (3M ESPE)

↓

Self-Etch (No Rinse):
  Sixth generation
    Late 1990s—Type I—2 bottles. Primer applied, and then adhesive resin
    Early 2000s—Type II—2 bottles. Primer and adhesive mixed and applied
    Products: Sixth generation
  Type I—*AdheSE* (Ivoclar Vivadent), *Clearfil SE Bond* (Kuraray America), *UniFil Bond* (GC America), *ONE-STEP PLUS with Tyrian SPE* (BISCO), *OptiBond Solo Plus self-etch adhesive* (Kerr Dental)
  Type II—*Adper Prompt L-Pop Self-Etch Adhesive* (3M ESPE), *Touch&Bond* (Parkell), *Tenure Uni-Bond* (DenMat), *Xeno III* (Dentsply International)

↓

    2002—One-bottle (all-in-one, seventh generation) systems—etching, priming, and bonding combined
    Products: *iBond* (Heraeus Kulzer)
    2011 (approximately) Universal adhesives were introduced—capable of bonding to both tooth structure and many dental materials. Two-bottle systems were introduced first: *Futurabond DC* (VOCO), *Xeno IV Dual Cure* (Dentsply), *Clearfil DC Bond* (Kuraray America), Later, one-bottle systems were introduced: Scotchbond Universal Adhesive (3M ESPE), All-BOND Universal (BISCO), Prime&Bond Elect (Dentsply).

Data from Nazarian A: The progression of dental adhesives [online continuing education]. *Dental CE Digest,* 2007. PennWell Publications.

Separate steps for etching with phosphoric acid and rinsing and drying were eliminated with the self-etching primers. These systems had primer and bonding resin in separate bottles (sixth generation).

In the early 2000s, improvements were made in self-etching materials so that components were contained in one bottle ("all in one" adhesives—seventh generation) and did not require mixing. Around 2010, another class of bonding resins was developed that could not only bond to tooth structure but also to restorative materials such as ceramics and metal and these have been called universal bonding agents.

CLASSIFICATION OF BONDING SYSTEMS

Each generation of adhesive systems has consisted of better materials or simpler procedures. The variety of combinations of primers and adhesives has gotten simpler but can still be confusing to the beginner until some experience in using the materials is gained. An easier way to view the current adhesive systems rather than by their generations is to categorize them into one of three basic groups: **etch-and-rinse bonding systems**, **self-etch bonding systems** and **universal bonding systems** (Table 5.1). These three bonding systems all have an acidic etchant, a primer for the dentin and a resin adhesive. HEMA (hydroxyethyl methacrylate) is

used in the dentin primer because it is a hydrophilic monomer that can very effectively penetrate etched dentin, facilitate formation of the hybrid layer and enhance bond strength. It is soluble in acetone, ethanol and water, which are the solvents used commercially for the resin adhesives.

All Bonding Systems Have These Things in Common

- An acid etchant
- A dentin primer
- A bonding resin (adhesive resin)

ETCH-AND-RINSE BONDING SYSTEMS (GENERATIONS 4 AND 5)

Etch-and-rinse (also called *all-etch* or *total etch*) refers to phosphoric acid etching of both enamel and dentin with a separate step that includes rinsing off the acid. After the acid is rinsed off, the dentin is left slightly moist (glistening but no water puddles), so that the collagen fibrils stay fluffed up. The etch-and-rinse technique became successful when hydrophilic resin monomers (HEMA) were added to the primer and adhesive. The hydrophilic monomers facilitated the penetration of the adhesive resin into the moist

TABLE 5.1	Etch-and-Rinse and Self-Etch Bonding Systems: Application and Commercial Products		
ETCH-AND-RINSE		**SELF-ETCH (NO RINSE)**	
Fourth generation: 2 bottles (3 steps)	Fifth generation: 1 bottle (2 steps)	Sixth generation: 2 bottles or chambers (2 steps)	Seventh generation: 1 bottle (1 step)
Step 1. Etch, rinse, and gently air dry. Leave dentin moist	Step 1. Etch, rinse, and gently air dry. Leave dentin moist	Step 1. Etch and prime, apply acidic monomer, lightly air dry	Step 1. Etch, prime, and bond (all in one bottle), gently air dry, light cure
Step 2. Apply primer, gently air dry	Step 2. Apply primer/ bonding resin, gently air dry, light cure	Step 2. Apply bonding resin, gently air dry, light cure	
Step 3. Apply bonding resin, gently air dry, light cure			
Strongest, most reliable bonds to enamel and dentin	Strong bonds to enamel and dentin	Strong bonds to dentin	Strong bonds to dentin
Reliably etches enamel	Reliably etches enamel	Bonds to enamel are not strong, especially uncut enamel. "Selective etch" advisable	Only a few products reliably etch enamel. "Selective etch" advisable
Scotchbond Multi-Purpose (3M ESPE) ALL-BOND 3 (BISCO) Bond-It (Pentron) DenTASTIC All-Purpose (Pulpdent) Gluma Solid Bond (Heraeus Kulzer) OptiBond FL (Kerr) Perma/Quick (Ultradent) Syntac (Ivoclar Vivadent)	Adper Single Bond Plus (3M ESPE) Bond-1 (Pentron) DenTASTIC UNO (Pulpdent) ExciTE (Ivoclar Vivadent) Gluma Comfort Bond (Heraeus Kulzer) IntegraBond (Premier) ONE-STEP PLUS (BISCO) OptiBond Solo Plus (Kerr) PQ1 (Ultradent) Prime & Bond *NT* (Dentsply)	AdheSE (Ivoclar Vivadent) Adper Prompt L-Pop (3M ESPE) ALL-BOND SE (BISCO) Brush&Bond (Parkell) Clearfil SE Bond (Kuraray America) Nano-Bond (Pentron) OptiBond Solo Plus SE (Kerr Corporation) Peak SE (Ultradent) Xeno III (Dentsply)	AdheSE One (Ivoclar Vivadent) Adper Easy Bond (3M ESPE) Clearfil S^3 Bond Plus (Kuraray America) Futurabond DC (VOCO) G-Bond (GC America) iBond (Heraeus Kulzer) OptiBond All-In-One (Kerr Corporation) Xeno V+ (Dentsply)

Adapted from Anusavice KJ, Shen C, Rawls HR: Table 12-1. In: *Phillips' Science of Dental Materials*, ed 12, St. Louis, 2013, Elsevier.

dentinal tubules and peritubular dentin. Drying with air is done at this stage to remove the volatile solvents from the resin and any remaining water. The resin is then light-cured (or chemical-cured).

Hybrid Layer

The layer that is formed by the intermixing of dentin bonding resin with collagen fibrils and the etched dentin surface is called the **hybrid layer** (first described by Japanese researchers Fusayama in the late 1970s and Nakabayashi in the early 1980s), because it is a combination (or hybrid) of dentin components and resin. The resin-rich hybrid layer facilitates bonding of the composite resin to the tooth through a chemical resin-to-resin bond (Fig. 5.11).

All of the current bonding systems work by micromechanically locking into etched enamel and by forming a hybrid layer with dentin.

Because the serous-like fluid in the dentinal tubules neutralizes the etching acid, the walls of the dentinal tubules are etched mostly around the opening and not very far into the tubules. As a consequence, long resin tags extending into the tubules do not add much to the retention of the resin because they are not bonded to the walls. Most of the retention comes from penetration into the etched mineral of the intertubular (between tubules) and peritubular (surrounds a tubule) dentin and around the collagen fibrils. Most systems use light-cured resins.

Two-Bottle Adhesive Systems (Fourth Generation)

The two-bottle systems have three basic steps in their procedure: (1) acid etch (and rinse), (2) application of primer, and (3) application of bonding resin. After the etch procedure, the primer is applied, dried, and light-cured. Then, the bonding resin is applied over the

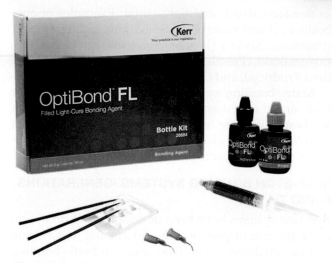

FIG. 5.12 Two-bottle etch-and-rinse bonding system. Components: primer, adhesive resin, etchant in syringe with delivery tips, micro-tip brushes and disposable mixing well. (OptiBond FL, Courtesy Kerr Corp.)

primer, and it is light-cured. The two-bottle etch-and-rinse systems provide the strongest bonds to dentin of all the bonding systems, assuming the technique is followed carefully. If over-etching, under-etching, over-drying or under-drying of the dentin occurs, then the bond strength can be diminished. Examples of two-bottle total-etch systems include Scotchbond Multi-Purpose Plus (3M ESPE), OptiBond FL (Kerr Corporation) seen in Fig. 5.12, ALL-BOND 2 (BISCO), and ProBOND (Dentsply Caulk/Dentsply International).

One-Bottle Adhesive Systems (Fifth Generation)

With one-bottle systems, after etching the primer and bonding resin are already mixed together and applied

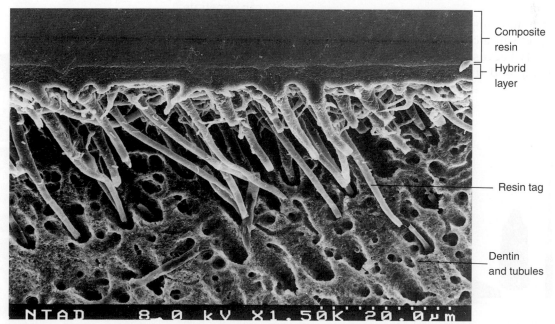

FIG. 5.11 When a bonding resin is applied to etched dentin, it penetrates the exposed collagen matrix and dentinal tubules. An intermingling of resin with etched dentin forms a hybrid layer. This layer provides a resin-rich layer for bonding with other resins such as composite resin. (Courtesy of Jorge Perdigão, University of Minnesota School of Dentistry [Twin Cities, MN].)

in one step, dried, and light-cured. Examples of one-bottle etch-and-rinse bonding systems include Bond-1 (Pentron), ExciTE F (Ivoclar Vivadent) seen in Fig. 5.13, IntegraBond (Premier Dental Products), PQ1 (Ultradent Products), and ONE-STEP (BISCO).

Many bonding systems have a chemical activator that can be mixed with the bonding resin to allow it to chemically cure as well as light-cure. When both modes of cure are available at the same time, the material is called *dual-cure*.

SELF-ETCH BONDING SYSTEMS (GENERATIONS 6 AND 7)

Bonding systems have been developed that do not require the use of phosphoric acid etching and rinsing and partial drying steps. One- and two-bottle bonding systems incorporate acidic groups (typically carboxylic acid) in a resin primer that will etch enamel and dentin and at the same time, prime them with resin without the need for rinsing and drying. These are called *self-etching bonding systems*.

The primers use water as a solvent to ionize the acidic monomer. Etching of the dentin with acidic primers dissolves the smear layer without deeply demineralizing the dentin and opening the tubules. Etching is not as deep as with etch-and-rinse systems. The acid component gradually shifts in pH to neutral and is incorporated into the polymerized resin, as are the dissolved tooth mineral and the smear layer. When the solvent has evaporated, the adhesive layer is thin and not very strong. Applying two coats of adhesive resin can increase the bond strength. Self-etching adhesives need a longer drying time of at least 10 seconds after application in order to evaporate all of the water solvent. Water left behind will degrade the bond over time.

While etch-and-rinse systems have the highest bond strengths, self-etch systems have less postoperative sensitivity because they directly seal the dentin without rinsing and drying steps. Because self-etch systems use acidic primers to demineralize dentin and there is no rinsing, it is easier for the primer and adhesive resin to penetrate the full depth of demineralization. With etch-and-rinse systems, the phosphoric acid may be left on too long and the primer cannot penetrate the more deeply etched surface, or if the etched surface is dried too much, the collagen will collapse and prevent primer and adhesive penetration. The unsealed dentin can contribute to postoperative sensitivity.

Self-etching bonding systems by not needing rinsing and drying steps eliminate the risk of over- or under- rinsing or drying, factors that can adversely affect the bond and cause post-treatment sensitivity.

The acidic primers are categorized as mild (pH 2 or above), moderate (pH 1 to 2), and strong (pH 1 or less). Systems with primers that are mildly acidic have weak bonds to enamel, especially uncut enamel, but strong bonds to dentin. Studies using the scanning electron microscope have shown that the etching pattern on enamel is shallow, resulting in poor micromechanical retention of the resin. Systems with primers that are strongly acidic demonstrate bond strengths similar to those with etch-and-rinse bonding systems.

To ensure a good bond to uncut enamel, many manufacturers recommend *"selective etching,"* meaning that enamel only should be etched with phosphoric acid before the application of the self-etching bonding materials (Fig. 5.14). If dentin is also etched with phosphoric acid, and then a self-etching bonding system is used, a good seal with the dentin may not occur. The phosphoric acid will etch the dentin deeper than the primer and bonding resin from the self-etch system can penetrate.

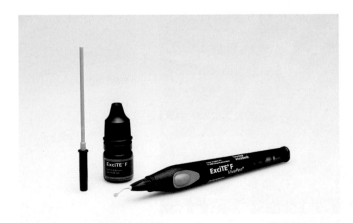

FIG. 5.13 One-bottle etch-and-rinse bonding system available in unit dose, bottle or pen dispenser (ExciTE F, Courtesy Ivoclar Vivadent).

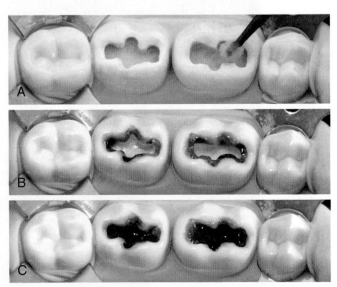

FIG. 5.14 Methods of etching (top to bottom): self-etch with acidic primers; selective etch of enamel and etch-and-rinse (total etch) with phosphoric acid (seen as blue gel). (Courtesy VOCO.)

Two-Bottle Self-Etch Bonding Systems

The two-bottle self-etching adhesive systems may be applied by two different methods depending on how they were manufactured. With type I self-etch adhesives, an acidic water-soluble primer is applied first, and then covered with a light-cured adhesive resin that contains nanosized filler particles (Fig. 5.15). Examples of type I self-etch adhesives include Clearfil Liner Bond (Kuraray America), Adper Scotchbond SE Self-Etch Adhesive (3M ESPE), and AdheSE (Ivoclar Vivadent). With type II self-etch adhesives, a drop of acidic primer from one bottle is mixed with one drop of adhesive resin from the other bottle and applied to the prepared tooth. Examples of type II self-etch adhesives include ALL-BOND SE (BISCO), and Xeno III (Dentsply Caulk/Dentsply International).

One-Bottle Self-Etch Bonding Systems

With one-bottle self-etch adhesive systems ("all-in-one" seventh generation), the adhesive resin is already combined with the acidic primer and does not require mixing (Fig. 5.16). Many of the self-etching primers

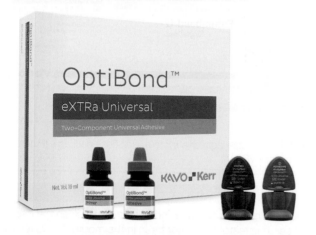

FIG. 5.15 Type 1 self-etching two-bottle adhesive system—bottle 1 is acidic primer and bottle 2 is bonding resin. Also available in unit-dose packaging. (OptiBond eXTRa, Courtesy Kerr Corporation.)

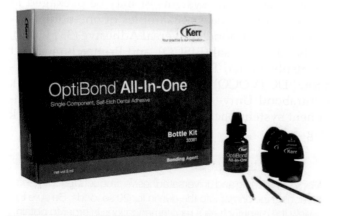

FIG. 5.16 All-in-one self-etching primer/adhesive seen in one bottle or unit-dose dispensing. (OptiBond All-In-One, Courtesy Kerr Corporation.)

require that two or more coats should be applied to the preparation, because they may not adequately cover the etched dentin with one coat. Many manufacturers also recommend scrubbing the primer into the dentin for 20 seconds. Follow the manufacturer's recommendations as to how many coats to apply and whether scrubbing into dentin is needed. Many one-bottle self-etching bonding systems require refrigeration to prevent the bonding agent from degrading. The bottle should be removed about 30 minutes before use to allow it to return to room temperature. Cooling of the material will affect the dynamics of polymerization and also make the material so viscous that it will not flow readily. Most of these systems are available in a bottle or unit-dose container. Examples of one-bottle bonding systems include Xeno V+ (Dentsply), Opti-Bond All-In-One (Kerr Corporation), iBond Self Etch (Heraeus Kulzer), All-Bond SE (BISCO), Adper Easy Bond Self-Etch Adhesive (3M ESPE), and AdheSE One (Ivoclar Vivadent). Fig. 5.17 illustrates self-etch adhesive systems.

Etch-and-rinse systems are preferred for indirect restorations (such as porcelain veneers) when mostly enamel is available for bonding, because phosphoric acid provides the most retentive etch in enamel. Self-etch systems are preferred for direct composites when mostly dentin is available, because they produce greater bond strength to dentin and reduce post-operative sensitivity.

 Clinical Tip

One-bottle systems (that combine primer and adhesive resin) whether they are etch-and-rinse or self-etch tend to produce a resin adhesive layer overlying the hybrid layer that is too thin. Applying at least two coats is recommended.

Universal Bonding Systems

Manufacturers continue to simplify and improve their bonding systems. In the past few years, they have developed bonding materials that are called universal bonding systems. While there is currently no consensus as to what constitutes a universal bonding system, in general, universal adhesives bond not only to tooth structure but also to a variety of restorative materials such as ceramics, noble and base metals and composites. While the universal adhesives can bond to these restorative materials, not all products develop a strong, lasting bond.

Universal adhesives are very versatile and most can be used with etch-and-rinse, self-etch and selective-enamel etch techniques. The key ingredient in all universal bonding systems is a phosphate ester that allows them to bond to tooth structure, ceramics and metals. Phosphate esters are also acidic and capable of etching tooth structure. Universal adhesives have a pH that ranges from 2.2 to 3.2 depending on the

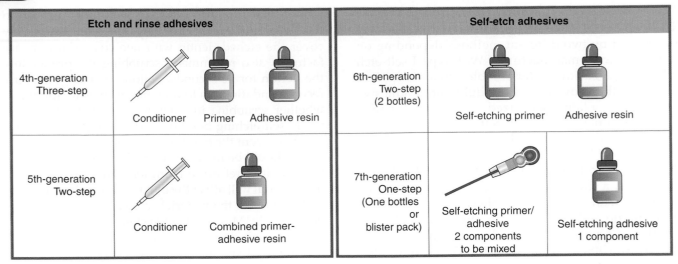

Etch and rinse adhesives				Self-etch adhesives		
4th-generation Three-step	Conditioner	Primer	Adhesive resin	6th-generation Two-step (2 bottles)	Self-etching primer	Adhesive resin
5th-generation Two-step	Conditioner	Combined primer-adhesive resin		7th-generation One-step (One bottles or blister pack)	Self-etching primer/ adhesive 2 components to be mixed	Self-etching adhesive 1 component

FIG. 5.17 Summary of self-etch adhesive systems. (Adapted from Cardoso MV, de Almeida Neves A, Mine A, et al: Current aspects on bonding effectiveness and stability in adhesive dentistry. *Aust Dent J*, 2011;56(Suppl 1):31–44.)

product. Products with a pH in this range are capable of etching and bonding to dentin. The ability to etch enamel adequately for bonding varies from product to product. To be safe, selective enamel etching may be used.

Some universal bonding systems require that an activator be added to the adhesive in order for it to be compatible with other manufactures' self- and dual-cured resin restorative materials and resin cements. The acidity of the adhesive can deactivate the chemicals needed for self-curing and will not permit the resins in the self-cure/dual-cure restorative materials or cements to cure properly without adding an activator.

Small quantities of microscopic filler particles composed of colloidal silica are added to increase the strength of the adhesive resin. The filler size ranges from 0.8 to 0.0007 μm. The smallest fillers are referred to as *nanofillers*. To put the size of these nanofillers into perspective, the following comparisons are made: the diameter of a human hair is approximately 40 μm, a bacterium is about 2 μm, and a virus is about 0.1 μm. See Chapter 6 for an in-depth discussion of fillers. Some universal adhesives also have fluoride compounds that are claimed by manufacturers to be released over time to aid in the prevention of recurrent caries at the margins of restorations. However, the quantities of fluoride released are generally too small to have a therapeutic effect.

Bonding to zirconia (a non-glass ceramic, see Chapter 9 Dental Ceramics) is challenging. Etching with hydrofluoric acid (8% to 10%) may create a powdery residue that is difficult to remove and may interfere with bonding. To aid bonding, some clinicians sandblast the internal surface (intaglio) of the ceramic restoration. The bond from some universal adhesive alone may prove to be less than desirable. Many clinicians and researchers think that a separate primer developed specifically for zirconia should be used, such as Z-Prime Plus (BISCO).

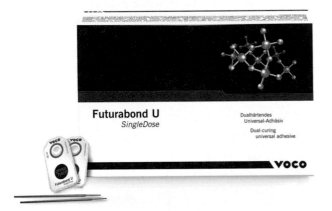

FIG. 5.18 Universal adhesive system. Unit dose package. (Futurabond U, Courtesy VOCO.)

> **💡 Clinical Tip**
>
> Some clinicians use *phosphoric acid* gel to clean the interior of ceramic restoration after try-in in the mouth. However, the etchant needed to create a surface roughness for bonding is 8% to 10% *hydrofluoric acid.*

Universal adhesives are manufactured as one-bottle or two-bottle systems or may be packaged in unit-dose blister packs. Examples of one-bottle systems are Scotchbond Universal Adhesive (3M ESPE), All Bond Universal (BISCO), and Prime&Bond Elect (Dentsply Sirona) Two-bottle systems include Futurabond DC (VOCO) and OptiBond XTR (Kerr Corp). Futurabond Universal Bond (VOCO) is a two component system packaged in a unit-dose blister pack (Fig. 5.18).

> **💡 Clinical Tip**
>
> Many self-etching and universal adhesive products recommend scrubbing the primer into the dentin for 20 seconds. Be sure to review the manufacturer's recommendations in order to obtain the best results with each product you use.

Clinical Application of Universal Bonding Adhesive

A universal bonding adhesive, when applied to a cavity preparation and to the interior (intaglio) of an indirect restoration, can provide resin-coated surfaces for cementation of the restoration with resin cement. The resin bonding adhesive on the tooth and restoration will bond chemically with the resin cement forming a durable bond.

The following sequence of clinical images (produced by Dr. Daniel Poticny, Grand Pairie, TX) in Fig. 5.19 depicts how the above scenario works. The maxillary first molar was treated for a fractured distolingual cusp. After the tooth was prepared a digital image was made and the restoration was designed and milled using CAD/CAM equipment (CEREC AC, Dentsply

Sirona)(CAD/CAM is discussed in Chapter 9, Dental Ceramics) and a resin-base ceramic material (Lava Ultimate Restorative, 3M ESPE) . The restoration was tried in to check margins, contours and proximal contacts. Next, the restoration was polished and internal surfaces were sandblasted for micromechanical retention. Selective etching of the enamel margins of the cavity preparation was done for 15 seconds with 37% phosphoric acid, then rinsed and dried, but leaving the dentin moist. Next, a universal adhesive was applied to the entire cavity preparation and scrubbed into the dentin surface for 20 seconds using a microtip brush. The same treatment was applied to the internal surface of the restoration. Silane treatment of the restoration was not needed because the universal

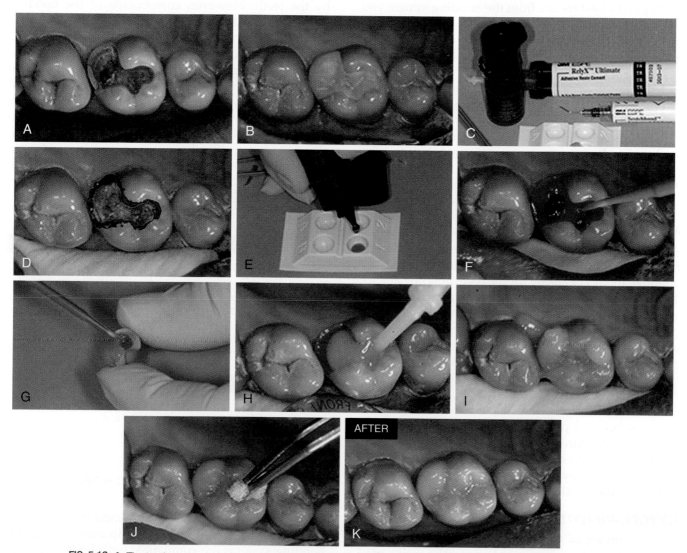

FIG. 5.19 A, The tooth was prepared and a digital impression was made with the CEREC AC (Sirona Dental Systems) CAD/CAM system. **B,** The CAD/CAM restoration was milled in-office using a Lava Ultimate Restorative block (3M ESPE) (shade A3 HT), and then tried-in for fit. **C,** The universal bonding adhesive, adhesive resin cement (RelyX Ultimate), etchant, dispensing well and microbrush applicators as set-up prior to the procedure. **D,** Selective enamel etching with phosphoric acid was done for 15 seconds. Bonding adhesive (Scotchbond Universal Adhesive [3M ESPE]) was dispensed into the well. **F,** Universal adhesive was scrubbed into the cavity preparation with a microtip applicator. **G,** Universal adhesive was scrubbed into the intaglio surface of the restoration. **H,** Adhesive resin cement [RelyX Ultimate, 3M ESPE]) was injected into the preparation. **I,** Cement flowed evenly from the margins upon seating. **J,** Excess cement was cleaned with a mini-sponge and removed from the interproximal with knotted floss. **K,** The final restoration after polishing. (Courtesy of Dentistry Today and Dr. Daniel Poticny.)

adhesive contains silane.(Silane is a coupling agent that helps to bind the ceramic to resin.) Adhesive resin cement (Rely X Ultimate Adhesive Resin Cement, 3M ESPE) was used to cover all surfaces of the preparation and the restoration was seated under pressure to force out excess cement and assure complete seating. Excess cement was removed with a mini-sponge and the proximal contact area was cleared with floss. Occlusal high spots were adjusted and final polish was accomplished with diamond polishing paste.

 Clinical Tip

Many of the self-etch systems recommend "selective etching" of the enamel with phosphoric acid in order to ensure a good etch and bond to enamel.

To get the best results from the bonding system you are using:

- Review the manufacturer's instructions
- Be meticulous in your technique
- Maintain good isolation
- Use enough drying time with an air stream to evaporate the solvent and remove water from "wet" dentin—at least 10 seconds
- Use fresh material. Refrigeration may extend the shelf-life. Remove from the refrigerator half an hour before use.
- Use unit-dose packaging when possible. If using bottles, recap immediately after dispensing materials.

MODES OF CURE OF ADHESIVES

Adhesive systems are cured (polymerized) by methods similar to those used for composite resins. There are three modes of curing for the resin bonding agents. The most commonly used mode is a light-cure process that uses a light in the blue wave range to activate a chemical (a photosensitizer, camphorquinone) that reacts with an initiator (a tertiary amine) to set off the polymerization reaction (see Chapter 6 for an in-depth discussion of resin polymerization). The second mode is a self-cure process in which a chemical reaction occurs when two resins are mixed together, one of which contains benzoyl peroxide as an initiator. The third mode is a dual-cure process that uses a combination of self-cure and light-cure ingredients. Dual-cured resins can be activated by light or can cure chemically without application of the curing light.

OXYGEN-INHIBITED LAYER

On the surface of the polymerized bonding resin is a very thin coating of uncured resin. The resins used for composites and sealants will also form this layer of uncured resin on their surfaces. Polymerization is inhibited where the surface is exposed to oxygen in the air (this layer is called the **oxygen-inhibited layer**, or *air-inhibited layer*). Once the composite resin is placed over the bonding resin, its presence will exclude air, and that uncured layer on the bonding resin will cure

when the composite is cured. The uncured layer will actually help facilitate a chemical bond between the bonding resin and the composite resin. When the oxygen-inhibited layer is exposed to the mouth as with sealants, many clinicians prefer to wipe it off because it can impart an unpleasant taste.

BIOCOMPATIBILITY

Acid etching dentin is unlikely to cause pulpal irritation because it is limited in its depth of penetration. The hydroxyapatite is etched less than 7 μm in depth and acid entering the dentinal tubules is buffered to neutral by components of dentinal fluids and hydroxyapatite. However, acid and acidic primers should not be placed directly on a pulpal exposure.

Bonding and restorative materials are well tolerated by the teeth. However, components of the bonding systems can irritate the skin, mucosa, and eyes. Acidic components can cause burns. Some dental personnel develop allergies to the materials, especially HEMA. Personal protective equipment should be used when handling these materials. Use of the rubber dam will minimize contact with the patient's oral mucosa. Any area of contact with the skin should be washed with soap and water. An eyewash station should be available to treat accidental exposure to the eyes. Most of the undesirable effects are the result of contact with the unpolymerized components. Once the materials are polymerized the risks of untoward reactions are much less.

 Caution

Resins, solvents, and acids in the bonding systems can irritate the skin, mucosa, or eyes, and therefore caution should be taken when these materials are applied. Materials on skin or mucosa should be washed thoroughly. Eye protection should be worn by the patient and PPE worn by the operator and assistant.

 Caution

A small portion of the population may have an allergic response to acrylate resins. Precautions are to be followed because these resins may penetrate commonly used gloves.

COMPATIBILITY WITH OTHER RESINS

Etch-and-Rinse Systems

Two-bottle bonding systems are compatible with light-cure, self-cure, and dual-cure composites. One-bottle bonding systems are compatible with light-cure composites. They are not compatible with self-cure composite core materials or resin cements, because the bonding agents are acidic and that interferes with the set of the composite or resin cement. One-bottle bonding systems require that an activator be mixed with the bonding resin in order for it to be compatible with self-cure and dual-cure composites and resin cements.

Self-Etch Systems

Type I self-etching bonding systems (primer applied first followed by bonding resin) are generally compatible with light-cure, self-cure, or dual-cure composites, but the type II bonding systems (primer and bonding resin mixed together, then applied) are not. Light-cured all-in-one bonding systems are also not compatible with self- and dual-cured composites, but dual-cured all-in-one systems are compatible.

  Clinical Tip

Before placing a composite core for a crown preparation, check the manufacturer's fact sheet for compatibility of the bonding system with self-cured and dual-cured composite core materials.

Three Main Steps of Bonding Systems

All bonding systems have three main steps in common:
- Etching with either phosphoric acid or an acidic primer
- Priming with hydrophilic monomers in a solvent that penetrates etched surfaces
- Bonding with hydrophobic bonding resins to seal etched surfaces and to chemically bond to composite resin or resin luting cements

MICROLEAKAGE

Restorations can leak when they are not completely sealed at their margins (junction of the restoration with the tooth surface). Leakage usually occurs at the microscopic level (called **microleakage**) and permits fluids, bacteria, and debris to enter the cavity preparation (Fig. 5.20). Microleakage can contribute

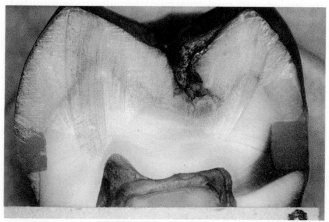

FIG. 5.20 Seen is a longitudinal section through a molar that has cervical composite restorations on the right- and left-hand sides. When a good bond is not formed between the tooth and the composite, fluids and bacteria can seep between them, a process called *microleakage*. The tooth was soaked in a dark dye to show areas of microleakage. The restoration on the right shows leakage, as indicated by dye penetration; the one on the left does not. (Courtesy of Larry Watanabe, University of California School of Dentistry [San Francisco, CA].)

to decay under the restoration and increase sensitivity of the tooth. Pulpal irritation comes more from bacteria entering from microleakage than from chemical components of the bonding or restorative materials.

Contaminants are substances that interfere with the enamel or dentin bonding, such as saliva, blood, the smear layer, or oils from the dental handpiece or from prophy pastes. Contaminants can contribute to microleakage when they are not properly removed before and during the bonding process. Microleakage can have other causes, such as shrinkage of composite resins when they cure (see Chapter 6) or restorations placed without bonding, such as conventional amalgam restorations (see Chapter 10). When restorative materials expand and contract with temperature variations (the change in volume of the restoration is called the *coefficient of thermal expansion*) at a different rate from the tooth structure, **percolation** can occur, in which fluids and bacteria percolate or flow into and out of the gap at the interface of the restoration and the tooth. Cold foods such as ice cream or beverages cause contraction of the restoration and widening of the gap, and hot foods or beverages cause expansion of the restoration and reduction of the gap. Percolation can lead to (1) pulpal irritation with tooth sensitivity, (2) staining at the margins, and (3) recurrent caries.

CONTAMINATION OF BONDING SITE

For successful bonding, good isolation and soft tissue management are essential. Saliva and blood are the most common sources of **contamination** in the oral cavity. If the newly etched surface becomes contaminated, rinse it thoroughly and re-etch for 10 to 15 seconds.

Astringents and hemostatic agents (e.g., aluminum chloride and ferric sulfate; see Chapter 15 [Impression Materials] for more detailed information) used to control bleeding from the gingiva can interfere with bonding, lower bond strengths and lead to microleakage. Instead, the soft tissues can be infiltrated with a local anesthetic containing epinephrine (in patients who can tolerate epinephrine) to constrict the local blood vessels and capillaries and stop the bleeding.

Avoid using a temporary cement containing eugenol for provisional restorations. Eugenol interferes with the set of resins and will cause a drop in bond strength. Clean the teeth with a slurry of pumice to remove residual eugenol before bonding. Do not use prophy paste because it may contain flavoring oils that can interfere with bonding.

Carbamide peroxide and hydrogen peroxide whitening agents can leave residual oxygen in the tooth structure that interferes with the bond. Wait 1 to 2 weeks after whitening before performing bonding procedures.

Factors That Prevent Good Bonding

- A surface that is overly wet does not allow good penetration of the bonding resins into the etched enamel and dentin.
- An overly dry etched dentin surface causes the collagen fibrils to collapse and cover the dentin surface so that the bonding resins cannot penetrate to reach the etched dentin and the tubules.
- Blood or saliva on the etched enamel or dentin will interfere with the ability of the bonding resin to penetrate the surface.
- Failure to saturate dentin with a bonding resin will result in voids and incompletely sealed dentin. This can result in reduced bond strength and sensitivity because tubules are open.
- Failure to adequately cure the bonding resin will cause the resin to separate from the enamel or dentin.
- Moisture from the air-water lines can wet the enamel and dentin at the wrong step in the bonding process, resulting in loss of a proper bond and seal.
- Oil lubricants expelled from the handpiece onto the tooth during preparation will prevent the bonding resins from adhering to the etched enamel and dentin.
- Recently applied whitening or topical fluoride agents can affect the enamel so that it is more difficult to etch or to bond to. Studies have shown that the bond to recently whitened enamel is not as strong. Fluoride makes the surface of the enamel more resistant to being etched by acid.
- Eugenol in cements for provisional restorations will interfere with the set of resin bonding agents and composite resins.
- Aluminum chloride– and ferric sulfate–containing astringents (e.g., Gingi-Aid [Belport] and Astringedent or ViscoStat [Ultradent]) used to control gingival bleeding will interfere with the set of the bonding agents.

POSTOPERATIVE SENSITIVITY

Some patients may experience transient tooth sensitivity after a bonded restoration is placed (also see Chapter 6). This usually occurs for only a short time—a few hours to a few days. The pain response comes from odontoblasts that lie in the pulp at its junction with the dentin. The odontoblasts have processes that extend about one third of the way up the dentinal tubules, and the tubules contain a column of pulpal fluid. The odontoblastic processes have pressure receptors that can only interpret in a painful response any change in pressure in this column of pulpal fluid. One primary reason for the sensitivity is unsealed dentinal tubules. Phosphoric acid etching removes the smear layer and smear plugs in the tubules leaving open tubules. If they are not properly sealed during the dentin bonding process, a number of things can influence the pressure on the fluid in the tubules and elicit a pain response. This dentinal fluid movement caused by pressure changes is called the **hydrodynamic theory of tooth sensitivity** and was described by M. Brännström.

The following conditions can contribute to this sensitivity:

- The tooth has been over-dried (desiccated) during the bonding process, trapping air in the dentinal tubules; when the patient bites down, the restoration compresses the dentin, putting pressure on the air in the tubules.
- The dentin has been over-etched and is not adequately sealed with priming and bonding resins. Open tubules allow pressure on the column of fluid within the tubules.
- The composite resin restoration is cured in increments that are too large, causing contraction stress on the tooth cusps or causing the composite resin to leak as it pulls away from the walls and floor of the cavity preparation as it shrinks (see Chapter 6).

Less postoperative sensitivity is found with self-etching bonding systems compared with etch-and-rinse bonding systems. Self-etching bonding systems have the advantage of eliminating separate etching, rinsing, and drying steps that might introduce errors of over-etching or under-etching and over-drying or under-drying that contribute to postoperative sensitivity. The acidic primer in the self-etch systems etches and primes the dentin with a hydrophilic resin in the same step. The depth of etching with acidic primer is shallower than with phosphoric acid and the primer penetrates to the depth of its etch, achieving a good seal of the dentin and its tubules.

For both etch-and-rinse and self-etch materials, it is important to carefully follow each manufacturer's instructions for use to ensure that the dentinal tubules are sealed and post-treatment sensitivity is avoided. These are technique-sensitive materials, and poor attention to detail can create a weak or inadequate bond that may lead to failure of the restoration and pain for the patient.

 Clinical Tip

When bonding to preparations with large areas of enamel remaining, etch-and-rinse systems are preferred. When bonding mostly to dentin, self-etch systems are preferred. Selective etching (with phosphoric acid) of enamel when using self-etching systems is recommended to ensure satisfactory enamel etch pattern for bonding.

CLINICAL APPLICATIONS FOR BONDING

BONDING OF RESTORATION

After the initial bonding resin is cured on the tooth, other adhesive bonding resins or resin cements can be used to attach restorations to the tooth by way of resin-to-resin chemical bonds (see Procedure 5.1). Restorations that are not made of resin, such as metal or ceramic products, require treatment of their surfaces to allow them to bond to the resin on the tooth (see Procedure 5.2). A description of bonding with composite restorations and glass ionomers can be found in Chapter 6. Glass ionomers do not require a separate bonding agent. After the smear layer is removed with a mild acid (typically 10% polyacrylic acid), the glass ionomer chemically bonds directly to the mineral component of enamel and dentin.

CERAMIC BONDING AND REPAIR

Ceramic restorations are retained much better if they are bonded to the tooth rather than if they are merely cemented (Procedure 5.2). Bonding also helps minimize microleakage that can contribute to sensitivity or recurrent caries. On occasion, ceramic restorations will chip and need repair instead of replacement. Techniques have been developed to permit repair of porcelain and other glass-based ceramics (see Chapter 9) in the mouth, usually when the repair will not be subjected to heavy chewing forces.

Clinical Technique. The process of bonding composite to glass-based ceramics is similar to bonding to enamel or dentin. The difference lies in the etchant used and the surface preparation completed on the ceramic restoration before application of the bonding resin. Some operators prefer to roughen the surface of the ceramic with a diamond bur or by sandblasting before applying the acid. To bond to ceramics, the acid most commonly used is hydrofluoric acid in a syringe designed for intraoral or extraoral use. After the surface of the ceramic is etched and rinsed, a solution of silane is applied for 60 seconds, and then the surface is dried to evaporate the solvent. Silanes are coupling agents that react with the glass in the ceramic and leave a coating of vinyl that will bond to the resin in the bonding agent. Next, the bonding resin is placed and light-cured, and the final composite restorative material is placed and finished (see Chapter 9).

This repair technique will not work with non-glass ceramics such as zirconia or alumina. They need special treatment.

! Caution

Hydrofluoric acid is used to etch porcelain and other glass-based ceramics for cementation or repair, and it is a highly caustic solution. Hydrofluoric acid also can etch adjacent ceramic, composite, and glass ionomer restorations, as well as tooth structure, and can burn soft tissues. Take precautions to properly isolate the area to be bonded. Protect the tissues and restorations adjacent to the area being etched.

METAL BONDING

Metal bonding is used to create better retention of metal to a tooth during the cementation (luting) of a restoration such as a crown. (See Chapter 11 Casting Metals, Solders, and Wrought Metal Alloys for a description of metals and Chapter 9 for porcelain-bonded-to-metal restorations.) Metal bonding is also used for placement of a composite veneer over metal for cosmetic reasons, or for covering metal exposed when porcelain fractures from a porcelain-bonded-to-metal crown.

Laboratory and clinical techniques. To bond to the metal of a crown or resin-bonded (Maryland) bridge, the metal surface is roughened by sandblasting or with a coarse diamond bur to create micromechanical retention. The surface of the metal can also be treated by electrochemical etching in the laboratory or by depositing a thin layer of tin through an electroplater. The latter two methods are often used for metal preparation before cementation of a resin-bonded bridge. Noble metals in particular, such as gold, need to be tin-plated for an effective bond to the resin. Although, in practice many clinicians simply sandblast the interior to provide micromechanical retention. Once the metal surface is prepared, it is cleaned and dried before it is coated with the bonding resin for cementation. These cements are usually self-cured or dual-cured (see Chapter 14 Dental Cement) because the metal blocks the curing light.

For repair of a porcelain-bonded-to-metal crown or bridge with fractured porcelain and exposed metal (see Figure 9-10 in Chapter 9 for an example), the porcelain and metal are prepared as described previously in the section Ceramic Bonding and Repair. Next, a one-step bonding resin is applied, thinned with air, and light-cured for 20 seconds. An opaque masking resin is then applied to the metal to keep it from showing through and causing a gray appearance of the overlying composite. It is light-cured for 20 seconds. Finally, a composite resin that matches the color of the porcelain is selected, applied, light-cured, finished, and polished.

AMALGAM BONDING

Traditionally, amalgam is retained in the cavity preparation by mechanical retention with undercuts and grooves placed in sound tooth structure. In the 1990s bonding of amalgam to the cavity preparation became popular because laboratory studies showed that microleakage could be reduced and the strength of the prepared tooth and retention of the restoration could be increased. With increased retention, cavity preparations could be more conservative because sound tooth structure did not need to be removed to create undercuts. However, clinical studies monitoring the bonded amalgams for as long as 6 years found no difference between bonded and non-bonded amalgams in terms of marginal integrity, recurrent caries and fracture of the tooth, or restoration. Few clinicians presently bond their amalgams.

COMPOSITE RESIN REPAIR

A large multi-surface composite restoration, a composite veneer, or a large incisal angle composite may have a minor defect of the margin, a small chip, or a small amount of recurrent caries. It may be more conservative and cost-effective to repair the existing composite rather than replace it. However, the older the composite is, the weaker will be its bond to new composite. In order to achieve a clinically acceptable union, the old composite surface to be repaired is roughened with a diamond bur or by sandblasting. Next, the composite surface and tooth structure involved in the preparation are etched with phosphoric acid before application of the bonding system. After the bonding resin has been applied and cured, new composite can be placed.

ORTHODONTIC BRACKET BONDING

Orthodontic brackets have replaced bands for many uses, especially in the anterior part of the mouth. Because brackets cannot be used with conventional cements, they must be bonded to the enamel using adhesive materials. Bonding of orthodontic brackets is done with plastic or metal brackets, which have a retentive mesh (see Fig. 5.32 in Procedure 5.3) or a series of knobs to lock in the resin adhesive, or with ceramic brackets that have a pre-etched bonding surface. The adhesive bonding resins are self-cured, light-cured, or dual-cured. Because the metal or ceramic material will not allow light to reach and cure the resin cement under the bracket directly, the light is cast from mesial, distal, and lingual, as well as facial, directions to cure the resin by light that has passed through the enamel.

Clinical Technique. Direct bonding of orthodontic brackets is explained and illustrated in Procedure 5.3. Some clinicians use an indirect method of application of brackets. With the indirect method, brackets are aligned on the diagnostic cast in the same position as they will be placed on the teeth and held with sticky wax. Then a matrix, often constructed from impression putty, is formed over the brackets and the teeth on the cast. The brackets are picked up in the matrix and, at the time of bonding, are oriented in the same manner on the teeth as they were previously on the cast.

BONDING OF CERAMIC VENEERS

Ceramic veneers are a relatively conservative means of achieving anterior esthetics. They can be used to change the shape and color of the teeth, close diastemas, straighten the alignment of teeth, and lengthen chipped or worn teeth. Usually, the tooth substrate that the veneer will be bonded to is mostly enamel. The etch-and-rinse bonding systems are preferred because

phosphoric acid develops a better etch pattern for a strong bond.

Clinical technique. Confirm that the bonding system is compatible with the resin cement that will be used. After the veneers have been tried in and any adjustments made, rinse off the try-in paste from the veneers and tooth surfaces and dry the surfaces.

Tooth preparation. Etch the prepared enamel for 30 seconds with 37% phosphoric acid. If dentin is exposed, etch it for 10 seconds only. Apply a bonding resin to the tooth and thin with the air syringe. Too thick a coat will not allow the veneers to seat fully.

Veneer preparation. Ceramic (glass-based) surfaces to be bonded are prepared by etching with hydrofluoric acid (5% to 10% concentrations are preferred) for 60 seconds, rinsing it off, and drying. The acid creates micromechanical retention in the surface of the ceramic. Silane is applied for 60 seconds and then dried. The bonding resin is applied in a thin coat and further thinned with the air syringe. Do not cure it. Apply the resin cement evenly to the veneers. If the veneers are thin, use the resin cement in the light-cure mode. If the veneers are thick or opaque, then use the cement in the dual-cure mode (mix base and catalyst). Some clinicians like to use flowable composite as the cement.

Seating the veneers. Seat the veneers starting with the two central incisors, next the laterals incisors, and finally the canines. Use a small brush to wipe away the gross excess cement but stay short of the margins to prevent removing cement from under the edge of the margin. Use a spot cure or wave cure (curing light is waved over the veneer surfaces) for 3 seconds to gel the resin cement without fully curing it to allow easy cleanup. Clear the cement from the interproximal areas with floss. Use a #12 scalpel blade or a narrow, sharp sickle scaler to remove excess cement from the margins. Complete the cure of the resin cement. Use extra fine finishing diamond burs to complete the finish of the margins. (Other techniques, materials, and instruments may be used. This is presented as an example of one technique.)

Note: Veneers made from ceramic materials, such as zirconia (e.g., Lava; 3M ESPE), will require special treatment and primers to prepare the veneer surface for cementation (see Chapter 9). See Table 5.2 for a summary of bonding for ceramic restorations.

BONDING OF ENDODONTIC POSTS

Posts are placed within the roots of endodontically treated teeth to retain dental materials used to build up the teeth (core buildup) when coronal tooth structure is inadequate for restoration with a crown. The posts are made of a variety of materials and can be

TABLE 5.2	Bonding to All-Ceramic Restorations: A Summary			
PROCEDURE STEPS	**FELDSPATHIC PORCELAIN**	**LITHIUM DISILICATE**	**ALUMINA**	**ZIRCONIA**
Etch ceramic	Hydrofluoric acid 60 seconds	Hydrofluoric acid 60 seconds	No etch Sandblast to roughen	No etch, Sandblast to roughen
Rinse	Yes	Yes	No	No
Silane	Yes (unless universal adhesive contains silane)	Yes (unless universal adhesive contains silane)	No, if universal adhesive contains silane	No, if universal adhesive contains silane
Bonding agent	Apply etch-and-rinse adhesives	Apply etch-and-rinse adhesives	Apply special primer and universal adhesive	Apply special primer and universal adhesive
Cement	Light- or dual-cured resin cement	Light- or dual-cured resin or self-adhesive resin cement	Self-adhesive resin cement; resin-modified glass ionomer; or special primer, universal bonding agent, and resin cement;	Self-adhesive resin cement; resin-modified glass ionomer; or special primer, universal bonding agent, and resin cement

Adapted from Farah JW, Power JM: Bonding Agents—2008. *The Dental Advisor*, 2008;25:1–9.

categorized into two general types: metal and non-metal. Metal posts are made of cast gold, stainless steel, titanium alloy, or pure titanium (see Chapter 11 Casting Metals, Solders and Wrought Metal Alloys). Nonmetal posts are made of fibers of carbon or glass encased in resin or zirconium-based ceramic. The posts are bonded to the root with dentin bonding resins and resin cements following the manufacturer's recommendations.

Clinical technique. When it is determined that an endodontically treated tooth needs a post, the dentist prepares one or more roots with specially shaped drills that shape the root canal to the shape of the post. The prepared canal is etched with phosphoric acid for 10 to 15 seconds. The acid is thoroughly rinsed off and excess water is removed with paper points. The dentin is left slightly moist (glistening but without puddles). A dentin primer is placed in the canal and air-dried to drive off any remaining water and the volatile solvents in the primer. (A universal system could be used on the tooth and post.) Next, self-curing or dual-curing composite resin cement is applied to both the canal and the post. (Make sure the bonding system and resin cement are compatible.) The post is inserted into the prepared canal and is held under hand pressure until the cement has cured. Self-etching bonding systems should not be used, because the acidity of the primers will prevent the resin cement from setting. However, self-adhesive resin cements (have a bonding resin within the cement) are popular alternatives to phosphoric acid etching and application of bonding resins.

If the post is manufactured (pre-formed) rather than a cast metal dowel with a core already attached, the buildup of missing coronal tooth structure may be done using amalgam or one of the bonded composite core materials (see Chapter 6). The operator will place the core buildup and then the tooth can be prepared for a crown once the buildup has set.

Metal and ceramic posts may be sandblasted to enhance the bond of the cement to the roughened surface of the post. Posts made of zirconia require a special primer to allow them to be bonded with resin cement. Fiber-reinforced resin posts chemically bond to the resin cement. Some clinicians suggest treating the resin post surface with silane to improve the bond with the resin cement.

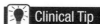 **Clinical Tip**

Resin cement remaining on the mixing pad cannot be reliably used as a guide for final set of the cement within the canal. Many of the resin cements will not set when they are in thin layers exposed to oxygen in the air. The cement in the canal is not exposed to air and will set readily, but the cement on the mixing pad may not.

SUMMARY

Bonding has a wide variety of uses in the modern dental practice. Present day bonding systems are similar in their basic bond to the tooth. They bond to enamel by micromechanical retention into the etched enamel surface, and they bond to etched dentin by formation of a resin-rich hybrid layer. This resin-rich layer allows other resins to bond to it by chemical resin-to-resin bonding. Thus composite resins can be retained by bonding to the hybrid layer and to the etched enamel that has been primed with resin. Non-resin materials such as ceramic and metal restorations can be bonded to the hybrid layer and to resin-primed enamel by resin adhesives (cements) after their surfaces have been appropriately prepared. The setting reactions of bonding resins can be self-activated by mixing components together, light-activated by stimulating photo-initiators with high-intensity blue light, or dual-cured (a combination of the two processes).

Bonding systems can be placed into three general categories: etch-and-rinse, self-etch and universal. Etch-and-rinse systems generally provide stronger bonds to enamel and dentin but are prone to postoperative sensitivity due to the technique requirements of the etching, rinsing and drying process. Self-etch systems initially had weaker bonds to uncut enamel and required selective etching, but some newer systems have solved that issue by using primers that are more acidic. The acidic primers seal the dentin as they demineralize the surface and no rinsing is required. As a result, the self-etching systems have less postoperative sensitivity. Universal systems can be used with etch-and-rinse, self-etch and selective etch techniques, and they can bond to most restorative materials. To get good results with any bonding system careful attention to the manufacturer's recommendations is required.

INSTRUCTIONAL VIDEOS

See the Evolve Resources site for a variety of educational videos that reinforce the material covered in this chapter.

Procedure 5.1 Enamel and Dentin Bonding Using the Etch-and Rinse Technique

See Evolve site for Competency Sheet.

Consider the following with this procedure: *safety glasses are recommended for the patient, PPE is required for the operator, ensure appropriate safety protocols are followed, and check your local state guidelines before performing this procedure.*

EQUIPMENT/SUPPLIES (FIG. 5.21)

- Rubber dam setup or cotton rolls and bibulous pads
- Dappen dishes or wells for bonding agents
- Disposable brushes for applying bonding agents and 37% phosphoric acid (if not in a dispenser)
- Bonding agent, curing light
- Restorative material—composite

PROCEDURE STEPS

1. Isolate the field.

   NOTE: Rubber dam is preferred because it can provide the best isolation for the longest time. Cotton rolls and bibulous pads can also be used. Moisture interferes with the formation of a good bond.

2. Etch cavity preparation with phosphoric acid: 10 seconds for dentin and 20 to 30 seconds for enamel (Fig. 5.22).

   NOTE: Start applying the etchant to the enamel first, and then to the dentin. Overetching dentin will open the tubules too much and remove too much mineral (hydroxyapatite) from the dentin surface.

3. Rinse with water for at least 10 seconds.

4. Blot or gently air-dry enamel and dentin for 2-3 seconds (removing any puddles).

   NOTE: Do not over-dry the dentin because the collagen matrix will collapse and prevent adequate penetration of the bonding resin into the tubules and etched dentin. Dentin should be glistening (moist) with no puddles. If only enamel is etched, it should be dried thoroughly and should appear frosty.

5. Saturate the etched surface with the bonding resin (Fig. 5.23).

   NOTE: Some bonding resins are administered as a one-bottle/one-step application and others require two bottles/two steps—with each component applied

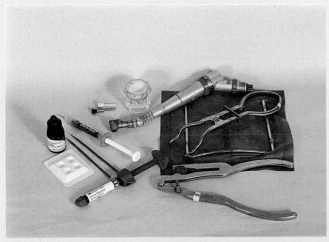

FIG. 5.21

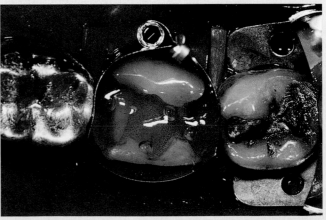

FIG. 5.22 (Courtesy of Alton Lacy, University of California School of Dentistry [San Francisco, CA].)

Procedure 5.1   Enamel and Dentin Bonding Using the Etch-and-Rinse Technique—cont'd

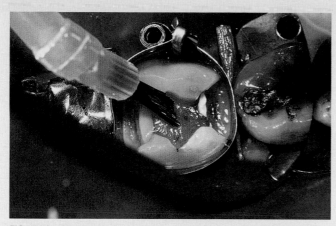

FIG. 5.23   (Courtesy of Alton Lacy, University of California School of Dentistry [San Francisco, CA].)

separately. If the bonding resin contains acetone as its solvent, it is particularly volatile. Do not dispense it until you are ready to apply it to the etched tooth or most of the solvent may have evaporated. Also, be sure to recap the bottle immediately to keep from changing the consistency of the bonding resin and its ability to penetrate moist etched dentin. Use of unit-dose ampules eliminates this problem.

6. Apply a gentle air stream to thin the resin and to remove volatile solvents and water.
   NOTE: The bonding resin is not as strong as the composite, so it should not be allowed to puddle in the preparation and cause weakness in the restoration. The solvent that the bonding resin was dissolved in must be removed by applying a stream of air, otherwise the resin may not set completely. Likewise, air is used to evaporate any remaining water from the moist dentin.
7. Light-cure for 10 to 20 seconds. The cavity preparation is now ready for placement of a restoration.
   NOTE: The tip of the light wand is usually held about 1 mm from the surface. The curing time may vary with newer, high-intensity curing lights. If the light tip cannot be placed close to the restoration surface, then a longer curing time may be needed. Follow the manufacturer's recommendations. The enamel and dentin surfaces have been physically bonded with resin bonding agent and will bond to resin restorative materials, such as composite, placed on top of them by resin-to-resin chemical bonding.

Procedure 5.2   Surface Treatment for Bonding Ceramic Restorations (Glass-Based) or for Ceramic Repair

See Evolve site for Competency Sheet.

Consider the following with this procedure: safety glasses are recommended for the patient, PPE is required for the operator, ensure appropriate safety protocols are followed, and check your local state guidelines before performing this procedure.

EQUIPMENT/SUPPLIES (FIG. 5.24)
- High- and low-speed handpieces with prophy attachment
- Dappen dish with flour of pumice and rubber prophy cup
- Isopropyl alcohol or acetone, hydrofluoric acid, silane, enamel and dentin bonding resin
- 37% phosphoric acid, resin luting cement, curing light

PROCEDURE STEPS
1. Isolate area to be bonded and clean tooth with slurry of flour of pumice. Try in ceramic restoration for fit.
   NOTE: Isolation is necessary to prevent moisture contamination of the surfaces during bonding. Pumice removes any plaque or pellicle that might interfere with etching and bonding.
2. Clean the internal surface of the ceramic with alcohol or acetone to remove salivary contaminants from the try-in.

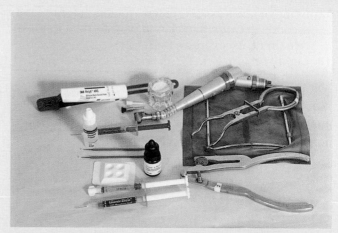

FIG. 5.24

NOTE: For ceramic repair, roughen the surface with a coarse diamond bur or sandblasting at low pressure to enhance micromechanical retention. Follow steps 3 through 5.

3. Apply hydrofluoric acid to the cavity side of the ceramic for 1 minute to etch it.
4. Rinse with water for 10 seconds and dry with air (Fig. 5.25).

Continued

Procedure 5.2   Surface Treatment for Bonding Ceramic Restorations (Glass-Based) or for Ceramic Repair—cont'd

5. Apply silane to etched ceramic for 60 seconds, and then dry with air to remove alcohol solvents.

   NOTE: Silane allows bonding of resins to the treated ceramic surface. Some ceramics may require special primers for bonding. Check the manufacturer's recommendation.

6. Apply bonding resin to ceramic, but do not light-cure it.

   NOTE: The thickness of the bonding resin may prevent proper seating of the restoration if cured at this stage. For ceramic repair, the bonding agent should be light-cured for 20 seconds.

7. Steps 7 to 10 are the same as in Procedure 5.1 for enamel and dentin preparation for bonding. Etch the tooth surfaces to be bonded with 37% phosphoric acid: 20 to 30 seconds for enamel and 10 seconds for dentin.

8. Rinse with water for 10 seconds.

   NOTE: If the surface is enamel only, dry thoroughly. If dentin is to be bonded, leave both enamel and dentin slightly moist. Trying to dry the enamel may overdry the dentin.

9. Apply enamel-dentin bonding resin (Fig. 5.26). Blow the bonding resin thin with air.

   NOTE: Do not allow it to pool in the preparation or it will interfere with seating of the restoration.

10. Light-cure for 20 seconds.

11. Apply resin cement to the restoration and seat it (Fig. 5.27).

12. Remove gross excess cement, then light-cure for 3 seconds to cause the resin to partially set. Remove remaining excess resin (Fig. 5.28).

13. Light-cure for 40 to 60 seconds or longer if needed for final set.

   NOTE: Self-cured or dual-cured resins are used for cementation of inlays, onlays, or crowns because the thickness of the restoration prevents adequate penetration of the light. With thin veneers, a light-cured resin can be used. For ceramic repair, apply composite resin and build up to full contour in increments. Light-cure each increment for 40 seconds. Some high speed curing lights with high light intensity might alter these recommended curing times. Check manufacturer's recommendations.

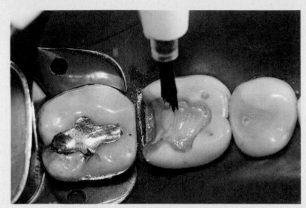

FIG. 5.26 (Courtesy of Alton Lacy, University of California School of Dentistry [San Francisco, CA].)

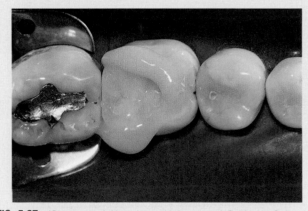

FIG. 5.27 (Courtesy of Alton Lacy, University of California School of Dentistry [San Francisco, CA].)

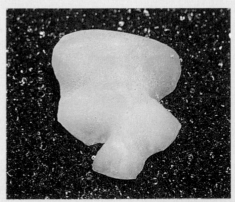

FIG. 5.25 (Courtesy of Alton Lacy, University of California School of Dentistry [San Francisco, CA].)

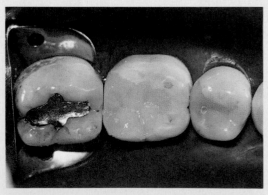

FIG. 5.28 (Courtesy of Alton Lacy, University of California School of Dentistry [San Francisco, CA].)

Procedure 5.3 Bonding Orthodontic Brackets

See Evolve site for Competency Sheet.

Consider the following with this procedure: safety glasses are recommended for the patient, PPE is required for the operator, ensure appropriate safety protocols are followed, and check your local state guidelines before performing this procedure.

EQUIPMENT/SUPPLIES (Fig. 5.29)

- Basic setup
- Low-speed handpiece, prophy angle, rubber cup, and slurry of pumice
- Etchant (37% phosphoric acid), light-cured bonding resin
- Curing light, lip retractors
- High-volume evacuator (HVE) tip, cotton rolls
- Orthodontic brackets, bracket placement pliers, scaler

PROCEDURE STEPS

1. Inform the patient of the procedures to be done. Clean the facial surfaces of the teeth to be bonded with pumice slurry in a rubber cup.

   NOTE: Pumice removes adherent plaque and organic pellicle that might interfere with proper etching and bonding.

2. Place lip retractors or cotton rolls to isolate the anterior teeth for bracket placement.

   NOTE: Moisture from the lip mucosa will interfere with bonding.

3. Apply etching solution or gel for 30 seconds to that portion of the enamel that will receive the bracket.

4. Rinse the etchant off with water and thoroughly dry the enamel (Fig. 5.30).

   NOTE: Properly etched enamel should appear frosty or chalky white. Because no dentin is involved, the enamel is dried thoroughly.

5. Apply a thin coating of liquid bonding resin to the etched enamel and light-cure for 20 seconds (Fig. 5.31).

NOTE: This bonding resin acts to prepare or prime the enamel to allow adhesion of the resin adhesive paste that holds the bracket in place. The bonding resin and the adhesive resin chemically bond to each other.

6. Apply light-cured adhesive resin to the metal mesh on the back of the bracket (Fig. 5.32), and place the bracket in the location prescribed by the dentist, using bracket placement pliers. An orthodontic scaler can be used to adjust the position of the bracket and remove excess resin.

NOTE: The resin adhesive does not chemically bond to the bracket, but it will physically lock into the

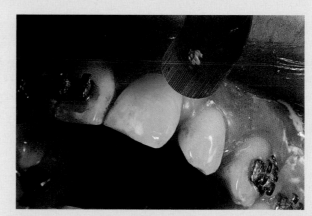

FIG. 5.30

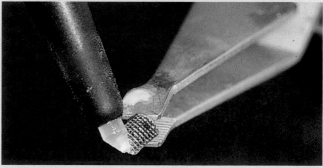

FIG. 5.31

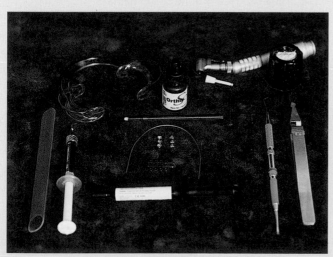

FIG. 5.29

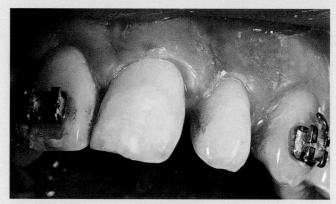

FIG. 5.32

Continued

Procedure 5.3 Bonding Orthodontic Brackets—cont'd

mesh on the back of the bracket. Some brackets are manufactured with the adhesive applied at the factory and are covered with a plastic cover that is stripped away at the time of placement.

7. Light-cure the adhesive resin for 40 to 60 seconds, directing the light from mesial, distal, incisal, cervical and lingual toward the bracket.

NOTE: Although the metal of the bracket blocks penetration of the light directly, the translucency of the enamel allows light to transmit through it to cure the resin underlying the bracket. High intensity curing lights may alter the curing times.

8. Repeat the procedure to complete the placement of all of the brackets (Fig. 5.33).

NOTE: Typically, the six anterior teeth are all etched and primed at the same time. Brackets may be bonded individually or placed together and light-cured individually.

9. The arch wire and elastic or wire ligatures can be placed after all brackets are bonded (Fig. 5.34).

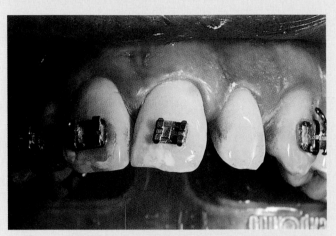

FIG. 5.33

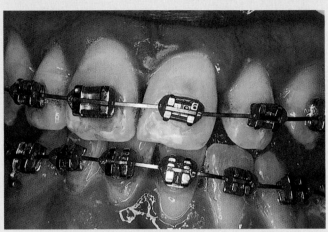

FIG. 5.34

Get Ready for Exams!

Review Questions

Select the one correct response for each of the following multiple-choice questions.

1. The acid used most commonly to etch tooth structure for bonding procedures is
   a. Citric
   b. Hydrochloric
   c. Hydrofluoric
   d. Phosphoric

2. Which one of the following statements about bonding to **enamel** is true?
   a. Bonding is achieved by micromechanical retention.
   b. Bonding is achieved by chemical bonds.
   c. Bonding is achieved by resin tags penetrating the collagen matrix.
   d. Bonding to enamel is less reliable than bonding to dentin.

3. Bonding to **dentin** by the etch-and-rinse technique
   a. Is best on dentin that has been etched with 37% phosphoric acid for 30 seconds
   b. Is stronger when the dentin is well dried after etching
   c. Is inhibited by formation of the hybrid layer
   d. Is best accomplished when the dentin is kept moist after etching

4. One of the following statements about etch-and-rinse bonding resins is true. Which one?
   a. Water is the most common solvent used with these bonding resins.
   b. They form the best hybrid layer with dry dentin.
   c. They chemically bond to the composite resin.
   d. They chemically bond to the dentin.

5. Self-etching bonding systems
   a. Use 37% phosphoric acid as the etchant
   b. Use acidic primers to etch the tooth structure
   c. Require rinsing after etching
   d. Generally etch enamel equally as well as dentin

6. Etch-and-rinse bonding systems
   a. May result in tooth sensitivity caused by overdrying or overetching
   b. Do not require a separate etching and rinsing step
   c. Do not require drying of the primer
   d. Do not provide a good etch of uncut enamel

7. With the etch-and-rinse system when bonding to dentin, one of the following statements is true. Which one?
   a. The dentin surface should be thoroughly dried after etching and rinsing.
   b. The surface of the etched, rinsed, and lightly dried dentin should be "glistening."

Get Ready for Exams!—cont'd

   c. The surface of prepared dentin should have visible water droplets.

   d. Once you have dried the etched surface, it cannot be rewetted.

8. Dentin sensitivity can be caused by

   a. Pressure changes in the column of fluid within the dentinal tubules

   b. Stimulation of odontoblastic processes within the dentinal tubules

   c. Open (unsealed) dentinal tubules

   d. Overetching or overdrying of the dentin

   e. All of the above

9. The smear layer

   a. Is a tenacious layer of cut tooth debris on the surface of enamel and dentin

   b. Is easily removed by rinsing with water

   c. Is necessary for good bonding

   d. Is not removed when bonding by the etch-and-rinse technique

10. All of the following statements about bonding to repair fractured porcelain on a crown are true *except* one. Which one is this *exception*?

   a. The surface is cleaned and roughened.

   b. 10% phosphoric acid is used to etch the porcelain.

   c. Silane is applied after etching to enhance the bond of adhesive resins to the porcelain.

   d. Composite resin is usually used to restore the fractured portion.

11. Which one of the following does *not* interfere with the formation of a good bond?

   a. Saliva on the etched enamel or dentin

   b. Oil lubricant from the handpiece

   c. Moist dentin after rinsing etchant off and lightly drying

   d. Flavoring agents in prophy paste

12. Which type of bonding system has been shown to consistently provide the greatest bond strengths to enamel and dentin?

   a. Three-step, two-bottle etch-and-rinse (fourth generation)

   b. Two-step, one-bottle etch-and-rinse (fifth generation)

   c. Two-step, two-bottle self-etch (sixth generation)

   d. One-step, one-bottle self-etch (seventh generation)

13. When endodontic posts are bonded into root canals, the bonding resin should not be

   a. Self-curing

   b. Light-curing

   c. Dual-curing

   d. Applied in a thin layer

14. All of the following are correct steps for bonding orthodontic brackets *except* one. Which one is this *exception*?

   a. The tooth surface is cleaned with pumice.

   b. The enamel is etched with 37% phosphoric acid for approximately 30 seconds.

   c. The enamel is rinsed and left slightly moist.

   d. A resin adhesive may be used to bond the bracket.

15. When bonding composite resin to metal that is exposed after the overlying porcelain has fractured, which one of the following is *false*?

   a. Retention to the metal is enhanced by roughening the surface with a coarse diamond bur, by sandblasting, by electrochemically etching, or by tin-plating.

   b. Bonding agents are not needed because the composite resin sticks to the metal.

   c. An opaque resin is applied before the composite resin to mask the metal and prevents a gray color from showing through the slightly translucent composite resin.

   d. Light-curing materials can be used.

For answers to Review Questions, see the Appendix.

Case-Based Discussion Topics

1. A 24-year-old graduate student needs two occlusal sealants on his lower first molars and a composite resin restoration to repair toothbrush abrasion on the facial root surface of his maxillary left canine.

Discuss the similarities and differences in bonding to enamel for the sealants and to dentin for the composite resin.

2. A 50-year-old female attorney is in need of a ceramic onlay on her mandibular left first premolar.

Discuss the differences in the mechanisms and procedural steps used to bond to enamel and dentin as opposed to bonding to a glass-based ceramic (lithium disilicate) onlay.

3. A 42-year-old male factory worker comes to the dental office with a chief complaint of tooth sensitivity after recent placement of a class II posterior composite resin restoration on the lower right second molar. He complains that the tooth hurts when he bites on it and when cold drinks or cold air hits the tooth.

Discuss the likely causes of the sensitivity and the measures that can be taken to prevent postoperative tooth sensitivity after bonding procedures.

4. A 65-year-old retired schoolteacher needs restoration of both mandibular first molars, which have root caries on the facial root surfaces. The caries extends beneath the crest of the gingiva so that isolation with a rubber dam is not possible. The patient wants tooth-colored restorations.

Discuss the requirements for ensuring a good bond.

5. A 35-year-old female stockbroker comes to the dental office with a chief complaint of having chipped the mesial corner off her right maxillary central incisor porcelain-fused-to-metal crown by accidentally biting on a fork. Examination reveals a 2 mm × 1 mm loss of porcelain without exposure of underlying metal.

Discuss the materials and procedures in their proper sequence of use to repair the crown in the office.

6. A 23-year-old college student comes to the dental office complaining of sensitivity to cold foods and air on her lower right first molar. The pain is limited to the cervical part of the tooth at the gingival crest, which has receded 3 mm. The problem appears to be caused by toothbrush abrasion of the root from brushing too hard. The patient is a needle phobic and does not want an injection of local anesthetic. The dentist wants to apply a bonding resin to the area.

Why is the area of abrasion sensitive? Discuss which bonding materials to select. Which technique (etch-and-rinse or self-etch) will likely cause the patient the least amount of pain? How do these materials work for root sensitivity?

BIBLIOGRAPHY

Alex G: Universal Adhesives: the next evolution in adhesive dentistry? *Compendium of Continuing Education in Dentistry*, 2015.

Anusavice KJ, Shen C, Rawls HR: Bonding and bonding agents. In *Phillips' Science of Dental Materials* (ed 12). Philadelphia, 2013, Saunders.

Bird DL, Robinson DS: Dental liners, bases and bonding systems. In *Modern Dental Assisting* (ed 12). St. Louis, 2018, Elsevier.

Farah JW, Powers JM: Bonding agents—2008. *The Dental Advisor*, 25(1–9), 2008.

Ferracane JL: Direct esthetic anterior restoratives. In *Materials in Dentistry*. Philadelphia, 2001, Lippincott Williams & Wilkins.

Heymann HO, Swift EJ, Ritter AV: Fundamental concepts of enamel and dentin adhesion. In *Sturdevants's Art and Science of Operative Dentistry* (ed 6). St. Louis, 2013, Mosby.

Lane JA, Hughey SJ, Gregory PN, et al.: Is your dental adhesive forgiving? How to address challenges. *Compend Contin Educ Den*, 37(10), 2016.

Nakabayashi N, Nakajima K, Masuhara E: The promotion of adhesion by resin infiltration of monomers into tooth structure. *J Biomed Mater Res*, 16:265, 1982.

Nazarian A: The progression of dental adhesives [online continuing education]. *Dental CE Digest*. 2007, PennWell Publications.

Ozer F, Blatz MB: Clinical applications of self-etching and etch-and-rinse adhesive systems. *Inside Dentistry*, 2013.

Phillips RW, Moore BK: Adhesion and elasticity. In *Elements of Dental Materials for Dental Hygienists and Dental Assistants*. Philadelphia, 1994, Saunders.

Poticny DJ: Adhesive systems continue to evolve: a case report. *Dentistry Today*, 2013. Available at http://www.dentistrytoday.com/dental-materials/9217-adhesive-systems-continue-to-evolve-a-case-report.

Powers JM, Wataha JC: Bonding agents. In *Dental Materials: Foundations and Applications* (ed 11). St. Louis, 2013, Elsevier.

Retief DH: Effect of conditioning the enamel surface with phosphoric acid. *J Dent Res.*, 52:333, 1973.

Sakaguchi RL, Powers JM: Materials for adhesion and luting. In *Craig's Restorative Dental Materials* (ed 13). Philadelphia, 2012, Mosby.

Silverstone LM: The acid-etch technique: In vitro studies with special reference to the enamel surface and the enamel-resin interface. In *Proceedings from the International Symposium on Acid Etch Technique*. St. Paul, MN, 1975, North Central Publishing.

Strassler HE: Contemporary resin adhesives. *Inside Dentistry*, October 2014.

Composites, Glass Ionomers, and Compomers

Chapter Objectives

Upon completion of this chapter, the student should be able to:

1. Describe the various types of composite resin restorative materials.
2. Discuss the advantages and disadvantages of each type of composite resin.
3. Discuss the similarities and differences among chemical-cured, light-cured and dual-cured composite resins.
4. Describe how fillers affect the properties of composites.
5. Explain why incremental placement of composite resin is recommended.
6. Describe the factors that determine how long an increment of composite resin should be light-cured.
7. Place a sectional matrix for a class II composite.
8. Select an appropriate type of composite for a class II cavity preparation.
9. As permitted by state law, place a composite in a class II cavity preparation.
10. Light-cure a composite resin restoration following recommended exposure times and use proper precautions for eye/retina protection.
11. As permitted by state law, finish and polish a class III composite restoration.
12. Discuss the procedural differences between direct and indirect composite restorations.
13. Describe the composition of glass ionomer restoratives and their uses, advantages and disadvantages.
14. Explain the effects of fluoride-releasing, resin-modified glass ionomer restorations in the prevention of recurrent caries.
15. List the components of compomers.
16. Describe the uses of compomers.
17. Compare the clinical applications of composite resin restorative materials with glass ionomer cement restorative materials

Key Terms

Direct-Placement Esthetic Materials tooth-colored materials that can be placed directly into the cavity preparation without being constructed outside of the mouth first

Composite Resins direct-placement, tooth-colored materials composed of an organic resin matrix, inorganic filler particles, a coupling agent, and coloring pigments

Organic Resin Matrix thick liquids made up of two or more types of organic molecules (polymers) that form a matrix around filler particles

Inorganic Filler Particles fine particles of quartz, silica, or glass that give strength and wear resistance to a material

Silane Coupling Agent a chemical that helps to bind the filler particles to the organic matrix

Pigments coloring agents that give composites their color

Monomers high molecular weight molecules that act as building blocks to link by covalent bonds to form larger, complex molecules known as polymers

Polymerization the joining of monomers end-to-end to form chains or networks of polymers often causing a material to harden

Self-Cured Composites composites that polymerize by a chemical reaction when two filled resin pastes are mixed together

Light-Cured Composites single-paste composites that polymerize when a photosensitive chemical is activated by light in the blue wave range

Depth of Cure the depth to which light from a curing unit can penetrate and cure composite resin

Dual-Cured Composites composites that contain components of light-activated and chemically activated materials. When the two parts are mixed together, it polymerizes by a chemical reaction that can be accelerated by blue light activation

Incremental Placement a technique for composites that places and cures small increments individually to reduce the overall polymerization shrinkage and shrinkage stress in the restoration and permit curing throughout the increment

Elastic Modulus a measure of the stiffness of a material; the higher the elastic modulus the stiffer the material

Macrofilled Composites an early generation of composites that contained large filler particles ranging from 10 to 100 microns (μm)

Microfilled Composites composites that contain very small filler particles averaging 0.04 μm in diameter

Hybrid Composites composites that contain both fine fill (2 to 4 μm) and microfill (0.04 to 0.2 μm) particles to obtain the strength of a macrofill and the polishability of a microfill

Microhybrids hybrid composites that contain fillers that are smaller fine-particle (0.04 to 1 μm) and microsized fillers

Nanohybrids microhybrids to which nanosized fillers have been added

Universal Composites composites that have physical and mechanical properties such as strength and polishability that allow them to be used in both the anterior and posterior parts of the mouth

Nanocomposites composites that contain all nanosized fillers to enhance physical properties

Flowable Composites light-cured, low-viscosity composite resins

Bulk-Fill Composites composites with greater depth of cure that permit placement in large increments up to 4 mm thick instead of the standard 2 mm; their use speeds up the filling process

Indirect-Placement Esthetic Materials tooth-colored materials that are used to construct restorations outside of the mouth in the dental laboratory or at chairside on replicas of the prepared teeth. They are later cemented to the teeth

Glass Ionomer Cements (GICs) self-cured, tooth-colored, fluoride-releasing restorative materials that bond to tooth structure without an additional bonding agent

Resin-Modified (or Hybrid) Glass Ionomer a glass ionomer to which resin has been added to improve its physical properties

Nano-Ionomers glass ionomers that contain nanosized filler particles to enhance their physical properties

Compomer composite resin that has polyacid, fluoride-releasing groups added

Bioactive Dental Materials materials that interact with living tissue and are used to remineralize and repair dentin.

Composites have for some time overtaken amalgams as the most frequently placed direct restorations. The use of composites has grown exponentially over the past three decades. In 1999 approximately 86 million composites were placed in the USA. By 2006 approximately 146 million composites were placed in the USA (ADA Survey of Dental Services). Manufacturers have continually improved composites by making them easier to handle, more durable, esthetic, and color stable. Other esthetic materials such as glass ionomer cements and compomers have also been developed and improved upon, providing the dental team with a wide selection of esthetic materials and colors for the restoration of carious or damaged teeth and for cosmetic enhancement. With the capability of bonding restorative materials to tooth structure, advances in esthetic materials and techniques have improved the ability of the dental team to deliver the esthetic results that patients demand. The dental team must keep current with the rapid changes that occur with materials and techniques. Good listening skills are needed to determine the types of esthetic services the patient is requesting so that the dental team and the patient are working in concert toward the same goal. Esthetic materials must be carefully selected so that their properties are compatible with the patient's oral condition and occlusion. Dental hygienists and dental assistants must understand the properties of these materials, so that as important members of the dental team they can help the dentist to assess the performance of the restorations and can alert the dentist when they perceive that a restoration may be failing. They need to be familiar with the physical properties of the materials so that they do not damage the restorations during routine oral hygiene, coronal polishing, and preventive procedures. They need to know the handling characteristics of the esthetic materials so that they can assist the dentist in their placement or can perform steps in their placement, finish and polish as permitted by state dental practice acts.

This chapter describes the physical and mechanical properties, clinical applications, advantages, and shortcomings of directly placed esthetic materials. These materials include composite resins, glass ionomer cements, resin-modified glass ionomer cements, and compomers. Indirectly placed composite resin restorations are discussed as well. Guidelines for selection of the shade of these materials to obtain satisfactory cosmetic results also are discussed.

HISTORY OF THE DEVELOPMENT OF COMPOSITE RESIN FOR DENTISTRY

For the first half of the twentieth century, amalgam and gold were the primary restorative materials for posterior teeth. Some anterior teeth also had metal restorations that were visible when the patient smiled in the form of gold margins of three-quarter crowns, class III and V gold foils and inlays, or amalgams. Silicate cement, introduced in 1873, was the first tooth-colored restorative material but was not widely used until the early 1900s. Although it was somewhat esthetic, it was relatively soluble in the mouth and washed out over time. In the latter half of the twentieth century, various direct-placement tooth-colored restorative materials were introduced. Initially, chemical-cured, unfilled acrylic resins were used, but they leaked, wore down quickly, and became discolored.

In 1955, Michael Buonocore introduced the acid etch technique for bonding the acrylic to enamel. In 1962 Rafael L. Bowen developed bis-GMA resin monomer that is still used in many composites today. Silica particles were added to bis-GMA to reinforce it and make it more wear resistant, and this became the basis of the composite resin used in dentistry. In 1963, chemical-cured composite resin (Addent, 3M Dental Products) was introduced. The early composite resins were available in a very limited number of shades, were rough and worn out quickly, discolored, and shrank excessively when they cured. Resin bonding agents had not been developed yet, so the restorations leaked and postoperative sensitivity and recurrent caries were common occurrences. In an effort to have more control over the working time, composites cured by ultraviolet light were developed. Later, composites cured by visible light were introduced. Most of the improvements that have occurred in composites to the present have been related to reducing shrinkage, using smaller fillers to enhance polishing and wear resistance, improving the selection of colors, increasing durability, improving handling properties, and delivery methods.

DIRECT-PLACEMENT ESTHETIC RESTORATIVE MATERIALS

Esthetic materials are those that are tooth colored. Direct-placement esthetic materials are those that can be placed directly into the cavity preparation or onto the tooth surface by the clinician without first being constructed outside of the mouth. The direct-placement esthetic materials used most commonly are as follows:

- Composite resin
- Glass ionomer cement
- Resin-modified glass ionomer cement (also called *hybrid ionomer*)
- Compomer

COMPOSITE RESIN

A composite is a mixture of two or more materials with properties superior to any single component. **Composite resins** are tooth-colored restorative materials that are used in both the anterior and posterior parts of the mouth. They are composed mainly of an **organic resin matrix** and **inorganic filler particles** joined together by a **silane coupling agent** that sticks (adheres) the particles to the matrix. Also added are initiators and accelerators that cause the material to set and **pigments** that give color to the material and match tooth colors. Composite resins are commonly called *composites* and also can be referred to in the dental literature as *resin composites*.

COMPONENTS

Resin Matrix

The most commonly used resin for the matrix of composites is bis-GMA (bisphenol-A-glycidyl dimethacrylate), produced by reacting glycidyl methacrylate with bisphenol-A. Another resin that is used for the composite matrix is urethane dimethacrylate (UDMA). These resins are thick liquids made up of two or more types of organic molecules called *oligomers*. To reduce viscosity and allow loading with filler particles, a low molecular weight monomer, such as TEGDMA (triethylene glycol dimethacrylate), is added.

Monomers are organic molecules (that make up the oligomers) with double carbon bonds that link together by an addition reaction to form a polymer. When the **polymerization** reaction goes to completion, the result is a cured composite resin.

Filler Particles

The addition of filler particles to the organic resin has several functions. Fillers make the composite stronger and more wear resistant. By reducing the amount of resin, fillers help to reduce the amount of shrinkage that occurs when the resin matrix polymerizes, or sets. Fillers can also be used to control the translucency of the composite by their effect on the scattering of light. The amount of filler and the size and shape of the filler will affect the viscosity of the composite and how it handles. Reducing the amount of resin by adding filler reduces thermal expansion and contraction and decreases water sorption (uptake) that softens the resin and makes it more likely to wear.

The fillers used in many composite resins are composed of glass, quartz, silica, or ceramic. Fillers may be modified with ions to improve their characteristics. To make the composite resin restoration show up (appear radiopaque) on radiographs, heavy metal ions may be added to the filler particles. Nanosized filler particles are synthesized from zirconia (a ceramic material) and silica. Glass fillers are the least inert of the fillers. They are leached slowly from the composite by dietary acids and by application of acidulated phosphate fluoride in the dental office.

Important factors for the durability of the composite resin are the size of the filler particles and the ratio or weight of the filler to the matrix. As a general rule, the higher the filler content, the stronger and more wear resistant the restoration will be and the less it will shrink when polymerized. The amount of filler in a composite resin usually is reported by the manufacturer as the percent of filler by weight (weight %) in the resin.

Composites can be classified by the size of the filler particles they contain (Fig. 6.1). Wear of the composite is related to the filler particle size, the amount of filler

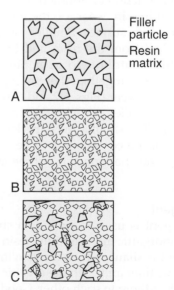

FIG. 6.1 Variety of filler sizes that are combined in the composite resins and contribute to their classification names. **A,** Macrofilled; **B,** microfilled; **C,** hybrid—a combination of micro fillers (about 0.4 μm) and small fillers (about 1-4 μm).

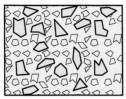
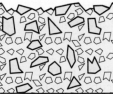

Smooth surface at time of placement and surface polish | Irregular surface due to erosion and loss of filler particles

FIG. 6.2 Wear of composite surface. At left, smooth surface at the time of placement and surface polish. At right, rough surface caused by wear and loss of filler particles at the surface.

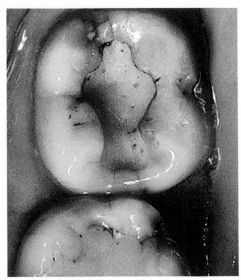

FIG. 6.3 Worn composite with staining at the margins indicative of microleakage. Opposing occlusion has worn the composite down, and numerous pits have developed as bits of the composite have fractured out.

in the resin, and the amount of resin between particles. Large filler particles tend to get pulled from the resin matrix at the surface (called *plucking*) when the restoration is under function or abraded by food and tooth brushing, resulting in wear of the remaining resin matrix and a rough surface. Smaller particles are not as easily plucked from the resin and therefore cause fewer voids that contribute to wear. Smaller particles can be packed closer together, thereby exposing less of the resin matrix to wear (Figs. 6.2 and 6.3) and increasing the number of filler particles that can be added to the resin matrix. The smaller the particles, the smoother the surface of the composite will be after finishing and polishing and the longer it will be able to retain its luster.

Coupling Agent

A coupling agent is used to provide a stronger bond between the inorganic fillers and the resin matrix. This coupling agent is silane, which reacts with the surface of the inorganic filler and with the organic matrix to allow the two to adhere to each other. Good adhesion of the two is necessary to minimize loss of filler particles and to reduce wear. The silane is applied to the filler surface before the filler is added to the resin monomer.

Pigments

Inorganic pigments are added in varying amounts to develop a variety of colors that approximate the basic colors of teeth or specialized colors. Pigmented resins (also called *coloring resins*) can be used to cover discolorations or dark dentin, or to hide the graying effect of a metal post in a root canal–treated tooth. Pigments are also used to characterize a restoration when the tooth being restored or adjacent teeth have white spots as with mild fluorosis (see Chapter 7 Preventive and Desensitizing Materials) or other special characteristics. Coloring resins are usually lightly filled and come in a variety of colors including blue, white, orange/yellow, pink, light and dark brown, ochre, and clear. An example is Vit-l-escence Colors (Ultradent Products).

POLYMERIZATION

Polymerization is the chemical reaction that occurs when low molecular weight resin molecules called *monomers* join together end-to-end to form long-chain, high molecular weight molecules called *polymers*. For composite resins, activation of the polymerization process can be done chemically (chemical-cured), or by light (light-cured), or by a combination of the two (dual-cured). During polymerization, regardless of method, an activator (chemical or light) causes an initiator molecule to form free radicals (highly charged molecules that have unpaired electrons). The monomers (called *dimethacrylates*; e.g., bis-GMA) have carbon-to-carbon double bond (C=C) functional groups. The free radicals break one of the carbon-to-carbon double bonds to form a single bond and another free radical. That free radical can cause the same reaction with another monomer to add to the polymer chain (called *addition polymerization*). As the monomers link together into chains, the volume of resin decreases, so the net result is shrinkage (called *polymerization shrinkage*).

Cross-linking of polymer chains. Polymer chains have small groups of atoms (called *branches*) hanging off their sides. When side groups of adjacent polymer chains share electrons, they form covalent bonds that link (called *cross-linking*) the chains together (Fig. 6.4). Cross-linking of polymers produces a much stronger, stiffer material than is formed with single-chain polymers. (See Chapter 17 for a more detailed description of polymer formation and properties.)

Modes of Cure

Chemical cure. Chemically cured composite resins, or **self-cured composites**, are two-paste systems supplied in screw-type syringes or cartridges. One paste, called the *base*, contains composite and benzoyl peroxide as an initiator. The other paste, called the *catalyst*, contains composite and a tertiary amine as an activator. Equal parts of these two pastes are mixed together, and the polymerization reaction begins. The reaction could go to completion very quickly, but chemicals

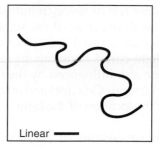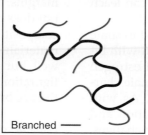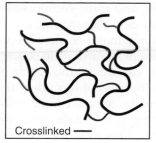

Linear ——   Branched ——   Crosslinked ——

FIG. 6.4 Diagrams of linear, branched, and cross-linked polymers. Adjacent linear polymer chains are linked by covalently bonded atoms from short side chains (branches). (From Anusavice KJ, Shen C, Rawls HR: *Phillips' Science of Dental Materials* (ed 12). St. Louis, 2013, Elsevier.)

called *inhibitors* are added to each paste to slow down the reaction. The operator has a limited amount of time (working time—usually about 2 minutes in the mouth) to place the restoration before it becomes too stiff to manipulate. Once the initial set occurs, the material should not be manipulated or the properties of the restoration will be degraded. Disposable mixing sticks are usually supplied with the composite contained in screw-type syringes. Because the two pastes must be manually mixed, air can be incorporated into the material, causing voids or porosity in the restoration.

Composites in cartridges come with mixing tips that automatically mix the two pastes as they are extruded from the cartridge (see Fig. 6.12). This "automixing" greatly reduces the introduction of air into the mixed composite and provides the correct proportions of each material. The composites most commonly found in cartridges are those used as core materials for crowns.

Light cure. **Light-cured composites** are the most common type of composite resin used in private practice. Many clinicians prefer light-cured composite resin, because it requires no mixing and the operator can control the working time by deciding when to apply the curing light. An intense visible light in the blue wave range activates these materials. Blue light with a wavelength of about 470 nanometers (nm) activates an initiator (camphorquinone) that, in the presence of an accelerator (an organic amine), causes the resin to polymerize. These components are both present in the composite but do not react until the light triggers the reaction. Inhibitors are also present to reduce the effects of the operatory light on a premature setting. However, some manufacturers' materials are still sensitive to direct operatory light. The operator may choose to turn the operatory light away from the mouth when placing the composite.

Depth of cure. The ability of the light to penetrate the composite and cure it (called the **depth of cure**) is limited in depth. Just how far the light can penetrate and cure is affected by several factors: the length and intensity of the light application, the distance the composite is located from the light, the thickness of the composite, the color of the composite, the amount and type

of filler used, and the type of material the light must pass through to reach the composite (such as enamel, dentin, ceramic). A composite restoration that is not completely cured can lead to microleakage and recurrent caries.

Dual cure. **Dual-cured composites** are two-paste systems that contain the initiators and activators of both light-activated and, to a lesser extent, chemically activated materials. The advantage is that when the two pastes are mixed together and placed in the tooth, the curing light is used to initiate the setting reaction, and the chemical setting reaction continues in areas not reached by the light to ensure a complete set. This dual-cure process is very helpful when one is building up an endodontically treated tooth and placing composite core material into the canal space. The curing light might not reach the material in the canal, but the composite material will cure chemically on its own.

PHYSICAL AND MECHANICAL PROPERTIES OF COMPOSITE RESINS

Important properties of composites include the following:
- Biocompatibility
- Strength
- Wear
- Polymerization shrinkage
- Degree of conversion
- Thermal conductivity
- Coefficient of thermal expansion
- Water sorption
- Elastic modulus
- Radiopacity

Biocompatibility

Newly placed composite resins can release chemicals that, in deep cavity preparations, could pass through the dentinal tubules into the pulp, causing an inflammatory reaction. When the tubules are sealed by dentin bonding agents or protected with a base or liner, there is no problem. Composites can release components into the oral cavity as well. Water or other solvents in the diet can dissolve out unbound monomers and other additives, and some components can leach out as the composite degrades over time.

Bisphenol A is a polymer that can be found in some composites and fissure sealants. The concern with bisphenol A is that it can mimic the effects of estrogen and cause the development of secondary female characteristics or stimulate certain cancer cells. As with most chemicals there is a certain concentration and repeated exposure needed to induce cellular changes. Research reports suggest that the level of bisphenol A released by composites is very low and does not represent a health threat to individuals. Researchers continue to investigate this issue.

Polished composites are well tolerated by surrounding soft tissues. A very few individuals may be allergic to one or more of the components of the material, and for these individuals another restorative material must be chosen. Formaldehyde may be formed as a byproduct of polymerization and may cause soft tissue reactions that resemble lichen planus which can affect mucous membranes causing white striations that may be accompanied by erythema (redness from irritation) and are called *lichenoid reactions*.

Strength

Most of the composites commonly used today are similar in compressive strength. They are not as strong in compression as amalgam but are stronger than glass ionomers. In terms of tensile and shear strength, microfill composites are weaker than hybrids and nanocomposites.

Wear

Composites wear faster than amalgams. Recent improvements have made the latest generation of composites more wear resistant than early composites, and they are beginning to approach the wear rate of amalgams under normal function. Filler content has an effect on the wear rate. Composites with a lower volume of filler (microfills and flowables) wear faster than more heavily filled materials. Wear can result from abrasion by foods or toothbrushing or by contact with opposing teeth during eating or bruxing. The wear from the opposing teeth is much more destructive. Bruxers (people who grind their teeth) will wear down composites at a much faster rate than amalgam. Therefore, it is recommended that posterior composites not be used for very large restorations that are not protected in the functional occlusal range by surrounding tooth structure.

Polymerization Shrinkage

Polymerization shrinkage refers to the shrinkage that occurs when the composite is cured (polymerized). It was once thought that light-cured composites shrank toward the curing light, and a great effort was made to correctly place the light probe in order to draw the material toward the cavity wall to minimize leakage at the margins. More recent research indicates that the material does not shrink toward the light. Chemical-cured composites cure toward the center of the bulk of the material; light-cured materials have this tendency as well, but are also influenced by the cavity shape (configuration factor or C-factor) and size with minimal influence by the location of the light.

Clinical consequences of polymerization shrinkage. As composite polymerizes and shrinks it tends to pull toward the walls of the cavity preparation that are bonded. When an increment of composite is placed in contact with two opposing walls (like a class I or II preparation with buccal and lingual enamel walls) and cured, the shrinking composite will stress the bonds to the two walls and may end up pulling away from one of the walls. This will cause a gap at the margins that allows microleakage (leakage on a microscopic level) of fluid and bacteria at the margins with possible tooth sensitivity or future staining at the margins and recurrent caries. Shrinking composite that is well bonded to buccal and lingual cavity walls can also put tension on the cusps of the tooth, pulling them slightly toward each other. This causes discomfort when the patient bites down. The bond to enamel is a strong one. When the composite shrinks near the cavosurface margins in enamel, occasionally some of the enamel rods pull away from the tooth. The result of this microscopic cracking of the enamel can be seen as a white line around the margin.

Reducing the effects of polymerization shrinkage. The greater the resin content of the composite, the greater the shrinkage will be. One way to reduce polymerization shrinkage is to place more filler in the composite so there will be less resin. Microfill composites and flowables have more resin monomer and therefore shrink more than hybrids and nanocomposites. Hybrids have a combination of larger filler particles and smaller ones. The smaller particles fill in the spaces between the larger particles. There is a limit as too how much filler can be placed into the resin matrix. Too much filler will make the composite too stiff to manipulate, and some of the physical and mechanical properties may be diminished.

Another way to reduce polymerization shrinkage is to use pre-polymerized filler. To make these fillers, high concentrations of microfillers and nanofillers are forced into a resin matrix under pressure and heat, and then cured. The highly filled clumps of resin are then ground into large filler particles (about 30 to 60 μm). These large particles already have undergone polymerization shrinkage. They are loaded into a resin matrix along with other micro- or nanofillers to make a micro- or nanohybrid composite. This composite when polymerized will shrink less because a portion of its volume has already been polymerized by way of the pre-polymerized particles.

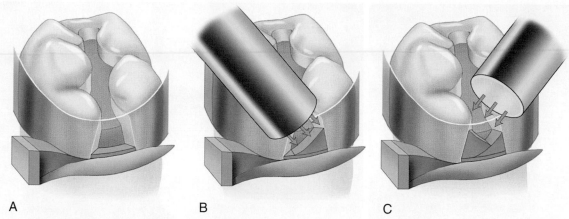

FIG. 6.5 Incremental placement of composite to minimize polymerization shrinkage and ensure complete cure of composite. **A,** First increment has been placed horizontally *(gray area)* in a thin layer on the gingival floor and light-cured. **B,** Second increment has been placed diagonally and light-cured. **C,** Third increment has been placed diagonally on the opposite wall and light-cured. (From Anusavice KJ, Shen C, Rawls HR: *Phillips' Science of Dental Materials* (ed 12). St. Louis, 2013, Elsevier.)

The effects of polymerization shrinkage can be minimized by placing the restoration in small incremental layers, avoiding joining opposing walls with one increment, and curing each layer separately. For most moderately sized or large cavity preparations, the composite resin should be placed in increments about 2 mm thick; this is referred to as **incremental placement**. The benefits of this are twofold. First, it minimizes polymerization shrinkage, because the shrinkage of the first increment is made up for by the application of the next increment and continues with each successive increment. Second, it permits light from the curing unit to adequately penetrate and thoroughly cure each increment (Fig. 6.5).

Another way to manage shrinkage in the cavity is to do an indirect composite restoration (one that is prepared and cured outside of the mouth). The shrinkage occurs in the restoration before it is placed in the tooth; then the restoration is cemented in place with a thin layer of a low-viscosity resin cement such as that used to cement veneers. This thin layer of cement will have minimal shrinkage.

Last, polymerization shrinkage can be reduced by using low-shrinking monomers. Several products are undergoing testing and one resin, silorane, is commercially available in Filtek LS (3M ESPE). Its polymerization shrinkage is less than 1%. However, it takes twice as long to polymerize and requires its own bonding agent. It is not compatible with most methacrylate-based bonding agents. Another low shrinkage composite using a dimer-based material is N'Durance (Septodont). Its polymerization shrinkage is less than 2% and it is compatible with most bonding agents.

Degree of Conversion

The degree of conversion of a resin indicates the percentage of carbon-to-carbon double bonds that have undergone conversion to single bonds during formation of the resin polymer. The composite resin transitions from a paste to a solid mass. As the composite polymerizes most of the resin monomer is converted into polymer, but some remains unconverted. With a higher rate of conversion the physical and mechanical properties of the resin improve: the resin will be stronger, resist wear better, and be more color stable.

Thermal Conductivity

Composite resin will transmit hot and cold temperatures much like the natural tooth structure. So, its thermal conductivity is compatible with the teeth and much lower than that of metal, such as amalgam or gold. It is therefore a biologically protective material for the dental pulp.

Coefficient of Thermal Expansion

Ideally the coefficient of thermal expansion (CTE) of the filling material would be the same as that of the tooth structure. In the case of composite, the CTE is greater, and therefore it will undergo a greater change in dimension than will the adjacent tooth structure. This can result in debonding and leakage of the restoration. The greater the filler content, the lower the CTE; the greater the resin content, the greater the CTE. Microfilled composites and flowable composites have a higher CTE than do packable or hybrid varieties.

Elastic Modulus

The **elastic modulus** (also referred to as the *E-modulus* or *Young's modulus*) is a measure of the stiffness of a composite and is determined by the amount of filler. The greater the volume of filler, the stiffer (higher elastic modulus) and more wear resistant the restoration will be. This is an important consideration for selection of the type of composite. For example, an occlusal restoration on a posterior tooth must have greater wear resistance than a class V gingival restoration. In fact, the stiffer material is probably contraindicated at the gingival margins, because it does not have the flexibility needed in that area. Microfilled and flowable

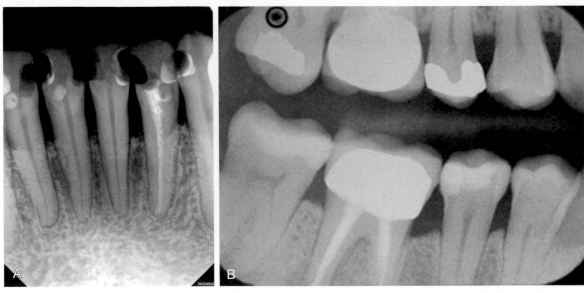

FIG. 6.6 X-rays of two types of composites **A,** Older anterior composites that lacked heavy metals in the filler particles so they are radiolucent and appear to be missing. **B,** A class II composite on tooth #29 DO that is radiopaque.

composites have fewer particles and more resin. They deform more readily under function and therefore can break more easily. Microfills generally are used in non–stress-bearing restorations.

Water Sorption

The resin matrix absorbs water from the oral cavity over time. The greater the resin content, the more water is absorbed. Therefore, microfills and flowables tend to have greater water sorption. The water can soften the resin matrix, leading to gradual degradation of the material (called *hydrolysis*). Water also causes some expansion (hydroscopic expansion) of the composite over the first week after placement.

Radiopacity

Metals such as lithium, barium, or strontium are added to the filler to make a restoration more opaque when viewed on a radiograph. However, some older composite materials do not have any of these additives and might appear radiolucent on radiographs (Fig. 6.6). Clinicians may have a difficult time determining whether there is recurrent caries around such radiolucent composites, because the caries also appears somewhat radiolucent on radiographs.

Quartz is not radiopaque, but it is sometimes used as filler for composites used in the anterior part of the mouth, because it has good optical properties that can enhance the color match to the tooth. It allows light to be transmitted through the restoration more readily and to pick up coloration from the surrounding tooth structure, making for a better color match.

CLASSIFICATION OF COMPOSITES BY FILLER SIZE

Composite resins have undergone a steady progression in their development to improve their properties.

Over time, the filler particle size has become smaller and smaller, the number of filler particles placed in the resin has increased, and polymerization shrinkage has decreased. As a result, composite restorations have become more durable, leak less, polish better, and match the teeth better. One way to classify composites is by the size of the filler particles they contain.

Macrofilled Composites

The first generation of composite resins used relatively large particles as fillers, ranging in size from 10 to 100 microns (μm). These composites are called **macrofilled composites**. The large particles make these composites difficult to polish, and they become rough as filler particles are lost at the surface under function or the resin wears, exposing the large particles. They are generally stronger than composites with smaller particles. Because of their roughness and rapid wear, macrofilled composites are no longer widely used. The first two macrofilled composites on the market were Adaptic (Johnson & Johnson) and Concise (3M ESPE).

Microfilled Composites

Microfilled composites were developed to overcome the problems that arose with larger particle size. They became commercially available in the late 1970s. As the name implies, microfilled composites have fillers that are much smaller than those in macrofilled composites. Microfill particles average about 0.04 μm in diameter and range in size from 0.03 to 0.5 μm. Several small particles have a larger total surface area than one large particle of similar weight. It is difficult to load a large volume of microfillers in the resin matrix because of this large surface area. Therefore the volume of filler in microfilled composites is only 35% to 50%, as opposed to 70% to 85% with many other composites. A lower filler volume results in a composite with poorer physical properties (i.e., weaker, with greater polymerization shrinkage, and more wear). To help overcome these shortcomings, some manufacturers mix microfillers into a resin, polymerize (cure) it, and grind the hardened material into particles ranging from 10 to 20 μm. Then they use these particles (consisting of pre-polymerized resin and microfillers) as the filler so that they can get more microfillers into the resin and improve its physical properties. Alternative methods to increase the numbers of microfillers that can be loaded into the resin include clumping the microfillers together by heating them or by condensing them into large clumps.

When polished, the microfilled composites produce a very smooth, shiny surface, unlike the rougher macrofilled composites. However, because of their poorer physical properties, they are not suitable for stress-bearing sites such as for class I, II, and IV (incisal edge repair) restorations (Table 6.1). Microfilled composites include Renamel Microfill (Cosmedent), Heliomolar (Ivoclar Vivadent), and EPIC-TMPT (Parkell).

Hybrid Composite

In the late 1980s, the next generation of composites was introduced. They are called **hybrid composites**, because

they contain both large fillers (2 to 4 μm) and 5% to 15% microfine fillers (0.04 to 0.2 μm). The combination of the two filler sizes produces a strong composite that polishes well. The microfine particles fill in between the larger particles to allow higher filler content (70% to 80% by weight). These composites have universal application in that they can be used well in both the anterior and posterior parts of the mouth. Most manufacturers have stopped making hybrid composites because improved products have reduced the demand for them. However, 3M ESPE still has its hybrid, Z100, available.

Microhybrids

The hybrids were improved on by the use of even smaller particles (75% smaller than 1 μm). These hybrids are called **microhybrids**, because they contain a mixture of small particles (0.04 to 1.0 μm) and microfine particles (0.01 to 0.1 μm). Microhybrids can contain high filler content (70% by volume), because microfine particles fill in spaces between small particles. Popular microhybrids include Esthet-X (Dentsply Sirona), Venus (Heraeus Kulzer), Point 4 (Kerr Dental), Tetric Ceram (Ivoclar Vivadent), and Filtek Supreme (3M ESPE).

Table 6.1   Classification of Dental Caries (or Cavity Preparations)

CLASS OF CARIES	LOCATION OF CARIES
Class I	Pits & fissures –posterior teeth; lingual of maxillary incisors
Class II	Proximal surfaces of posterior teeth
Class III	Proximal surfaces of anterior teeth
Class IV	Proximal surfaces of anterior teeth & the incisal angle
Class V	Cervical third of anterior & posterior teeth
Class VI	Incisal edges of anterior teeth; cusp tips of posterior teeth

CLASSES	ILLUSTRATION OF CARIES LOCATION
Class I	
Class II	
Class III	
Class IV	
Class V	
Class VI	

Nanohybrids

Soon after the microhybrids, the nanohybrids were introduced. **Nanohybrids** are microhybrids with nano-sized particles added. Their particle sizes range from 0.005 to 0.020 μm. The ability to add increased numbers of filler particles reduces the amount of resin. With less resin, these composites shrink less when polymerized. Shrinkage has been reduced from roughly 2% to 3% with earlier composites to about 1% with some of the nanohybrids. They are strong composites that can be polished to a high shine, and they retain that shine better than earlier composites. Examples of nanohybrids include Esthet-X HD (Dentsply Sirona), Aelite Aesthetic Enamel (BISCO), Filtek Supreme Ultra (3M ESPE), Tetric EvoCeram (Ivoclar Vivadent), Clearfil Majesty ES-2 (Kuraray), and Premise (Kerr Dental).

The nanohybrid composites are called **universal composites** because they are esthetic, wear resistant, and strong and therefore can be used in both the anterior and posterior parts of the mouth.

Nanocomposites

Nanofilled composites, or **nanocomposites**, have filler particles that range in size from 5 to 75 nanometers (nm). They are about a thousand times smaller than conventional fillers, which are approximately 1 μm. It is difficult to imagine how small these particles are. One nanometer is one billionth of a meter. These particles are so small that they cannot be produced like the other fillers, by grinding down larger chunks of glass, quartz, or ceramic materials. Instead, they are produced synthetically by a chemical building up of the fillers from molecular-size structures of zirconia and silica.

Nanocomposites have a combination of individual spheroidal particles and clusters of these particles produced by fusing the particles together at their edges (Fig. 6.7). The spaces between the particles in the cluster are filled with silane, which helps bind the clusters to the resin matrix. Nanoclusters range in size from 0.6 to 1.4 μm. The extremely small size of the filler particles allows many more of them to be packed into the resin and more closely together than in the other types of composites. This high filler content (about 78% by weight) reduces polymerization shrinkage (1.4% to 1.6%) and provides strength (and fracture toughness) so that they can be used in both anterior and posterior applications. They have excellent polishability and with improved wear resistance will maintain their

luster long-term. They have handling characteristics and physical and mechanical properties similar to micro- and nanohybrids.

Optically, the nanocomposites are very esthetic. They are more translucent, because the filler particles are smaller than the wavelength of visible light, and the light passes through rather than being absorbed. Light is also scattered by the multitude of particles, so the composite tends to blend in better with the surrounding tooth structure. Examples of nanocomposites are Filtek Supreme Ultra and Filtek Supreme XTE, both from 3M ESPE.

Continuing improvements. Each generation of composite represents some improvement in physical, mechanical, or chemical properties, handling characteristics, polishability, or ability to match the teeth. Research on other methods to improve the properties of the composite resins includes the use of fibers embedded in the resin to reinforce it and the use of crystals to increase strength.

Composite kits may contain anywhere from 10 to 30 or more shades (colors). Most kits have shades that are slightly translucent to mimic enamel and shades that are more opaque to mimic dentin. Shades that are more translucent are available to mimic incisal translucency, and opaque shades are available to block out or hide discolorations or darker dentin. Very light shades have been made to match teeth that have been whitened.

OTHER COMPOSITE TYPES

Flowable Composites

Flowable composites are low-viscosity, light-cured resins that may be lightly filled (about 40%) or more heavily filled (up to 70%). Initially, the particle size was in the range of those for hybrid composites. However, nanosized fillers are also being used in flowable composites.

Delivery. These composites flow readily and can be delivered directly into cavity preparations by small needle cannulas attached to the syringes in which they are packaged. Because of their low viscosity, they adapt well to cavity walls and flow into microscopic irregularities created by diamond and carbide burs.

Uses. They are well suited for use in conservative dentistry (i.e., minimal preparations), where they readily flow into the narrow preparations created with small diameter burs, diamonds and lasers. Many dentists use them in place of conventional pit and fissure sealants. They are more wear resistant than most lightly filled sealants, because their filler content is higher. They are useful as liners in large cavity preparations, because they adapt to the preparation better than more viscous materials such as hybrid and packable composites.

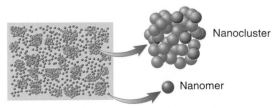

FIG. 6.7 Illustration of nanofilled composite with nanomers and nanoclusters. (From Sakaguchi RL, Powers JM: *Craig's Restorative Dental Materials* (ed 13). St. Louis, 2012, Elsevier.)

Flexibility. Their low elastic modulus allows them to cushion stresses created by polymerization shrinkage

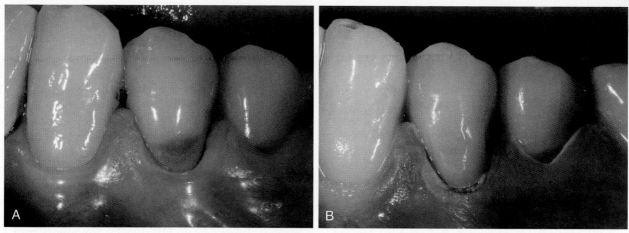

FIG. 6.8 Restoration of class V erosion lesion. **A,** Erosion lesion pretreatment. **B,** Lesion restored with flowable composite. (From Powers JM, Wataha JC: *Dental Materials: Properties and Manipulation* (ed 10). St. Louis, 2013, Elsevier.)

TABLE 6.2	Four Classification Methods for Composites			
CLASSIFICATION METHOD	**MICROFILL**	**MICROHYBRID**	**NANOCOMPOSITE**	**FLOWABLE HYBRID**
1. Filler amount (volume %)	30-50	60-70	78	30-55
2. Particle size (μm)	Macro (10-100)	Fine (0.1-10)	Micro (.01-0.1)	Nano (0.001-0.01)
3. Matrix composition	Bis-GMA	Bis-GMA or UDMA	Silorane(low shrinkage)	Bis-GMA or UDMA
4. Polymerization method	Self- or light-cured	Self- or light-cured	Light-cured	Light-cured

Bis-GMA, bisphenol-A-glycidyl dimethacrylate; *UDMA*, urethane dimethacrylate.

or heavy occlusal loads when they are used as an intermediate layer under hybrid and packable composites. (The lower the elastic modulus, the more flexible the material; the higher the elastic modulus, the stiffer the material.) They are useful for restoration of cervical noncarious lesions caused by toothbrush abrasion, acid erosion, or abfraction (from occlusal stresses, such as bruxing [grinding of teeth], which lead to flexing of the tooth) (Fig. 6.8). In cervical restorations flowable composites tend to flex when the tooth flexes. Stiffer composites often fall out when the tooth flexes. For toothbrush abrasion lesions, the patient should have the heavy toothbrushing habits corrected first. Otherwise, the flowable composites may wear rapidly if the patient continues to brush too hard. Examples of microhybrid flowable composites are Point 4 Flowable (Kerr Dental), Filtek Supreme Plus Flowable (3M ESPE), Gradia Flowable (GC America), and Virtuoso Flowable (DenMat). Examples of nanohybrid flowable composites are Herculite Ultra Flow (Kerr Dental), Nexcomp Flow Nano Hybrid (Meta Dental Corp), and Filtex Supreme Plus Flow (3M ESPE).

Properties. Lightly filled flowable composites wear more readily, are weaker, and shrink more (about 4% to 6%) when polymerized than hybrid composites (<3%), However, flowable composites too are being improved to make them stronger and more durable with less shrinkage. Some manufacturers have developed self-adhesive flowable composites (Vertise Flow [Kerr Dental] and *Fusio* Liquid Dentin [Pentron]) that

bond directly to dentin without the need for a separate bonding agent, since the bonding agent is incorporated into the composite. See Table 6.2 for classification of composites by four different criteria.

Pit and Fissure Sealants

Pit and fissure sealants are low-viscosity resins that vary in their filler content from no filler to more heavily filled resins that are essentially the same as flowable composites. They are used to prevent dental caries in pits and fissures of teeth (see Chapter 7 Preventive Materials).

Bulk-Fill Composites

Bulk-fill composites were developed to speed up the placement process of the composite restoration. Instead of having to place and cure multiple increments, the clinician can place one large increment and cure it. This is a significant time savings and is the main reason these materials have quickly become popular.

Depth of cure. The challenges of the bulk-fill composite are to have a depth of cure that permits increments of 4 mm or more, to not shrink excessively, to flow well into all aspects of the preparation without voids, to have acceptable physical and mechanical properties, and to be esthetic with good polishability. To achieve a greater depth of cure manufacturers have done one or more of the following: increased the translucency, reduced the amount of filler, or changed the chemical makeup to enhance polymerization when curing is initiated.

Because the bulk-fill composites are more translucent, they do not match the tooth shade very well. Additionally, with reduced filler they wear more readily. For these two reasons, translucency and reduced filler, bulk-fill composites may need to be covered with a veneer of a more wear resistant and color matching composite such as a micro- or nanohybrid.

Bulk-fill has limitations on its use in the proximal box of class II restorations, because the depth of the box is often 6 or 7 mm, far beyond its curing capability. In this case, more than one increment should be used in the proximal box.

Polymerization shrinkage. Polymerization shrinkage of bulk-fill composites has been reduced by adding special modifiers that relieve stress in the restoration during curing or by adjusting the size, number, and composition of the filler. The shrinkage for bulk-fill composites is in the range found with other high-viscosity composites (about 1.3% to 2.4%).

Formulations. Bulk-fill composites are found in two consistencies—flowable and viscous nanohybrids. Flowables adapt well to the internal portions of the preparations, whereas viscous nanohybrids must be carefully manipulated into the line angles and undercut areas. One manufacturer uses a sonic device to manipulate the composite (SonicFill; Kerr Dental) into the preparation. The sonic energy makes the composite less viscous, so that it flows readily and adapts to all aspects of the preparation. When the sonic device is turned off, the composite regains its thicker viscosity and can be sculpted and carved. Other common brands of bulk-fill composites include Tetric EvoCeram Bulk Fill (Ivoclar Vivadent), QuiXX (Dentsply Sirona), Reveal HD Bulk (BISCO), and Filtek Supreme Ultra (3M ESPE). Flowable versions include HyperFIL-DC (Parkell), SureFil SDR flow (Dentsply Sirona), and Venus Bulk Fill (Heraeus Kulzer). In general, shade selection is very limited, with most manufacturers offering only one to four shades.

Light-curing bulk fill composite. To achieve the desired depth of cure, the curing light must be used for the recommended time. Check the light wand tip to make sure it is free of residual composite debris that could limit the transmission of light. Light exposure times for fast-curing lights such as an argon laser or plasma arc curing light, typically suggested as 5 to 10 seconds for curing, may be too short to adequately cure a bulk-fill composite to its depth; curing times may need to be extended.

Packable Composites

Packable composites are highly viscous materials that contain a high volume of filler particles (as much as 90% by volume). The filler particles are long, rough, irregular fibers (about 100 μm in length) that bind on each other as the composite is packed into the preparation giving them a stiff consistency and make them less likely to stick to the composite placement instrument. They are used in posterior teeth for class I and II restorations, because they are slightly stronger and more wear resistant than most hybrids that contain less filler. They were marketed as substitutes for amalgams because of their stiffness and were also called condensable composites. However, packable is the preferred term since they cannot truly be condensed like amalgam. Their physical properties show no significant improvement over traditional universal composites. They are not widely used but are still available as QuiXX (Dentsply Sirona), Solitaire 2 (Heraeus Kulzer), SureFil (Dentsply Sirona), Tetric Ceram HB (Ivoclar Vivadent), and Alert (Pentron).

Core Buildup Composites

Core buildup composites are heavily filled composites used in badly broken-down teeth needing crowns. They replace missing tooth structure lost from dental caries or tooth fracture so that there is adequate structure to retain a crown. These composites can be light-cured, self-cured, or dual-cured. They often contain pigments that colorize them so that they can be easily differentiated from natural tooth structure (Fig. 6.9). Dentin-colored core materials are used when all-ceramic crowns are to be placed. An amalgam core buildup would create an esthetically unacceptable dark discoloration under the all-ceramic crown, as light passes through the porcelain and reflects off the amalgam.

Core composites are strong and can be bonded to tooth structure to minimize bacterial leakage and increase retention. However, mechanical retention in the remaining tooth structure is necessary, because bonding alone is not strong enough to resist the forces placed on the crown. The tooth can be prepared immediately after the composite core is placed and polymerized.

The materials are packaged in compules (also called "ampoules"), syringes, and cartridges with automixing tips similar to impression materials (see Fig. 6.12).

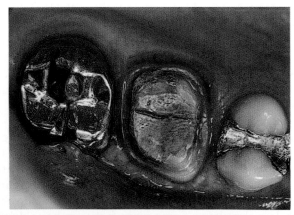

FIG. 6.9 Composite core material with color contrasting to the tooth structure for easy identification during crown preparation. (Courtesy of Dennis J. Weir [Novato, CA].)

Some core materials are supplied in syringes that have two chambers (one for base and one for catalyst). An automixing tip is attached to the syringe to mix the material. A small delivery tip can be added to the mixing tip to deliver the mixed composite directly into the preparation.

Examples of composite core materials include Build-It FR (Pentron), Clearfil Photo Core (Kuraray America), CompCore AF (Premier Dental), CoreRestore2 (Kerr Dental), FluoroCore 2+ (Dentsply Sirona), and ParaCore Automix (Coltène/Whaledent).

> **Clinical Tip**
>
> Not all light-cured bonding agents are compatible with chemical-cured composites, so follow the manufacturer's recommendations when selecting a bonding agent for the core material.

Provisional (Temporary) Restorative Composites

Provisional (temporary) crowns and bridges hold the prepared teeth in position so they do not drift and change their proximal contact position or occlusal relation with the opposing teeth (see Chapter 18). Provisional restorations also have the following functions: (1) they provide esthetics in the smile zone, (2) maintain proper speech, (3) allow proper function for chewing, (4) maintain proper form for oral hygiene, (5) protect exposed dentin, and (6) provide a good marginal seal.

Until the last decade or so, acrylic resins (polymethylmethacrylates) were widely used for the construction of provisional onlays, crowns, and bridges. They are inexpensive, but they exhibit wear, shrink significantly on polymerization, and release heat as they cure. They have an unpleasant odor and taste, can discolor, and are messy to use.

Newer provisional materials made with bis-acrylics and rubberized urethane have improved physical and mechanical properties. Bis-acryl composite resin is easy to handle and comes in a two-tube cartridge with automixing tips. It can be dispensed directly into the matrix (or carrier) for a provisional restoration. It exhibits very little shrinkage on curing and is radiopaque. It is more brittle than acrylic resin and tends to break more easily with longer-span bridges. Common brands include Protemp 3 Garant (3M ESPE), Luxatemp (Zenith/DMG America), and Integrity (Dentsply Sirona).

Rubberized urethane is a new type of provisional composite resin that is similar to bis-acrylic in its setting characteristics, radiopacity, and curing shrinkage. However, many of its properties have been improved because of the addition of a rubber molecule to the diurethane resin. It has increased flexural strength and is less brittle, so it holds up better for longer-span bridges. It is more impact resistant under occlusal loading and is more flexible, so it is easy to insert and remove. It is commercially available as Tuff-Temp (Pulpdent).

Both bis-acrylic and rubberized urethane materials are available in several shades. They are dual-cured materials, so they can be chemically cured (about 90 to 120 seconds); if a clear matrix is used, they can be light-cured as well. They can be repaired easily with flowable composites to add to contact areas and margins. They can be shaped and adjusted with acrylic burs, abrasive disks, and finishing diamonds. They can be polished with abrasive rubber points or wheels and polishing pastes or painted with a resin glaze to provide a smooth, shiny surface.

See Table 6.3 for a description of composite resin types on the basis of their properties.

CLINICAL HANDLING OF COMPOSITES

Uses of Composite Resins

Composites are used in all classes of restorations, from class I through class VI. Although previously used mostly for class III and class V esthetic restorations, these materials are very popular for posterior as well as anterior restorations. Advantages and disadvantages of the various types of composites can be found in Table 6.4. Composite materials are also used for provisional restorations, core buildups, fiber-reinforced posts, and laboratory-fabricated onlays and bridges.

Selection of Materials

Several criteria can be used for the selection of composite resins for restorations. When used in the anterior part of the mouth in non–stress-bearing areas, selection is usually based on the ability of the material to match the color of the teeth and to achieve a high polish. Microfills and microhybrids and nanohybrids are well suited for this purpose. When incisal edges or other stress-bearing areas are being restored, one of the

TABLE 6.3	Comparison of Properties of Composite Resins				
COMPOSITE	POLYMERIZATION SHRINKAGE	FLEXURAL STRENGTH	COMPRESSIVE STRENGTH	POLISHABILITY	WEAR RESISTANCE
Macrofills	Low	High	High	Low	Low
Microfills	Moderate	Moderate	Moderate	High	Low
Hybrids (nano)	Low	High	High	High	High
Bulk fill	Low	High	High	Moderate	Moderate
Flowables	High	Low	Low	High	Low

TABLE 6.4	Posterior Composite Resins: Advantages and Disadvantages	
ADVANTAGES	**DISADVANTAGES**
Durable (but not for as long as amalgam)	More costly than amalgam
Placed in one appointment	Wear is slightly greater than with amalgam
Good compressive strength	Shrinks when cured
Tooth colored	May leak, especially on root surfaces
Preparation more conservative than amalgam	Technique sensitive—patient may have sensitivity to cold or biting if restoration not properly placed
Bonding helps to support the surrounding tooth	Not a good choice for very large restorations

micro- or nanohybrids should be considered, because they are stronger than microfills. In the stress-bearing areas of the posterior part of the mouth, again, one of the hybrid composites is usually chosen for its strength and wear resistance. Flowable composites should not be used in areas subjected to stress or abrasion, because they are relatively weak and wear more rapidly.

HOW TO MATCH THE SHADE
Selecting the Shade
The dental assistant or hygienist may be asked to assist the dentist in obtaining the appropriate shade for a restoration. Selection of an inappropriate shade will result in a mismatch to the patient's dentition. A poorly chosen shade will likely result in a re-make of the restoration to satisfy the patient's esthetic expectations. This is disappointing for all involved and usually results in additional chair-time and possibly an additional appointment. Therefore, it is important for all clinical members of the dental team to have an understanding of what goes into the perception of color and how to match the variation of shades within a single tooth.

Color Characteristics: Hue, Chroma, and Value
When teeth are viewed for shade taking, three characteristics should be taken into consideration: hue, chroma, and value (see Chapter 2, section on Esthetics):

- **Hue** is the color of the tooth and may include mixtures of colors, such as yellow-brown. It is determined by the wavelength of light that is reflected from or transmitted through the tooth. On a color wheel, the wavelengths of light range progressively from the shorter violet wavelengths to blue, green, yellow, and red at the long end of the wavelength range.
- **Chroma** is the amount or intensity of color present; for example, a bold yellow has more chroma than a pastel yellow. The more chroma, the more intense the color (hue) will be.
- **Value** is the amount of lightness or darkness of the tooth (some describe it as the grayness of the tooth). A tooth with low value is darker and one with high value is brighter. Also, as the chroma increases, the value will decrease.

Patients tend to notice differences in value (or brightness) more than differences in hue or chroma when they assess how well a restoration matches their own teeth. So, if a restoration is the same value as the natural dentition but is slightly off in its color or chroma, it will be better accepted by the patient than if the restoration is too dark or too light.

Involving the Dental Assistant/Hygienist and the Patient
The dentist often relies on the chairside assistant or hygienist to help obtain a good color match for restorations with composite or ceramics. Three pairs of eyes (doctor, assistant, and patient) are usually better than one. Each person may interpret color differently. In addition, color-blindness (or the inability to correctly perceive certain colors) is more common in males (about 8% of males) than females. Involving the patients in shade taking helps the clinician in determining whether their expectations can be met. Matching shades can be very difficult, because many teeth do not match the standard shade guides.

Lighting for Shade Taking
The lighting in which the shade is viewed is very important. Shade matching should be done in two different types of light, because the perception of shade may vary in different lights, a phenomenon called *metamerism*. Most dental offices have fluorescent or incandescent lights (or both). Fluorescent lights emit more blue light, and incandescent lights emit more yellow light. Some dentists install color-corrected light bulbs (at color temperature 5500 K) to help in shade taking. Ideally, the laboratory should also have color-corrected lighting. A natural north light is considered a good light for shade taking. However, early morning and late afternoon natural light contains more yellow and orange light and less green and blue. If possible, the shade should also be taken while in the type of lighting that the patient is in most often. The bright light from the dental unit will tend to increase the perceived brightness of the shade and decrease the color intensity, so it should be turned off or moved away from the mouth.

Matching the Shade
A neutral background is important, so that the colors do not distract the eye and alter the perceived shade. A pastel-blue patient bib is a good color for shade taking. Female patients should be requested to remove lipstick

and colorful makeup, because these colors may influence the shade. Colorful clothes should be covered. The room in which the shade is selected should not have brightly colored walls or decorations. The ideal color for the area in which the shade will be matched is a neutral gray.

In general, the shade should be taken before the tooth is prepared and before a rubber dam or other isolation is placed. The color of the rubber dam can interfere with accurate matching, and teeth dry out and become lighter when under the dam or when isolated with cotton rolls. For best shade matching, the teeth should be clean, free of stain, and moist.

💡 Clinical Tip

Prior to Taking the Shade:
- Have the patient remove lipstick and colorful makeup
- Cover bright, colorful clothing with a neutral colored bib such as pastel blue
- Place the patient in a neutral colored room
- Remove debris and surface stain from the teeth
- Do not isolate the teeth; keep them moist
- Move the dental unit light away from the mouth

Shade Guides

Select the appropriate shade guide for the material that will be used. Many manufacturers of composites include a shade guide with color tabs that can be used to help in shade selection. Sometimes these color tabs are not an exact match to the composites they represent. Therefore, it is a good practice to apply and cure a small quantity of the composite selected onto the clean, moist tooth before the tooth is isolated and dried. Some practitioners prefer to make their own custom shade guides directly from the composite material, because these will be more accurate representations of the true composite colors.

The shade tab should be moist and held in the same plane as the surface of the teeth being matched, not in front of the teeth or behind them; otherwise the light reflected off the tooth and the tab will be slightly different (Fig. 6.10). The tab should be viewed under different lighting conditions. Do not stare at the color for longer than a few seconds at a time, because the retina adjusts for red and yellow colors, and the brain's perception of the color will be off. Looking at a pastel-blue object (such as a pastel-blue patient bib) after each shade tab was once recommended, but it causes blue color retinal fatigue. Instead, look at a neutral gray color for a few seconds.

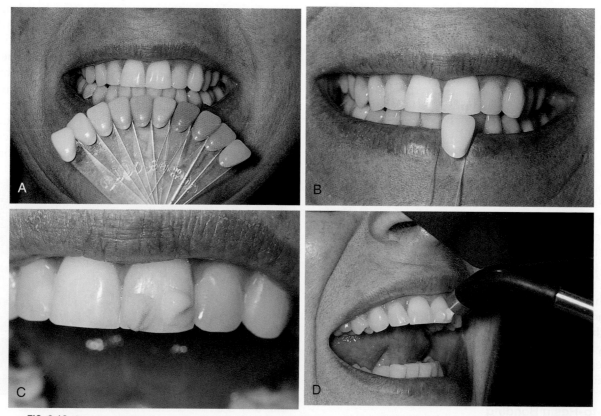

FIG. 6.10 Shade selection for composites. **A,** Hold shade guide up to the teeth and look for the shade that is the closest match. **B,** Hold that shade tab next to the tooth to be restored to confirm the match. **C,** If unsure of an exact match, place a small amount of composite in the two closest shades on the tooth. **D,** Light-cure the composite so that its final shade can be compared with the tooth. Select the closest match. On occasion, a couple of shades will need to be mixed together to get a good match.

The patient, dentist, and assistant should view the tabs and rank them as to the closest match for lightness or darkness (value) and color intensity (chroma). If the color intensity of the tooth is low, it may be more difficult to determine the color. In this case, the cervical area of a tooth with a more intense color, such as a maxillary canine, should be used to help pick the initial color. It is often necessary to take separate shades for the cervical portion of the tooth, for the occlusal surfaces of posterior teeth, and for the incisal edges of anterior teeth.

Some clinicians find it helpful to arrange the shade guide tabs by value from lightest to darkest, and then they select the three shades closest to the tooth in value. From there, they narrow the selection to the one that most closely matches the tooth color.

 Clinical Tip

A good use of time is to take the shade after the injection of local anesthetic, while you are waiting for the patient to get numb.

PLACING THE COMPOSITE

Thickness of Composite Increments

Most composites should be placed in small increments about 2 mm thick. Bulk fill composites can be placed in increments about 4 mm thick.

Light-Curing the Increments

If the composite resin is placed in too thick an increment, the light might not penetrate completely, and the composite might not cure all the way to the bottom. Longer curing times may be required for increments greater than 2 mm thick. Even with a long curing time some light-curing units may not have the output needed to cure to the bottom of large increments (>4 mm). More powerful curing lights might be able to cure greater thicknesses of material. Interproximal areas may need additional time to cure completely because of the more difficult access of the area to the direct path of the light. It is good practice to cure the interproximal composite restoration again from both facial and lingual surfaces after the metal matrix band is removed to ensure complete curing in the bottom of the box form of the preparation. Darker shades also require a longer curing time, because the light is more readily absorbed by the dark color and does not transmit through the material as readily as through lighter-colored materials. Composites that are heavily filled also will take longer curing times because the filler tends to disperse the light rather than allowing it to transmit through the composite to its full thickness.

Resin-to-Resin Bonding

Etched enamel and dentin are infiltrated with resin bonding agents to form a resin-rich layer. The resin-infiltrated dentin is called the *hybrid zone* or *hybrid layer* (see Chapter 5 Principles of Bonding). The initial increment of composite resin will chemically bond to the resin bonding agent on the enamel and dentin. Each additional increment will bond to the previously placed increment of composite as long as good isolation is maintained and no contaminants are introduced. When resins polymerize, there is a thin layer of unpolymerized resin on the surface because contact with oxygen in the air inhibits the cure. This "air-inhibited" layer looks shiny and feels slippery. This thin, unset layer facilitates chemical bonding with the next layer of composite. It will set when the layer placed over it excludes air and then is cured. The completed restoration comprises a series of layers of resin-based materials that are all chemically bonded to each other and micromechanically (mechanically locking into microscopic irregularities created by acid etching) bonded to the tooth structure. Starting from the dentin side of the restoration and progressing toward the composite, there are resin tags in the tubules, the resin-rich hybrid layer, the adhesive resin layer, and the composite resin restoration (Fig. 6.11). In most cases, the final thin, air-inhibited layer on the surface of the composite is removed during finishing and polishing. It may have an unpleasant taste and should be wiped off with gauze before the patient leaves if finishing and polishing are not required (as with pit and fissure sealants).

Contaminants

Newly etched dentin is kept moist for "wet" dentin bonding. However, before and after bonding, any form of extraneous moisture (water, saliva, fluid from the gingival sulcus [i.e., space between the gum and tooth], or blood) should be kept away from the tooth until the restoration has been completed. Contamination requires removal of the contaminant and re-etching for 10 to 15 seconds. Alcohol should not be used to wet the composite placement instrument to keep the composite from sticking, because it weakens the composite. Use of a little of the bonding agent or other

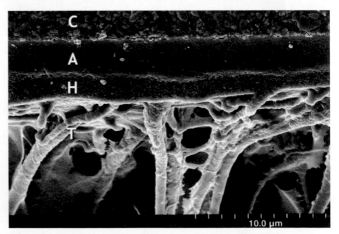

FIG. 6.11 Scanning electron micrograph of a traverse section of bonded composite restoration after the tooth has been dissolved away. Layers from the top are *(C)* composite, *(A)* adhesive layer, *(H)* hybrid layer, and *(T)* resin tags that had gone into the dentinal tubules. (From Sakaguchi RL, Powers JM: *Craig's Restorative Dental Materials* (ed 13). St. Louis, 2012, Elsevier.)

unfilled resin on the instrument to prevent sticking can dilute and thin the composite, making it weaker and more likely to wear. Special composite instruments are made with a coating of nonstick materials to help with the stickiness problem. They should be reserved for composite placement, because once they get scratched they lose their nonstick quality. IRM, which contains eugenol, and liners, bases, or temporary cements containing eugenol should not be used with composites, because eugenol inhibits the set of resins.

Layering (Stratification) of Composite

Many dentists prefer to apply layers of composite of different shades or degrees of opacity or translucency to obtain a good match to the natural teeth. This process is called layering or stratification. Teeth are usually not one color throughout, but a variety of colors and can be described as three general areas. (1) The cervical part of the tooth is closest to the dentin color. This is because the translucent enamel is thinnest in the cervical part of the tooth, and light passing through it reflects back the color of the dentin. The dentin color is the bulk of the color of the tooth and can range from yellow to orange to red or mixtures of those colors. The dentin color of composite is usually the most opaque and is useful for blocking out stains from amalgam or tooth discolorations. (2) The middle of the tooth is called the *body area*. Its color is a result of light interacting with both enamel and dentin. The enamel in this area is thicker than in the cervical area. (3) The incisal part of the tooth is mostly enamel and will be more translucent. Often the interplay of the light with the translucent enamel will produce a bluish tint to the enamel. Cusp tips of posterior teeth are not translucent like anterior teeth but will appear lighter in color than the cervical or body areas.

Dentists can select dentin, body, and enamel shades and apply them in layers to simulate the natural tooth colors with their opacities and translucencies. When faced with a challenging color match, dentists may choose to do a trial run or mock-up on the unetched tooth. The colors selected are applied in the desired layers and light-cured. The results can be seen and modified, if necessary, before the tooth is restored. Because the tooth has not been etched, the mock-up material will come off easily. The restoration can be characterized to replicate white spots, stains in occlusal fissures, or bluish incisal translucency. Special tints or stains made for composite can be used.

Shelf Life

The shelf life of composites varies with the type of resin used and the manufacturer. In general, avoiding heat and light can extend shelf life. Manufacturers usually recommend refrigerating the material. The average shelf life is 2 to 3 years if stored properly. Check the label on the container that the composite came in to see the expiration date.

Dispensing and Cross-Contamination

Light-cured composites are supplied in compules or syringes. All of these containers are opaque so that the material is not affected by light. Some offices prefer single-use (unit-dose) items such as composite compules (small containers of composite resin that fit into a delivery gun) that can be disposed of after the procedure to minimize the risk of cross-contamination. Reusable syringes require careful handling to ensure that they are not contaminated during the procedure. The delivery tip on syringes of flowable composites should be disposed of in a sharps container after use, and the syringes should be recapped and sprayed or wiped with disinfectant. Composite in screw-type syringes should be dispensed after the shade is selected and covered in a light-protected container until use (Fig. 6.12). Chemical-cured composites come in screw-type tubes or two-container cartridges. They require similar dispensing measures to prevent cross-contamination.

If the composite is stored in the refrigerator, it should be removed an hour or more before its planned use to allow it to return to room temperature. Cold composite will be stiff, less likely to stick to the placement instruments but more difficult to adapt to the wall of the cavity preparation. Composite syringes or compules can be placed in warm water to increase the flow of the material. Devices (e.g., Therma-Flo; Vista Dental Products) are commercially available for warming the composite. Manufacturers claim it makes highly filled composites flow like flowable composites.

> **💡 Clinical Tip**
>
> Placing a composite syringe or compule in warm water will increase its flow. Putting it in the refrigerator before use will make it stiffer; consequently, it will not stick to the placement instrument as much.

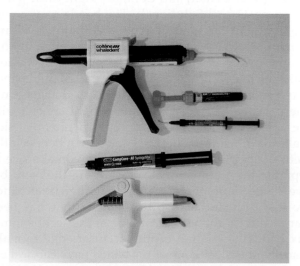

FIG. 6.12 Dispensing systems for composites. *Clockwise from top to bottom:* Dual cartridges with auto-mixing tip, screw-type syringe, injection-type syringe, dual syringe with auto-mixing tip and compules delivered by a dispensing gun.

MATRIX SYSTEMS

Matrix systems for operative dentistry are comprised of components such as metal or plastic bands, wedges, and pressure rings (also called separator rings) that help to adapt and shape the restorative material. The matrix is used most often when restoring the proximal surface of a tooth. It is also used for extensive direct restorations such as complex composites or amalgams and crown build-ups. On occasion, a matrix is used when restoring cervical lesions with composite or glass ionomer cement.

Matrix Bands

The purpose of the matrix band is to help contain the restorative material within the preparation during placement and to develop natural contours and contact areas. Matrix bands for anterior teeth are usually clear plastic (polyether or celluloid), and they may be pre-contoured (e.g., Bioclear; Bioclear Matrix Systems) to help shape the proximal surface of the restoration or straight strips (Mylar Strips; Keystone Industries). Pre-contoured forms are also available for repairing a proximal surface involving an incisal angle.

Whole crown forms (e.g., Strip Crown Forms; 3M ESPE) can be used when the entire crown must be built up. The stock crown form is trimmed to fit the remaining tooth structure, and then filled with composite. After etching and application of bonding agent, it is pressed onto the remaining tooth structure and cured. The crown form is slit and peeled away.

Matrix bands for posterior teeth are made of soft metal (typically stainless steel in thicknesses ranging from 0.02 to 0.045 mm) that is flat or pre-contoured or of clear pre-contoured polyester (e.g., SuperMat Matrix [Kerr Dental] and Composi-Tight Clear Bands [Garrison Dental Solutions]). The bands may go entirely around the tooth (circumferential) or just on a proximal surface (sectional). Sectional bands fit only on one proximal surface at a time, as with mesiocclusal or distocclusal cavities. Circumferential bands may be difficult to fit around a tooth that has only one proximal surface prepared. A tight contact with the adjacent tooth on the unprepared proximal side makes it difficult to slip the band down between the teeth. Placing a wedge in the interproximal space to separate the teeth can help in slipping the band between the unprepared teeth. Circumferential bands are also difficult to use on a tooth that has been clamped for a rubber dam. Some of the sectional matrix bands have a tab on the occlusal edge to make placement easier. Some of the bands have cervical extensions used for proximal boxes that extend subgingivally. Circumferential metal bands can also be pre-welded into loops (Denovo Dental) or spot-welded

in the office to the desired diameter. With the T-band (Pulpdent), flanges of metal that form the T shape can be folded and crimped around the band at the desired diameter. T-bands are thin, soft brass or stainless steel and have been used in pediatric dentistry for decades (Fig. 6.13).

The curing light is placed from the occlusal surface with metal bands for initial curing; then it is placed from the facial and lingual surfaces after the matrix band is removed. Any of these matrices can be used with chemical-cured composites as well.

Wedges

Wedges are placed interproximally and hold the matrix band against the tooth to seal the gingival margin, so that the restorative material does not extend out of the cavity preparation and cause an overhang. Wedges are usually placed from the lingual side, because the lingual embrasure is usually the widest. On occasion, wedges will need to be placed via both buccal and lingual approaches to secure the band against the tooth without gaps at the gingival margin. Wedges are usually inserted with pressure to create some separation of the teeth to make up for the thickness of the matrix band. Otherwise, when the band is removed from the interproximal area after placement of the restoration, a space will exist between the restoration and the adjacent tooth (an open contact) leading to food impaction and periodontal disease. Placing a wedge before cavity preparation will help protect the gingival papilla and prevent bleeding during the preparation. It also initiates separation of the teeth.

Wedges are made of wood or plastic and are color-coded for their size. Plastic wedges may be opaque or transparent. The newer generations of plastic wedges (Wedge Wands [Garrison Dental Solutions]; V4 Wedge [Ultradent Products]) have an advantage over the wooden wedges, because they are shaped to conform better to the embrasure space and to the tooth. The Wedge Wand has a long handle attached to the end of the wedge to facilitate placement. The handle can be bent at 90 degrees to aid in placement from the lingual side in the molar region. After the wedge is put firmly into place, the handle can be twisted off. Transparent wedges are used on proximal surfaces when a clear matrix band is used for restoration of light-cured composites. The clear wedge allows light transmission to cure the material at the gingival margin; an opaque wedge would block the light (Fig. 6.14).

Sectional Matrix Systems

Sectional matrix systems used for class II composite resins usually are equipped with a selection of pre-contoured sectional bands of various widths appropriate for premolars or molars, a pressure

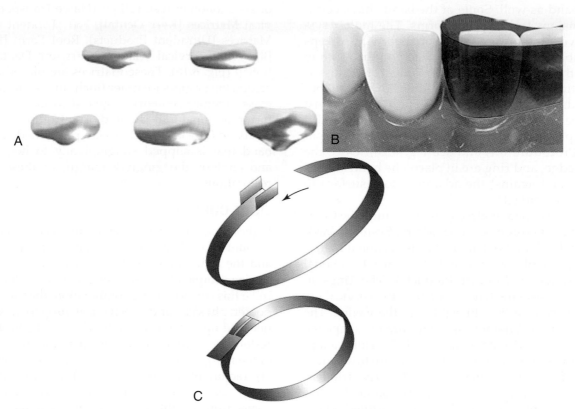

FIG. 6.13 Matrix bands. **A,** Sectional metal matrix bands with some having cervical extensions. **B,** Clear plastic band. **C,** T-Bands. (**A** and **B,** Courtesy of Garrison Dental Solutions, Spring Lake, MI; **C,** From Bird DL, Robinson DS: *Modern Dental Assisting* (ed 11). St. Louis, Elsevier.)

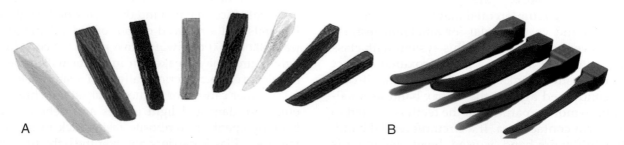

FIG. 6.14 Wedges. **A,** Wooden anatomic wedges. **B,** Plastic contoured wedges. (**B,** Courtesy of Garrison Dental Solutions, Spring Lake, MI.)

ring, and ring placement forceps. Some systems supply plastic wedges and forceps for handling the matrix band as well. Some of the bands have cervical extensions for deep box forms. The matrix systems have a metal ring that is opened with forceps like a rubber dam clamp and placed on the tooth to engage the interproximal embrasures of a class II preparation. The ring has metal tines or soft rubber that holds the sectional matrix band firmly against the buccal and lingual surfaces of the tooth, and it applies pressure to the teeth to cause some separation (Procedure 6.1; and see Fig. 6.26). Once the band, wedge, and ring are in place, the band should be burnished against the adjacent tooth surface to ensure firm contact.

Popular sectional matrix systems include the Composi-Tight 3D Fusion Sectional Matrix System (Garrison Dental Solutions), Palodent Plus Sectional Matrix System (Dentsply Sirona), and Triodent V4 Sectional Matrix System (Ultradent Products). The rings in these newer systems have a notch in the cervical extent of the ring so they fit right over the wedge. The matrix bands are anatomically contoured to shape the contact areas and embrasures, and the rings adapt them to the tooth while applying pressure to separate the teeth for a solid contact (Fig. 6.15). The Triodent V4 system has a novel metal matrix band that has hundreds of tiny windows that are resin-filled. These windows allow light to transmit to the composite during light-curing.

If more than one proximal surface on a tooth is to be restored (i.e., a mesio-occluso-distal [MOD] restoration), a sectional band could be placed on each proximal surface and pressure rings could be stacked one over the other. Otherwise, one proximal surface could be restored, and then the other.

Circumferential Matrix Systems

The Tofflemire circumferential matrix system is well established and very popular for amalgam restorations. It is very difficult to use this system with class II composites and achieve a good proximal contact area. Composite shrinks when it cures, and it cannot be condensed against the matrix band as amalgam can, so more separation of the teeth is needed to create a firm contact area. If a circumferential band, like the Tofflemire band, is used, heavy wedging is required to create enough separation of the teeth to make up for the thickness of the band in both mesial and distal interproximal spaces. In addition, the band is flat and needs to be contoured to the adjacent tooth to help form an anatomic contact area. Pressure rings could be placed on mesial and distal embrasures to help with separation of the teeth, but it is more difficult to place where the Tofflemire retainer is connected to the band. Tofflemire bands and retainers are discussed in depth in Chapter 10 Dental Amalgam.

Cervical Matrices

Plastic matrices are available for cervical composite or glass ionomer restorations (Hawe Transparent Cervical Matrices [Kerr Dental], 360° Triodent Cervical Matrices [Ultradent Products], Root Form [Directa], BlueView Cervical Matrix [Garrison Dental Solutions]) (Fig. 6.16). These matrices are placed over the composite or glass ionomer (including resin-modified glass ionomer cement) to give it form and then the restorative material is cured. The Contour-Strip Matrix Band (Ivoclar Vivadent) is a preformed, U-shaped band that is slipped subgingivally to help contain and contour the gingival margin of these cervical restorations.

LIGHT-CURING

Light-cured composite resins must receive the correct amount of radiant energy at the right exposure time and the right wavelength in order for them to polymerize completely. If the composite resin does not receive this correct curing combination, then it will have poorer physical and mechanical properties and will not hold up as well clinically. The result could be (1) a restoration with a shorter life span due to breakdown of the margins, (2) recurrent caries, (3) excessive wear, (4) fracture of the restoration, (5) discoloration of the composite, or (6) lack of retention. The light source comes from a light-curing unit that may be built into the dental unit or free-standing. Free-standing units have a handheld light guide (also called a wand) attached to a base by a cord or may detach from a recharging base and contain a battery pack.

Light Factors Affecting the Cure

Among the factors that can affect the cure of a restoration are the following: (1) short curing times, (2) inadequate light output, (3) the wrong wavelength of light, and (4) an incorrectly positioned light guide. Surveys of dental offices have found that many of the light-curing units had a reduced output of radiant energy. (At least 300 to 400 milliwatts [mW]/cm^2 is needed.) The light source may weaken in intensity with time and should be checked periodically with a radiometer (Fig. 6.17). Other causes for reduced output are chipped or otherwise damaged light guides and debris such as bonding agent or composite resin stuck to the tip of the guide. Plastic barriers put over the light guide may also reduce the output, particularly if the seam of the plastic cover is across the tip. Test the light output with a radiometer with the barrier in place to see what effect it might have.

 Clinical Tip

Periodically check the output of the curing light with a radiometer to make sure it has not diminished. Inadequate output will adversely affect the composite restoration.

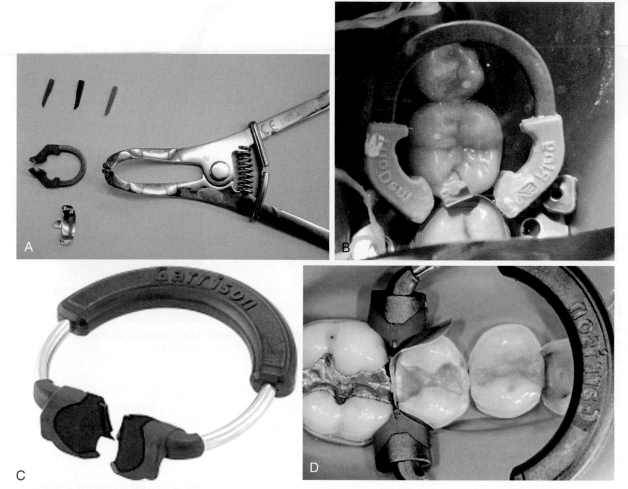

FIG. 6.15 Sectional matrix systems. **A,** Sectional matrix set up with wedges, pressure ring (Triodent V3, Dentsply Caulk), sectional matrix band, and ring forceps. **B,** Sectional matrix system applied clinically. **C,** Pressure ring (Composi-Tight 3D XR, Garrison Dental Solutions), for sectional matrix to create slight separation of the teeth to ensure a firm contact. **D,** Pressure ring and sectional matrix band in place. (Courtesy of Garrison Dental Solutions, Spring Lake, MI.)

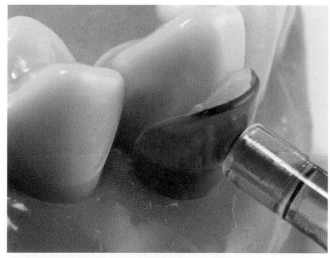

FIG. 6.16 Cervical matrices. (BlueView Cervical Matrix, courtesy of Garrison Dental Solutions, Spring Lake, MI.)

Position of the Light Guide

The technique used to light-cure composite resin may also affect the amount of radiant energy that reaches the restoration. The light guide should be held about 1 mm away initially and then almost in contact after a second or two. The tip of the light guide should be positioned at 90 degrees to the composite surface so the light shines directly on the composite. However, it is not always possible to position the guide at this angle or close to the composite surface. The shape and size of the light guide may be a limiting factor in the ability to position the tip ideally. When restoring molars in patients who cannot open fully or if matrix bands are in the way, the closeness to the restoration and the light guide angulation may be compromised.

Curing in proximal box. A proximal box may be 6 to 7 mm deep; most light guides cannot reach the bottom of such a box, and therefore the tip will be several millimeters away from the increment of composite on the gingival floor. Therefore, the curing time should be increased when (1) the light guide angulation is compromised, or (2) it is positioned further away from the composite than is ideal. In

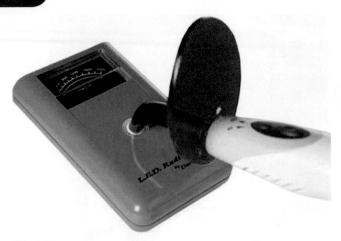

FIG. 6.17 Radiometer used to test the output of the curing light. (Courtesy Kerr Dental.)

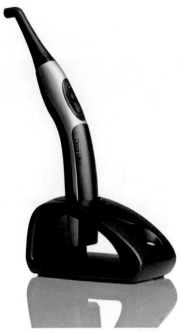

FIG. 6.18 LED wand-type recharging curing light. (Demi Ultra, courtesy of Kavo Kerr Group, Charlotte, NC.)

addition, the composite in a proximal box should be cured through the enamel from the buccal and lingual sides after the matrix band is removed. Class III restorations should also be cured from the facial and lingual surfaces. It is thought that the high level of recurrent caries (much higher than with amalgam) seen at the gingival margin of the proximal box in a class II composite may be due, in part, to incomplete curing of the composite or bonding agent at the bottom of the box. Therefore, an increased curing time is recommended (time will depend on the light intensity of the unit).

Types of light-curing units. Light-curing units are of four different types (Fig. 6.18):
- Quartz-tungsten-halogen (QTH or *halogen,* as they are commonly called)
- Light-emitting diode (LED)
- Argon laser
- Plasma arch curing (PAC)

These four types of curing lights can vary in their light intensity and the light spectrum (range of wavelengths) they produce.

Simple LED curing units have the lowest intensity of light and do not generate heat. The diodes can last as long as 5000 hours, and rechargeable batteries ensure portability and convenience. LED units emit blue light (within the visible light range) at 450 to 490 nm in wavelength. Newer versions of the LED units can generate an energy output of about 1000 mW/cm^2. At present, they are the most popular curing light units.

Halogen lights are next to lowest in light intensity. The halogen light bulb delivers a blue light that ranges from 400 to 500 nm in wavelength. The initiator, camphorquinone, absorbs light between 460 and 480 nm. The halogen bulb generates heat so an internal fan is built into the unit. The bulb lasts about 100 hours but deteriorates over time; the intensity therefore needs

to be checked periodically with a radiometer to make sure it will provide an adequate cure. The bulb output should be 400 to 800 mW/cm^2 so if it drops below 300 mW/cm^2, it should be replaced. Halogen units with special turbo tips may generate as much as 1300 mW/cm^2.

For curing lights with a heat output, a stream of cool air should be directed across the restoration while it is being cured to minimize heating the pulp.

> **Clinical Tip**
>
> To test the halogen curing light for heat output, put the light tip on your fingernail and turn on the light for 20 seconds. If you can feel your nail getting hot, then your unit produces enough heat to cause some pulpal sensitivity in deep preparations. Use a stream of cool air on the composite during curing to help reduce the heat delivered to the tooth.

Rapid curing. Rapid curing greatly speeds up the procedure, because conventional curing of many small increments each for 20 to 40 seconds increases the total time required. PAC and argon laser lights provide the fastest cure, but they also transmit heat to the composite and the tooth. PAC lights are very intense (about 1000 mW/cm^2) and are filtered to reduce heat. Argon laser lights are the most intense and are marketed as high-speed curing units requiring only 5 seconds for up to a 5-mm increment of composite. Rapid curing will occur in the upper 2 to 3 mm of the composite increment. Much of the composite resin below that level will not cure completely, because the light is scattered and absorbed and the intensity greatly diminishes. Thus, additional curing time will be needed to achieve a complete cure beyond 2 to 3 mm.

Match the curing light to the composite. Composites that use camphorquinone (CQ) as the photoinitiator are usually well matched with the curing units. However, some composites use different photoinitiators. The narrow light wave spectrum of argon lasers (490 nm) and most LED units (450 to 490 nm) may be a mismatch for these non–CQ-initiated composites, so they will not cure completely. Broadband LED units that have a broad light spectrum and a higher intensity have been made to correct this problem. Halogen lights have a broad light spectrum (400 to 500 nm) and will cure all of the current composites. PAC light units are the least common of the four types. They have a very intense light, are filtered to reduce heat, and have a broad spectrum of light (400 to 500 nm).

Typical curing times for LED and halogen lights for thin layers are 20 to 40 seconds for each 2-mm increment. Longer curing times are needed for (1) thicker increments, (2) bulk-fill composites, (3) very light bleaching shades, (4) darker composites, (5) opaque composites, (6) heavily filled composites, or (7) composites located farther from the light probe than is ideal. The amount of additional time depends on the type and intensity of the light being used. The intensity of the light diminishes rapidly the farther away the composite is from the tip of the light guide.

> Factors requiring longer curing times for composite resins:
> - Increments thicker than 2 mm (or 4 mm for bulk-fill composites)
> - Very light shades for whitened teeth
> - Opaque shades
> - Darker shades
> - Heavily filled composites
> - Composites located farther from the light tip than ideal

Areas of composite that lie just outside the borders of the light guide tip (typically 8 mm in diameter) should be cured separately. Wider tips are available and may be useful when curing broad areas such as occlusal composites or sealants or anterior veneers. The wider the tip, the more divergent the light beam will be, so longer curing times may be needed. Some manufacturers provide narrow diameter tips for reaching into proximal box preparations or other tight spaces.

The light guide on the curing unit is often glass, glass encased in metal, or a type of plastic. Some curing units are in the configuration of a wand; others are in the shape of a gun. Many units have the capability of being used remotely rather than being plugged into an electrical outlet, because they have rechargeable batteries.

Light-Curing Methods

There are many representatives in the marketplace of the four types of light-curing units mentioned, and there are many "bells and whistles" available with each type. In addition, several methods are used for curing composite restorations with these lights. These methods are used in an attempt to minimize the stress on the bond created by polymerization shrinkage. One method is called *soft-start curing*. The theory is that a slow rate of curing will allow the resin to flow as the polymer chains are being formed and, thereby, reduce the curing shrinkage stress. There are three forms of soft-start curing: (1) ramped, (2) stepped, and (3) pulse-delay. Ramped curing starts with low light intensity, gradually increases to high intensity over a 10-second interval, and then remains constant for the rest of the exposure. Stepped curing starts at low intensity for 10 seconds, and then immediately goes to maximal intensity for the rest of the exposure. Pulse-delay curing starts with a brief low-intensity exposure, then delays for shaping the restoration, and finally completes the exposure with a long exposure at high intensity. Some clinicians want to speed up the curing process and use very fast curing called *turbo curing*. However, high-intensity exposure even for short intervals will generate higher stress during curing. Newer high-speed or variable-intensity light units should use the curing times recommended by the manufacturers. Only recently have some manufacturers started to give guidance on curing times for their materials.

> Desirable Features for Your Curing Light
> - Easy to use
> - Simple infection control procedures
> - Broad spectrum output to cure all composites
> - High output for effective polymerization
> - Has a radiometer to test output
> - Wide curing tip angled at 90° with short height for access in the posterior
> - Durable

Eye protection. The blue light emitted from a curing unit can be damaging to the retina of the eye. With curing units increasing in their light intensity the risk for damage becomes greater if precautions are not taken. A prolonged blast of blue light directly into the eye can cause immediate and irreversible damage to the retina. Repeated low-level exposure over time can accelerate aging of the retina and contribute to macular degeneration. Protective glasses with filters that block the blue light should be worn by those in the operatory—the operator, assistant, and patient. Some offices use an orange filter shield that is held between the operator and the light. Some units have a filter that attaches to the light guide. Looking directly at the light, even briefly, should be avoided.

Infection control methods. In many offices the light guide and handle (or the entire unit, depending on the type) are covered with a disposable barrier such as a clear plastic cover. The cover will also prevent bonding agent, composite resin, blood, and other debris from sticking to the tip of the guide. The ideal unit is one with a removable light guide that can be autoclaved and has smooth surfaces that can be wiped down with disinfectant. Autoclaving may cause some residue to accumulate on the tip of the light guide, but it can be polished off. Some disinfecting solutions may cause clouding of glass-fibered light guides and can discolor the plastic casing of the unit. Check with the manufacturer for the recommended disinfectant.

Guidelines for Light-Curing

- Provide eye protection to those exposed to the light.
- Position the patient so as to provide best access for the light to the restoration.
- Check the light guide tip for damage or debris.
- Use curing times and output modes recommended by the manufacturer.
- Err on the side of using longer curing times than shorter.
- Direct the light at 90 degrees to the composite surface.
- Start curing with the tip about 1 mm from the composite surface and move closer after the surface has cured. Use longer curing times when the tip is farther away from the composite.
- When close access to the composite is limited (as with a class II proximal box), supplement with curing from buccal and lingual sides after the matrix is removed.
- With high-intensity curing units and extended exposure times, blow an air stream over the tooth to prevent overheating. Pause for a couple of seconds between curing cycles.

Adapted from Ferracane JL, Watts DC, Ernst C-P, et al: Effective use of dental curing lights: A guide for the dental practitioner. *ADA Professional Prod Rev,* 8:2–13, 2013.

 Caution

Do not look directly at the light when curing materials. Stabilize the light tip using finger rests before you look away from the light to prevent it from drifting away from the restoration.

Use a light shield or filtering eyewear to protect the eyes. Have the patient close his or her eyes, or provide filtering eyewear.

Precautions

- *Inadequate light output:* It is important to check halogen light–curing units frequently (monthly), because the light bulbs will deteriorate over time and will not produce an adequate cure. Other light units should also be tested periodically. In addition, light probes can darken with application of surface disinfectants or sterilization or can become chipped or scratched and may not transmit light as well. If composite or a bonding agent has come in contact with the light tip and hardened on it, this will impede the light output. Light output can be measured with commercially available radiometers (light meters). Some light units have a built-in light meter for periodic testing.
- *Premature set of composite:* The operatory light can cause an initial set of the surface of the composite as it is being placed. Once this has happened, the composite can no longer be manipulated, but it is not cured through the depth of the material. The operatory light should be moved farther from the composite or temporarily turned away from the field, so that the direct light is not shining in the patient's mouth. Operators using headlamps should turn them away or use a filter on the light. Some manufacturers have added chemicals to inhibit premature polymerization by ambient light.
- *Eye protection:* The operator is cautioned to use a light-shielding protective device to protect the eyes of the patient and the staff. Protective eyewear that filters the light should be used by the patient, assistant, and operator. The intense blue light has the potential to cause damage to the retina with direct exposure.
- *Heat generation:* Some curing lights (halogen, argon laser, and PAC) generate a certain amount of heat when applied to the tooth, and composite resins release heat (exothermic reaction) when they polymerize. The combination of the two heat sources has the potential to elevate the temperature of the pulp in deep cavities that have less than 1 mm of dentin over the pulp. An increase in pulpal temperature of about 6°C has the potential to cause an inflammatory reaction in the pulp and even death of the pulp. A protective liner or base may be needed before placing the composite.

FINISHING AND POLISHING

Finishing is the process used to correct irregularities in contour, remove excess material, and smooth the margins and external surfaces. Polishing takes the process a step further by removing scratches by the step-wise application of sequentially finer abrasives to produce a glossy, very smooth surface. The smooth surfaces produced with polishing resist plaque retention and make cleaning with floss and brush much simpler (see Chapter 13 Abrasion, Finishing, and Polishing).

Before starting the finishing and polishing process, the restoration should be dried and inspected for (1) integrity of margins, (2) surface voids, (3) over- or undercontoured surfaces, and (4) snug proximal contacts, if present. If a rubber dam is being used, the inspection should be done while the dam is still in place. This is a prime opportunity to make corrections to the restoration before the surface becomes contaminated. If surfaces have been contaminated with saliva or blood, re-isolation is needed and the surfaces should be rinsed and dried. The area of the composite to be repaired and the adjacent tooth surface are prepared. Then, start as though preparing to place the composite for the first time with acid etching, application of bonding agent and composite.

Finishing

Excess composite can be removed with multi-fluted carbide finishing burs, fine and ultrafine diamond burs, and abrasive disks. Small excesses at the gingival margin or interproximal can be removed with special composite knives, a #12 surgical scalpel blade, flame-shaped carbide or diamond burs, or abrasive strips. Carbide and diamond finishing burs and disks should be used at slow speeds with gentle, controlled (finger rest), intermittent strokes moving from tooth to restoration so as not to ditch the margins or flatten contours. With intracoronal restorations the surrounding tooth structure is the guide to developing the contours and shaping the occlusal anatomy. When using finishing strips to finish the gingival margin on the proximal surface, be sure the strip is not so wide as to engage the contact area. Otherwise, it may produce a weak or open contact. Narrow strips are commercially available, or wide strips can be cut in half lengthwise. When using abrasive disks on convex surfaces as with cervical restorations, smaller disks should be used and their angulation to the tooth should be changed to follow the tooth contours. Otherwise, the restoration may be flat rather than convex like the tooth. Some operators prefer flame-shaped diamonds to finish the convex surfaces. Egg-shaped or football-shaped carbide and diamond finishing burs can be used to finish and contour the occlusal surfaces of posterior teeth and the lingual surfaces of anterior teeth.

Finishing is considered complete when (1) all flash (excess composite extending over the cavosurface margins) has been removed, (2) the cavosurface margins are flush and smooth-feeling to the explorer, (3) the axial contours have been refined, (4) the occlusal anatomy shaped, and (5) the occlusion adjusted. Only when all of the surfaces have been properly finished and contoured should polishing be started.

Polishing

Polishing of composites can be achieved by the use of successively finer abrasive disks and interproximal finishing strips; rubber polishing points, cups, and disks impregnated with abrasives; and polishing pastes. A highly polished surface will not be achieved if steps are skipped in progressing from coarser to finer polishers. As with finishing, the polishers should be used by moving from tooth to composite using similar light and intermittent strokes to prevent the generation of heat. Polishing cups or points are used on the occlusal and other accessible surfaces. Some operators like to use polishing brushes (bristles are impregnated with

tiny abrasive silicon carbide polishing particles), e.g., Jiffy brush (Ultradent Products), to produce a high shine on occlusal surfaces. Very fine disks can be used on facial, lingual, and accessible proximal surfaces. Very fine abrasive strips can also be used on proximal surfaces. Some operators will give a final polish with a soft brush and polishing paste to gain a high luster (Fig. 6.19).

 Clinical Tip

The finishing process will be much easier if care is taken during composite placement to carefully develop contours and not grossly overfill the cavity preparation.

Surface Sealers

Some clinicians prefer to add an unfilled resin to the surface of the composite after finishing and polishing. This surface sealer is thought to reseal margins that might have been opened by polymerization shrinkage and to fill in any surface porosities created by small voids or air pockets in the composite that were uncovered by finishing. Finishing itself may introduce microcracks on the surface and the low-viscosity, unfilled resin can help fill and repair them.

To place the unfilled resin, the surface of the composite is rinsed and dried thoroughly; it and the surrounding enamel are etched for 15 seconds, and then a thin layer of the unfilled resin is applied and thinned further with a gentle stream of air and light-cured for 20 seconds. Thick layers might interfere with the occlusion. Interproximal contacts should be flossed to ensure that resin has not been trapped. Some manufacturers are marketing an unfilled resin as a replacement for polishing, because a smooth, glossy surface is obtained. However, the unfilled resin does wear off in about a year, leaving an improperly polished surface that can collect plaque and accelerate wear.

Composite resin has many applications in restorative dentistry. It is a versatile and very esthetic material, but it must be handled properly to maximize its longevity in the harsh environment of the mouth.

WHY COMPOSITES FAIL

It has been estimated that 60% of all operative dentistry work done is to replace failing restorations. Studies have shown that amalgam restorations outlast composite restorations in similar applications. Composite restorations are more technique sensitive than amalgam restorations. However, composite resins have gained in popularity for posterior applications because patients demand esthetic restorations, and they have concerns about metals, especially mercury.

The average lifespan for composite resin restorations (both anterior and posterior) is 5.7 years. Two of the most common reasons for failure of light-cured composites are (1) fracture of the restoration and (2) recurrent caries. Composites are also replaced because of excessive wear, breakdown and leakage at the margins,

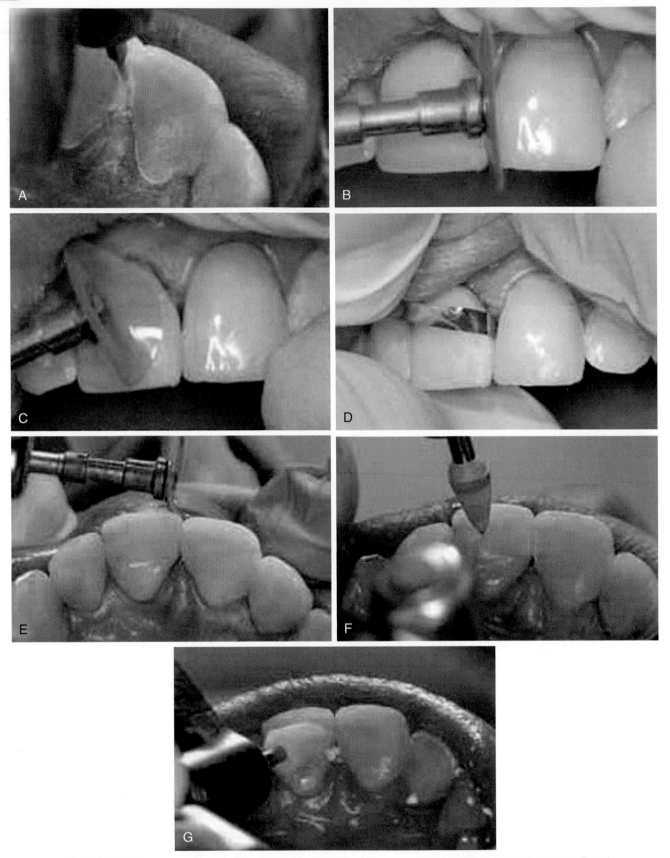

FIG. 6.19 Finishing and polishing. **A,** Fine diamond bur used to reduce excess composite and smooth margins. **B** and **C,** Fine disks used to smooth and contour the composite. **D,** Narrow metal finishing strip used to smooth margins and contour the embrasure surfaces. **E,** Very fine disk used to polish the facial surface. **F** and **G,** Rubber polishing points used to polish the facial and lingual surfaces. (From Contouring, Finishing and Polishing Anterior Composites, by K. William Mopper, DDS, from manuscript in *Inside Dentistry,* March 2011.)

discoloration, and fracture of the tooth. One of the major problems with class II composites is recurrent caries at the gingival margin of the proximal box. Certainly, patient factors such as poor diet, poor oral hygiene, and bruxism can contribute to recurrent caries and fracture, but also operator errors are important causes. Operator errors include poor cavity preparation, inadequate isolation, over- or underetching, improper rinsing and drying of the tooth, poor incremental placement techniques, open proximal contacts, overheating the pulp, and inadequate curing of the bonding agent or composite resin.

COMPOSITE REPAIR

Many clinicians who practice minimally invasive dentistry will attempt to repair existing composites rather than replace them when there are only minor defects at the margins or small areas of chipping. Usually, these are larger composites that are otherwise in good condition. There are no long-term clinical trials that indicate how effective the repair of an existing composite is in the oral environment. However, studies with 2- to 3-year follow-up show good success rates with repair of margins.

The protocol for repairing a newly placed composite differs from that for an older composite. A repair done at the same visit as the initial placement (e.g., the patient bites down and fractures a corner off the marginal ridge just after the restoration has been placed) will have a chemical union between the repair and the initial composite, because there will still be unreacted methacrylate to join with the new addition. However, the older the composite gets, the fewer unreacted methacrylate groups will be present. So, the repair will need to rely more heavily on mechanical retention than bonding. The bond of the new composite to the old composite in this case will be less than 50% of the initially placed composite. The most successful repairs occur when there is enamel rather than dentin on the tooth side of the repair.

INDIRECT-PLACEMENT COMPOSITE RESINS

Indirect-placement esthetic materials are tooth-colored materials that are constructed outside of the mouth (chair-side or in the laboratory), and then cemented in place. Composites can be used for indirect methods as well as direct. Some indirect-placement composite restorations are fabricated on a die (replica of the prepared tooth) and others are designed and milled from a block of composite material using CAD/CAM (computer-assisted design/computer-assisted machining) technology (see Chapter 9 Dental Ceramics). The finished restoration is tried in the mouth, adjusted, and bonded into place with bonding agent and resin cement. Indirect materials were developed to try to eliminate the problems associated with polymerization shrinkage, such as marginal leakage, post-treatment sensitivity, and recurrent caries, and to reduce the wear seen with direct composites.

LABORATORY-PROCESSED COMPOSITES

An impression of the preparation, opposing cast, bite registration (or digital versions of these items taken with an optical scanner) and a prescription with the proper shade are sent to the laboratory for construction of the restoration. There are several advantages to having the restoration constructed in the laboratory. The technician can process the composite material under heat and pressure. This creates a restoration that is denser, polymerized more completely, and is tougher. The polymerization shrinkage occurs outside of the mouth, and then the restoration is cemented with a thin layer of resin cement. Shrinkage from the thin layer of resin cement is much less than would have occurred with a composite that is cured in the tooth. Therefore, less stress is created internally on the composite and the walls of the cavity preparation. Microleakage should be reduced.

Blocks of composite for CAD/CAM milling have also been processed under heat and pressure to gain the advantages discussed for laboratory processed composites.

Materials for Indirect Composites

Different types of composite materials can be used:
1. Conventional composite
2. Fiber-reinforced composite, which contains a fiber mesh composed of carbon Kevlar (similar to the material used in bulletproof vests), glass fibers, or polyethylene for improved strength
3. Particle-reinforced composite, which is heavily filled (70% to 80% by weight) with particles of nano-sized ceramic filler. An advance in CAD/CAM composite blocks is Lava Ultimate (3M ESPE) (see the section CAD/CAM Technology in Chapter 9). Lava Ultimate is a composite that is composed of nanoceramic fillers in a heat-treated, highly cross-linked resin matrix. It has high flexural strength, increased wear resistance, long-lasting polish, and stain resistance. Its initial strength is greater than blocks of feldspathic or leucite-reinforced porcelain (see Chapter 9), is not as brittle, and is less prone to cracking under functional loads. It causes less wear of the opposing enamel than ceramic materials. It can be repaired with conventional nanohybrid composites. It can be used to fabricate onlays, inlays, and veneers. It is not recommended for full coverage crowns, because it is somewhat flexible under chewing forces causing the cement bonds to break. After adjustments it can be re-polished with rubber polishing points, and then with extrafine (5 µm) diamond polishing paste on a bristle brush for a high shine.

Indirect chairside technique. An impression is made of the prepared tooth with alginate. Immediately, a fast-setting die stone or a polyvinyl siloxane die material (e.g., Mach-2 Die-Silicone, Parkell) is injected

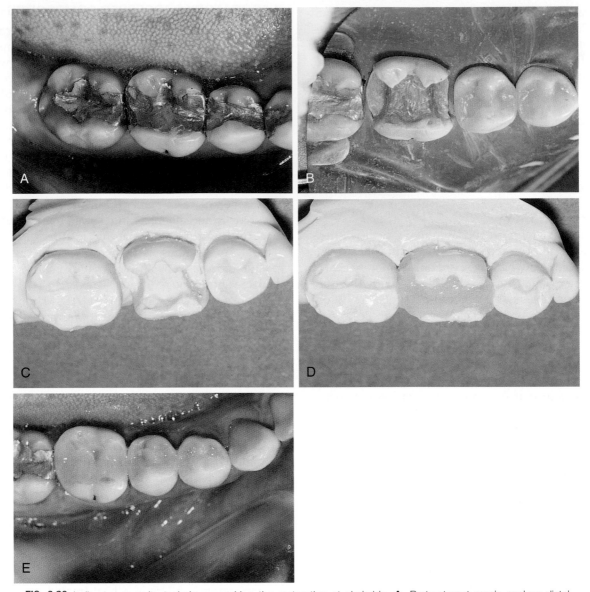

FIG. 6.20 Indirect composite technique—making the restoration at chairside. **A,** Pretreatment mesio-occluso-distal (MOD) amalgam restoration in the lower first molar. **B,** Tooth prepared for MOD composite inlay. **C,** Polyvinyl siloxane die of the preparation from an alginate impression. **D,** Composite inlay prepared outside of the mouth at chairside. **E,** Composite inlay after cementation with a resin cement. (Courtesy of Alton Lacy, University of California School of Dentistry [San Francisco, CA].)

into the impression. The resulting die is used to make the restoration with light-cured composite material at the chairside. The composite restoration is seated into the preparation and adjusted. It is removed from the mouth and polished on the die. Then it is cemented with resin cement in the same manner as laboratory-processed composite inlays (Fig. 6.20).

GLASS IONOMER CEMENTS

Glass ionomer cements are categorized in two main forms:
- Conventional glass ionomers
- Resin-modified glass ionomers (also called hybrid ionomers)

CONVENTIONAL GLASS IONOMER CEMENTS

Glass ionomer cements (GICs) were introduced in the early 1970s by Wilson and Kent. GICs are self-cured, fluoride-releasing materials that bond to tooth structure directly without a bonding agent. They are made by mixing a water-soluble polyacrylic acid (pH 1.0) with fluoroaluminosilicate glass powder (base). An acid-base reaction occurs when the liquid and powder are mixed. The acid is neutralized by the base and fluoride and other ions are released.

Several GIC materials have been developed and classified for use in dentistry:

Type I: Luting (cementation) agents
Type II: Restorative materials
Type III: Liners and bases for cavity preparations

The materials in these three types are similar in chemical composition, but the size of the powder particles and the ratios of powder and liquid are different.

PHYSICAL AND MECHANICAL PROPERTIES

Glass ionomers have some highly desirable characteristics, as well as some drawbacks:

Biocompatibility: Glass ionomers are tolerated well by surrounding soft tissues and are considered kind to the pulp.

Bond to Enamel and Dentin: GICs bond directly to the enamel and dentin. They are the only restorative materials that form an ionic (chemical) bond to tooth. The carboxyl group of the polyalkenoic acid chemically bonds to calcium in the tooth hydroxyapatite. With GIC there is no intermediate bonding agent that can hydrolyze over time as with composites. GICs shrink about 2% to 3%, but because they set gradually, they do not generate the great internal stresses that might break bonds to the tooth, as composite resins do with their rapid set. They absorb water over time and this helps to offset the contraction. Therefore, glass ionomers maintain their seal to the tooth better.

On a tooth surface that has been prepared with a carbide or diamond bur or hand instrument, a *smear layer* forms (see Chapter 5). As with resin bonding agents in order for the GIC to bond to the tooth, the smear layer must be removed. To remove only the smear layer and not the calcium in the surface of the preparation, a weak acid (usually 10% polyacrylic acid) is applied for 10 seconds, and then rinsed and lightly dried. Phosphoric acid used to etch the tooth before application of bonding agents should not be used on dentin. It is too aggressive and removes not only the smear layer but also removes a layer of hydroxyapatite from the dentin. That leaves collagen exposed. The GIC cannot bond to the collagen, and therefore no bond is formed. The restoration may leak, have postoperative sensitivity, and may fall out.

Although the bond strength of GIC to the tooth is about one-fourth that of composite, the bond in non-stressed areas is adequate. The seal to the tooth, however, is superior on dentin compared with that achieved with composite, and thus microleakage is minimized. On root surfaces where maximal esthetics is not necessary, GIC should be considered instead of composite. For noncarious cervical lesions (abrasion/abfraction/erosion) the root surface is usually very smooth and difficult to bond to. A carbide or coarse diamond bur should be used to roughen the surface before removing the smear layer and placing the GIC.

Fluoride release: GICs release an initially high level of fluoride for the first few days, and then the fluoride levels fall to low levels. They can absorb fluoride from in-office applications, fluoride rinses, or fluoride toothpaste and re-release it, thereby acting as a fluoride reservoir. The assumed caries-preventing effects of the fluoride released from glass ionomer cements have not been proved in clinical studies but are based on laboratory test results. Fluoride has some antibacterial properties as well, and it is thought to suppress the streptococci associated with tooth decay.

Solubility: Among the less desirable properties of GICs is their sensitivity to moisture uptake or loss during the first 24 hours after placement. They are highly soluble during this time and should be covered with a protective varnish. They also are prone to crack or craze (develop numerous shallow cracks on their surface) if dried too much during the first 24 hours. Earlier generations of the glass ionomers could not be finished until they had completely set after 24 hours. Newer materials can be finished within a few minutes of their set and are not as sensitive to moisture uptake or loss.

Thermal expansion and contraction: They have thermal expansion and contraction similar to tooth structure and stiffness (modulus of elasticity) comparable to dentin.

Thermal protection: They are good insulators against temperature extremes.

Compressive and tensile strength: They have a moderately high compressive strength but are weaker in tension and are relatively brittle in thin sections. New formulations that use modified polyacrylic acid have better fracture toughness, but they still should not be used in stress-bearing areas such as occlusal surfaces and incisal edges for permanent teeth.

Wear resistance: Glass ionomers wear faster than composite resins. Their surface gets rougher over time. They cannot be polished to as smooth a surface as composites.

Radiopacity: They are more radiopaque than dentin.

Color: Glass ionomers are more opaque than composites. Translucency and the number of colors available have improved over the years.

PACKAGING

GICs are supplied in three ways: (1) hand-mixed powder and liquid, (2) encapsulated powder and liquid, and (3) two-paste systems. The powder and liquid can be measured and mixed quickly (usually less than 30 seconds) at chairside on a paper pad, and then delivered on an instrument into the cavity preparation. The material also comes in capsules with premeasured powder and liquid. The capsule is activated by rupturing a membrane that separates the powder from the liquid. The capsule is placed in a triturator and is mixed at speeds and times recommended by the manufacturer. The capsule is then inserted into a gun-type applicator and delivered into the cavity preparation through a nozzle on the capsule. The third method of delivery is a paste-paste system. Very fine glass powder is used in the pastes to provide a creamy consistency to the mixed pastes. The two pastes are contained in a two-chambered cartridge and are dispensed in equal portions onto a paper pad. The pastes are quickly mixed together and applied to the preparation. A variation of the third delivery method uses a two-chambered cartridge with two pastes that are mixed with an automixing tip and delivered directly into the cavity preparation with a fine nozzle.

The GICs are manufactured in a variety of shades but not in the wide selection available with composites.

USES FOR GLASS IONOMER CEMENTS

Luting Cements

(See also Chapter 14 Dental Cement.) Glass ionomer luting cements were once very popular because they are pulpally kind, bond to tooth structure, release fluoride, and have a low film thickness, so crowns can be seated easily. Their use has decreased since the introduction of hybrid ionomer cements and resin cements that have better physical and mechanical properties (stronger and less soluble). These newer and stronger hybrid ionomer cements are also used to cement orthodontic brackets and have the advantage over resin cements of releasing fluoride into the surrounding enamel. The objective is to help prevent decalcification seen as white lines around brackets or bands, which often occurs when patients' oral hygiene efforts are poor.

Restorative Materials

Glass ionomer restoratives are used in non–stress-bearing areas, because they are weak in tensile strength and are not as wear resistant as composites. They are used for restoration of root caries, because they bond to the root better than composites and release fluoride to resist recurrent caries. They are useful for restoration of noncarious cervical lesions (such as toothbrush abrasion), because they can be placed conservatively without the need for cutting away sound tooth structure to create mechanical locks in the tooth to retain the restoration, as is necessary with amalgam. Studies show that they are better retained than composites in class V preparations. They can be used in anterior class III cavities when color match is not an issue. Encapsulated materials are desirable, because powder-to-liquid ratios are improved. Mixing is done in a triturator and provides a consistent mix with less trapped air than is seen with hand-mixing. The mixed material can also be dispensed directly into the cavity from the capsules, which have a dispensing tip attached (Fig. 6.21).

Cermets. In the 1980s GIC restoratives called *cermets* (e.g., Ketac Silver [3M ESPE]; Miracle Mix [GC America]) were developed to improve on the properties of GIC. These products have silver particles added to improve their wear resistance and strength. However, the gain in strength is still inadequate to use them in stress-bearing areas. Because they are dark gray in color, cermets are used in locations where esthetics is not a concern and as core buildup materials when the bulk of the subsequent crown will be supported by tooth structure.

Liners and bases. Glass ionomer liners are materials used to cover the dentin for pulpal protection from chemicals within other restorative materials or acid etchants. They have low powder content and are applied in thin layers that are relatively weak. Glass ionomer bases are used to rebuild missing dentin within the cavity preparation and provide thermal protection for the pulp, especially with metal restorations such as amalgam. They are usually much thicker layers than liners. They have a higher powder content and stronger mechanical properties.

Lamination or "sandwich" technique. On occasion, glass ionomer is used in combination with another restorative material to gain the best properties of each material. In 1985 John McLean described a lamination technique (called the "sandwich" technique) with GIC and composite resin. It is most commonly used when the proximal box of a deep class II cavity preparation has the gingival floor located on the root rather than enamel. GIC is placed as the first layer on the gingival floor of the proximal box. Glass ionomer can obtain a better seal to the root than composite and additionally will release fluoride into the surrounding root surface to resist secondary decay. Composite resin is used to complete the restoration (Fig. 6.22).

> **Clinical Tip**
>
> Before applying glass ionomer cement to a cavity preparation, remove the smear layer that forms when a preparation is cut. Use a conditioner (typically 10% polyacrylic acid) for 10 seconds on enamel and dentin. Rinse and lightly dry. The clean surface will allow the glass ionomer to bond to the calcium in the tooth surface. Do *not* use phosphoric acid. It is too aggressive on dentin and will remove the calcium from the surface and expose collagen. GIC cannot bond to collagen.

Glass ionomer cement (GIC) as fissure sealant. Glass ionomer cements have been used as fissure sealants because of their fluoride release. Some GICs (Fuji VII and Fuji Triage, GC America) have been formulated to have very high fluoride content (about six times as much as regular GIC). Studies have shown that they are not retained as well as resin sealants. GIC is fairly thick and does not penetrate fissures as well as resin sealants. However, those who advocate the use of GIC suggest that it will provide fluoride to

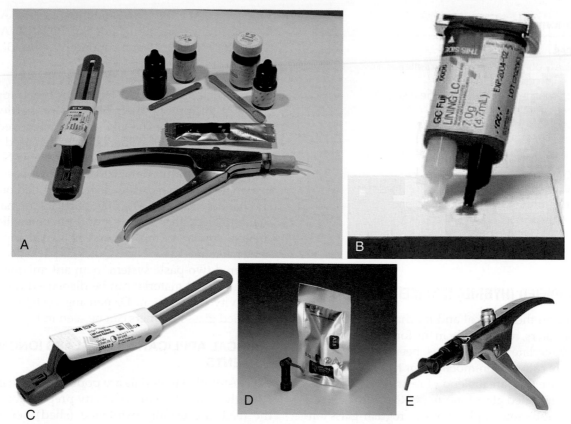

FIG. 6.21 Delivery systems for glass ionomer cements (regular and resin-modified). **A,** Glass ionomer may be supplied as powder and liquid in containers with powder measuring spoons (liner and luting at *top left* and *right,* respectively) or as powder and liquid premeasured in capsules. The encapsulated material is mixed in a triturator and delivered by a gun dispenser *(bottom).* **B,** Paste-paste resin-modified GIC dispenser. **C,** Glass ionomer may also come in a paste-paste system with a dispenser that distributes the proper proportions (the green clicker system). **D,** Packaging of single-unit automix capsule for two-paste resin-modified GIC. **E,** Two-paste capsule activated and in delivery gun with dispensing nozzle extended. (**B-E,** From Sakaguchi RL, Powers JM: *Craig's Restorative Dental Materials* (ed 13). St. Louis, 2012, Elsevier.)

Sandwich technique
in a Class II cavity preparation

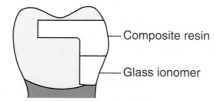

Composite resin

Glass ionomer

Glass ionomer (GI) is "sandwiched" between the tooth and composite. GI seals better on the root while composite is more wear resistant and esthetically pleasing.

FIG. 6.22 Sandwich technique with glass ionomer "sandwiched" between the tooth and composite restoration.

the newly erupted tooth surface and make it more resistant to future caries. Newly erupted enamel does not contain as much mineral, including fluoride, as enamel that has been exposed to saliva for some years. Saliva is a supersaturated solution of calcium and phosphate ions and contains fluoride from drinking water, toothpaste, and other sources. These high fluoride-containing materials are also used as provisional restorations in caries-active patients who need caries control measures before final restorations are placed.

Atraumatic restorative treatment. In developing countries with rural villages or in areas of high poverty in the United States where dental treatment is not available, dental caries often goes untreated, and serious and painful abscesses can occur. The atraumatic restorative treatment (ART) technique allows non–dentally trained personnel to help stop or slow down the progression of open carious lesions without the use of dental drills. The way it works is that treating personnel dig out as much decay as they can from frank open cavities with whatever implements they have. Next, they mix specially formulated high-viscosity GIC (e.g., Ketac Molar [3M ESPE] or Fuji IX [GC America]). The mix is rolled between the fingers into a ball and is pressed by hand into the cavity. The patient bites down while the material is still soft, to establish the occlusion. Excess material is wiped away. Although a less than ideal procedure, it helps to maintain teeth when no other options are available.

Glass Ionomer Cements

ADVANTAGES

- Chemically bond to enamel and dentin
- Release fluoride
- Take up fluoride to act as a fluoride reservoir
- Reduced microleakage on dentin
- Reduced postoperative sensitivity
- Biocompatible
- Expand and contract similar to tooth structure

DISADVANTAGES

- High wear rate
- Too weak for stress-bearing restorations
- Less esthetic (more opaque) than composites
- Cannot polish as well as composite—surface rough
- Initially sensitive to water loss or uptake

RESIN-MODIFIED (HYBRID) IONOMERS

To improve on the physical and mechanical properties of glass ionomers, resin mostly in the form of 2-hydroxyethyl methacrylate (HEMA) has been added. These materials are called **resin-modified (or hybrid) glass ionomers** because they are a blend of resin and glass ionomer. Resin-modified glass ionomers (RMGICs) are used for many of the same applications as regular glass ionomers. They have some properties of composites and many of the properties of glass ionomers. Resin makes them stronger, more esthetic, more polishable, and more wear resistant. They are more esthetic than GIC, because they are not as opaque. Once the resin polymerizes, it protects the material from exposure to moisture and drying while the acid-base reaction goes to completion. The polymerized resin makes the RMGIC less soluble and gives it early strength. RMGICs can be finished immediately after placement. They release fluoride into the surrounding tooth structure and into the saliva, and they can absorb fluoride from fluoride products to act as a fluoride reservoir and gradually re-release the absorbed fluoride. Their thermal expansion and contraction is similar to tooth structure.

Resin-modified glass ionomers are available as light-cured materials. Light polymerization of the resin component occurs in a similar fashion to composite resins. Most of these materials also have a chemical cure of the resin in the absence of light, as well as the acid-base reaction of the glass ionomer cement. The chemical cure allows for final curing in locations where light cannot reach, but it takes longer to cure than when light activated. For example, if the margin of a gold crown with caries was repaired with glass ionomer cement, the cement up under the margin would not be accessible to the curing light because of the gold but would chemically cure in a few minutes. Examples of restorative RMGICs are Fuji II LC (GC America), Riva Light Cure (SDI), and Photac Fil (3M ESPE).

RMGIC is formulated for use as lining cement and luting cement as well. Examples of GIC liners are Vitrebond (3M ESPE) and Fuji Lining LC (GC America). RMGIC luting cements include Fuji Plus (GC America), Nexus RMGI (Kerr Dental), and RelyX Plus (3M ESPE).

NANO-IONOMERS

Nanoparticle technology has also been applied to RMGICs to improve their physical properties. These **nano-ionomers**, or nano-GICs, have improved esthetics (they match tooth colors better), increased wear resistance, and improved polishability. Ketac Nano (3M ESPE) was introduced in 2007. It is a two-paste system in a dual-chamber cartridge that is extruded onto a pad and hand-spatulated. The filler particles are nanosized, silane-treated silica particles and zirconia-silica nanoclusters similar to those found in nanocomposites. A newer version (Ketac Nano Quick) is packaged as a premeasured two-paste system in an automixing capsule, and the mixed material can be dispensed directly into the cavity preparation. Dispensing systems for resin-modified glass ionomers can be seen in Fig. 6.21, A-D.

CLINICAL APPLICATION OF GLASS IONOMER CEMENTS

GIC restorative materials are popular for use in primary teeth for most classes of cavity preparation, because the teeth are usually exfoliated (shed) before excessive wear can become a problem. They can be used for crown buildups when half or more of the tooth structure remains to help support the crown. Otherwise, they lack the strength necessary to reliably support the crown on their own. They are very useful for restoring root caries because they provide a better seal to the root than composite resins (Fig. 6.23).

As previously mentioned, the smear layer must be removed from the prepared enamel and dentin to allow the formation of a chemical bond between the GIC and the calcium on the surface. After the smear layer is removed with a mild acid (polyacrylic acid conditioner), and rinsed off, the preparation is lightly dried, not totally desiccated. The GIC is applied to the clean surface and a chemical bond will form.

The GIC can be delivered to the cavity preparation directly from the nozzle of the capsule, or, if hand-mixed, it is picked up on an instrument and placed in the preparation. It can be contoured somewhat with a plastic instrument or with a cervical matrix. Unlike composite, GIC is not very viscous and cannot be readily shaped before it sets. Typically, the cavity preparation is slightly overfilled and final contouring is accomplished with carbide or diamond finishing burs under water spray.

It is important when placing the GIC to stop manipulating it when the initial gel stage begins. The gel stage can be identified by a loss of shininess of the material and an increase in viscosity. Working time varies from 1.5 to 3 minutes, depending on the manufacturer and whether or not the material is regular or fast set. Even light-cured hybrid GIC starts to gel in less than 3 minutes in the oral cavity when not exposed to the curing light. After

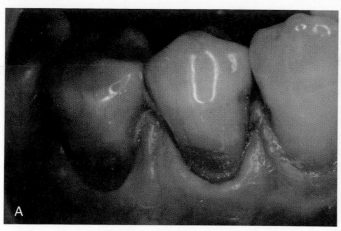
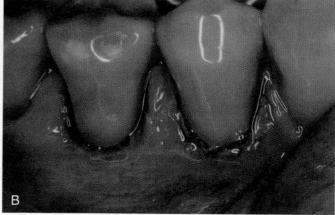

FIG. 6.23 Restoration of root surface lesion. **A.** Abrasion/erosion lesion on mandibular second premolar **B.** Lesion was restored with resin-modified glass ionomer cement. (Courtesy Dr. Thomas J. Hilton, Portland, OR.)

approximately 5 minutes, the new formulations of conventional GICs can be contoured and finished with carbide or diamond finishing burs or abrasive disks. Light-cured RMGICs can be finished right away. It is best to apply a protective varnish that is usually furnished with the material or to coat it with an unfilled resin surface sealer. Even though the material has gone to its initial set, an acid-base reaction still occurs for several hours within the material. The coating protects it from excessive uptake of moisture from the saliva. Core buildup GICs can be reduced as part of the crown preparation after the initial set. They will be protected by the provisional crown until the final crown is cemented. The glass ionomer cements have grown in popularity as their handling characteristics, esthetics, and ease of use have improved.

COMPOMERS

Compomers are essentially composite resins that have been modified with polyacid. The resin component contains polycarboxylic acid and methacrylates together. This provides methacrylate groups for cross-linking as with composites and carboxyl groups for the acid-base reaction as with glass ionomers, hence the name *compomers*. The idea was to join the good qualities of the composite (namely strength, wear resistance, esthetics, and polishability) with the fluoride release of the glass ionomer. Light-activation chemicals are included to make the compomers light-cured. The fillers (about 45% to 65% filled by volume) are glasses similar to those used in composites, along with some fluoride-releasing silicate glasses, and range in size from 0.8 to 5.0 μm. The release of fluoride, however, is not the same as with the glass ionomers, because the resin binds these fillers together as soon as the light activation starts the curing process. Fluoride release is delayed for some months and does not seem to be at all comparable to that of the self-cured or light-cured glass ionomers. Likewise, there is little or no recharging of the compomer with fluoride as with glass ionomers. Some compomers have fluoride-releasing monomers

added to enhance the level of fluoride release, but this is still much less than with glass ionomers.

Compomers for restorations are available as a light-cured single paste that is packaged in compules or syringes or in a flowable form much like flowable composites. Common brands include Dyract eXtra (Dentsply Sirona) (see Fig. 6.24) and Compoglass F (Ivoclar Vivadent). Compomers are made for luting as well and are manufactured as a powder and liquid or as a two-paste dual cartridge with automixing capability. Luting agents may be chemical-cured, light-cured, or dual-cured.

The setting reaction in restorative compomers occurs in two phases. Phase 1 is similar to that of the light-activated composite resins and forms a resin network encompassing the fillers. This causes the material to harden in the cavity preparation. Phase 2 is an acid-base reaction that occurs more slowly over several days as the restoration absorbs water.

Compomers do not bond to tooth structure through ion exchange as glass ionomers do. Acid etching and primer

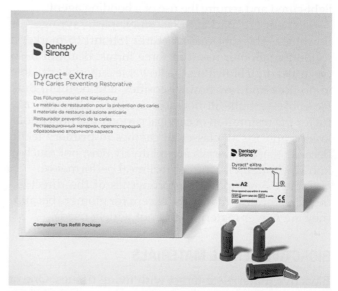

FIG. 6.24 Compomer restorative material. Dyract eXtra (Dentsply Sirona) in compules. (Courtesy Dentsply Sirona.)

TABLE 6.5	Comparison of Properties of Direct Esthetic Restorative Materials						
MATERIAL	**COLOR MATCH**	**BONDING AGENT NEEDED**	**FLUORIDE RELEASE**	**WEAR RATE**	**POLISHABILITY**	**COMPRESSIVE STRENGTH**	**FLEXURAL STRENGTH**
Glass ionomer	Low	No	High	High	Low	Low	Low
Hybrid ionomer	Medium	No	Medium	Medium	Medium	Medium	Medium
Compomer	High	Yes	Low	Medium	High	Medium	Medium
Microfill composite	High	Yes	No	High	High	Medium	Medium
Hybrid (nano) composite	High	Yes	No	Low	High	High	High

Adapted from Craig RG, Powers JM, Wataha JC: *Dental Materials: Properties and Manipulation*, ed 7, St. Louis, 2000, Mosby.

or adhesive are indicated during placement of the compomers. The bond strength to dentin is about the same as that of a hybrid glass ionomer. The bonding agents will reduce the chances of fluoride leaching from the material into the dentin. Research indicates that they have about the same cervical margin adaptation as composite resins. They can be used in most situations where a microfilled composite would be used, that is, mostly for low stress–bearing class III and V restorations. Finishing and polishing is accomplished the same as for composites.

GIOMERS

Giomers are relatively new hybrid restorative materials. The name "giomer" is derived from the words "glass ionomer" and "composite" as these new materials have some of the desirable properties of each. Giomers release fluoride but less of it and at a slower rate than glass ionomers. They can be recharged with fluoride from toothpaste or mouth rinse to act as a fluoride reservoir. They obtain their fluoride from fillers that are a product of the reaction between fluoroalumino silicate glass and polyalkenoic acid. These pre-reacted glass ionomer fillers are added to a urethane resin that has silica fillers. The filled resin component provides good handling properties, esthetics, and polishability. Like composites and compomers, they are light-cured and require the use of a bonding agent.

Giomers are packaged as single-paste syringes or flowables. The first manufacturer (Shofu) to market a restorative giomer has it in three forms: Beautifil II—a paste, Beautifil Flow Plus—a flowable material available in no-flow and low-flow viscosities, and Beautifil Bulk Flowable—a bulk-fill flowable material. They are useful for the restoration of cervical carious and noncarious lesions and for all classes of cavities in primary teeth. Because these materials are relatively new, not much is known about their long-term clinical performance.

Table 6.5 compares the properties of the direct esthetic restorative materials (except for giomers because they are newer materials and not widely used).

BIOACTIVE DENTAL MATERIALS

Bioactive materials interact with living tissues. One of the first bioactive materials was a bone grafting material, Bioglass, which formed chemical bonds with bone. Bioactive dental cements were introduced in the mid 1990s with ProRoot MTA (Dentsply, Tulsa Dental Specialties) for root sealing and repair.

In dentistry the term bioactivity has come to mean the ability of a material to form apatite-like substance on its surface when exposed to body fluid such as saliva. The dental biomaterials with this apatite-forming ability used in clinical applications fit into two groups: calcium silicates and calcium aluminates. When powders of these materials are mixed with water they undergo an acid-base reaction that culminates in an alkaline pH when set. The higher pH tends to stimulate more bioactivity. Their physical strength and mechanical properties are similar to conventional glass ionomer cement. Calcium aluminate– and calcium silicate–based cements have been shown to have some degree of bonding to dentin. These bioactive cements have been used primarily as liners and pulp capping materials (TheraCal LC, BISCO), bases (Biodentine, Septodont), and luting cements (Ceranir, Doxa) to remineralize and stimulate repair of dentin and as endodontic sealer (EndoSequence BC Sealer, Brasseler USA) or root repair materials (ProRoot MTA).

More recently, the bioactive materials have been added to resins to promote bioactivity. One product, Activa (Pulpdent), claims to be a bulk fill, bioactive composite that penetrates and seals dentin and stimulates apatite formation. Newer bioactive materials show promise but need to establish a sound clinical record before gaining widespread acceptance.

SUMMARY

Composite resins are very popular direct-placement esthetic materials. They have a wide variety of uses in both the anterior and posterior parts of the mouth. They are esthetically pleasing and durable restorative materials that are rapidly replacing amalgam as the material of first choice in posterior teeth. They have applications in all classes of cavity preparations and many cosmetic applications. They can be used to close anterior diastemas as a conservative alternative to porcelain veneers. Indirect composites also have applications where reduced shrinkage and added strength can be achieved by processing the material in the laboratory or by using preprocessed composite blocks for CAD/CAM technology. Glass ionomer cement restorative materials are not as esthetically pleasing and strong as composite resin and cannot be polished to a high shine, but they offer the advantages of bonding directly to the tooth without a bonding agent and providing a better seal to the root structure. They have wide applications in pediatric dentistry and for restoration of root caries in the elderly. Compomers are materials that are closer to composites than to glass ionomers but do not have the best qualities of either material. Like giomers, they are not widely used. Bioactive materials with the capability to repair and remineralize damaged dentin show much promise.

INSTRUCTIONAL VIDEOS

See the Evolve Resources site for a variety of educational videos that reinforce the material covered in this chapter.

Procedure 6.1 Placement of Class II Composite Resin Restoration

See Evolve site for Competency Sheet.

Consider the following with this procedure: *safety glasses are recommended for the patient, PPE is required for the operator, ensure appropriate safety protocols are followed, and check your local state guidelines before performing this procedure.*

EQUIPMENT/SUPPLIES (FIG. 6.24)
- Rubber dam setup
- Curing light and light shield
- Composite placement instruments
- Light-cured nanohybrid composite resin
- Bonding agent and finishing glaze
- Mixing wells or Dappen dish
- Finishing burs, diamonds, disks
- Articulating paper in paper forceps
- Local and topical anesthesia setup
- High-volume evacuator tip
- High- and low-speed handpieces
- Shade guide
- Etchant and applicator
- Matrix system and wedges
- Polishing points, cups, paste

PROCEDURE STEPS
1. Apply topical anesthetic. Local anesthetic is administered.
2. Take a composite shade. Hold the shade guide close to the patient's mouth and select two or three shade tabs that are close to the patient's tooth color. Moisten and check each tab individually against the tooth under room light (and natural light, if possible) (Fig. 6.25). Verify the shade by taking a

small amount of composite in the closest shade and light-curing it on the tooth for 20 seconds.

NOTE: Shade is taken before the rubber dam is applied, because the color of the dam might interfere with taking an accurate shade, and the teeth might dry out under the dam and appear lighter. Lipstick should be removed, and brightly colored clothing should be covered with a pale blue or gray patient bib to prevent the colors from influencing the perceived shade.

3. Apply the rubber dam.

NOTE: Cotton roll isolation can be used, but a rubber dam provides more reliable isolation. Moisture from the breath can affect the bond adversely.

4. Rinse and dry the cavity prepared by the dentist.
5. Apply a sectional matrix, wedge, and pressure ring (Fig. 6.26).

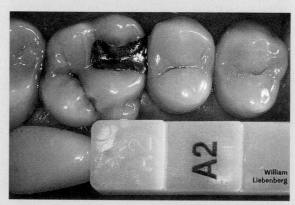

FIG. 6.26 (Courtesy of Dr. William Liebenberg. North Vancouver, BC, Canada.)

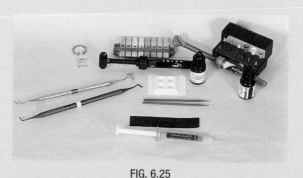

FIG. 6.25

NOTE: A Tofflemire matrix can be used, but it is much more difficult to obtain tight contact when both mesial and distal interproximal spaces have matrix band in them at the same time. The wedge helps close the matrix band at the gingival margin to prevent overhang of composite, and it helps separate the teeth to make up for the thickness of the matrix band so that firm contact with the adjacent tooth can be established. The pressure ring helps adapt the matrix against the facial and lingual surfaces of the tooth and helps separate the teeth slightly.

Continued

6. Apply etchant to enamel first for 10 to 20 seconds, and then apply it to dentin for 10 seconds (Fig. 6.27).

NOTE: Etching dentin for longer than 10 seconds will overetch it and contribute to weaker bond strength and postoperative sensitivity by opening the tubules excessively. A self-etching bonding system could be used instead, and no rinsing would be needed (see Chapter 5).

7. Rinse thoroughly and dry lightly so that the dentin remains slightly moist (glistening but no pooling of water).

NOTE: Drying the dentin will cause collapse of the collagen fibrils and interference with penetration of the dentin primer into the tubules and etched dentin surface (see Chapter 5).

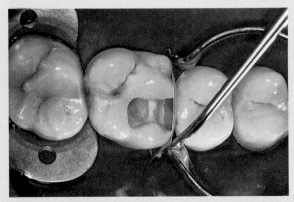

FIG. 6.27 (Courtesy of William Liebenberg. North Vancouver, BC, Canada.)

8. Apply dentin primer/bonding resin with a brush applicator as directed by the manufacturer (dentist's choice of one- or two-bottle bonding materials) and thin with a gentle stream of air (Fig. 6.28).

NOTE: See Chapter 5 for one- and two-bottle dentin primers and bonding resins. When the dentin primer and bonding resin are applied in separate steps, the dentin primer is usually light-cured for 10 to 20 seconds before placement of the bonding resin. Some dentists prefer to use a base or liner on the dentin before acid etching.

9. Dry gently and light-cure for 20 seconds.

NOTE: Drying at this step removes water and volatile solvents from the resin.

10. Apply composite resin in small increments, starting with the proximal box (Fig. 6.29). Each increment should be no more than 2 mm thick and light-cured for 20 to 40 seconds.

NOTE: Small increments are used to minimize the effects of polymerization shrinkage and to allow the light to cure the increment all the way through. Dark or opaque shades are more difficult for the light to penetrate and require longer curing times. Increase the curing time when the light probe is more than 1 mm from the composite. Some curing lights may have an initial low setting that ramps up to a high intensity to minimize shrinkage and stress within the material. Some very high intensity curing lights require less curing time. Manufacturers' recommendations should be followed.

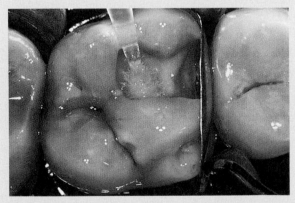

FIG. 6.29 (Courtesy of William Liebenberg. North Vancouver, BC, Canada.)

11. Remove the pressure ring, wedge, and matrix band after the cavity preparation is slightly overfilled with composite and cured. Cure the proximal box for an additional 20 to 40 seconds from the facial and the lingual sides. Contour the occlusal surface and remove excess material with finishing diamond and carbide burs. Disks and interproximal finishing strips are used on the proximal surfaces (Fig. 6.30). Check the contact area with floss to ensure solid contact and no overhang at the gingival margin.

NOTE: The composite in the proximal box should be cured again from the facial and lingual sides after removal of the matrix and wedge, because these

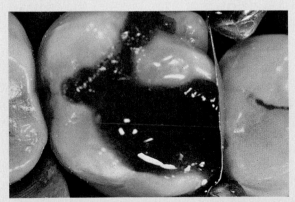

FIG. 6.28 (Courtesy of William Liebenberg. North Vancouver, BC, Canada.)

Procedure 6.1   Placement of Class II Composite Resin Restoration—cont'd

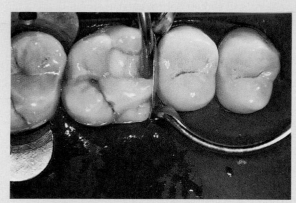

FIG. 6.30 (Courtesy of William Liebenberg. North Vancouver, BC, Canada.)

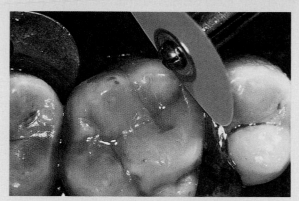

FIG. 6.31 (Courtesy of William Liebenberg. North Vancouver, BC, Canada.)

materials may have partially blocked light transmission to the floor of the box, causing an incomplete cure of the composite.

12. Remove the rubber dam. Check occlusal contacts with articulating paper and adjust.

NOTE: A high restoration can cause a sore tooth by stressing the periodontal ligament, or a tooth that is temperature sensitive.

13. Polish surfaces with polishing points, cups and brushes at low speed. A polishing paste can be used to produce a highly polished surface (Fig. 6.31).

NOTE: Some operators prefer to apply a finishing glaze to the composite. A finishing glaze is an unfilled resin that bonds to the composite resin. Its purpose is to reseal the margins if polymerization shrinkage has caused composite to pull away from the enamel margin, and it fills in any small voids in the surface that contribute to wear and staining. When the glaze is used, the tooth is isolated with cotton rolls, and the composite and adjacent enamel are etched for 10

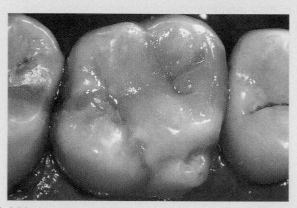

FIG. 6.32 (Courtesy of Dr. William Liebenberg. North Vancouver, BC, Canada.)

seconds, rinsed, and dried. A brush is used to apply a very thin layer of glaze so as not to interfere with the occlusion. It is light-cured for 20 seconds.

Get Ready for Exams!

Review Questions

Select the one correct response for each of the following multiple-choice questions.

1. The major components of composite dental materials include all of the following *except* one. Which one is this *exception?*
   a. Bonding agent
   b. Resin matrix
   c. Coupling agent
   d. Fillers

2. Composite resins are often classified according to their
   a. Strength
   b. Polishability
   c. Resin content
   d. Filler particle size

Continued

Get Ready for Exams!—cont'd

3. The shortcomings of flowable composites as compared with more viscous microhybrid composites include all of the following *except* one. Which one is this *exception?*
   a. They are weaker.
   b. They wear faster.
   c. They shrink more when polymerized.
   d. They are more difficult to polish.

4. The purpose of a silane coupling agent for composite resins is
   a. To improve the bond between the filler particles and the resin matrix
   b. To help the composite retain its color
   c. To reduce the oxygen-inhibited layer
   d. To help the various layers stick together

5. The curing light requires repair
   a. If it causes a slower set of a dark-color composite
   b. If it has not been tested
   c. If a 2-mm-thick piece of composite does not cure through the bottom at the recommended exposure time
   d. If the light appears blue

6. Polymerization shrinkage of a composite
   a. Is cause for alarm
   b. Is greater than 10% of the volume
   c. Can be minimized by placing and curing a series of small increments
   d. Has no effect on the final restoration

7. Fillers are composed of all of the following *except* one. Which one is this *exception?*
   a. Quartz
   b. Alumina
   c. Silica
   d. Glass

8. Which one of the following statements about a coupling agent is *false?*
   a. It minimizes the loss of filler particles.
   b. It reduces wear.
   c. It prevents filler from sticking to the resin.
   d. It is made of silane.

9. All of the following will increase the wear of a composite restoration *except* one. Which one is this *exception?*
   a. Use of large filler particles
   b. Incompletely curing the composite
   c. Use of small amount of filler particles
   d. Saliva contamination of the etched enamel

10. Which one of the following types of composites is the weakest and should not be used in stress-bearing tooth surfaces?
    a. Hybrid
    b. Microfill
    c. Nanofill
    d. Nanohybrid

11. Heavily filling the resin matrix with nanosized fillers particles will reduce which one of the following?
    a. Curing time
    b. Strength of the material
    c. The esthetics
    d. Polymerization shrinkage

12. Which one of the following composites is most difficult to polish to a high shine?
    a. Hybrid
    b. Microhybrid
    c. Nanohybrid
    d. Macrofilled composite

13. Which one of the following types of composites generally will shrink the most when polymerized?
    a. Bulk-fill composite
    b. Microhybrid
    c. Flowable composite
    d. Nanocomposite

14. Common effects of polymerization shrinkage of composites may include all of the following *except* one. Which one is this *exception?*
    a. Microleakage
    b. Death of the pulp
    c. Microcracking of enamel causing white lines around the margins
    d. Postoperative sensitivity

15. Methods used to minimize polymerization shrinkage include all of the following *except* one. Which one is this *exception?*
    a. Cure the composite rapidly with a high-intensity light.
    b. Use prepolymerized filler clusters.
    c. Use composite with a high filler content.
    d. Place composite using small increments.

16. All of the following circumstances may require a longer curing time for a composite *except* one. Which one is this *exception?*
    a. Use of an opaque shade
    b. Use of increments of composite greater than 2 mm
    c. Placement of the curing light tip 6 to 8 mm from the composite
    d. Composite placed in a class III preparation on #8 mesial

Get Ready for Exams!—cont'd

17. What allows a new increment of composite to stick to the previously cured increment?
    a. Mechanical retention
    b. Chemical resin-to-resin bond
    c. Addition of a bonding agent to the cured increment
    d. The silane coupling agent

18. The function of the wedge placed interproximally with a class II preparation includes all of the following *except* one. Which one is this *exception?*
    a. Stop bleeding
    b. Create slight separation of the teeth
    c. Seal the matrix band against the tooth at the gingival margin
    d. Protect the gingival papilla during cavity preparation

19. One of the advantages of glass ionomer compared to composite is
    a. The ability to finish it immediately
    b. That it has higher strength than composite because of the glass fillers
    c. That it uses the same bonding agents as composites
    d. That it has been shown to release fluoride

20. Which one of the following statements about glass ionomer cement (GIC) is *false?*
    a. GIC chemically bonds to the mineral of the tooth.
    b. GIC releases fluoride.
    c. GIC functions well for class II restorations in adults.
    d. GIC reduces microleakage at margins of a restoration on the root.

21. Resin-modified (hybrid) glass ionomers have all of the following advantages over conventional glass ionomers *except* one. Which one is this *exception?*
    a. Stronger
    b. Less sensitive to moisture when set
    c. Can be finished at the same appointment
    d. Contain quartz fillers like some composites

22. Nano-ionomers have all of the following properties *except* one. Which one is this *exception?*
    a. Improved esthetics
    b. Increased wear resistance
    c. Improved polish
    d. Greater strength than nanocomposites

23. Compomer restorative materials
    a. Release as much fluoride as glass ionomer materials
    b. Are only self-cure resins
    c. Are closer to composite resins in their makeup than to glass ionomers
    d. Are like glass ionomers in that they do not require a separate bonding agent

For answers to Review Questions, see the Appendix.

Case-Based Discussion Topics

1. A 24-year-old aspiring actress comes to the dental office seeking replacement of occlusal amalgams in her mandibular molars, because they are visible when she talks and sings. She does not grind her teeth.
From among the esthetic materials discussed in this chapter, which ones have properties that would make them suitable for use in this situation? Which ones are more suitable for anterior class III or V cavities?

2. A 75-year-old retired plumber who is taking medication to control his blood pressure is found on examination to have a dry mouth and numerous root caries.
Which types of direct-placement esthetic materials discussed in this chapter would have the greatest advantage for restoring root caries? Why? How do these materials bond to tooth structure?

3. A 43-year-old nurse comes to the office complaining of tooth sensitivity to air, cold, and sweets. Examination reveals several deep noncarious, cervical lesions caused primarily by heavy toothbrushing with stiff bristles. No dental caries is present.
Considering that resistance to wear is an important physical property, are lightly-filled, flowable composites suitable materials? Why or why not? What other materials could be used successfully in this situation?

4. A 57-year-old secretary comes to the dental office for a periodic examination and prophylaxis. She has maxillary anterior composite veneers and class V glass ionomers in her maxillary premolars.
What must the dental hygienist and dental assistant be concerned about when treating patients who have esthetic composite and glass ionomer restorations present in their mouths?

5. An 18-year-old volleyball player was hit in the mouth with an elbow by one of her teammates. Tooth #9 was fractured at the mesioincisal edge creating a 4 mm by 4 mm loss of tooth structure. The patient is being seen on an emergency basis and the dentist asked you to set up the operatory.
Which types of composites would work well for this situation? Why? Which type of composite should be avoided? Why?

BIBLIOGRAPHY

Anusavice KJ, Shen C, Rawls HR: Resin-base composites. *Phillips' Science of Dental Materials* (ed 12). St. Louis, 2013, Saunders.

Bird D, Robinson D: Restorative and esthetic dental materials. In *Modern Dental Assisting* (ed. 12). St. Louis, 2018, Elsevier.

Christensen GJ: Does your curing light have the most desirable characteristics? *Clinicians Report, Spring*, 1–2, 2017.

Donly KJ, Segura A, Weffel JS: Evaluating the effects of fluoride-releasing dental materials. *J Am Dent Assoc*, 130:819, 1999.

Ferracane JL: *Dental Composites in Materials in Dentistry* (ed 2). Philadelphia, 2001, Lippincott Williams & Wilkins.

Ferracane JL, Watts DC, Ernst CP, et al: Effective use of dental curing lights: A guide for the dental practitioner. *ADA Professional Prod Rev* 8:2–12, 2013.

Glazer HS, Lowe R, Strassler HE: Rubberized-urethane composite for provisional restorations. *Inside Dentistry*, 8(6):78–82, 2012.

Jefferies SR: Bioactive dental materials: composition, properties and indications for a new class of restorative materials. *Inside Dentistry*, 12(2), 2016.

Leinfelder KF, Bayne SC, Swift EJ: Packable composites: overview and technical considerations. *J Esthet Dent*, 11(5):234–249, 1999.

Marshall GW, Marshall SJ, Bayne SC: Restorative dental materials: scanning electron microscopy and x-ray microanalysis. *Scanning Microsc*, 2(4):2007–2028, 1988.

Mount GJ, Hume WR: Glass-ionomer materials, composite resins, and rigid materials used in tooth restoration. In *Preservation and Restoration of Tooth Structure*. Philadelphia, 1998, Mosby.

Mousavinasab SM: Biocompatibility of composite resins. *Dental Res J*, 8:S21–S29, 2011.

Nagaraja UP, Kishore G: Glass ionomer cement—the different generations. *Trends Biomater Artif Organs*, 18:158–165, 2005.

Powers JM, Wataha JC: Direct esthetic restorative materials. In *Dental Materials: Properties and Manipulation* (ed 10). St. Louis, 2013, Mosby.

Radz GM: Direct composite resins. *Inside Dentistry*, 7(7):108–114, 2011.

Roberson TM, Heymann HO, Swift EJ: Biomaterials. In *Sturdevant's Art and Science of Operative Dentistry* (ed 5). St. Louis, 2006, Mosby.

Sakaguchi RL, Powers JM: Restorative materials—composites and polymers. In *Craig's Restorative Dental Materials* (ed 13). St. Louis, 2012, Mosby.

Shah P: Composite roundup: the basics of bulk fill. *Dental Products Report*, 2013.

Wilson AD, Kent BE: A new translucent cement for dentistry: The glass ionomer cement. *Br Dent J*, 132:133–135, 1972.

Preventive and Desensitizing Materials

Chapter Objectives

Upon completion of this chapter, the student should be able to:

1. Describe the applications of fluoride in prevention.
2. Explain how fluoride protects teeth from caries.
3. Discuss the various methods of fluoride delivery.
4. Explain the benefit of using an antibacterial rinse in conjunction with fluoride.
5. Describe the antibacterial effects of chlorhexidine.
6. Apply topical fluoride gel, foam, varnish, or silver diamine fluoride correctly (as permitted by state law).
7. Describe how sealants protect pits and fissures from dental caries.
8. List the components of sealant material.
9. Recite the steps for applying sealants.
10. Apply sealants to teeth (as permitted by state law).
11. Recite causes of tooth sensitivity.
12. Explain how desensitizing agents work.
13. List the types of materials used to treat sensitive teeth.
14. Apply desensitizing agents to sensitive teeth (as permitted by state law).
15. Explain the process of remineralization of enamel.
16. Describe how products for remineralization work.
17. Explain how resin infiltration of the early white spot lesion works.
18. Apply remineralizing products (as permitted by state law).

Key Terms Defined within the Chapter

Antibacterial Mouth Rinse liquid used to rinse the oral cavity to reduce or suppress bacteria associated with dental caries or periodontal disease

Cariogenic substances or microorganisms that promote dental caries

Demineralization action that removes mineral from the tooth, usually caused by acids

Dental Caries a disease process whereby bacteria in plaque metabolize carbohydrates and produce acids that remove mineral from teeth and permit bacteria to invade the tooth and do further damage

Desensitizing Agent a chemical that seals open dentinal tubules in order to reduce tooth sensitivity to air, sweets, and temperature changes

Erosion loss of tooth mineral caused by dietary or gastric acids, not by bacterial metabolism (caries process)

Fluorapatite tooth mineral that results when fluoride is incorporated into the tooth

Fluoride naturally occurring mineral that helps protect tooth structure from dental caries

Fluorosis enamel condition caused by consumption of excessive levels of fluoride

Over-the-Counter (OTC) available in retail or drug stores without a doctor's prescription

Prevention/Preventive Aids chemicals, devices, or procedures that inhibit, reduce, or eliminate disease or tooth destruction in the oral cavity

Remineralization process that replaces mineral lost from the tooth by an acid attack

Sealant a protective resin that is bonded to enamel to protect pits and fissures from dental caries

Substantivity property of a material that has a prolonged therapeutic effect after its initial use

---

*CAMBRA (caries management by risk assessment) is now a common practice in many dental offices. Dental auxiliaries play important roles in assisting the dentist to prevent disease and maintain the health of patients. They can gather information about caries risk factors, and educate patients about the disease processes and the measures needed to prevent the disease. Materials needed to prevent dental diseases are widely used in the dental office. Fluorides, antibacterial mouth rinses, silver diamine fluoride, and sealants are important preventive measures for caries management and are discussed in detail in this chapter. Patients often ask dental assistants and hygienists about the prescription or over-the-counter (nonprescription) agents the dentist has recommended for the prevention of tooth decay and periodontal disease and, therefore, they must have a working knowledge of these products. In addition, the auxiliary is often asked by the dentist to dispense, apply, or fabricate devices such as fluoride trays for home use and to deliver these **prevention/preventive aids** or devices to the patient. In many states, the dental assistant or hygienist, when properly certified and/or licensed, can apply sealants and other preventive products prescribed by the dentist. The indications for sealants,* *application techniques, and troubleshooting guides are discussed. It is essential that all members of the dental team are familiar with the mechanism of action and application of these products. This chapter also presents information on desensitizing and remineralizing agents. Clinical and laboratory procedures for many of these topics are included.*

FLUORIDE

Fluoride is a naturally occurring mineral found in many forms in the modern world. It may be found in well water, in food that has absorbed fluoride from the soil, and as an additive in many over-the-counter dental products or those prescribed by dentists and physicians. Consumption of excess fluoride during tooth formation may lead to a condition known as **fluorosis**. Severe fluorosis can cause brown staining and pitting of the enamel surface (called *mottled enamel*) (Fig. 7.1) and is found where high levels (more than 2 parts per million [ppm]) of fluoride occur naturally in the drinking water. Mild or moderate fluorosis may create opaque white spots or bands on the teeth. High levels of fluoride in the water supply usually cause fluorosis, but it may also be caused by children swallowing excess amounts of fluoride toothpaste or by iatrogenic (doctor-induced) factors such as overly prescribed fluoride drops or tablets.

In fact, observations in 1901 by a young dentist, Frederick McKay, of unsightly brown stains on the teeth of residents of Colorado Springs eventually led to the discovery of the preventive effects of fluoride. Eight years after his initial observations, McKay was able to convince renowned dental researcher G.V. Black to collaborate with him on an epidemiological study to determine the cause of this stain. Black and McKay discovered that stained and mottled enamel occurred during the development of teeth, not afterward. They also discovered that teeth affected by the stain were surprisingly resistant to tooth decay. It took 30 years before it was discovered that the brown staining was the result of high levels of fluoride in the drinking water. The accepted optimal level of fluoride in drinking water for the US is 0.7 mg/L or ppm. The anti-caries effect of fluoride initiated the transformation of dentistry into a prevention-oriented profession.

TOPICAL AND SYSTEMIC EFFECTS

The enamel and dentin of the tooth are composed of tiny mineral crystals (hydroxyapatite) within a protein–lipid matrix. Microscopic gaps or pores between these millions of crystals are filled with protein, lipid, and water. It is in these matrix gaps that small molecules such as lactic acid and ions such as hydrogen, calcium, and phosphate are allowed to pass. There is a constant interchange of mineral ions between the tooth surface and the saliva. Usually, the minerals entering the surface balance the minerals coming out of the tooth surface.

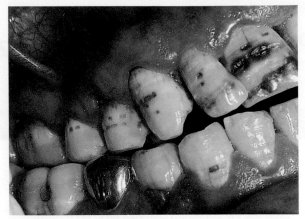

FIG. 7.1 Severe fluorosis. Note enamel defects and discolorations. (Courtesy of Steve Eakle, University of California, San Francisco [San Francisco, CA].)

The tooth crystals are not pure hydroxyapatite but contain inclusions of carbonate, which makes them much more soluble in acid. When bacteria in the plaque on the tooth surface metabolize cooked starches or sugars, they produce acids. The acids remove more mineral (**demineralization**) than the amount of mineral coming into the tooth from the saliva. When these acid attacks are repeated over time, the surface becomes more porous and allows bacteria to enter the tooth. This is the start of the caries process.

Ingested fluoride that enters the developing tooth bud can come from multiple sources such as drinking water, foods, beverages, or fluoride supplements prescribed by the dentist or pediatrician. For years it has been thought that fluoride incorporated into the teeth at the time of development was the main reason for the lowering of **dental caries** (tooth decay) rates seen in areas of water fluoridation. While fluoride incorporated into developing teeth does have a very important effect, work by Featherstone and others (1990) and epidemiological studies have shown that fluoride's greatest anticaries benefit is gained from topical fluoride exposure after the teeth have erupted. Fluoride in the saliva surrounding the teeth is incorporated into the surface of enamel crystals during **remineralization** (replacing minerals lost from the tooth surface) to form a surface veneer containing **fluorapatite**, which has much lower solubility than the original tooth mineral. The pH (a measure of acidity) at which tooth mineral dissolves is 5.5 (7.0 is neutral pH—neither acid nor base). However, when the tooth mineral is converted to fluorapatite, the pH at which it dissolves is lowered to 4.5 (a lower number indicates that it is more acidic; e.g., stomach acid has a pH of less than 1.0). Therefore fluoride makes it more difficult for the acids produced by **cariogenic** (decay-causing) bacteria in plaque to demineralize tooth structure and cause dental caries.

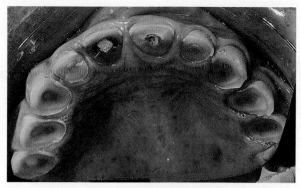

FIG. 7.2 Erosion from stomach acid. Note severe loss of enamel and dentin from the teeth due to chronic vomiting. (Courtesy of Steve Eakle, University of California, San Francisco [San Francisco, CA].)

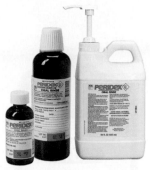

FIG. 7.3 Chlorhexidine oral rinse (Peridex). (From Darby ML, Walsh MM: *Dental Hygiene: Theory and Practice*, ed. 4, St. Louis, 2015, Elsevier.)

In a recent study published in *Langmuir,* the journal of the American Chemical Society (Loskill et al., 2013), researchers found yet another way in which fluoride helps to fight cavities. They tested how strongly *Streptococcus mutans* bacteria adhere to smooth hydroxyapatite before and after treatment with fluoride. They found that fluoride reduced the adhesive force of the bacteria to the hydroxyapatite surfaces.

Other than dietary sources, topical fluorides come from fluoride toothpastes and mouth rinses, and fluorides applied in the dental office in the form of liquids, gels, foams, and varnishes. There is evidence that fluoride from drinking water, toothpastes, mouth rinses, and some foods remains in the saliva for several hours and has a prolonged topical effect. Some of the fluoride that is ingested returns to the mouth by way of the saliva.

PROTECTION AGAINST EROSION

Highly acidic foods and beverages such as citrus fruits, sodas, and wine can contribute to loss of tooth mineral that is called **erosion**. Erosion differs from caries in that bacteria are not involved and most of the tooth mineral loss is at the surface. It is important to maintain a well-balanced diet to minimize excess acidic foods. Some medical conditions also cause erosion of the teeth by causing stomach acid to enter the mouth (Fig. 7.2). Examples are acid reflux (burping up stomach acid), anorexia nervosa (body wasting from extreme dieting and forced vomiting to purge food and keep from gaining weight), and bulimia (chronic forced vomiting to control weight gain after binge eating). By making the tooth structure less soluble in acids, fluoride provides some degree of protection against erosion, but repeated acid attacks will overcome the beneficial effects of fluoride.

BACTERIAL INHIBITION

Fluoride interferes with the essential enzyme activity of bacteria. Although the fluoride ion has been shown not to cross the bacterial cell wall, it can travel through it in the form of hydrofluoric acid (HF). As decay-causing bacteria produce acids during the metabolism of sugars and cooked starch, some of the fluoride present in the plaque fluid combines with hydrogen ions from the acid to become HF and rapidly diffuses into the cell. Once in the alkaline cytoplasm of the cell, the HF again separates into fluoride ions and hydrogen ions. These ions disrupt the enzyme activities essential to the functioning of bacteria and cause their death.

FLUORIDE AND ANTIBACTERIAL RINSES FOR THE CONTROL OF DENTAL CARIES

Studies have shown that fluoride alone is not as effective in managing dental caries as when it is used in conjunction with an **antibacterial mouth rinse**. Therapeutic mouth rinses help suppress bacteria associated with dental caries but are not meant to be substitutes for daily mechanical plaque removal.

Chlorhexidine gluconate is a bisbiguanide that is effective against a broad spectrum of microorganisms. In several European countries, it is used at a concentration of 0.2%, but in the United States, the maximum concentration allowed in an oral rinse by the U.S. Food and Drug Administration (FDA) is 0.12%. It is a prescription mouth rinse that is available commercially through several companies. The most common trade names are Peridex (3M ESPE) (Fig. 7.3), Periogard (Colgate-Palmolive), and Oris CHX (Dentsply International). It is one of the most effective agents for reduction of plaque (55%) and gingivitis (45%). Chlorhexidine kills bacteria by binding strongly to the bacterial cell membrane, causing it to leak and lose its intracellular components. It binds very strongly on many sites in the oral cavity, including the mucous membranes and plaque, and is released slowly, giving it a prolonged effect (called **substantivity**). The antibacterial effect from a single dose is greatest for several hours after use, but it may last for a few days. It is used in the management of many bacteria associated with periodontal disease and also is effective in suppressing *Streptococcus mutans* strains (*S. mutans*) associated with dental caries. The current recommended rinsing regimen to control dental caries, as suggested by an organization of western U.S. dental schools, is as follows: Rinse nightly for 1 minute with approximately 10 ml

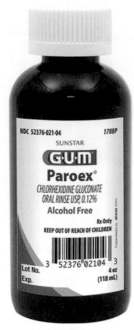

FIG. 7.4 Alcohol free Chlorhexidine oral rinse (Peroex). (Courtesy of Sunstar.)

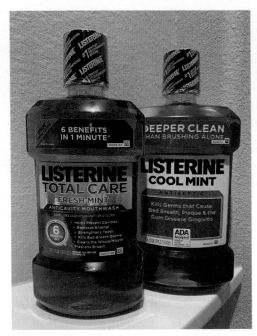

FIG. 7.5 Listerine antiseptic mouthrinse available over-the-counter (OTC).

of 0.12% chlorhexidine for 1 week each month. Repeat the cycle monthly until the dentist, who is monitoring bacterial cultures of *S. mutans* strains and lactobacilli, determines that further rinsing is not needed.

The side effects associated with this product are the formation of a brown stain (see Chapter 8, Fig. 8.3) on the teeth and tongue; on glass ionomer, compomer, and composite restorations; and on artificial teeth. It has a bitter taste and may affect the taste of some foods. Some flavoring agents have been introduced to offset the bitter taste. The solution contains alcohol, which might be harsh for individuals with sensitive mucous membranes. A non-alcohol version is available (GUM Paroex chlorhexidine gluconate oral rinse from Sunstar Inc.) (Fig. 7.4). Staining seems to be more rapid in some individuals. Diet and brushing habits are thought to play an important role in how rapidly staining occurs. More frequent professional teeth cleaning and polishing is usually necessary for patients who use these compounds routinely.

The longest-used antibacterial mouth rinse agents are the phenolic compounds, also called essential oils. The best-known product is Listerine (Johnson & Johnson) (Fig. 7.5), which has received the American Dental Association (ADA) Seal of Acceptance. It is a combination of phenol-related essential oils (thymol, eucalyptol, and menthol) mixed in methylsalicylate in a 26.9% hydroalcoholic vehicle. The antibacterial action of these compounds is a result of their alteration of the bacterial cell wall. Listerine now has products on the market which do not contain alcohol and only contain essential oils (Fig. 7.6). These products are best for patients who cannot use alcohol products or have xerostomia as alcohol can dry the oral tissues.

Listerine has not been shown to be an effective anticaries rinse, but clinical studies have shown reduction

of plaque scores by about 25% and gingivitis by 30% with use of these compounds. In some patients, these compounds cause a burning sensation in the tissues and a bad taste. Flavoring agents have been added in an attempt to overcome the taste problem.

METHODS OF DELIVERY

Dietary Fluoride Supplements

Fluoride may be obtained through drinking water, either naturally occurring or in fluoridated water supplies. In non-fluoridated communities, dentists and physicians may prescribe fluoride supplements for children in the form of tablets, drops, or lozenges (Fig. 7.7). Consideration should be given to the total fluoride exposure the child receives from other sources, such as school rinse programs, toothpaste, or prepared foods with fluoride. There is a schedule that recommends daily doses of fluoride supplements based on the child's age and the fluoride content of the community water supply. Supplements are not desired when the community water supply has a fluoride content that is higher than 0.6 ppm. Tablets and lozenges should be sucked to gain a topical effect. A portion of systemically ingested fluoride, including that in drinking water, is returned to the oral cavity by way of the saliva, thereby contributing to a topical effect.

In small communities where fluoridation of the water supply is not economically feasible, an alternative is to add fluoride to table salt. This type of fluoridation has been used for more than five decades in Switzerland. This method has been endorsed by the World Health Organization. Potassium fluoride and sodium fluoride are added to table salt at a concentration of 250 to 300 ppm. The salivary fluoride levels of the individuals using the fluoridated salt is similar to individuals drinking fluoridated water. This form of fluoridation can be used in areas of the world where other preventive measures for oral health are not available.

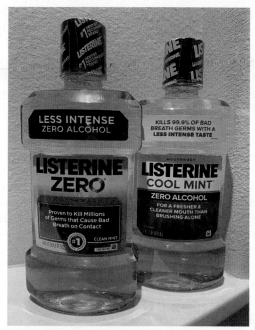

FIG. 7.6 Listerine Zero antiseptic mouthrinse without alcohol available over the counter (OTC).

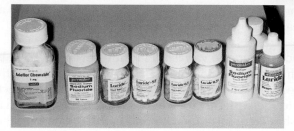

FIG. 7.7 Fluoride tablets. (From Bird DL, Robinson DS: *Modern Dental Assisting*, ed 12, St. Louis, 2018, Elsevier.)

In-Office Fluoride Applications (Topical)

Children with newly erupted permanent teeth and children and adults at high risk for caries are good candidates for professionally applied fluorides. The dental hygienist is most often the professional applying the fluoride in conjunction with dental prophylaxis. In some states properly trained dental assistants can also play this important role.

Silver diamine fluoride. Silver diamine fluoride (SDF) was approved in 2014 by the FDA for use in treating dentinal hypersensitivity. SDF has been used in other countries for over 80 years and silver alone has been used for over 100 years in healthcare. Fluoride has an anti-cariogenic effect while the silver has antimicrobial effects. The combination of fluoride and silver together as active ingredients in silver diamine fluoride produces a product which allows fluoride to strengthen and remineralize the tooth while the antimicrobial silver kills bacteria to prevent biofilm from forming on the tooth. This discovery has caused dental professionals to use SDF off label for these benefits. Current evidence indicates SDF is effective in arresting caries in over 90% of lesions when applied two times annually.

SDF is supplied as a colorless liquid in an 8 ml bottle (Advantage Arrest) or unit dose container (Fig. 7.8). Both contain silver at 25%, fluoride at 5%, ammonia at 8%, and water at 65%. The label indicates the SDF is a 38% solution which is established by combining the silver, fluoride, and ammonia percentages. Ammonia is added to the solution to stabilize the high concentration of fluoride suspended in the water. The pH of SDF is very basic at 10 on the pH scale. The average shelf-life is three years.

SDF is a trauma free and inexpensive method to arrest dental caries in all populations. It is frequently

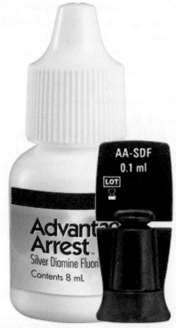

FIG. 7.8 Advantage Arrest Silver Diamine Fluoride in bulk and single dose containers. (Courtesy of Oral Science.)

used in children, geriatrics, and vulnerable populations (Table 7.1).

Application. One drop of SDF will treat 1-5 teeth. The solution should be applied using a microbrush and placed on the identified area for 60 seconds (Fig. 7.9; Procedure 7. 3).

Only areas of decay are to be treated with SDF. Good isolation is required as the silver in the solution will stain soft tissue and rough or unfinished margins of composites and crowns. It should also be noted that the silver will stain surfaces, clothing, and skin. Upon application SDF, the area of decay will turn dark brown or black in color (Fig. 7.10).

For this reason SDF is recommended in posterior regions or on deciduous teeth where esthetics are not a concern. Some clinicians cover the area treated with SDF with a composite or glass ionomer to lighten the darkness caused by the treatment.

There are no established guidelines for the number of applications or frequency of application. The manufacturer recommends waiting one week between repeated applications. Current research has evaluated effectiveness after one application versus two applications two times a year. After one application SDF effectively arrested more than 65% of active caries the while two applications annually resulted in a caries arrest rate over 90%.

Sodium fluoride varnish. Fluoride varnishes have become the most common form of fluoride application used in the dental office. Varnishes are applied directly onto the surfaces of teeth (Procedure 7.1). These varnishes were introduced more than 30 years ago, their advantage being that they would hold the fluoride against tooth surfaces longer than other products. The FDA has approved varnishes for use in treating dentin hypersensitivity; however, they are primarily used worldwide as an in-office topical fluoride treatment to prevent caries. They are available as 5.0% sodium fluoride (22,600 ppm fluoride) in a resin carrier or as 1% difluorsilane (1000 ppm fluoride) in polyurethane. They remain on the teeth for 1 to 3 days if the patient brushes gently. Varnishes are particularly useful for direct application to early dental caries that can remineralize (Fig. 7.11). They supply a high concentration of fluoride to the porous demineralized enamel. They can be applied directly around orthodontic bands and brackets to help prevent the formation of white spots (evidence of demineralization) caused by inadequate plaque removal. Fluoride varnishes have replaced the use of foams and gels in the dental office, because they can be applied rapidly and do not have the unpleasant side effects of nausea, vomiting, and gagging often seen with tray application of foam or gel. Fluoride varnish has been shown to be an effective caries preventive agent, with caries reduction of 18% to 77% depending on frequency of application, oral hygiene and diet of the individual, and other factors.

Gels and foams. Topical gels or foams (Fig. 7.12) that are applied for 4 minutes in disposable trays (Procedure 7.2) were historically the most commonly used fluorides in the dental office; however, varnishes have now taken their place as the most common. This is due to the quick application of varnishes and the continual fluoride release over an extended period of time. Some manufacturers market topical fluorides suggesting they can be applied for only 1 minute. A 1-minute application is not recommended by the ADA. Evidence-based dentistry indicates the 1-minute application delivers approximately 85% of the fluoride that a 4-minute application delivers. However, a 1-minute application is appealing to clinicians managing small children with active tongues and profuse salivary flow, and patients who tend to gag easily. This is another reason varnishes have increased in popularity.

Table 7.1	Indications and Contraindications for use of Silver Diamine Fluoride	
INDICATIONS	**CONTRAINDICATIONS**
Active carious lesions	True silver allergy
Lack of access to dental care	Ulcerations or sores on soft tissues
Inability to tolerate conventional dental care	Concern for esthetics
Multiple lesions requiring extensive dental treatment over a period of time	Pregnancy

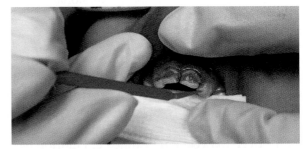

FIG. 7.9 Areas of decay on deciduous teeth being treated with Silver Diamine Fluoride (SDF). (Courtesy of Affiliated Children's Dental Specialists.)

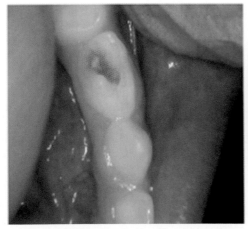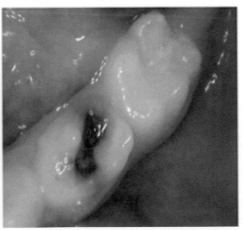

FIG. 7.10 Picture A (on left) area of decay. Picture B (on right) staining on of tooth structure after application of Silver Diamine Fluoride (SDF). (Courtesy of Oral Science.)

Fluoride varnish 2-4 times a year for high-risk children and adults

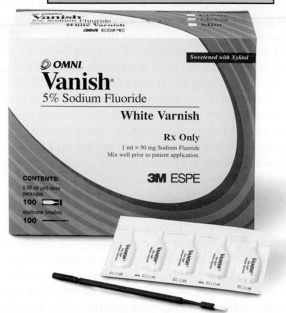

FIG. 7.11 Fluoride varnish with tri-calcium phosphate. (From Darby ML, Walsh MM: *Dental Hygiene: Theory and Practice*, ed. 4, St. Louis, 2015, Elsevier.)

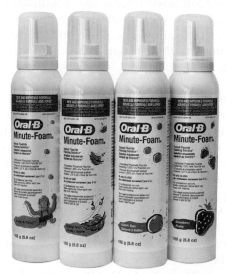

FIG. 7.12 In-office fluoride foams. (Courtesy of Procter & Gamble.)

When used once or twice a year, topical fluoride treatments have been shown to produce 20% to 26% caries reduction. Before fluoride varnish became popular, acidulated phosphate fluoride (APF) was once used frequently with children, because it contains 12,300 ppm fluoride and has good uptake in the enamel. Two percent neutral sodium fluoride (NaF) contains 9000 ppm fluoride and is used more often with adults, because the phosphoric acid in APF tends to etch the surface of restorations made of porcelain, composite resin, glass ionomer, or compomer. The phosphoric acid will also worsen root sensitivity in those patients who are experiencing it by dissolving plugs that block the dentinal tubules.

Self-Applied Topical Gels and Pastes

Self-applied fluoride gels and pastes are recommended for individuals who are at high risk for dental caries. They are also used for orthodontic patients to prevent caries and decalcification around brackets and bands that cause permanent white spots and lines on the enamel. These white spots are unsightly and represent the early stages of the caries process (demineralization of enamel by bacterial acids). Elderly patients who take medications that dry up their salivary flow are at very high risk for caries, especially on exposed root surfaces, and can receive benefit from gels used at home. Self-applied gels are available by prescription as 1.1% neutral sodium fluoride (5000 ppm fluoride) or 0.4% stannous fluoride (900 ppm fluoride) (Fig. 7.13 & Fig. 7.14).

Stannous fluoride may cause some staining of the surfaces of the teeth, and it delivers less fluoride ion to the teeth.

Fluoride gels can be brushed on the teeth or applied in custom fluoride trays. Custom fluoride trays can be made with the same thermoplastic material as whitening trays (see Procedure 8.2 Clinical Procedures for Home Whitening in Chapter 8 Teeth Whitening Materials and Procedures). Four minutes of use in a custom tray is much more effective than 1 minute of brushing with the gel, because the tray prevents saliva from quickly diluting the gel and removing it

High concentration 5000 ppm fluoride toothpaste/gel for caries high-risk clients from age 6 years and older

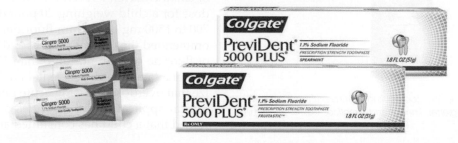

FIG. 7.13 Sample prescription fluoride products. (From Darby ML, Walsh MM: *Dental Hygiene: Theory and Practice*, ed. 4, St. Louis, 2015, Elsevier.)

from contact with the teeth. The custom trays, however, involve some additional expense for the time required to make impressions, pour casts, and construct the trays. Children younger than 6 years of age should not use these gels, because they tend to swallow too much of the gel. In place of a brush-on gel, some manufacturers have made prescription toothpastes containing 1.1% neutral sodium fluoride. The idea is that the prescription toothpaste will aid compliance, because the patient will not have to brush the teeth first and then brush again with a gel, but can achieve both at the same time. Self-application by school-aged children has produced significant caries reduction (about 24%).

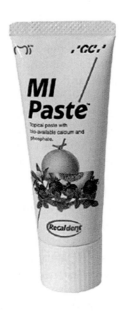
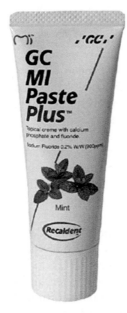

FIG. 7.14 MI paste, calcium and phosphate product for home use. (From Darby ML, Walsh MM: *Dental Hygiene: Theory and Practice*, ed. 4, St. Louis, 2015, Elsevier.)

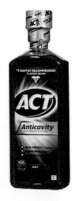

FIG. 7.15 Sample of over the counter fluoride rinse. (From Darby ML, Walsh MM: *Dental Hygiene: Theory and Practice*, ed. 4, St. Louis, 2015, Elsevier.)

Over-the-Counter Fluoride Rinses

Over-the-counter (OTC) fluoride rinses have been demonstrated to provide 28% caries reduction when used in a daily rinse program. Rinses are available as 0.05% sodium fluoride (225 ppm fluoride) (Fig. 7.15). Patients typically are instructed to rinse with 10 ml for 30 to 60 seconds, spit out the excess, and not rinse, eat, or drink anything for at least 30 minutes. Fluoride rinse is often used just before bedtime so that a residue of fluoride can remain in the saliva during sleep. Parents should supervise children using these rinses to prevent the child from swallowing them. Prescription rinses contain 0.2% sodium fluoride or 0.63% stannous fluoride.

Fluoride-Containing Toothpaste

Studies with Crest toothpaste conducted in the 1950s first established the caries-preventive capability of fluoride in toothpaste. Many studies conducted since then have shown sodium monofluorophosphate (MFP) and sodium fluoride to be more effective and chemically stable than stannous fluoride. The fluoride content of most toothpastes is about 1000 ppm. Children younger than 6 years of age should be supervised when brushing and should be given only a pea-sized amount of toothpaste once a day. Toothpaste for children is available with much lower fluoride content. They tend to swallow the paste and run the risk of mild fluorosis of the permanent teeth if they consume too much.

Fluoride-Containing Prophylaxis Pastes

Prophylaxis pastes contain pumice as an abrasive to remove surface stains and plaque/biofilm from the teeth. In the process, they remove a small amount of the fluoride-rich enamel surface. It is thought that some of the lost fluoride can be regained by incorporating fluoride in the paste. The most common fluoride additive is 1.23% APF. These pastes have not received the ADA Seal of Acceptance as effective for caries prevention, because studies have not shown them to be effective for this purpose. In some dental offices, polishing the teeth after prophylaxis is not routinely done, to avoid removing that fluoride-rich surface layer.

SAFETY

All fluorides should be used as directed and kept out of small children's reach for safety reasons. The lethal dose for a child weighing 20 pounds is approximately 700 to 1500 mg of sodium fluoride. Therefore, it is recommended that prescriptions for dietary supplements of fluoride contain no more than 120 mg to avoid the risk of a fatal overdose. Dental auxiliaries should realize that overdoses causing acute illness can occur from topical applications of fluoride as well. If it is determined that a child has consumed an excessive amount of fluoride, vomiting should be induced and milk of magnesia should be given to bind to the fluoride ions. Cow's milk could be given to slow absorption from the stomach. The child should be taken to the emergency room of the nearest hospital. The most common reaction seen in the dental office or shortly after leaving the office when a child has swallowed fluoride gel is nausea and vomiting. The fluoride, particularly with the acidulated gel, irritates the stomach (see Procedure 7.2 for the clinical technique for in-office topical fluoride application). Table 7.2 lists common in-office and home-use fluoride products.

 Caution

Parents with children under age 6 years should be advised to carefully supervise their children when brushing with fluoride-containing toothpaste. Children at this age tend to swallow the paste and over time could consume enough fluoride to cause mild fluorosis. Only a pea-sized portion of paste should be used.

PIT AND FISSURE SEALANTS

PURPOSE

Sealants are unfilled or lightly filled resins (see Chapter 6) that are used to seal the noncarious pits and fissures of deciduous and permanent teeth. The sealant is a preventive measure to reduce or eliminate dental caries in the pits and fissures. The widespread use of fluoride has caused a significant reduction in dental caries in children who receive regular dental care, but not necessarily in low-income children. Although the overall caries rate has dropped, the greatest benefit from fluorides has been seen on smooth enamel surfaces. Most caries (about 88%) in children is found in pits and fissures. The nature of the shape of the pits and fissures makes them vulnerable to dental caries. Pits and fissures are often deep, narrow channels in the enamel surface that can extend close to the dentinoenamel junction (Fig. 7.16). They collect bacteria and food debris that cannot be removed by toothbrushing, so dental caries can occur readily in these locations. Sealants are not as widely used as they should be. Increasing sealant placement is part of the national health initiative and included as part of "Healthy People 2020." Among low-income children, use of sealants is only about 30%, and this is the high caries risk group that could benefit most from sealants.

Sealants have been shown in numerous studies to be an effective and conservative means of preventing caries in pits and fissures by blocking bacteria and food products from entering them. The American Dental Association encourages sealant application because sealants have been shown to effectively reduce caries. Caries is often difficult to detect in its early stages in pits and fissures. For this reason, some dentists are reluctant to use sealants for fear of sealing undetected caries. There is ample evidence in the dental literature to indicate if caries is inadvertently sealed in the pits and fissures, the caries process stops, because bacteria are cut off from their nutrients. Going and co-investigators found mostly negative bacterial cultures (no growth) in teeth with carious dentin that has been sealed with Nuva-Seal for 5 years. Treatment of carious teeth with sealants resulted in an 89% reversal from a caries-active to a caries-inactive state. Those sites that remained carious had significantly fewer viable bacteria than unsealed carious control sites. Handelman and co-investigators demonstrated a decrease of 2000-fold in viable bacteria that could be recovered from carious dentin in pits and fissures that were sealed for 2 years compared with unsealed control teeth. They demonstrated that small caries inadvertently sealed in the tooth and monitored on radiographs for 2 years not only did not progress, but in some cases partially repaired. However, only incipient enamel caries should be considered for the sealant procedure. If a sealant leaks because it is not properly placed, caries can occur beneath it. More advanced caries should be treated by conservative restorative procedures rather than with sealants.

INDICATIONS

The lack of an accurate means of predicting where caries will occur has complicated the process of selecting which teeth should be sealed and which should not. Because some individuals will remain caries-free throughout their lifetime, it is not indicated to seal all posterior teeth. The dentist should use his/her clinical judgment based on specific criteria to determine which teeth should be sealed. Consideration should be given to the age, oral hygiene, caries risk, diet, fluoride history, and tooth type and morphology.

Although the main thrust of sealant therapy is aimed at permanent teeth, primary molars may also be sealed to reduce the caries rate and prevent premature tooth loss. Approximately 44% of caries in primary teeth occurs in the pits and fissures of the molars. Although the occlusal morphology of primary molars is flatter and less fissured than that of permanent molars, sealants are still indicated if deep or stained fissures are found and if the child has a high incidence of caries or high caries risk.

Permanent teeth should be sealed if there is/was evidence of caries susceptibility in the primary dentition or the patient has a high caries risk. Teeth with steep cuspal inclines and deep, sticky fissures are more likely candidates for sealants than teeth with shallow cusps and highly coalesced (fused together) pits and fissures (Fig. 7.17). Molars decay three to four times more frequently than premolars, undoubtedly as a result of the more complex occlusal morphology. Premolars are not generally high-risk teeth, and sealants should be

TABLE 7.2	Common In-Office and Home-Use Fluoride Products				
USE	PRODUCT	FLUORIDE CONTENT (ppm)	COMMON BRANDS	FREQUENCY OF USE	PRECAUTIONS
In-office treatment	1.23% APF gel or foam	12,300	NUPRO APF Gel, Foam (Dentsply) DentiCare Gel, Foam (Medicom) Topex 60 Second Fluoride Gel, Foam (Sultan Healthcare)	Twice a year	Gastrointestinal upset, vomiting if swallowed; may etch esthetic restorations; not for children younger than age 3 yr
	2.0% NaF	9,000	Oral-B Neutra-Foam (Procter & Gamble) NUPRO Fluoride Oral Solution (Dentsply) DentiCare Foam (Medicom) Topex Neutral pH Fluoride Gel, Foam (Sultan Healthcare)	Twice a year	Gastrointestinal upset, vomiting if swallowed; not for children younger than age 3 yr
	38% SDF	44,800	Advantage Arrest (Elevate Dental Care)	Twice a year	Staining of soft tissues and margins of restorations, discoloration of tooth after application to carious lesion
	5% NaF varnish	22,600	Duraflor Halo (Medicom) Colgate Duraphat (Colgate-Palmolive) Flor-Opal (Ultradent) NUPRO White (Dentsply) Vanish (3M ESPE) DuraShield (Sultan Healthcare)	2-4 times per year depending on caries risk	Nausea with extensive application in patients with sensitive stomachs
Prescription home use	1.1% NaF gel or toothpaste	5,000	Colgate PreviDent (Colgate-Palmolive) Oral-B NeutraCare (Procter & Gamble) DentiCare Gel (Medicom) Fluoridex (Philips Oral Healthcare) Topex Take Home Care (Sultan Healthcare)	Daily	Not for children younger than age 6 yr
	0.4% SnF$_2$ gel	900	Colgate Gel-Kam (Colgate-Palmolive) Oral-B Stop (Procter & Gamble) DentiCare Gel (Medicom) Perio Plus (Oral Dent Pharma) Topex (Sultan Healthcare)	Daily	May cause surface staining of teeth; not for children younger than age 6 yr
	0.2% NaF rinse	900	Oral-B Fluorinse (Procter & Gamble) Colgate PreviDent Dental Rinse (Colgate-Palmolive) NUPRO Fluoride Rinse (Dentsply)	Weekly	Not for children younger than age 6 yr
Over-the-counter home use	0.05% NaF	250	ACT (Chattem) Colgate FluoriGard (Colgate-Palmolive)	Daily	Not for children younger than age 6 yr
	0.02% NaF	100	Listerine Smart Rinse (Johnson & Johnson) Crest Pro-Health (Procter & Gamble)	Daily	Not for children younger than age 6 yr
	Toothpaste 0.24% NaF	1,100	Numerous brands and manufacturers	Daily	Not for children younger than age 6 yr
	Toothpaste 0.8% MFP	1,000	Numerous brands and manufacturers	Daily	Use pea-sized amount with children younger than age 6 yr

APF, acidulated phosphate fluoride; *SDF,* silver diamine fluoride; *MFP,* sodium monofluorophosphate; *NaF,* sodium fluoride; *SnF$_2$,* stannous fluoride.

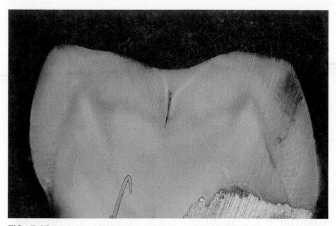

FIG. 7.16 Section of tooth showing a long, narrow fissure containing debris. A sealant is present and covers the opening of the fissure. (Courtesy of Steve Eakle, University of California, San Francisco [San Francisco, CA].)

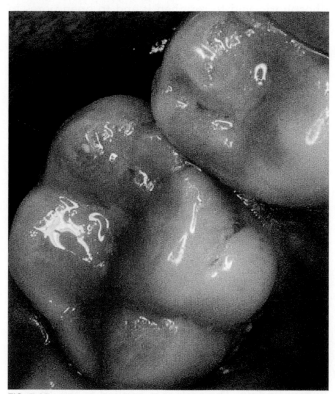

FIG. 7.17 Enamel without significant fissures (well coalesced). (Courtesy of Steve Eakle, University of California, San Francisco [San Francisco, CA].)

applied selectively when specific indications are present. On occasion, maxillary central and lateral incisors have deep lingual pits that require sealing. However, emphasis is placed on sealing first and second molars as a priority.

SUSCEPTIBILITY OF TEETH TO FISSURE CARIES

Teeth most susceptible to pit and fissure caries are listed in the order of their risk for decay:
- Lower molars—about 50% of the caries occurs in these teeth
- Upper molars—about 35% to 40%

TABLE 7.3	Filler Content and Color of Commercial Sealants	
FILLER CONTENT, % BY WEIGHT	**BRAND NAME (MANUFACTURER)**	**COLOR**
No filler	Conseal Clear (SDI)	Clear
	Delton (Dentsply Sirona)	Clear, white, amber
	Helioseal (Ivoclar Vivadent)	Clear, white
Lightly filled (6%-8%)	Clinpro (3M ESPE)	White when set
	Conseal F, (SDI)	
	Natural Elegance (Henry Schein)	White
	Seal-Rite Low Viscosity (Pulpdent)	White
		Off-white
Heavily filled (30%-70%)	Delton Plus (Dentsply)	White
	Embrace WetBond (Pulpdent)	Off-white, tooth-colored
	Guardian Seal (Kerr Dental)	White
	Helioseal F (Ivoclar Vivadent)	White
	Grandio Seal (VOCO)	Pearly white
	Ultraseal XT plus (Ultradent)	White, tooth colors A1, A2, clear

- Upper and lower second premolars
- Upper laterals and upper first premolars
- Upper centrals and lower first premolars

Taken as a group, caries occurs most often in upper and lower molars, accounting for 85% to 90% of pit and fissure caries.

COMPOSITION

Sealants are chemically similar to composite resins. Their resin component is based on a dimethacrylate monomer that is either bisphenol A-glycidyl methacrylate (bis-GMA) or urethane dimethacrylate (UDMA). Polymerization of the resin occurs either solely by chemical reaction (self-cure) or by light activation (light-cure) (see Chapter 6). Self-cure is by the conventional peroxide-amine system, which requires the mixing of two components. Light-cured sealants are one-component systems that are polymerized by blue light. The vast majority of sealants in use today are light-cured. Many manufacturers add very small filler particles to the sealants to make them more wear resistant. Sealants are not as heavily filled (see Table 7.3 for sealant filler content) as most composites, because they would be too viscous to flow into the narrow fissures. Some of the filler particles used in sealants may be radiopaque and may allow the sealants to be seen on x-rays. Many sealants, however, are radiolucent (see Chapter 6).

In 1996 a study done at the University of Granada (Granada, Spain) called into question the safety of dental sealants because of the presence of bisphenol A (BPA) in the saliva of patients after placement of sealants. Bisphenol A can interfere with estrogen (a hormone that regulates reproduction and development) and may have other adverse health effects. In this study only one sealant was tested, but the resin in that sealant (bisphenol A dimethacrylate) is not representative of the resins used in most sealants (bis-GMA or UDMA). Bis-GMA releases very little bisphenol A and UDMA has none. In 2008 the ADA issued a statement indicating that peer-reviewed evidence shows that dental resin materials leach out only very low levels of BPA and do not constitute a health risk for patients. (See also Chapter 6 regarding concerns about bisphenol A.)

 Caution

Do not stare directly at the curing light. There is potential for damage to the retina with repeated exposures. An appropriate filter should be used to protect the eyes.

WORKING TIME

Self-cured sealant polymerizes to final set within approximately 2 minutes from the start of mixing of the two components, the initiator and the accelerator. An experienced operator can apply the material to one or two quadrants of posterior teeth with one mix of material, so it has the advantage of being applied faster than light-cured material on a comparable number of teeth. Light-cured material requires a 20-second application of light on each tooth to polymerize the sealant if a standard halogen light is used. LED and laser curing lights can be much more intense and require less curing time (see Chapter 6 Light Curing Units). Follow the manufacturer's recommendations for curing times. Light-cured material has the advantages of allowing the operator to place and cure the material when the operatory is ready and not requiring mixing prevents the incorporation of bubbles into the material.

COLOR AND WEAR

Manufacturers provide sealants in a variety of colors. Sealants may be clear, amber, tooth colored, or opaque white. Patients usually prefer the clear or tooth-colored sealants, but it is easier for the dental team to identify the presence of the sealants at the time of placement and at subsequent examination visits if they contrast with the tooth color. Sealants are subject to wear from the occlusion. Sealants that contain no inorganic filler particles will wear faster than those that have filler particles added. Some clinicians use flowable composites as sealants, because they are more heavily filled and therefore more resistant to wear, while at the same time having adequate flow to enter the fissures. Wear does not create much of a problem as long as the fissure remains sealed. If part of the fissure is uncovered, repair is recommended.

Sealants seldom flow to the bottom of long, narrow fissures because of the presence of debris (see Fig. 7.16)

and trapped air. Some clinicians prefer to open the fissures with a small-diameter carbide or diamond bur to look for decay, remove debris, and allow better penetration of the sealant.

PLACEMENT

The ADA Council on Scientific Affairs does not recommend routine opening of fissures with cutting instruments before sealant placement. The technique of placement of sealants requires attention to detail (see Procedure 7.4). This technique has many steps in common with the placement of other bonded restorations (see Chapter 5 Principles of Bonding and Chapter 6 Composites, Glass Ionomers, and Compomers). The surface must first be cleaned with pumice to remove any surface debris that would interfere with acid etching or bonding. Retention of the sealant is obtained by etching the enamel with 37% phosphoric acid to roughen it and to open pores in the enamel for penetration of the resin sealant. After etching, rinsing, and drying of the enamel, isolation of the field is very important. Etching enlarges the size and volume of pores in the enamel and roughens the surface so that the sealant can penetrate and mechanically lock into these spaces. Some clinicians like to use a drying agent after etching and rinsing to remove any remaining water in the fissures held there by capillary action. Drying agents usually consist of alcohol. They will mix with the water, and when they evaporate, they will carry off the excess water with them.

Use of Bonding Agent

Studies have shown that application of an enamel bonding resin before placement of the sealant enhances the retention and seal. Bonding resins are low-viscosity resins that can flow readily into the fissures and microscopic porosities created by acid etching (see Chapter 5). Resin-containing sealant will then adhere to the bonding resin by a chemical resin-to-resin bond. However, many clinicians have not yet started using bonding agents with sealants, because this is a relatively new finding. The sealant is applied to the pits and fissures and surrounding enamel and is cured.

 Clinical Tip

Application of a resin bonding agent after etching the enamel will increase the retention of sealants!

 Caution

Place etchant with care to avoid etching adjacent teeth or restorations. Matrix strips could be placed between adjacent teeth, but careful application will prevent inadvertent etching. Avoid contact with the patient's eyes or skin. Protective eyewear should be used by all.

Oxygen-Inhibited Layer

The cured sealant will have a very thin film of un-cured resin on its surface. The surface will appear shiny and will be wet to the touch, because the set of the resin at its surface is inhibited by contact with oxygen in the air. This film is called the *oxygen-* or *air-inhibited layer*. It should be wiped off with gauze or a cotton roll, because it might have an unpleasant taste to the patient.

 Caution

Recap sealant and bonding agent bottles promptly to prevent loss of volatile monomers that would create a very viscous liquid that cannot penetrate fissures and etched enamel.

Any moisture on the tooth could result in failure of the sealant. Moisture could come from saliva, an air-water syringe that leaks water into the air stream, or even moisture from the patient's breath. Failure may be seen as immediate loss of the sealant, complete or partial loss of the sealant seen at subsequent visits, or retained sealants that are leaking and could result in dental caries beneath the sealant. Maxillary and mandibular second molars are the teeth that most frequently lose sealants, probably because they are the ones for which it is difficult to maintain isolation when a rubber dam is not used. In addition, moisture from the patient's breath could coat the etched enamel and interfere with the bond of the sealant.

 Clinical Tip

Maintaining good isolation is critical to the success of sealants. Moisture from saliva or even the breath can affect their retention. The most common sites where sealant is lost in the first 6 months are the maxillary and mandibular second molars, and these are the sites where isolation is most difficult to maintain.

Remineralization of Etched, Unsealed Enamel

One concern that has been raised about etching enamel surfaces for placement of sealants is that if the sealant comes off, the exposed surface is more caries susceptible. Studies have shown that the etched enamel begins remineralization after a 24-hour exposure to saliva by deposition of calcium phosphate salts. In areas where sealants wear away, resins tags remaining in the enamel provide some caries protection.

Etching Precautions

Care should be taken in placement of the acid etchant so that adjacent teeth are not etched and the soft tissues are not exposed to the acid. Mylar matrix strips or metal matrix bands can be placed in the interproximal spaces to prevent etching of adjacent

teeth, but careful application of etchant will prevent this from occurring. Care should also be taken to avoid contact of the acid with the eyes and skin of the patient and operator. Both should wear protective eyewear.

Bite Interference by Sealant

If a sealant layer is too thick (often described as "high sealant"), it might cause interference with the bite of the patient. Unfilled sealants that are too high will wear down in a few days or weeks. Sealants with filler particles are much more wear resistant. Ideally, all high sealants should be adjusted to be compatible with the patient's bite. Otherwise, sore teeth or jaws may result. Articulating paper should be used to identify the high spots, and an appropriate carbide or diamond bur can be used to adjust them.

PATIENT RECORD ENTRIES

The sealant procedure should be carefully documented in the patient's chart. Chart entries should include the following:

- The date
- Patient (18 years of age or older) or parental consent as obtained
- Type of isolation
- Teeth and surfaces sealed
- Materials used including percentage of phosphoric acid (etchant) and brand of sealant used
- Statement that the patient or parent was informed of the need for periodic inspection and maintenance of the sealants
- Any adverse events, such as acid splashed on the oral tissues or face, causing a burn, or difficulty with isolation or patient management that may lead to sealant failure

Sealant Retention Studies have shown that retention rates are better when four-handed techniques are used for the placement of sealants. Having an extra pair of hands to help maintain isolation and place or cure the sealants is a definite bonus. In many states, dental hygienists and dental assistants can be licensed or certified to place sealants. State dental practice act guidelines must be followed as to the oral health care providers permitted to place sealants and adjust the occlusion on a high sealant. The dental hygienist can play an important role in the maintenance of sealants by carefully checking them at hygiene visits.

 Clinical Tip

Avoid placing sealant on adjacent unetched enamel. After the sealant is cured it will look sound, but leakage will occur under the unetched portion of the sealant. When the patient returns for the periodic oral examination there will be dark staining under the sealant in those areas and the leakage may lead to the development of caries.

Table 7.4   Advantages and Disadvantages of Chemical-Cured and Light-Cured Sealants

CHEMICAL-CURED (SELF-CURED OR AUTOPOLYMERIZING) SEALANTS	
ADVANTAGES	**DISADVANTAGES**
• No need for curing light. • No risk of damage to the retina from the curing light. • Sealants can be applied to several teeth without having to go back and individually cure each one with a light.	• Setting time can vary greatly with variations in room temperature; the warmer the material, the faster the set. • Setting time of 2 minutes may be too long if there is trouble maintaining a dry field or controlling a hyperactive child. • Mixing two liquids together introduces bubbles into the material that could produce voids in the completed sealant. • The viscosity (thickness) of the material increases continuously from the start of mixing. When the material is applied to several teeth, the ability of the material to flow well into tight fissures diminishes with time and a new mix may be needed.
LIGHT-CURED SEALANTS	
ADVANTAGES	**DISADVANTAGES**
• Material sets in a short period of time (typically 20 seconds). This is particularly useful when one is working on an active child or is trying to control heavy salivary flow. • Time for application Is not limited as with chemical-cured sealants. • Mixing is not required, so fewer bubbles are introduced into the material. • Viscosity remains low throughout the application period until light is applied.	• The curing light can cause damage to the retina if protection is not used. • The curing light and filter are added expenses. • Only the material directly under the light tip is completely cured, so that when several teeth are done, the total curing time may be significantly increased and it may be difficult to manipulate the light tip to reach the distal pits of maxillary second molars in small mouths.

EFFECTIVENESS

Carefully placed sealants are very effective at preventing decay in the pits and fissures. Simonsen (1991) monitored sealants for 15 years after placement and found them to be highly effective (Table 7.4).

In that study, sealants were placed on permanent posterior teeth; this procedure was followed by periodic examinations. If sealants were completely or partially lost, they were not replaced or repaired. (In dental practice, lost sealants would be replaced.) At the end of 15 years, more than 68% of teeth were caries free compared with 17% in a control group with no sealants. A much greater reduction in caries could have been obtained by replacement of lost sealants.

TROUBLESHOOTING PROBLEMS WITH SEALANTS

Most sealant failures occur within the first 3 to 6 months, and all or part of the sealant comes off. The worst failure is a sealant that leaks but remains in place. The leak can go undetected and can decay significantly underneath the sealant before it is detected. Placing too much sealant can result in excess material flowing into the embrasure space between adjacent teeth (Fig. 7.18). Once the sealant is cured, the contact area is blocked and the patient would not be able to floss it. See Table 7.5 for potential problems and their causes and ways to solve the problems.

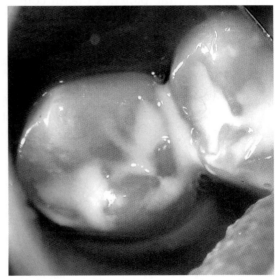

FIG. 7.18 Too much sealant was applied and excess blocks the proximal embrasure. (Courtesy of Steve Eakle, University of California, San Francisco [San Francisco, CA].).

GLASS IONOMER CEMENT AS A SEALANT

Glass ionomer cements have been used as sealants because of their adhesion to enamel and their release of fluoride into the surrounding tooth structure. However, the retention rate for glass ionomer sealants is rather low. One rationale for their use is to provide protection from caries by sealing the fissures and providing fluoride to the surface of the enamel while the

Table 7.5

TABLE 7.5 Troubleshooting Problems with Sealants

PROBLEM	CAUSE	SOLUTION
Sealant has come off when retention is checked at placement visit	Surface contamination (likely saliva)	Maintain good isolation and re-etch and apply the sealant
Sealant blocks the contact area	Too much sealant was appliedLack of finger rest to control placement	Use just enough sealant to cover fissure and 1 mm beyond. Use good finger rest. Remove excess material before curing it. Remove hardened sealant in contact area with a scaler
Sealant has holes in surface	Air bubbles in wet sealantVigorous scrubbing with application brush	Carefully dispense material to avoid bubbles. Gently work sealant into fissures with brush or explorer. Repair by working fresh sealant into holes with explorer tip (re-etch first if isolation was lost)
Sealant layer is too high, interfering with bite	Too much sealant was applied	Do not puddle the sealant. Use just enough to cover the fissure and 1 mm beyond

tooth is going through the eruption process, which can be somewhat slow for molars. Then, after the tooth is fully erupted, a resin sealant could be placed. Current recommendations from the ADA Council on Scientific Affairs after a review of the dental literature indicate that resin-based sealants are the preferred materials for pit and fissure sealants.

DESENSITIZING AGENTS

Many patients experience sensitivity in their teeth to cold foods or beverages, sweets, or cold air. Professionally applied or OTC materials applied to the teeth by the patient to reduce or eliminate the sensitivity are called **desensitizing agents**. Dental hygienists and assistants may be called on to apply certain types of desensitizing agents or to explain to the patient the causes of the sensitivity.

MECHANISM OF TOOTH SENSITIVITY

Teeth may become sensitive when the gingiva has receded and dentinal tubules are exposed to the oral cavity. Ordinarily, the root surface has a thin protective coating of cementum. When the cementum gets worn away, the dentinal tubules are exposed. Odontoblasts (cells in the pulp that lay down dentin) line the pulp and have extensions within the dentinal tubules that contain nerve endings. When some stimulus causes the fluid within the tubules to move, the sensitive nerve endings are deformed, causing them to fire and produce a quick, localized sharp pain (this is the hydrodynamic theory of dentin sensitivity). Temperature, usually cold, and sugars and acidic foods are common offenders.

Common Causes of Sensitivity

Common causes of exposed dentin include the following: (1) roots abraded by improper toothbrushing (see Chapter 13 Abrasion, Finishing, and Polishing, Fig. 13.14), (2) loss of enamel and dentin through the work of dietary or stomach acids (erosion), (3) loss of tooth structure in the cervical part of the tooth by abfraction (grinding of the teeth, which can cause bending of the teeth at the microscopic level with breaking away of enamel and dentin in the cervical area), and (4) scaling and root planing procedures. It is estimated that 15% of the population experiences tooth sensitivity. If the dentinal tubules become plugged, the sensitivity stops. Acidic foods and beverages, toothbrushing, or scaling and root planing procedures can remove the plugs and create sensitivity again. Citrus fruits and their juices can readily remove mineral from the surface of the teeth and open plugged dentin tubules. Besides being acidic they contain citrate that binds and removes calcium from the teeth and saliva, so remineralization is slowed. Desensitizing agents (Fig. 7.19) have been developed to treat sensitivity. However, not all causes of tooth sensitivity respond to desensitizers. Causes of tooth sensitivity such as dental caries, a cracked tooth, a high restoration, or a leaking restoration cannot be treated by desensitizers and need corrective measures.

Common Causes of Root Sensitivity

- Root caries
- Toothbrush abrasion
- Erosion by acids
- Abfraction associated with bruxism
- Scaling and root planing
- Leaking restoration on the root

TREATMENT

Treatment is currently centered around two main modalities: (1) occluding (plugging) the open tubules and (2) desensitizing the nerve endings. Plugging the open ends of the dentin tubules will reduce fluid movement

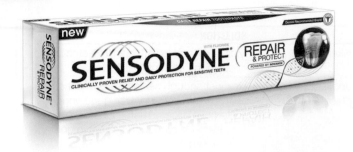

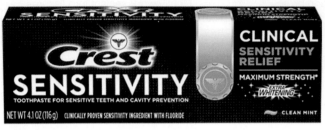

FIG. 7.19 Various desensitizing agents. (Courtesy of GlaxoSmith-Kline [Brentford, UK]; courtesy of Procter & Gamble Co. [Cincinnati, OH].)

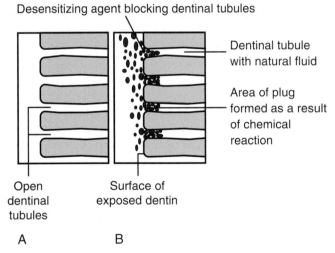

Desensitizing agent blocking dentinal tubules

Dentinal tubule with natural fluid

Area of plug formed as a result of chemical reaction

Open dentinal tubules

Surface of exposed dentin

A   B

FIG. 7.20 Illustration of **(A)**, open dentinal tubules and **(B)**, a desensitizing agent that forms a precipitate that occludes the dentinal tubules.

and stop pressure on the nerve endings. This may be done by a chemical or mechanical blocking process. Fluoride compounds in toothpastes, gels, or solutions are applied to the sensitive teeth. Ferric or potassium oxalate solutions are used to precipitate oxalate crystals in the open tubules (Fig. 7.20). Chemical solutions containing resin are also applied to block the tubules. Some materials actually create a bond with the dentin (dentin bonding agents) or mineralize the openings of the exposed tubules (amorphous calcium phosphate pastes). Some desensitizing agents, potassium nitrate in particular, work by passing through the dentinal tubules to the pulp and acting directly on the nerve. Potassium depolarizes the nerve so it cannot fire and cause pain.

Desensitizing agents are used in several different ways. They may be used at the time of placement of a restoration, prior to or after a prophylaxis or scaling and root planing procedure, or for teeth with gingival recession and exposed root surfaces that are hypersensitive to touch or temperature. One of the side effects of teeth whitening can be tooth sensitivity during the whitening process. Some whitening products include chemicals, such as potassium nitrate or fluoride, that reduce or eliminate the sensitivity during whitening.

CATEGORIES AND COMPONENTS OF DESENSITIZING AGENTS

Various desensitizing agents are available. They may be categorized as (1) toothpastes, (2) fluoride gels and varnishes, (3) inorganic salt solutions, (4) resin primers and bonding agents, (5) mineralizing agents, and (6) glass ionomer surface sealer (Table 7.6). Desensitizing toothpastes usually require repeated use over several days or weeks to achieve some relief. The relief will only continue as the toothpaste is used. If the patient discontinues the use of the desensitizing toothpaste, the sensitivity will return. Fluorides also may take a while before results are seen. Some of the inorganic salts that precipitate into the open dentinal tubules and seal their openings will have immediate results; others may take repeated applications. The resin desensitizing agents will have immediate results if all of the open tubules are sealed. A reduced level of sensitivity may remain if some of the tubules are still open. Desensitizing systems using bonding resins may require etching of the surface first, sometimes creating additional temporary sensitivity, particularly with rinsing and application of air. However, self-etching dentin primers are available that do not require rinsing after etching (see Chapter 5). The duration of relief varies greatly, from a few days to close to 1 year. None of these agents provides permanent relief. The duration of relief can be prolonged if the original cause of the sensitivity is eliminated. That is, the poor toothbrushing habit, the acidic diet, or the teeth grinding must be curtailed; otherwise, the desensitizing agent will be removed and the tubules reopened. If a patient has a history of sensitivity, the dental hygienist must provide the patient with one of the desensitizing agents after scaling and root planing. Chronically sensitive root surfaces may require restoration with glass ionomers, compomers, or composites to provide definitive relief.

REMINERALIZATION

Remineralization is the process of repairing the surface of tooth structure that has lost mineral because of exposure to dietary, environmental, gastric, or bacterial acids.

PRODUCTS

Some of the products used to treat tooth sensitivity can also be used to help remineralize the tooth. As previously discussed, fluorides are helpful in the remineralization

TABLE 7.6   Desensitizing Agents

PRODUCT CATEGORY	PRODUCT NAME	MANUFACTURER	ACTIVE INGREDIENT
Toothpastes	Sensodyne Deep Clean	GlaxoSmithKlIne	Potassium nitrate
	Sensodyne True White		Potassium nitrate
	Sensodyne Rapid Relief		Stannous fluoride
	Sensodyne Complete Protection		Stannous fluoride
	Sensodyne Repair and Protect		Stannous fluoride
	Colgate Sensitive	Colgate-Palmolive	Potassium nitrate
	Crest Sensi-Relief Whitening	Procter & Gamble	Potassium nitrate
	Colgate PreviDent 5000	Colgate-Palmolive	1.1% sodium fluoride
	Colgate Duraphat 5000 ppm	Colgate-Palmolive	1.1% sodium fluoride
	Clinpro 5000	3M ESPE	1.1% sodium fluoride
	Colgate Gel-Kam	Colgate-Palmolive	0.4% stannous fluoride
Fluoride varnish	FluoroDose	Centrix	5% sodium fluoride
	Vanish	3M ESPE	5% sodium fluoride
	NUPRO Fluoride Varnish	Dentsply	5% sodium fluoride
	Colgate Duraphat	Colgate-Palmolive	5% sodium fluoride
	Duraflor	Medicom	5% sodium fluoride
	Fluor Protector	Ivoclar Vivadent	Fluorsilane compound
Inorganic salts	D/Sense Crystal	Centrix	Calcium oxalate, potassium nitrate
	BisBlock	BISCO	Oxylates
Potassium nitrate	UltraEZ	Ultradent	3% potassium nitrate plus 0.11% sodium fluoride
	Relief ACP	Philips Oral Healthcare	Potassium nitrate, amorphous calcium phosphate
Resin agents	Gluma Desensitizer	Heraeus Kulzer	5% glutaraldehyde, 35% HEMA
	MicroPrime B	Danville Materials	HEMA, 0.5% sodium fluoride
	HurriSeal	Beutlich	HEMA, 0.5% sodium fluoride
	Pain-Free F	Parkell	4-META resin, fluoride (3000 ppm)
	All-Bond DS	BISCO	NTG-GMA and BPDM primers
	Seal & Protect	Dentsply	Prime & Bond NT with 7% filler
Mineralizing agents	SootheRx	3M ESPE	Calcium sodium phosphosilicate
	Teeth Mate	Kuraray America	Calcium phosphates
	MI Paste	GC America	Amorphous calcium phosphate
Glass ionomer surface sealer	Vanish XT	3M ESPE	Glass ionomer cement

BPDM, biphenyl dimethacrylate; HEMA, 2-hydroxyethyl methacrylate; 4-META, 4-methacryloxyethyl trimellitate anhydride; NTG-GMA, N-(p-tolyl)glycine glycidyl methacrylate.

process. Because tooth mineral is largely calcium and phosphate, products that contain calcium and phosphate can help replace lost tooth mineral. The main ingredients of these products are amorphous calcium phosphate or calcium sodium phosphosilicate. One product combines fluoride and amorphous calcium phosphate in a varnish (MI Varnish; GC America) (Fig. 7.21). The varnish will prolong the exposure of the covered tooth surfaces to both components. Glass ionomer cements, because they release fluoride, are also helpful.

RESIN INFILTRATION

A novel approach to halting progression of the early smooth surface white spot carious lesion is to infiltrate the lesion with a low-viscosity resin. As bacterial acids attack the enamel the surface and the body of the developing carious lesion become more porous. The objective for this new approach is to prevent caries progression by blocking the porosity in the enamel with a high-penetration resin (Icon-Infiltrant; DMG America). First, the right type of lesion is selected. The lesion should be on accessible smooth surfaces of the enamel, with no break or cavitation of the surface of the carious lesion. Interproximal early lesions can be treated but are more difficult technically, because they are not readily accessible. Next, the area is isolated and the surface of the lesion is cleaned with pumice. Then 15% hydrochloric acid is applied for 2 minutes, extending 2 mm beyond the borders of the lesion. The acid is washed off, the surface is dried, and an ethanol drying agent is applied for 30 seconds followed by air drying. Next, the penetrating resin is applied in two applications, totaling 4 minutes, and light-cured after each application. Not only does the resin obliterate porosities in the enamel, it makes the white spot lesion much less visible (Fig. 7.22). Although long-term clinical trials have not been done with this technique, the available research supports this conservative approach.

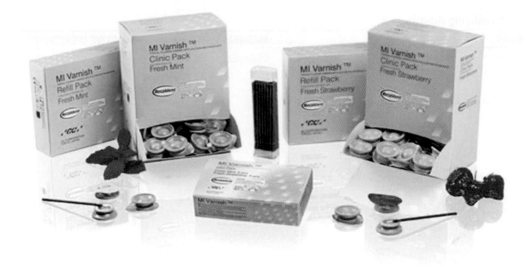

FIG. 7.21 Sample of MI Varnish. (Courtesy of GC Corporation.)

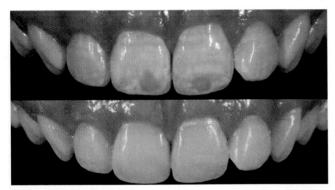

FIG. 7.22 Before and after images of white spot lesions and their improvement after the use of resin infiltration (Icon-infiltrant). (Courtesy of DMG America.)

 Clinical Tip

A current list of desensitizing agents approved by the ADA can be found at the public information section of the ADA website at www.ada.org under the topic ADA Seal of Acceptance. Many of the products available in drugstores have not yet received the ADA Seal of Acceptance.

SUMMARY

Conservative dentistry mandates that the allied oral health practitioner be familiar with the use of the various preventive materials available. By performing caries risk assessment and using topical applications of fluoride, as well as fluoride and antibacterial rinses, early caries can be arrested and tooth structure can often be remineralized. Sealants placed to protect pits and fissures of teeth are recognized as being effective in the prevention of tooth decay. Desensitizing agents are more important now than ever before, because people are retaining their teeth longer, and as a result are subject to the factors that produce root sensitivity. These agents provide relief to patients whose teeth have gingival recession and exposed dentin that subjects them to chronic or episodic pain.

INSTRUCTIONAL VIDEOS

See the Evolve Resources site for a variety of educational videos that reinforce the material covered in this chapter.

Procedure 7.1 Applying Sodium Fluoride Varnish

See Evolve site for Competency Sheet.

EQUIPMENT/SUPPLIES

- Basic examination set-up
- Sodium fluoride varnish
- Applicator brush
- 2×2 gauze squares
- Air water syringe tip
- Disposable cup

PROCEDURE STEPS

1. Open fluoride varnish container and mix solution with applicator brush if slight separation has occurred.

   NOTE: Product does expire. Clinician should inspect product and discard if past manufacturer's expiration date.

2. Hand patient cup for use at conclusion of application of varnish.

3. Remove excess fluids from the mouth prior to application of varnish.

4. Dry excess saliva from teeth by wiping dentition with 2×2 gauze square or lightly blowing air with air-water syringe.

5. Apply small amount of varnish to each tooth using applicator brush (Fig. 7.23).

   NOTE: Read manufacturer's instructions for recommended application. Some manufacturers recommend painting one surface of the tooth (i.e., facial or lingual).

6. Once all teeth have been painted, have the patient rub their tongue along all surfaces of the teeth to assist in distribution of varnish into the interproximal areas.

7. Have patient expectorate into disposable cup.

NOTE: Do not use saliva ejector or high-volume evacuation to gather excess fluids or varnish from the patient's mouth. The varnish will clog the suction lines over time.

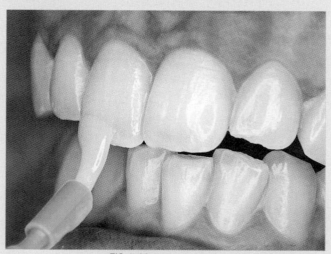

FIG. 7.23 (Courtesy of Dentistry Today.)

8. Instruct the patient to refrain from eating foods which are extremely hot, crunchy, or contain alcohol as all can remove the varnish from the tooth surface.

9. Instruct the patient to brush their teeth normally to remove all varnish from the tooth surface.

   NOTE: Varnish may remain on the teeth for 1 to 3 days if the patient brushes gently.

10. Provide patient with the homecare instructions sheet available from the manufacturer.

    NOTE: Each manufacturer provides homecare instruction sheets with their products to be distributed to the patient at the conclusion of treatment.

Procedure 7.2 Applying Topical Fluoride

See Evolve site for Competency Sheet.

EQUIPMENT/SUPPLIES (Fig. 7.24)

- Disposable trays of various sizes
- Topical fluoride foam or gel
- Air-water syringe
- Watch or timer
- Cotton rolls
- Saliva ejector
- High-volume evacuation (HVE) tip

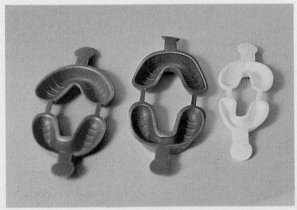

FIG. 7.24

PROCEDURE STEPS

1. Select appropriate disposable tray for the size of the patient's mouth (Fig. 7.25).
2. Examine the patient for the presence of calculus.

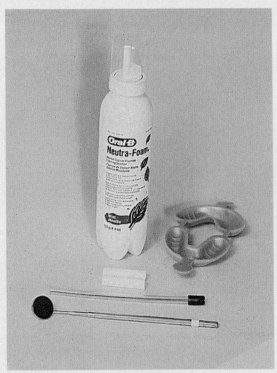

FIG. 7.25

If present, perform scaling procedure before proceeding.

   NOTE: Do not polish teeth with premanufactured prophylaxis paste. Flavoring oils deposited on the surfaces of the teeth may reduce the absorption of fluoride.

3. Seat the patient upright.

   NOTE: This reduces the amount of gel going down the patient's throat.

4. Load trays with fluoride (Fig. 7.26). Do not overfill, because that will cause excess fluoride to run into the patient's mouth.

   NOTE: Follow appropriate guidelines for the age of

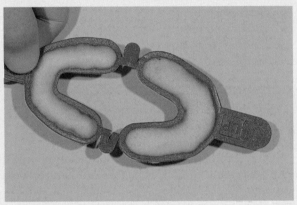

FIG. 7.26

the patient.

5. Place trays in the patient's mouth (Fig. 7.27). Place cotton rolls between the trays and have the patient close on the cotton rolls to keep the trays in place.
6. Place the saliva ejector in the mouth on the cheek

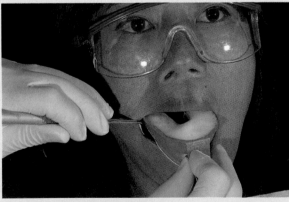

FIG. 7.27

side or between the trays, in the space created by the cotton rolls (Fig. 7.28).

   NOTE: The taste of the gel or foam and the presence of the trays will greatly increase the flow of saliva.

7. Time the fluoride application.

Procedure 7.2 Applying Topical Fluoride—cont'd

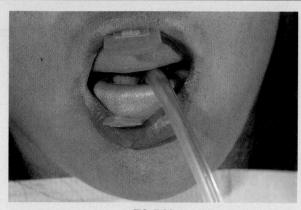

FIG. 7.28

8. Remove the trays after the appropriate time has passed. Remove excess gel/foam and saliva from the patient's mouth by HVE.
9. Instruct the patient not to rinse, eat, or drink for 30 minutes.

NOTE: Fluoride circulating in the saliva will continue to have a topical effect for a few hours after treatment.

Procedure 7.3 Applying Silver Diamine Fluoride (SDF)

See Evolve site for Competency Sheet

EQUIPMENT/SUPPLIES

- Basic examination set-up
- Silver diamine fluoride
- Lubricant ie: Palmer's Cocoa Butter or Vaseline to prevent staining of tissues
- Plastic dappen dish
- Microbrush
- Air-water syringe
- Watch or timer
- Cotton rolls, dry angles
- 2×2 gauze squares
- Saliva ejector
- High-volume evacuation (HVE) tip
- Super floss
- Bite block

PROCEDURE STEPS

1. Dispense one drop of SDF into plastic dappen dish.
   NOTE: One drop of solution will treat 1-5 teeth.
   NOTE: Glass dappen dish may react with the SDF.
2. Isolate area to be treated with SDF.

NOTE: Dental dam, cotton rolls, or dry angles can be used to isolate the area being treated.
3. Dry area with 2x2 gauze square
   NOTE: Drying area with air-water syringe is not recommended as this may cause the patient sensitivity.
4. Place microbrush into dappen dish to absorb a small amount of SDF.
5. Apply SDF to area of caries (see Fig. 7.9).
   NOTE: Keep SDF from touching unwanted areas such as gingival tissues and face as it will stain. If staining of the face occurs, immediately wipe face with hydrogen peroxide. This will reduce the staining that occurs on the face; however, the stain will subside on its own without wiping with peroxide.
6. Keep isolated and allow to dry for 60 seconds.
7. Remove excess with 2×2 gauze square.
   NOTE: Some patients complain of a metallic aftertaste due to the silver content in the solution.
8. Inspect areas of decay to ensure all susceptible areas have absorbed the SDF (see Fig. 7.10).
   NOTE: Glass ionomer can be placed over the tooth treated with SDF to reduce the discoloration that occurs. (See Chapter 6 for benefits of glass ionomer.)

Procedure 7.4 Applying Dental Sealants

See Evolve site for Competency Sheet.

EQUIPMENT/SUPPLIES (FIG. 7.29)

- Basic examination setup
- Prophy setup: slow-speed handpiece with prophy angle, prophy cup, or bristle brush
- High-volume evacuation (HVE), saliva ejector tips, and air-water syringe tip
- Dental dam setup (check for latex allergy); alternative isolation: cotton rolls and holder
- Flour of pumice or special prophy paste without fluoride or oils
- Dappen dish for pumice and mixing well for sealant, if supplied in bulk
- Curing light if using light-cure sealant, and light shield
- Sealant material: Self-cure or light-cure
- Etching solution/gel: 35% phosphoric acid
- Applicator brush or tips (some sealant materials have an applicator)
- Articulating paper, dental floss
- Bullet-shaped finishing bur or polishing stone

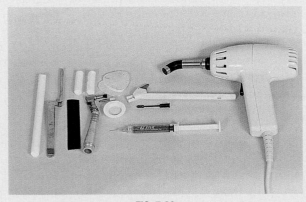

FIG. 7.29

PROCEDURE STEPS

1. Place dental dam or cotton rolls and saliva ejector to isolate teeth to be sealed.

   NOTE: Moisture contamination with saliva or water can cause a loss of or leaking sealant.

2. Clean the surfaces of the teeth to be sealed with pumice or oil/fluoride-free paste (Fig. 7.30).

3. Use three-way syringe and HVE to rinse and dry teeth thoroughly. Remove any retained polishing paste (Fig. 7.31).

   NOTE: Some dentists prefer to clean out the fissures with a small round or needle-shaped bur or diamond rotary instrument. This allows them to inspect the fissures for the presence of caries.

4. Place etchant on enamel to be sealed for 20 to 30 seconds (Fig. 7.32).

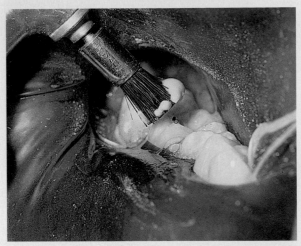

FIG. 7.30

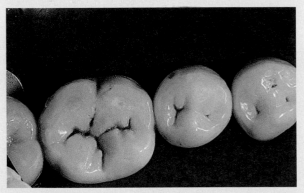

FIG. 7.31

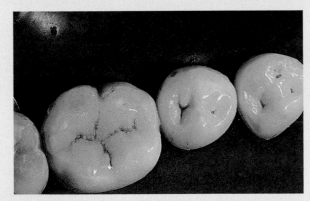

FIG. 7.32

NOTE: Some teeth need longer etching times, such as primary teeth and teeth with fluorosis.

5. Rinse with water for 10 to 15 seconds.

6. If using cotton rolls, carefully replace them or dry them out with the HVE.

   NOTE: Be certain that saliva does not contaminate the freshly etched surfaces or the enamel will need to be re-etched for 15 seconds.

Procedure 7.4   Applying Dental Sealants—cont'd

7. Dry the teeth thoroughly.

NOTE: Properly etched enamel should appear frosty (Fig. 7.33). If not adequately etched, re-etch for an additional 30 seconds. The fissures in Fig. 7.33 were opened minimally with a small bur before etching.

8. Apply sealant according to the manufacturer's instructions.

NOTE: Sealant should be gently worked into the pits and fissures to displace trapped air. It should cover the entire fissure but should not overfill the groove pattern because that will probably interfere with the occlusion.

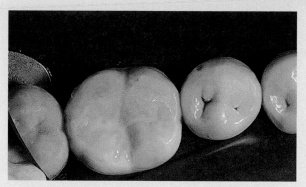

FIG. 7.34

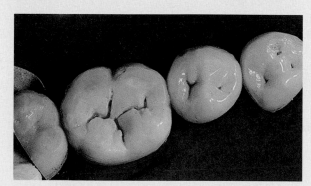

FIG. 7.33

9. Cure appropriately for the required length of time (self-cure or light-cure) (Fig. 7.34).

NOTE: If light-curing, each area under the light probe should be cured for at least 20 seconds. High-powered curing lights may require less time. Follow the manufacturer's recommendations.

10. Check with an explorer to ensure that all fissures and pits are covered, no holes in the material exist, and sealant is well retained. Apply more material, if needed.

11. Remove dental dam or cotton rolls and thoroughly rinse.

12. Check occlusion with articulating paper and adjust sealant where needed.

NOTE: Follow state laws as to which health care practitioners are allowed to do adjustment.

13. Check contact areas with floss.

NOTE: Excess material may have blocked these areas.

14. Check retention at each subsequent visit.

NOTE: Sealants should be checked for partial or complete loss. Make sure fissures are still covered. With retained sealants, check periphery for staining that may indicate leakage. Extensive decay can occur under leaking sealants if not detected early. Replace lost or leaking sealants.

Get Ready for Exams!

Review Questions

Select the one correct response for each of the following multiple-choice questions.

1. Fluoride helps to protect the teeth from decay by which one of the following?
   a. Neutralizing bacterial acids
   b. Making the enamel more resistant to bacterial acids
   c. Deflecting sugars from the tooth surface
   d. Removing bacterial plaque from the tooth surface

2. When tooth enamel first begins to demineralize, what is one of the corrective measures that can be taken to stimulate remineralization?
   a. Stop eating foods with proteins and amino acids
   b. Use a daily rinse containing fluoride
   c. Brush with baking soda and salt
   d. Check the labels on food packages to determine whether they contain fluoride

3. When enamel is remineralized with fluoride,
   a. It is a different color
   b. The fluoride contains a poison that kills all bacteria associated with dental caries
   c. The resultant remineralized crystal is more resistant to acids
   d. All of the calcium is replaced

4. Fluorosis is always considered to be:
   a. Destructive to the teeth
   b. Very unsightly
   c. A sign that the person has ingested more than the optimal amount of fluoride
   d. A sign that the person will need to have whitening and restorations

5. Nightly home fluoride treatment with 1.1% sodium fluoride as a brush-on gel or in custom trays is indicated for:
   a. Children younger than 6 years of age
   b. Adolescents with one or two pit and fissure caries

Continued

   c. Middle-aged women going through menopause

   d. Elderly patients taking medications that cause dry mouth

6. Sealant material is:
   a. Indicated for all permanent molars
   b. Used for protection of smooth surface caries
   c. An unfilled or lightly filled resin
   d. Never in need of replacement once it is placed

7. When a dental sealant is placed, the technique:
   a. Is exactly the same as bonding to dentin
   b. Requires the field to be kept dry
   c. Can be done by dental hygienists and assistants in all states
   d. Always requires the use of a curing light

8. Which one of the following is the best candidate for a sealant?
   a. A newly erupted tooth with numerous deep fissures
   b. A tooth with shallow pits and fissures
   c. A tooth with decay into the dentin
   d. A molar with stained fissures in a 50-year-old patient

9. If caries in a fissure is undetected and is inadvertently covered by a well-placed sealant, what will happen?
   a. Caries will progress rapidly
   b. Caries will progress slowly
   c. Caries will stop progressing

10. Very small filler particles are added to sealant material for which purpose?
   a. To improve the esthetics
   b. To decrease wear of the sealant
   c. To increase adhesion to the enamel
   d. To block the opening of the fissure

11. How is the surface of the tooth prepared before acid etching for sealant placement?
   a. The patient is asked to brush her/his teeth
   b. The teeth are wiped with gauze
   c. A fluoride gel is applied
   d. The surfaces are cleaned with pumice

12. The acid most commonly used to etch the enamel for sealant placement is which one?
   a. Citric acid
   b. Phosphoric acid
   c. Hydrochloric acid
   d. Nitric acid

13. The tip of the light wand of the curing light should be held how close to the sealant?
   a. In contact with the sealant
   b. Very close—about 1 mm away from the surface
   c. About 0.5 inch away
   d. With a good light it doesn't matter how far away you are

14. All of the following *except* one are reasons why pits and fissures are so susceptible to caries. Which one is the *exception*?
   a. The enamel lining them is always very thin
   b. They retain bacteria and food debris
   c. Toothbrush bristles cannot reach into the fissures to clean them
   d. They are often deep and narrow

15. After placement of a sealant, which of the following should be checked?
   a. The sealant surface for voids or porosities

   b. The occlusion
   c. The contact areas with adjacent teeth
   d. All of the above

16. The most common reason for loss of a sealant shortly after placement is which of the following?
   a. Inadequate etching time
   b. Inadequate curing time
   c. The sealant material was bad
   d. Saliva contamination after acid etching

17. How should the surface of the enamel appear after acid etching?
   a. Frosty white
   b. Shiny
   c. Bright gray
   d. Slightly yellow

18. What does acid etching do to the surface of the enamel?
   a. It creates a roughened, irregular surface
   b. It leaves a smooth, clean surface
   c. It evenly removes about half the enamel
   d. None of the above

19. The most important requirement for successfully bonding sealants to enamel is:
   a. Good isolation to prevent saliva contamination
   b. A high concentration of acid for etching
   c. Long etching times (60 seconds or longer)
   d. Long drying times (20 to 40 seconds)

20. Studies show caries to occur in pits and fissures most often in which group of teeth?
   a. Permanent maxillary incisors
   b. Permanent premolars
   c. Permanent molars

21. How does a sealant adhere to the etched enamel surface?
   a. Micromechanical retention
   b. Chemical bond to the surface
   c. By shrinking; when polymerized it tightly grips the surface
   d. The sealant is very sticky and adheres to the surface like glue

22. The main purpose of most desensitizing agents:
   a. Is to close the openings of the enamel rods to prevent temperature and osmotic changes in the enamel fluids
   b. Is to help the dental hygienist keep the patient comfortable during the dental prophylaxis procedure
   c. Is to plug the openings of the exposed dentinal tubules
   d. When added to toothpaste, is to improve the taste and keep it from burning the gingiva

23. What ingredient in Silver Diamine Fluoride stains the decayed portion of the tooth and anything it comes in contact with?
   a. Fluoride
   b. Ammonia
   c. Silver
   d. Water

24. Application of Silver Diamine Fluoride _____ times per year has shown to arrest caries at 90%.
   a. 1
   b. 2

Get Ready for Exams!—cont'd

c. 3
d. 4

25. Fluoride varnish can remain on the teeth for _____ days with light brushing.
   a. 1 to 3
   b. 1 to 2
   c. 1

For answers to Review Questions, see the Appendix.

Case-Based Discussion Topics

1. A 14-year-old female high school student with no restorations comes to the dental office with poor oral hygiene and early caries in the fissures of her mandibular first molars. An analysis of her diet reveals frequent consumption of sodas and between-meal snacking on sugary foods.

Discuss preventive measures that should be recommended for this young woman and the rationale for their use. What diet recommendations would you recommend for her?

2. A 75-year-old retired plumber who takes medication for hypertension comes to the dental office with moderate marginal gingivitis, root caries, and a complaint of dry mouth.

Discuss which of the antibacterial rinses this man should use. Discuss the type of fluoride regimen he should be using. Explain the rationale for each of these recommendations.

3. A 56-year-old business executive comes to the dental office for her annual examination and cleaning. Her chief complaint is that her front teeth are yellowing and thinning on the incisal edges. She also notes sensitivity to cold, sweets, and air on the roots of her maxillary premolars in areas of gingival recession. Questioning reveals that she loves lemons. She eats about five lemons each week and uses lemon juice frequently in cooking and on her salads.

Discuss the origin of her complaints and preventive and therapeutic measures that should be recommended for her.

4. A 3-year-old girl is brought to the dental office with baby bottle tooth decay on the maxillary anterior teeth. The mother said the girl does not complain about the teeth being sore but her mother does not want her to be in pain if teeth are left untreated.

Discuss how the teeth can be treated and how the decay can be prevented in the future. Explain how you would describe the necessary treatment to the parent and what post-op instructions would be provided.

BIBLIOGRAPHY

American Dental Association (ADA): Council on scientific affairs: evidence-based clinical recommendations for the use of pit-and-fissure sealants, *J Am Dent Assoc* 139:257–267, 2008.

Azuma Y, Ozasa N, Ueda Y, et al: Pharmacological studies on the anti-inflammatory action of phenolic compounds, *J Dent Res* 65:53–56, 1986.

Bird DL, Robinson DS: Oral health and prevention of dental disease. In *Modern Dental Assisting*, ed 12, Missouri, 2018, Elsevier.

Collins FM, Florman M: *Fluoride Guide*, Penwell Continuing Education Course, 2010.

Crespin, Shuman I: *Fluoride and Other Preventive Therapies; Maintaining Oral Health at Each Stage of Life*, Penwell Continuing Education Course, 2017.

Darby ML, Walsh MM: Dental caries management by risk assessment. In *Dental Hygiene Theory and Practice*, ed 4, St. Louis, 2015, Elsevier Saunders.

Eakle WS, Featherstone JD, Weintraub JA, et al: Salivary fluoride levels following application of fluoride varnish or fluoride rinse, *Community Dent Oral Epidemiol* 32:462–469, 2004.

Featherstone JD: Prevention and reversal of dental caries: role of low-level fluoride, *Community Dent Oral Epidemiol* 27:31–40, 1999.

Going RE, Loesche WJ, Grainger DA, et al: The viability of microorganisms in carious lesions five years after covering with a fissure sealant, *J Am Dent Assoc* 97:455–462, 1978.

Griffin SO, Jones K, Gray SK, et al: Exploring four-handed delivery and retention of resin-based sealants, *J Am Dent Assoc* 139:281–289, 2008.

Handelman SL, Leverett DH, Espeland MA, et al: Clinical radiographic evaluation of sealed carious and sound tooth surfaces, *J Am Dent Assoc* 113:751–754, 1986.

Healthy People 2020. Available at: Healthypeople.gov

Idon Pl, Esan TA, Bamise CT, Mohammed ASA, et al: Dentine hypersensitivity: review of a common oral health problem, *J AM Dent Assoc* 2:16, 2017.

Li Y: Dentin hypersensitivity: diagnosis and strategic approaches, *Inside Dentistry*, 2013.

Loskill K, Zeitz C, Grandthyll S, et al: Reduced adhesion of oral bacteria on hydroxyapatite by fluoride treatment, *Langmuir* 29:5528–5533, 2013.

Mandel JD: Chemotherapeutic agents for controlling plaque and gingivitis, *J Clin Periodontol* 15:488–498, 1988.

Oong E, Griffin SO, Kohn WG, et al: The effect of dental sealants on bacteria levels in caries lesions, *J Am Dent Assoc* 139:271–278, 2008.

Paris S, Meyer-Lueckel H: Inhibition of caries progression by resin infiltration in situ, *Caries Res* 44:54–57, 2010.

Robinson DS, Bird DL: Preventive dentistry, *Modern dental assisting*, ed 12, St. Louis, 2017, Elsevier.

Simonsen RJ: Retention and effectiveness of dental sealant after 15 years, *J Am Dent Assoc* 122:34–42, 1991.

Strassler HE: Dentin hypersensitivity: an update on diagnosis and etiology, *Inside Dentistry*, 2014.

Trushkowsky RD, Garcia-Godoy F: Dentin hypersensitivity: differential diagnosis, tests, and etiology. *Compend Contin Educ Dent*, 2014

8

Teeth Whitening Materials and Procedures

Chapter Objectives

Upon completion of this chapter, the student should be able to:

1. Describe how whitening materials penetrate the tooth.
2. Compare and contrast the whitening materials used for in-office, take home, and OTC home use.
3. Describe the precautions to take to protect the oral tissues when applying in-office power whitening products.
4. List the steps in the procedures for in-office power whitening.
5. List the potential side effects of in-office power whitening.
6. List the potential side effects of home whitening.

7. Describe the methods to whiten nonvital teeth.
8. Discuss the relative effectiveness of whitening products and whitening toothpastes in removing stains from teeth.
9. Demonstrate proper fabrication of home whitening trays.
10. Explain to a patient how home whitening products are used.
11. Identify clinical situations in which enamel microabrasion might be used.
12. Explain how enamel microabrasion works.

Key Terms

Whitening a cosmetic process that uses chemicals to remove discolorations from teeth or to lighten them

Extrinsic Stains stains occurring on the tooth surface

Intrinsic Stains stains that are incorporated into the tooth structure, usually during the tooth's development

Vital tooth has a living pulp, which produces response to temperature change or electrical stimuli

Power whitening in-office whitening procedure that uses strong whitening agents and may use a high-intensity light source to accelerate the whitening process

Nonvital tooth: no longer has a living pulp and ceases to give response to electrical stimuli or temperature changes

Walking bleach technique whitening technique for nonvital teeth in which whitening materials are sealed inside the tooth crown for a few days and the patient "walks" around with the whitening material in place

Enamel Microabrasion a process that uses hydrochloric acid and an abrasive such as pumice to remove shallow discolorations of the enamel

---

Teeth darken as part of the aging process; although, some teeth are discolored from medications or chemicals incorporated into the developing enamel and dentin. In a society where many strive to maintain their youthful appearance, patients desire to regain their brighter, whiter smiles. This has caused an explosion in the demand for cosmetic dental services. The use of whitening products has increased dramatically over the past quarter century. Whitening of teeth has become a significant part of many dental practices. Whitening can be done as an in-office procedure or as a home procedure supervised by the dentist. The dental auxiliary, depending on the state dental practice act, can perform many of the procedures associated with the whitening process, such as making impressions and custom trays, delivering and demonstrating use of the home whitening materials to the patient, providing home use instructions and precautions, and helping with various steps in the in-office whitening procedure. They can answer questions patients have about whitening. This team effort can help in the growth of the practice as pleased patients tell their friends and relatives

about the excellent services they have received from a knowledgeable, caring staff.

TEETH WHITENING (BLEACHING)

Controlled research and case studies indicate that **whitening** with peroxide products is safe and effective. Many stains and discolorations of the teeth can be removed or lightened by whitening procedures. However, some stains are more difficult to remove than others.

TYPES OF STAINS

Teeth may be discolored by **extrinsic stains** on the tooth surface, **intrinsic stains** incorporated internally into the tooth structure (often when the tooth is developing), or a combination of both (Table 8.1). Long standing extrinsic stains can penetrate the enamel to become intrinsic stains which makes the removal of the stain more difficult.

TABLE 8.1 Causes and Colors of Extrinsic and Intrinsic Discoloration

CAUSE	COLOR
Extrinsic Stain	
Poor oral hygiene	Yellow, brown, green, black
Coffee, tea, red wine, colored cola drinks, foods	Brown to black
Tobacco products and betel leaf chewing	Yellow-brown to black
Antimicrobial rinse (chlorhexidine)	Brown
Intrinsic Stain	
Medications during Tooth Development	
Tetracycline	Brown, gray, black bands
Fluoride	White, brown spots or bands
Medications after Tooth Development	
Minocycline (tetracycline-type drug)	Brown, gray
Diseases/Conditions during Tooth Development	
Conditions such as purpura (a blood disorder)	Red, brown, purple
Trauma	Blue, black, brown
Pulpal Changes	
Pulp canal obliteration	Yellow
Pulp necrosis with hemorrhage	Gray, black
Pulp necrosis without hemorrhage	Yellow, gray-brown
Other Causes in Nonvital Teeth	
Trauma during pulp extirpation	Gray, black
Tissue remnants in the pulp chamber	Brown, gray, black
Restorative dental materials	Brown, gray, black
Endodontic materials (not currently in use in USA)	Gray, black
Combination Intrinsic/Extrinsic Stains	
Aging	Yellow

Adapted with permission from Hayward VB: Current status and recommendations of dentist-prescribed, at home tooth whitening. *Contemp Esthet Rest Pract* 1999;3(suppl):2—9.

Extrinsic Stains

Some common foods or drinks that are known to contribute to extrinsic staining of the teeth include coffee, tea, red wine, colored cola drinks, grape juice, and berries. Poor oral hygiene accompanied by pigment-producing bacteria and food stains can also produce extrinsic stains of varying colors (Fig. 8.1). Tobacco products and betel leaf chewing also contribute to staining of the teeth (Fig. 8.2).

Antimicrobial mouth rinses such as chlorhexidine can contribute to surface staining (Fig. 8.3). Some extrinsic stains limited to the surface can be removed, in part, by toothbrushing, whitening dentifrices, and whitening mouth rinses. The dental hygienist can remove other stains by (1) hand or ultrasonic scaling, (2) coronal polishing, or (3) air polishing (using a spray of sodium bicarbonate or aluminum trihydroxide under air pressure). More stubborn stains that have penetrated the enamel surface cannot be polished or scaled away. These may require whitening products (peroxides) to remove them.

Intrinsic Stains

Intrinsic stains are internal and may be a result of developmental disturbances of the teeth during

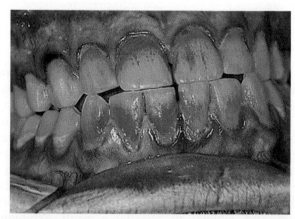

FIG. 8.1 Extrinsic stain on the teeth. Greenish stain as a result of accumulation of plaque, pellicle, food debris, and pigment-producing bacteria. (Courtesy of Dr. Steve Eakle, University of California, San Francisco, CA.)

development or hereditary conditions, or they may be age-related. Developmental disturbances can result from trauma to the developing teeth, illness with high fever, and excessive intake of fluoride or certain medications. Intrinsic stains such as age-related discolorations that are yellow or light brown are easier

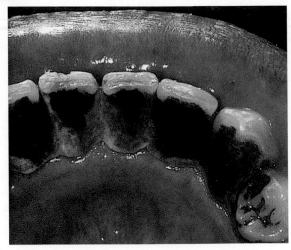

FIG. 8.2 Extrinsic stains on the teeth. Dark brown stains are the result of poor oral hygiene due to frequent smoking. (Courtesy of Dr. Steve Eakle, University of California, San Francisco, CA.)

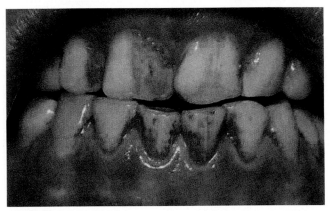

FIG. 8.3 Extrinsic stains on the teeth. Light brown stains on the teeth are a result of chlorhexidine antimicrobial mouthrinse. (From teethandmouth.blogspot.com. Courtesy of Asanka.)

to whiten than blue-gray and black stains. Blue-gray, gray-black, and yellow-brown stains are often caused during tooth development by chemicals or drugs, such as tetracycline or doxycycline (see Fig. 8.11). As a consequence, they are incorporated deep within the dentin and are also found in the enamel. Other antibiotics that are cycline derivatives can cause discoloration of teeth in adults as well. Externally applied, vital whitening usually takes much longer to lighten tetracycline stains and achieve an acceptable result. Whitening may make white spots from mild fluorosis less apparent by making the whole tooth whiter.

A single dark tooth should be radiographed and tested for vitality: even if the tooth is symptom free, the pulp may have died. Stains associated with endodontically treated teeth may require internal whitening. Some stains such as those caused by amalgam or dental caries are resistant to whitening. For stains that cannot be removed by whitening, tooth-colored restorative means such as veneers, crowns, or

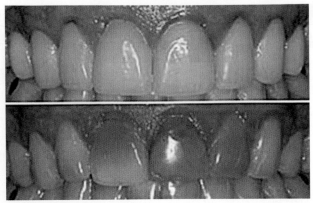

FIG. 8.4 Discolored teeth restored with Porcelain Veneers. (Courtesy of Huefner Sensational Smiles.)

composites must be used to eradicate the discoloration (Fig. 8.4).

HISTORY OF PEROXIDE WHITENING

In the mid-1960s some periodontists began applying peroxide in strips to aid in healing of gingival tissues following periodontal treatment. Soon after, orthodontist Bill Klusmier began using that approach by having his patients apply Gly-Oxide (GlaxoSmith-Kline) containing 10% carbamide peroxide to the interior of their orthodontic positioners to reduce gingival inflammation. Quite by accident he discovered that their teeth were also whiter. The discovery was largely ignored until the 1980s when general dentist John Munro directing his patients to use a 10% carbamide peroxide solution to reduce gingival inflammation noticed that their teeth became whiter. He developed a technique to fabricate a vacuum-formed plastic tray to contain the peroxide solution. He collaborated with a manufacturer resulting in the first commercial whitening preparation in 1988. Heymann and Haywood in 1989 introduced the technique of "nightguard bleaching" using a much more viscous solution to which Carbopol, a thickening agent, was added. It allowed the whitening agent to remain in the tray much longer and increased the whitening time. Later in 1989 Dan Fischer created a very thick whitening gel of carbamide peroxide called Opalescence (Ultradent Products) and the use of night guard whitening became wildly popular.

HOW WHITENING WORKS

The enamel of the tooth crown is composed almost entirely of mineral (97% by weight) with microscopic spaces between the enamel rods that contain water and organic material (Fig. 8.5). Stains accumulate within these small spaces in the enamel over time that may also penetrate to the dentin. Whitening occurs when a type of peroxide or other whitening material passes through the spaces in the enamel and reaches the dentin, where it releases oxygen free radicals that oxidize the stains and subsequently lighten the color of the dentin. This process can be accelerated by the use of low-intensity heat or high-intensity light, such as with a conventional composite curing light, a laser, or a high-intensity plasma arc light. Open carious lesions and leaking restorations can allow the whitening agents to penetrate too deeply into the tooth and pulpal irritation may result.

Some manufacturers have suggested that acid etching the enamel before application of the whitening chemical may enhance the penetration of the whitening material by increasing the permeability of the enamel. Research has shown that this does not improve whitening, and it can contribute to additional complications, such as increased sensitivity and surface wear. Etching may necessitate polishing the enamel before the patient is dismissed, because of the surface roughness it creates.

Whitening Materials

Depending on the manufacturer, current whitening products are based on either hydrogen peroxide or carbamide peroxide. Some products also contain additives such as potassium nitrate, amorphous calcium phosphate (ACP), casein phosphopeptide-ACP, calcium sodium phosphosilicate, arginine calcium carbonate, tri-calcium phosphate, and fluoride to help reduce sensitivity.

Hydrogen Peroxide. Hydrogen peroxide products are available as a liquid, varnish, or gel in concentrations ranging from 5% to 40%. Gels usually stay put best due to viscosity while liquids can more readily seep under a rubber dam and cause tissue burns. Varnishes typically remain in place for a specific period of time due to a clear protective coating placed over them. Personal protective equipment (PPE) should be worn by patients, operators, and auxiliaries when performing in-office hydrogen peroxide whitening procedures.

Carbamide Peroxide. Carbamide peroxide products are popular for home whitening and are available as liquids or gels in concentrations ranging from 10% to 35%, but some 44% gels are also available. Carbamide peroxide is a weaker oxidizing agent than hydrogen peroxide. A 10% carbamide peroxide gel breaks down into 3.35% hydrogen peroxide and 6.65% urea. The urea further breaks down into ammonia and water and increases the pH value of the solution, subsequently providing beneficial side effects of slowing demineralization by bacterial acids as part of the caries process. Carbamide products also contain either carbopol or glycerine base which slows the release of hydrogen peroxide making it work for a longer period of time.

Pretreatment Evaluation. Prior to starting the whitening process a thorough evaluation must be done that includes radiographs and a clinical examination to determine the following: cause of the stains, other treatment needs before whitening, alternatives to whitening, and the ideal whitening procedures for the specific patient's problem. Dental caries, leaking restorations, abscessed teeth, and root resorption should all be addressed before starting the whitening process. If gingival recession has occurred and root surfaces are exposed, the patient should be informed that it is more difficult to whiten the root surface and whitening may not be successful on these surfaces. White spots such as mild fluorosis will not be removed by whitening but may be less noticeable when the surrounding tooth surfaces are whitened.

Treatment Methods. There are three main treatment options for patients who wish to whiten their teeth. Treatment may be done as follows:
1. In the dental office, by the dentist and staff
2. At home, with the dentist prescribing and dispensing whitening materials for the patient to use
3. At home, with the patient purchasing over-the-counter whitening products and using them without professional supervision

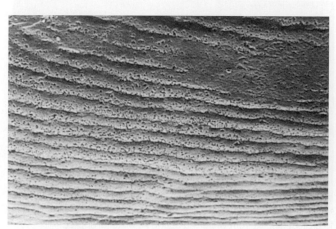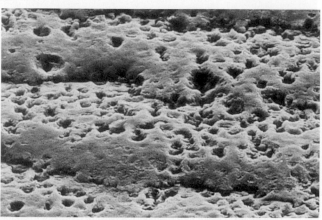

FIG. 8.5 The porosity of the enamel surface may be seen by scanning electron microscopy. An enlargement of the same image is seen on the *right*. (Courtesy of Dr. Ole Fejerskov, Aarhus University, Denmark.)

IN-OFFICE WHITENING

Whitening of Vital Teeth

In-office whitening is ideal for patients who want results quickly. Advantages of treatment in the dental office include direct supervision by the dentist and the staff, elimination of patient compliance issues, control over the whitening process, and ability to discontinue treatment if a problem arises. Whitening is done in the dental office for both vital and nonvital teeth. A **vital tooth** has a living pulp, which produces response to temperature change or electrical stimuli.

Whitening involves the use of various strengths of hydrogen peroxide solutions and gels or carbamide peroxide gels. For years whitening was done by means of a liquid consisting of 35% hydrogen peroxide and the application of a heating lamp. This method can be effective for single-tooth whitening, but it is a time-consuming process and is technique sensitive. If any of the liquid contacts the soft tissues, it can cause a chemical burn that will turn the affected tissue white, cause sloughing of the tissue and may be painful (Fig. 8.6). If gingival tissue is affected, Vitamin E oil (obtained by breaking open a vitamin E capsule) should be applied

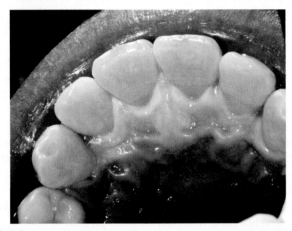

FIG. 8.6 Chemical burn of gingiva from contact with high-concentration hydrogen peroxide. (Courtesy of Dr. Steve Eakle, University of California, San Francisco, CA.)

to the site as soon as it is discovered. Many manufacturers of in-office whitening provide Vitamin E oil as part of the kit.

A high-concentration gel of 35% (or 45%) carbamide peroxide is more controllable than liquid hydrogen peroxide. All of these high-concentration products require the use of isolation consisting of a dental dam and gingival protection with petroleum jelly, or paint-on light-cured dental dam materials (such as Opal-Dam; Ultradent Products) (Fig. 8.7). Prior to completing a whitening procedure, it is best to record the starting shade of the patient's teeth via a Classic Vita shade guide (Fig. 8.8). Intra-oral before and after photos should be taken for in-office and take-home whitening procedures (Procedure 8.1). Vita also has a guide for bleaching purposes—see image below the classic guide. Also the classic guide can be arranged by value so that shades go from light to dark to make comparisons easier.

VITA BLEACHING GUIDE 3D MASTER

Power Whitening

In-office **"power whitening"** (use of strong whitening agents which may be activated by high-intensity light) has become a popular procedure, because it can be completed in one visit, and there is no need to rely on patient compliance as with home-use systems. Many patients simply do not want to spend the time to whiten their teeth at home for several hours a day over a period of two or more weeks. Special curing lights, light-emitting diode (LED) light, plasma arc light, or argon laser light may be used with the power whitening in-office systems. Some older systems utilized ultraviolet (UV) lights and the clinician must be aware if this type of light is being utilized as there are additional precautions to take with the patient. When using a UV light additional protection is needed on the patient's lips and nose. It would be best to have the patient provide a sunscreen of choice to limit allergies or breakouts. (Fig. 8.9); the treatment time is usually 45-60

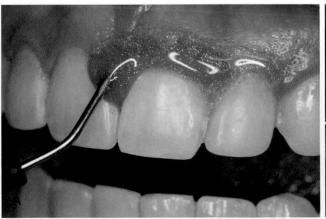
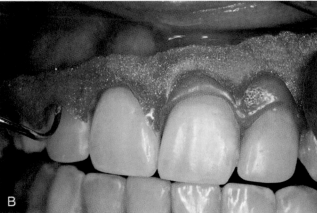

FIG. 8.7 Resin dam material (OpalDam; Ultradent Products) to protect gingiva from whitening agent. **A,** Material applied from syringe with needle cannula, then light cured. **B,** Material peels right off after use. (Courtesy of Ultradent Products, Inc. [South Jordan, UT].)

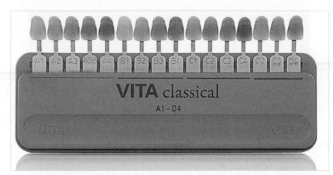

FIG. 8.8 Classic Vita Shade Guide. (Courtesy of Vita.)

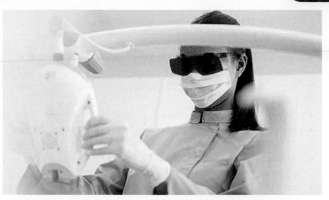

FIG. 8.9 In-office "power" whitening. Patient has protective barriers for oral tissues and eyes. High-intensity light (Zoom, Philips Oral Healthcare) is used to speed whitening. (Courtesy of Philips Oral Healthcare, Stamford, CT.)

minutes. Systems that use light activation of hydrogen peroxide products include Zoom (Philips USA) and LaserSmile (Biolase Technology),

Research shows that the use of high intensity light is not necessary for whitening to occur and at best it may hasten the process. The important factors are the concentration of the whitening material and the contact time with the tooth surface. Due to the high intensity light not being essential to successful whitening, there are products which have been developed that do not use a high-intensity light. Systems using these products include Perfection White (Premier Dental Products), Opalescence Xtra Boost (Ultradent Products), Illumin (Dentsply), and Niveous (Shofu Dental). Whitening materials should be stored in the refrigerator to prolong their limited shelf life.

Newer whitening systems are available which utilize an electrical current to activate the whitening gel or accelerate the whitening process. A special mouthpiece is required to deliver the electrical current without a light or heat. Hydrogen peroxide gels utilized in dental whitening systems must be maintained at a lower pH (5.5) in order to stabilize the materials and increase their shelf-life. The systems that use the electrical current to activate the whitening gel and increase the whitening process work by increasing the pH (10.8) of the hydrogen peroxide whitening gel with the electrical current produced in the whitening tray, thus allowing the whitening gel to lighten stains in the teeth more quickly. As with other in-office whitening systems the tissues must be protected from the peroxide gel as a chemical burn can occur. The paint-on light-cured dental dam materials are the most user friendly with the design of the mouthpiece used to deliver the electrical current.

Some patients may need a longer whitening time or additional visits depending on the type of discoloration they present with. Patients who desire maximal whiteness may need additional treatments or home whitening to achieve the shade they desire. Most systems recommend home tray whitening to complement in-office treatment. Power-whitening systems have a recommended number of applications per visit which is established by the manufacturer and usually fall into a range of 2 to 3 applications. Applications may need to be repeated until the desired whiteness is achieved; however, the maximum number of applications should not be exceeded in one visit as the patient will develop sensitivity. Some patients need more than one visit to achieve the whiteness they desire.

 Caution

High intensity whitening lights and lasers may generate heat that can irritate the pulp and contribute to post-treatment sensitivity.

It is important to remember that teeth dehydrate when they are isolated for a period of time and appear whiter than they will be after several hours when they have rehydrated. Dehydration of the teeth can also contribute to an increase in sensitivity during the procedure. It typically takes at least 2 weeks for the shade to stabilize. So, if a patient is to have cosmetic restorative treatment after whitening procedures, waiting a minimum of 2 weeks before matching the shade of whitened teeth is recommended. Bonding procedures including the placement of composite restorations should not be attempted on newly whitened teeth, because residual whitening materials may still be present in the tooth structure which can prevent proper bonding. Again, a 2-week wait is recommended before bonding.

Whitening results from in-office procedures will not last indefinitely. Manufacturers of in-office whitening recommend supplying patients with custom trays and whitening materials for home use when a "touch up" is desired. One study found that home whitening for 5 days, 8 hours per day, with 10% carbamide peroxide was equivalent to 1 hour of treatment in the office with 25% hydrogen peroxide.

In-Office Power Whitening Process

- Isolate teeth with a rubber dam or liquid-dam
- Retract the lips and use a dental napkin to protect skin around the mouth
- Provide the patient with protective eye wear, ideally with side shields
- Deliver the peroxide whitening gel to the teeth
- Spread the gel over the facial surfaces of the teeth with an applicator brush
- Activate the whitening gel with the recommended light source
- After 20-30 minutes remove the gel with suction and apply a new coating of gel
- Repeat this process for a total of 2-3 times
- Once the process is complete, thoroughly remove all gel, remove barriers, inspect tissues, and apply vitamin E oil as needed
- Apply desensitizing agents supplied with the whitening kit
- Provide the patient with post-treatment instructions

 Caution

The teeth must not be anesthetized during whitening procedures in order for the patient to provide feedback to the clinician pertaining to sensitivity. If the teeth are anesthetized painful stimuli produced by heat or the peroxide solutions does not occur and permanent pulp damage may result.

 Caution

With the use of high-concentration whitening materials the patient and chairside personnel should all wear PPE and avoid splashes to the skin that could cause burns.

Whitening Varnish

As with in-office power whitening, whitening varnish has become a popular procedure. It can be completed in one visit, it is not as technique sensitive as power whitening, and only remains on the teeth for 30 minutes rather than an hour like the power whitening. The teeth are isolated and the gingiva protected with a resin dam material (see Fig. 8.7). After isolated the teeth are painted with a 20% hydrogen peroxide whitening varnish. Once all the teeth on the maxillary and mandibular arches have been painted with the varnish, a sealant layer is painted over the varnish to keep it in place. After 30 minutes the teeth can be brushed or the varnish can be wiped off. Teeth whitening can be continued at home with whitening gel used in custom trays. The whitening varnish is considered a jump start to home-whitening procedures or may be used as a touch-up.

Whitening of Nonvital Teeth

A **nonvital tooth** no longer has a living pulp and ceases to give response to electrical stimuli or temperature changes. When the pulp of a tooth dies, the necrotic

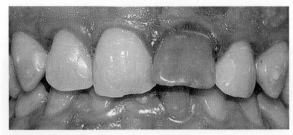

FIG. 8.10 Intrinsic stain in a maxillary central incisor as a result of trauma leading to pulpal death. Staining is due to blood products entering the dentinal tubules. (Courtesy of Dr. Steve Eakle, University of California, San Francisco, CA.)

breakdown products of the pulpal tissue or hemoglobin from blood in the pulp escapes into the surrounding dentinal tubules. Chemicals from these tissues (e.g., iron sulfide from hemoglobin) cause intrinsic staining of the dentin which can turn the tooth dark (Fig. 8.10). Whitening of nonvital teeth in the dental office typically involves teeth that have undergone root canal therapy. Whitening of nonvital teeth requires removing the restoration from the endodontic access cavity (the hole through which the root canal therapy was performed) and whitening internally through this access. The tooth is isolated with a rubber dam to prevent whitening solutions from contacting and burning soft tissues. A 30% to 35% hydrogen peroxide solution or gel is placed in the pulp chamber on a saturated cotton pellet. A hot instrument is plunged into the cotton several times to activate the peroxide.

An alternative approach is the **"walking bleach"** technique, in which a commercially prepared bleaching (whitening) gel or paste made in the office from sodium perborate monohydrate (e.g., Oral-B Amosan; Procter & Gamble) and 30% hydrogen peroxide is sealed into the pulp chamber with a temporary restoration. With the paste, both the sodium perborate monohydrate and hydrogen peroxide products release oxygen that helps whiten the tooth. When the patient returns in 2 to 7 days, the whitening material is removed, and a composite or amalgam restoration is placed in the endodontic access cavity.

Risk of Root Resorption. All internal whitening procedures require that a seal be established at the base of the endodontic access preparation just coronal to the level of gingival attachment to the tooth. This is done to prevent whitening material from leaking out through open dentinal tubules or accessory canals into the periodontal ligament. There have been cases of external root resorption that occurred when the whitening agent activated an inflammatory reaction in the periodontal tissues. External root resorption is an attack on the root surface by cells and enzymes in the periodontal tissues. It can actually eat a hole through the root, and the patient may lose the tooth.

HOME WHITENING (PRESCRIBED BY THE DENTIST)

Home whitening (also called *night guard bleaching*) is a popular and cost-effective means of whitening the teeth, but the treatment interval is much longer compared with in-office treatment (Procedure 8.2). The chemical that is used in home whitening systems is either 10% to 45% carbamide peroxide or 6% to 15% hydrogen peroxide. Carbamide peroxide products break down into two active ingredients, hydrogen peroxide and urea (an aqueous solution). Hydrogen peroxide breaks down into oxygen and water. Some whitening products have potassium nitrate added to reduce tooth sensitivity. Amorphous calcium phosphate (ACP) may be added to home whitening to increase tooth whitening efficacy and decrease dentinal hypersensitivity. Non-peroxide gels are also available and claim not to cause tooth sensitivity or gingival irritation, as peroxide products may do with some patients.

HOME WHITENING PROCESS

The gel is placed in a custom-formed soft, thin plastic tray and is worn by the patient for periods as short as 15 minutes twice daily or as long as overnight. The higher the concentration of the whitening material, application time is decreased. Trays may or may not have spaces, called *reservoirs,* built into them to hold the whitening material. Many offices use reservoirs, but some studies suggest that they may not be needed. Trays should be trimmed to follow the contour of the gingival crest on the facial aspect of the dentition to avoid contact of the gel with the gingiva, because gingival irritation may result (Procedure 8.3). Trimming the tray to follow the contour of the gingival crest on the lingual is not necessary, as the lingual aspect of the teeth will not be whitened.

The home whitening process is as effective as the in-office process but takes much longer and is sometimes used as a follow-up to the in-office procedure, which "jump-starts" the whitening process. Home whitening trays are recommended to be worn daily to achieve optimum results. Hydrogen peroxide solutions oxidize stain more quickly reducing wear time to 15 minutes to 1 hour according to the percentage of solution. Carbamide peroxide solutions oxidize stain slower increasing wear time to 30 minutes to 8 hours according to the percentage of solution. The whitening gels used in custom trays are most effective during the first 2 to 4 hours of use and gradually diminish in effectiveness. The recommended time for follow-up visits during treatment is every 2 to 3 weeks, and the procedure is performed under the supervision of the dentist. At the follow-up appointment, the auxiliary will ensure the

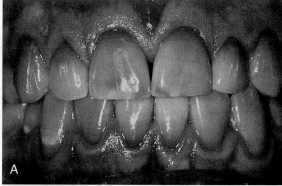
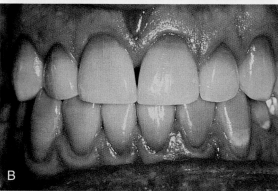

FIG. 8.11 Intrinsic stains. Teeth with tetracycline stains: **A,** before home whitening; **B,** after home whitening. (Courtesy of Ultradent Products, Inc. [South Jordan, UT].)

custom whitening trays still fit appropriately, no gingival burning has occurred, and take a new shade to verify progress.

Whitening agents suggested for night-time application include Nupro White Gold (Dentsply), Nite White Turbo (Philips USA), and Opalescence PF (Ultradent Products) which is for day- or nighttime whitening and another daytime product is Natural Elegance (Henry Schein).

Length of Treatment

The length of treatment varies for each patient depending on his or her discoloration and sensitivity. Yellow and light brown stains that are caused by aging or foods can usually be whitened more easily in about 2 to 4 weeks. Brown or orange stains caused by systemic or development disturbances are more difficult to whiten resulting in a 1 to 3 month whitening time period. The dark gray, brown, or bluish stains of tetracycline are the most resistant to whitening and may take as long as 6 months to whiten (Fig. 8.11). Intrinsic stains in bands or striations may not whiten evenly or at the same rate. Sometimes this difference will make the defect become more apparent.

Informed Consent

Whether whitening procedures are performed in the office or prescribed for home use, it is essential that the patient be informed of the risks and benefits of

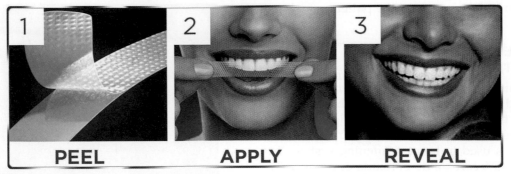

FIG. 8.12 1 – Removal of whitestrip from plastic backing. **2** – Placement of strip on facial aspect of dentition. **3** – Appearance of teeth upon removal of strip. (Courtesy of Proctor & Gamble.)

treatment and the alternatives to whitening, such as restorative procedures. Standardized informed consent forms can be used or the dentist can create one. The patient should sign the informed consent only after potential detrimental side effects and limitations of treatment have been presented and all the patient's questions have been answered. The signature of the patient should be witnessed and then the consent signed by the dentist or staff member. A copy should be given to the patient and one copy entered into the patient's record.

 Caution

Side effects from home whitening include irritation of oral tissues and throat from contact with the gel, hypersensitive teeth, and sore muscles and jaw joints if trays are worn overnight.

Indications for Whitening

- Discolored teeth
- Surface staining
- Isolated white or brown discoloration which is shallow in the enamel

Contraindications for Whitening

Not everyone is a candidate for whitening procedures. Here are some reasons why:
- Allergy to the products
- Pregnant or nursing
- Open carious lesions
- Cracked enamel
- Excessive dental work on front teeth unless patient is prepared to replace restorations that will no longer match the whitened teeth
- Actively leaking restorations
- Sensitive teeth
- Use of medications causing photosensitivity (light-activated systems could not be used)
- Inability to follow directions
- Unrealistic expectations
- Under the age of fifteen (15)
- Inability to provide informed consent

OVER-THE-COUNTER PRODUCTS

Over-the-counter (OTC) teeth whitening products are of four basic types:
1. Whitening strips
2. Paint-on whitening pastes
3. Whitening gels applied in stock trays
4. Rinses

With the use of over-the-counter products, professional supervision is not provided during whitening. In addition, no professional evaluation is done before whitening to ensure that decay and leaking restorations are repaired. Individuals with preexisting sensitive teeth might worsen their condition.

Whitening Strips

Whitening strips (e.g., Crest 3D Whitestrips; Procter & Gamble and Rembrandt Fast Whitening; Ranir) have become very popular and are the most widely used OTC whitening products (Fig. 8.12). They do not require the construction of whitening trays. The product typically consists of clear, flexible strips containing 10% peroxide gel and special polymers that help them adhere to the teeth. They are placed over the teeth and worn for 30 minutes at a time, once or twice daily. The shorter treatment time may be beneficial for patients who have developed sensitivity with longer treatment times when using trays. The strips are thin and do not interfere with speech. Research indicates that OTC whitening strips are just as effective as whitening with carbamide peroxide in custom trays, at a considerable reduction in cost. Early versions of whitening strips covered only the anterior six teeth in each arch; patients who wanted to whiten additional teeth needed to resort to night guard whitening or they would use multiple whitestrips to extend the whitening to the back of the mouth. However, more recent versions of whitening strips are longer and cover more teeth.

Paint-On Whitening Materials

Paint-on materials are viscous liquids applied directly to the enamel surface of the tooth with a brush. First, the user must air or towel-dry the teeth. Then the solution is painted onto the teeth and in 30 seconds to 1 minute, the liquid solidifies. The patient needs to keep the mouth open until the material dries. Some products are applied during the day and should be left on for at least 30 minutes. It is recommended that these materials be applied twice a day to achieve maximal benefit. Because it is directly exposed to saliva (unlike the gel in strips or trays), the whitening material may be diluted or may come off. Although paint-on products work, they are not known to be as effective as tray-applied whitening products or whitening strips.

Over-the-Counter Tray Whitening Systems

Several tray whitening systems are sold directly to the public by manufacturers. The trays in these systems are preformed stock trays or thermoplastic trays that are heated in boiling water and adapted to the teeth, much like "boil and bite" sports guards (see Chapter 19 Preventive and Corrective Oral Appliances). These trays are often poorly fitting and are not properly trimmed to prevent excess material from contacting the gingiva. Ill-fitting trays can irritate the gingiva. The whitening agent in these OTC systems is usually 10% to 22% carbamide peroxide gel.

Tooth Whitening Toothpastes

Most of the toothpastes on the market that claim to whiten teeth do so by removing surface stains with abrasives such as hydrated silica or calcium carbonate rather than penetrating the enamel to reach the dentin and whitening the teeth. In addition to mild abrasives some manufacturers add peroxides to their dentifrices to help with the whitening effect.

Tooth Whitening Rinses

Whitening rinses on the market (i.e. Crest 3-D White, Listerine Healthy White, and Colgate Optic White) contain hydrogen peroxide as the active ingredient. The use of the product on a long-term basis is intended to remove surface stains. The whitening rinses are still fairly new with limited clinical studies to back up their claims.

NON-DENTAL OPTIONS

Whitening has become so popular that it is now an offered whitening services in retail settings, such as mall kiosks, salons, and spas. These venues have come under scrutiny by the dental community in several states resulting in actions to limit delivery of whitening services by licensed dental healthcare providers. The rationale for limiting these non-dental professionals from providing whitening services is due to the fact that they are not educated in disease screening, infection control, or emergency procedures.

> **! Caution**
>
> The U.S. Food and Drug Administration (FDA) does not require testing for OTC bleaching and whitening products. Manufacturers are not regulated for these products.

ROLE OF THE DENTAL AUXILIARY

The dental auxiliary can play an important role in the delivery of whitening services to patients. In addition to chairside assisting for in-office whitening, assistants and hygienists can be active oral health providers for home whitening. They can help assess the patient for oral conditions that would contraindicate whitening procedures. They can perform several important clinical procedures, such as obtaining a shade, (see Procedure 8.2) making alginate impressions, and pouring casts, as well as fabrication of the whitening trays (see Procedure 8.3). As permitted by state dental practice acts, they may provide whitening services in the office. They can discuss home care remedies for tooth hypersensitivity, and advise the patient on foods and beverages that cause staining.

It is important that the patient be fully informed of the pros and cons of whitening. The assistant or hygienist can provide this information to the patient before the dentist completes the informed consent. In addition, the auxiliary can provide the patient with instructions for proper use of the whitening agent and care of the trays.

POTENTIAL SIDE EFFECTS OF TEETH WHITENING

Sensitivity

Tooth sensitivity is usually short term and can occur from the whitening process. The sensitivity can be managed by shortening the whitening time each day, using a lower concentration of whitening agent, or by stopping the whitening process for a few weeks. The sensitivity is likely caused by whitening agent penetrating through the enamel to the dentinal tubules or by passing through open dentinal tubules on exposed root surfaces and into the pulp, causing irritation. Studies have shown that peroxides can penetrate enamel and dentin and reach the pulp within a matter of minutes. Reversible pulpitis may occur with whitening procedures; however, the pain associated with the inflamed pulp will subside as whitening procedures are discontinued. Hydrogen peroxide can be damaging to cells with prolonged exposure or high concentrations.

Foods and beverages such as citrus fruits and their juices, sodas, vinegar, and other acidic foods should be avoided as long as the teeth are sensitive. Acids tend to open dentinal tubules in exposed root surfaces by dissolving plugs of salivary mucins and debris. Desensitizing products such as fluoride, potassium nitrate, amorphous calcium phosphate (ACP), casein phosphopeptide-ACP, calcium sodium phosphosilicate, arginine calcium carbonate, tri-calcium phosphate, or other desensitizing agents as previously described (see Chapter 7 Preventive and Desensitizing Materials) can be useful to reduce symptoms. In some cases brushing with desensitizing toothpaste for two weeks before whitening is started will reduce sensitivity.

Other Side Effects

Other possible side effects include irritation of the gingiva, mucosa, and throat from excess whitening material coming out of the trays. Gingival irritation can occur if the trays are not trimmed appropriately and the trays rub the tissues. If patients wear the whitening trays overnight, they may experience some soreness of the muscles of mastication and temporomandibular joints if the trays cause them to clench or grind or slightly displace the condyles (heads of the mandible) from the joints.

Home Whitening Instructions Given in the Dental Office

AT THE WHITENING SESSIONS

1. Brush and floss.
2. Place a small amount of whitening gel in the front of each tooth section of the tray. Too much gel in the tray will be displaced by the teeth and may irritate oral tissues and throat.
3. Place the tray over the teeth and seat it gently. Remove excess gel with a toothbrush or paper towel.
4. Wear the tray for the time prescribed by the dentist.
5. At the end of the whitening session, remove the tray, rinse the mouth with water, and use a toothbrush to remove residual gel.
6. Clean the tray under running water with a toothbrush. Liquid soap may be used. Shake off water. Place the tray in a storage container with the lid open to allow the tray to air-dry. Keep out of the reach of children and pets.

ADDITIONAL INFORMATION

1. Store whitening gel in a cool dry location, out of direct sunlight.
2. Whitening is not recommended while pregnant or nursing.
3. Avoid coffee, tea, red wine, colored cola drinks, berries, and tobacco, because they can cause staining of teeth.
4. Whitening results usually last 1 to 3 years. Gradual re-staining may necessitate occasional re-whitening.
5. Keep the whitening trays for future use; it should only be necessary to buy additional whitening agent for re-whitening.
6. If tooth sensitivity or other problems develop, call the office for guidance.

RESTORATIVE CONSIDERATIONS

Before the whitening process is started, cavities should be filled and leaking restorations replaced to prevent excessive penetration of whitening agent through the dentinal tubules, which might irritate the pulp and cause sensitivity. Whitening may be done as a pre-restorative procedure to whiten the teeth before composite bonding procedures, veneers, or porcelain crowns. However, research has shown that bonding to newly whitened surfaces will be weaker than if the teeth are allowed to stabilize for a couple of weeks. Prior to whitening procedures patients need to be informed that the color of existing restorations will not lighten with whitening of the teeth. If they have tooth-colored restorations in visible areas of the mouth that match the teeth before whitening, the restorations will appear darker after whitening the teeth, because the surrounding tooth structure will be lighter. Some patients have whitened their teeth so much that the shades found in regular composite kits may not be light enough to match the color of the whitened teeth. Several manufacturers have now developed whitening shades for composite materials. Some whitening gels that are mildly acidic may cause slight roughness of the surface of some composites, compomers, or glass ionomers. Most whitening materials available now are pH balanced, and therefore concerns about etching certain restorative materials are diminished. During the whitening process, patients should be advised to limit their intake of foods and beverages that can stain the teeth, including coffee, tea, red wine, colored cola drinks, and berries or berry juices. Smoking can also contribute to staining of the teeth.

 Clinical Tip

A period of at least 2 weeks is needed after whitening to allow the color of the teeth to stabilize before esthetic restorations are placed. Also, the bond to newly whitened surfaces is weaker than when the teeth are allowed to stabilize.

Contraindications: Whitening Is Not for Everyone

The following people should not attempt to whiten their teeth:
- People allergic to whitening or tray materials
- Pregnant or nursing individuals
- People with open carious lesions, leaking restorations, or cracked teeth
- People with hypersensitive teeth
- People with many tooth-colored restorations who do not want to replace them when whitening of the teeth make them look darker
- People taking medications that make them photosensitive should not have light-activated whitening as they may get skin irritation or burns
- People with unrealistic expectations about what whitening can do
- Adolescents under 15 years of age with recently erupted permanent teeth whose enamel is still porous and would allow too much penetration of whitening material causing sensitivity
- People who are mentally incapable of giving informed consent

RETREATMENT

Both in-office and home whitening will fade with time. One study found a relapse of approximately 40% at 1 year with in-office whitening. While another study evaluating at-home tray whitening found a 26% relapse at 18 months. Some offices provide home whitening kits to their patients who have undergone in-office whitening in anticipation that they will want to re-whiten or touch-up their teeth over time as retreatment may be required to maintain the whiteness. Typically, patients may find that in 1 to 3 years they will want to do some additional whitening. With in-office whitening, this often means that patients will have to pay the full bleaching fee again. With home tray whitening, patients need only purchase additional whitening solution if they keep their custom whitening trays.

ENAMEL MICROABRASION

A variety of noncarious discolorations can occur in the enamel. They may be caused by mild fluorosis, hypermineralized spots that occurred during enamel development, or previous carious white spot lesions that have remineralized but are still whiter than the surrounding enamel. When these discolorations are of concern to the patient one conservative approach to their removal is called enamel microabrasion. The lesions should be shallow to leave an adequate thickness of enamel after discoloration removal. The surface of the lesion is cleaned with pumice. Then an acid slurry made of flour of pumice and 6% hydrochloric acid (diluted from muriatic acid purchased at a hardware store or a commercial preparation such as PREMA [Premier] or Opalustre [Ultradent]) is applied to the discoloration for 1 minute. Next, the slurry is agitated with a ribbed rubber cup (prophy angle) revolving slowly (about 500 rpm) for an additional 1 minute. The acid slurry is then rinsed off the tooth. Repeat the process if the spot is not gone. Do not repeat more than three times as too much enamel will be removed. If the spot still remains, another approach, such as covering the spot with composite, might be needed (Fig. 8.13).

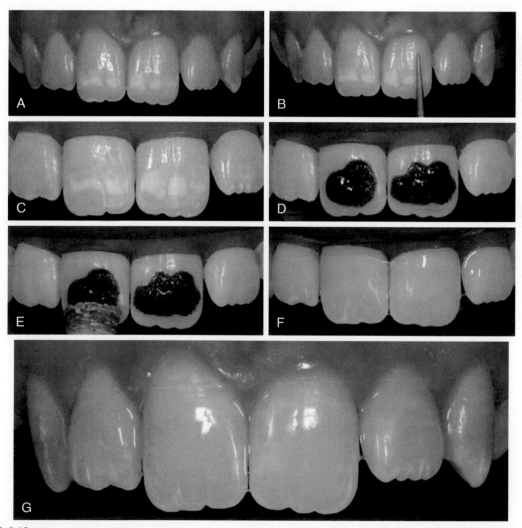

FIG. 8.13 Microabrasion. **A,** Before treatment: white enamel discoloration. **B,** Preparation (roughening) of tooth with bur. **C,** Isolation of teeth with dental dam. **D,** Application of microabrasion compound. **E,** Application of microabrasion at slow speed. **F,** Removal of microabrasion compound. **G,** After treatment: staining is considerably reduced. After microabrasion, a course of home whitening can further reduce the staining. (From *J Appl. Oral Sci*, 22(4):347–354, 2014.)

ADVERSE OUTCOMES

Care must be taken when performing microabrasion to prevent burns to the soft tissues from the acid. If treatment is too aggressive or too prolonged, so much enamel will be removed that the yellow dentin will show through the thinned enamel and the teeth will look much yellower than before treatment was initiated. The pulp may be irritated by penetration of acid, or by heat generated if the rubber cup is used with too much pressure and speed. As with any dental procedure, the established treatment protocol must be followed as recommended to avoid adverse outcomes.

SUMMARY

Whitening of teeth for cosmetic reasons is a popular aspect of cosmetic dentistry. To be effective in providing whitening services and advice to patients, clinicians must be knowledgeable about in-office, prescribed home whitening, and OTC products, including their indications and contraindications and potential side effects. Staining of the teeth caused by tetracycline or blood products from nonvital teeth can be the most difficult to remove. Patients need to be advised of potential limitations of treatment and other pros and cons before providing their informed consent to treatment. Dental assistants and hygienists are important team members in providing these popular cosmetic procedures.

INSTRUCTIONAL VIDEOS

See the Evolve Resources site for a variety of educational videos that reinforce the material covered in this chapter.

Procedure 8.1 In-Office Whitening

See Evolve site for Competency Sheet.

EQUIPMENT/SUPPLIES (FIG. 8.14)

- Basic examination setup
- Prophy setup: Low-speed handpiece with prophy angle, prophy cup, flour of pumice
- Tooth shade guide
- Dental dam setup (check for latex allergy)
- Tissue-protective material (petroleum jelly or manufacturer's coating or foam)
- High-strength whitening material (varies with manufacturer)
- High-intensity light, curing light, laser, or heat source (depending on whitening material type)
- Appropriately tinted safety lenses or light shield
- Timer or watch
- Three-way syringe and high-volume evacuation

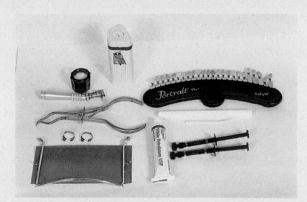

FIG. 8.14

(HVE) with disposable tips
- Waxed dental floss, 2 × 2 gauze
- Optional: Extraoral or intraoral camera for taking photographs

PROCEDURE STEPS

1. Obtain informed consent: One copy for the patient and one for the chart.
2. Clean the teeth with flour of pumice or nonfluoride/oil polishing paste.
3. Determine the starting shade and record. A photograph may also be taken, if desired.
4. Place tissue protection on the gingiva and interdental papillae according to the manufacturer's directions.
   NOTE: The gingiva is often coated with petroleum jelly or other protective layer under the dental dam in case the dam leaks.
5. Place the dental dam, isolating the teeth to be whitened (Fig. 8.15).

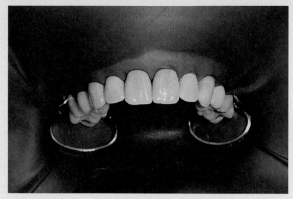

FIG. 8.15

NOTE: Holes must be of appropriate size and spacing to prevent leakage. Invert the edge of the dam around each tooth to form a seal, so that whitening material will not contact the gingiva.

6. Use waxed floss to help tuck in the dam interproximally. Use a hand instrument to invert the dam around each tooth.
7. Place high-strength whitener as provided by the manufacturer (usually 35% hydrogen peroxide) and follow specific directions as to time and light/heat source application (Fig. 8.16 and 8.17). Be aware of developing tooth or gum sensitivity during the procedure. Respond accordingly.

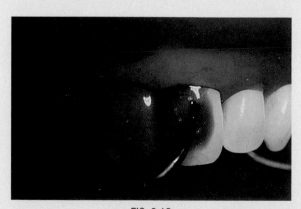

FIG. 8.16

NOTE: Tooth sensitivity may be due to overheating of the tooth, previously exposed root areas, or penetration of strong whitener into vital dentin. Gum sensitivity may be caused by a chemical burn from the whitening agent. Mild sensitivity usually goes away in a few days. Severe burns to the gingiva or mucosa can be painful and cause tissue necrosis that may take weeks to heal. Mild burns with surface whitening of the gingiva heal quickly.

Continued

Procedure 8.1 In-Office Whitening—cont'd

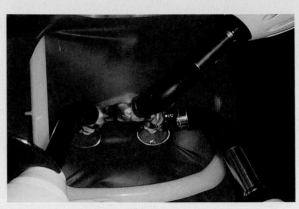

FIG. 8.17

8. Rinse off the whitener, wipe clean with 2 × 2 gauze, and examine for shade. Repeat the application of whitener as needed to achieve the desired shade.

NOTE: Teeth appear whiter with the dental dam in place because of the contrast in color and the dehydration that occurs under the dam. The true color appears after the teeth are rehydrated with saliva. Color stability is achieved 2 weeks after whitening.

9. Additional appointments may be needed to achieve the tooth whiteness goal.

NOTE: Desired results cannot always be achieved. Some stains are more resistant to whitening.

Procedure 8.2 Clinical Procedures for Home Whitening

See Evolve site for Competency Sheet.

EQUIPMENT/SUPPLIES (Fig. 8.18)

- Basic setup for examination
- Rubber mixing bowl and spatula
- Alginate, measures for water and powder
- Dental plaster or stone
- Alginate impression trays
- Tooth shade guide and camera (optional)
- Home whitening kit and instructions

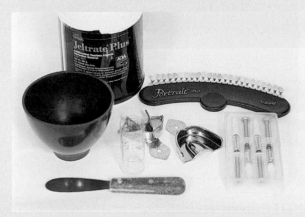

FIG. 8.18

PROCEDURE STEPS
First Appointment

1. Dentist examines the teeth and arches for type of discoloration and oral conditions that might influence the success of whitening. Potential areas of concern are corrected or planned for correction.

NOTE: Dental caries, sensitive teeth, and leaking restorations may need correction before whitening to prevent further sensitivity or pulpal problems.

2. Discuss the pros and cons of whitening. Obtain informed consent.

NOTE: A signed informed consent form signifies that the patient fully understands what is involved, has had his or her questions answered, and agrees to the treatment.

3. Record the patient's tooth shade (Fig. 8.19). Take photographs with a shade tab next to the teeth, if desired.

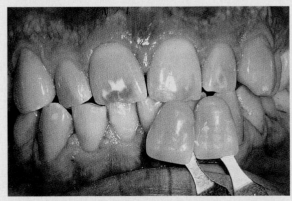

FIG. 8.19 (Courtesy of Ultradent Products, Inc. [South Jordan, UT].)

NOTE: Many manufacturers include a shade card that can be used to match the initial shade and later to compare it with the whitened shade at future visits.

4. Select impression trays of the correct size and make alginate impressions.

5. Rinse the impressions, spray with disinfectant or immerse in suitable disinfectant for 15 minutes,

Procedure 8.2 Clinical Procedures for Home Whitening—cont'd

wrap in wet paper towel, and seal in zippered plastic bag.

6. Pour impressions with dental stone using a vibrator to minimize bubbles. (Block out the tongue and palatal area with a wet paper towel to make trimming the casts easier when making trays.) Trays are fabricated in the office (see Procedure 8.3) or sent to a commercial laboratory.

Second Appointment

7. Insert trays for fit and comfort.
8. Demonstrate loading of trays with gel, tray insertion, and removal of excess gel (Fig. 8.20 through 8.22).

9.

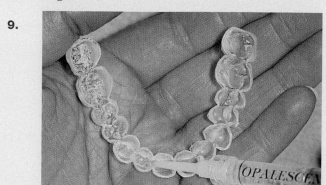

FIG. 8.20 (Courtesy of Ultradent Products, Inc. [South Jordan, UT].)

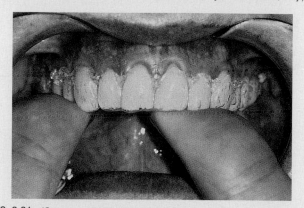

FIG. 8.21 (Courtesy of Ultradent Products, Inc. [South Jordan, UT].)

Demonstrate cleaning of trays after a whitening session.

10. Give verbal and written instructions. Review possible side effects. Dispense home whitening kit.

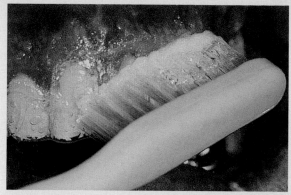

FIG. 8.22 (Courtesy of Ultradent Products, Inc. [South Jordan, UT].)

NOTE: Written instructions are important because patients sometimes forget what they have been told.

11. Schedule a follow-up appointment in 2 to 3 weeks following initial delivery. Determine and record tooth shade at each subsequent visit (Fig. 8.23). The procedure should be continued until the desired shade is achieved.

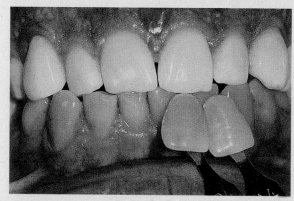

FIG. 8.23 (Courtesy of Ultradent Products, Inc. [South Jordan, UT].)

NOTE: Whitening will not change the color of existing tooth-colored restorations (composite, glass ionomer, compomer, or porcelain). The patient must understand that these restorations will appear darker than the surrounding whitened teeth and may need to be replaced to achieve the desired cosmetic result. Not all stains respond to whitening, and patients may not achieve the desired results. Cosmetic restorative procedures are done after whitening has stabilized for a period of 2 weeks or longer.

Procedure 8.3   Fabrication of Custom Whitening Trays

See Evolve site for Competency Sheet.

EQUIPMENT/SUPPLIES (FIG. 8.24)

1. Casts (models) of patient's dentition
2. Whitening reservoir material: Light-cured block-out resin
3. Vacuum former
4. Two sheets of 6 × 6-inch by 0.02- or 0.035-inch-thick thermoplastic vinyl tray material
5. Fine-tipped scissors for trimming the trays

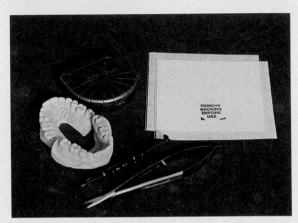

FIG. 8.24

PROCEDURE STEPS

1. Trim casts to eliminate much of the facial peripheral border. If the maxillary cast has a palatal area, drill a hole in the deepest part of the palate or grind away most of the palatal area (Fig. 8.25).

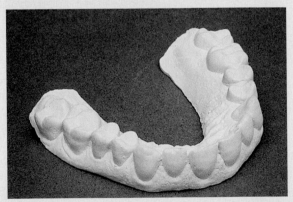

FIG. 8.25   (Courtesy of Ultradent Products, Inc. [South Jordan, UT].)

NOTE: Ledges or concave areas on the casts that trap air when the molten tray material is lowered over the casts will prevent good adaptation of the tray to the cast and result in a poorly fitting tray that leaks whitening gel into the patient's mouth. Before pouring stone into the alginate impressions, block out the tongue and palate areas with a wad of wet paper towel. This will save time trimming stone away from these areas later.

2. Allow the casts to dry, and then apply reservoir material (e.g., LC Block-out Resin, Ultradent Products) to the facial surfaces of the teeth (on the cast) to be whitened.
3. Light-cured block-out resin is applied to the facial surfaces of the teeth to be whitened in a thin layer about 1 mm thick. It should extend 1 mm short of the gingival crest and the interproximal embrasures (Fig. 8.26).
4. Resin on each tooth should be cured for 10 seconds with a curing light, or the entire cast can be placed in a Triad light-curing unit (Dentsply Sirona) for 1 minute.

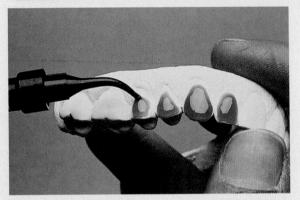

FIG. 8.26   (Courtesy of Ultradent Products, Inc. [South Jordan, UT].)

NOTE: The reservoir is left short of the gingival crest so the tray will seal in that area and prevent whitening agent from contacting the gingiva.

5. Clamp a sheet of thermoplastic vinyl tray material in the frame of the vacuum-forming unit (Fig. 8.27). Raise the frame until it is just below the heating element. Turn on the heating element.

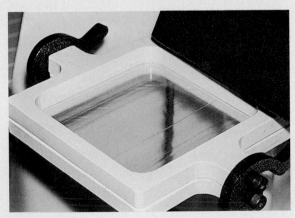

FIG. 8.27   (Courtesy of Ultradent Products, Inc. [South Jordan, UT].)

6. Place one cast in the center of the platform (it contains many holes) of the vacuum former.

Continued

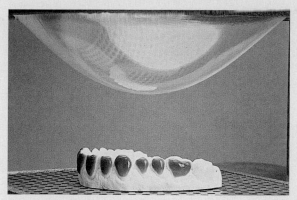

FIG. 8.28   (Courtesy of Ultradent Products, Inc. [South Jordan, UT].)

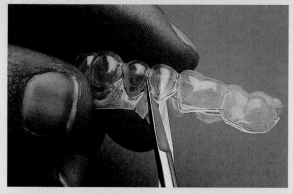

FIG. 8.29   (Courtesy of Ultradent Products, Inc. [South Jordan, UT].)

7. When the vinyl material has heated and sagged an inch or more (Fig. 8.28), lower the frame to the platform and turn on the vacuum. The molten material will be pulled down tightly over the cast.

   NOTE: If a pocket of air is trapped under the vinyl, push it out by adapting the tray to the cast by hand with a wet paper towel while the material is still soft and the vacuum is on.

8. Allow the tray material to cool for at least 1 minute before removing it from the frame. Place it under cold running water to cool thoroughly.

9. Trim excess material away from the cast with scissors. Remove the cast from the tray.

10. Use fine scissors to trim the tray so that it extends over the teeth just to the gingival crest (Fig. 8.29). It should have a scalloped appearance as it traces the outline of the gingival crest (Fig. 8.30).

    NOTE: If the tray extends over the gingiva on the facial surfaces, whitening agent can contact the gingiva and irritate it.

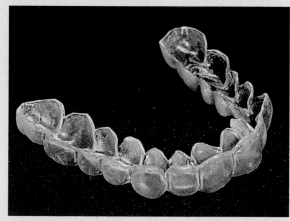

FIG. 8.30   (Courtesy of Ultradent Products, Inc. [South Jordan, UT].)

11. Repeat the process for the other cast.
12. Wash the trays with soap and water. Spray the trays with surface disinfectant and store until delivery in a zippered plastic bag marked with patient's name.

Get Ready for Exams!

Review Questions

Select the one correct response for each of the following multiple-choice questions.

1. What type of whitening solution is painted on the tooth structure and held in place for thirty minutes with a sealer?
   a. Power whitening
   b. Home whitening
   c. Whitening varnish
   d. Whitestrips

2. Whitening of teeth works:
   a. By removing surface stains
   b. By penetrating both enamel and dentin and oxidizing the stain
   c. By sealing surface porosities so that stain cannot enter the tooth surface
   d. By creating a white coating on the surface of the enamel

3. In-office whitening:
   a. Is superior in results to home whitening
   b. Produces equivalent results to home whitening but is faster
   c. Does not cause tooth sensitivity
   d. Has no effect if the whitening agent contacts the gingiva

4. The active ingredient in most in-office and OTC whitening products is:
   a. Sodium bicarbonate
   b. Ammonia
   c. Phosphoric acid
   d. Peroxide

5. Which one of the following can remove intrinsic stains?
   a. Prophy cup with polishing paste
   b. Hydrogen peroxide
   c. Air polishing with sodium bicarbonate powder
   d. Ultrasonic scaling

6. Whitening procedures should be avoided if the patient has any of the following *except* one. Which one is the *exception?*
   a. Open carious lesions
   b. Gingivitis
   c. Hypersensitive teeth
   d. Inability to give informed consent

7. Undesirable outcomes from home whitening include all of the following *except* one. Which one is the *exception?*
   a. Soft tissue irritation
   b. Root abrasion
   c. Sore muscles of mastication or TMJs
   d. Temperature sensitivity

8. The most difficult stains to remove are:
   a. Coffee stains
   b. Chlorhexidine stains
   c. Red wine stains
   d. Tetracycline stains

9. After whitening, how much time should the patient wait until a shade is selected for permanent restorations?
   a. 1 week
   b. 2 weeks
   c. 3 weeks

10. Which one of the following statements about whitening strips is true?
   a. Strips are less effective than paint-on whitening products
   b. Strips are typically worn for 4 to 6 hours at a time
   c. Strips interfere with speech
   d. Strips are just as effective as home tray whitening with 10 to 15% carbamide peroxide

For answers to Review Questions, see the Appendix.

Case-Based Discussion Topics

1. A 35-year-old housewife has been using an over-the-counter whitening system with trays adapted to the teeth after the material is boiled in water. She has been wearing the trays while she sleeps. She comes to the dental office complaining of sensitivity in her teeth, inflamed and painful gingivae, and sore jaw muscles.

   Discuss possible causes for each of her complaints and make recommendations to treat the problems and prevent their recurrence.

2. A 16-year-old high school student has just become a cheerleader. She wishes to have a brighter smile for her public appearances.

   Which whitening systems would be appropriate? What are the potential side effects on patients this young? What measures can be employed to minimize the side effects?

3. A 45-year-old plumber has high caries activity because he snacks on Snickers bars while he is out on house calls. He has a new girl friend and wants to whiten his dull teeth.

   What things should be considered before he starts whitening procedures? If he has anterior composites placed to restore carious teeth, should they be done before or after whitening? Why?

BIBLIOGRAPHY

American Dental Association (ADA): Council on Scientific Affairs: Statement on the Safety and Effectiveness of Tooth Whitening Products. Available at: https://www.ada.org/en/about-the-ada/ada-positions-policies-and-statements/tooth-whitening-safety-and-effectiveness.

American Dental Association (ADA): Council on Scientific Affairs: Tooth Whitening/Bleaching: Treatment Considerations for Dentists and Their Patients. Available at: https://www.ada.org/~/media/ADA/About%20the%20ADA/Files/whitening_bleaching_treatment_considrations_for_patients_and_dentists.ashx.

Bird DL, Robinson DS: Preventive, restorative and cosmetic dentistry. In *Modern Dental Assisting*, ed 12, St. Louis, 2018, Elsevier.

Darby ML, Walsh MM: Stain management and tooth whitening. In *Dental Hygiene Theory and Practice*, ed 4, St. Louis, 2015, Elsevier.

Haywood VB: Current Status and Recommendations for Dentist-Prescribed, at-home Tooth Whitening, *Contemp Esthet Rest Pract* 3(1):2-9, 1999.

Kugel G: Effective tooth bleaching in 5 days: using a combined in-office and at-home bleaching system, *Compend Contin Educ Dent* 18(4):378, *380-3,* 1997.

Kwon SR: Innovation in tooth whitening, *Dimensions of Dental Hygiene* 16(01):18, *21-23,* 2018.

Magid KS: In-office power bleaching with a plasma arc curing light, *Contemp Esthet Rest Pract* (9):14-20, 1999.

Mennito AS, Austin M, Wright M: Academy of Dental Learning and OSHA Training. Tooth Whitening: Comprehensive Review and Clinical Guidelines, 2012.

Dental Ceramics

9

Chapter Objectives

Upon completion of this chapter, the student should be able to:

1. Discuss the attributes and shortcomings of dental porcelains.
2. Compare the clinical applications of restorations made from porcelain with those made from lithium disilicate.
3. Explain why crowns made from zirconia can be used to restore molars.
4. Describe the methods used to process ceramic restorations.
5. Present a rationale for the selection of ceramic materials for restorations used in the anterior and posterior parts of the mouth.
6. Describe how porcelain bonds to metal for porcelain-fused-to-metal (PFM) crowns.
7. Select the appropriate cement for use with glass-based ceramic materials.
8. Describe common causes for failure of ceramic restorations.
9. Finish and polish ceramic restorations without generating too much heat or stress in the material.
10. Compare the relative strengths of feldspathic porcelain, lithium disilicate, and zirconium.
11. Explain how CAD/CAM technology is used to fabricate a ceramic crown.
12. List the clinical applications for all-ceramic restorations.
13. Prepare the ceramic rest **Lithium Disilicate Ceramics** oration for bonding with resin cement.
14. Assist the dentist in cementing an all-ceramic crown or veneers.
15. Properly prepare the conditions in the operatory for shade taking.
16. Assist the dentist in shade taking.

Key Terms

Ceramics materials composed of inorganic metal oxide compounds, including porcelain and similar ceramic materials that require baking at high temperature to fuse small particles together

Crown an indirect restoration that covers all or part of the coronal tooth structure (extracoronal) and is composed of metal, ceramic, or a combination of the two. It can also cover an implant

Fixed Bridge a dental prosthesis that replaces one or more missing teeth and is cemented to adjacent natural teeth or implants. It is composed of the same materials as crowns

Inlay an indirect restoration composed of ceramic, composite resin, or metal that is fitted to a cavity preparation that is within the crown of a tooth (intracoronal)

Onlay restoration that is similar to an inlay but covers or replaces one or more cusps

Veneers thin layer of ceramic or composite resin that is bonded to the facial surfaces of teeth to improve their color, shape, size, or length

Glass-Based Ceramics ceramic materials with a silica (glass) matrix with or without fillers such as leucite or lithium disilicate

Non–Glass-Based Ceramics crystalline-based ceramics without a glass matrix

All-Ceramic Restoration ceramic restoration with no metal core

Porcelain a tooth-colored ceramic material composed of crystals of feldspar, alumina, and silica that are fused together at high temperatures to form a hard, uniform, glasslike material

Lithium Disilicate Ceramics glass-based ceramics with lithium disilicate fillers to enhance physical and mechanical properties, especially flexural strength

Zirconia a non-glass polycrystalline ceramic that is the strongest ceramic used in dentistry

Flexural Strength strength required to resist bending of a bar of ceramic material to its point of fracture

Fracture Toughness material's ability to resist fracture from crack propagation

Sintering fusion of ceramic particles at their borders by heating them to the point that they just start to melt

Slip-Casting process whereby ceramic powder is mixed with a water-based liquid to form a mass or slip. The slip is pressed into a form and baked at high temperature

Heat-Pressing pressing molten ceramic material into a mold at high temperature and pressure

CAD/CAM computer-assisted design/computer-assisted machining that uses a scanning device to capture an image of the preparation and is integrated with computer software to design and a milling device to cut restorations from blocks of restorative dental material

Porcelain-Metal Restoration restoration that has a metal core over which porcelain is fused at high temperature. Commonly referred to as porcelain-fused-to-metal (PFM) or porcelain-bonded-to-metal (PBM)

Amalgam and gold were the main restorative materials until **ceramics** were introduced into dentistry over a hundred years ago. Ceramics were first used for the fabrication of denture teeth, and then Charles Land introduced porcelain jacket crowns and inlays in the 1900s. Land's porcelain jacket crowns were very esthetic but the porcelains of the time were brittle and tended to crack when used in high-function areas of the mouth. In the late 1950s porcelain was fused to a metal core to make esthetic crowns much stronger. In Europe in the 1970s, the first computer-aided design/computer-aided manufacturing (CAD/CAM) system was developed using ceramic blocks to produce inlays and onlays. In 1987 the first chairside CAD/CAM system (CEREC 1, Siemens Dental) was introduced. Also in the 1980s, the introduction of a castable glass-based ceramic launched numerous innovations in ceramic processing.

Within the past three decades all-ceramic materials have been introduced that are much stronger than the original porcelains, and with some improvements in esthetics. As a result, the use of all-ceramic restorations has dramatically increased while the use of the less esthetic porcelain-fused-to-metal crowns has decreased. At present, ceramic materials are used for a variety of restorations, such as **crowns, fixed bridges, inlays, onlays,** and **veneers**. Selection of the type of material to be used depends, in part, on the extent of damage to the tooth, the stresses that will be placed on the restoration, and the esthetic requirements of the patient.

By enhancing the ability to bond restorative materials to metal and tooth structure, advances in esthetic materials and techniques have assisted the dental team in delivering the esthetic results that patients demand. The dental team must keep current with the rapid changes that occur in materials and techniques. Good listening skills are needed to determine the types of esthetic services the patient is requesting, so that the dental team and the patient are working in concert toward the same goal. Esthetic materials must be carefully selected, so that their properties are compatible with the patient's oral condition and occlusion.

Dental hygienists and dental assistants must understand the properties of these materials, so that as important members of the dental team, they can help the dentist to assess the performance of the restorations and alert the dentist when they perceive that a restoration may be failing. The dental auxiliary needs to be familiar with the physical properties of materials, so that they do not damage the restorations during routine oral hygiene, coronal polishing, and preventive procedures. Dental assistants need to know the handling characteristics of esthetic materials, so that they can either assist the dentist in their placement or perform steps in their placement as permitted by state dental practice acts. In addition, they will be called on to assist in shade taking for the restorations and steps in CAD/CAM procedures if used in the office.

This chapter describes the physical and mechanical properties, processing methods including computer-assisted design/computer-assisted machining (CAD/CAM) technology, clinical applications, attributes, and shortcomings of esthetic ceramic materials. The rationale for the selection of ceramic materials for various clinical applications is presented. The principles for adjusting, finishing, polishing, and cementation of ceramic restorations are reviewed. Guidelines for selection of the shade of these materials to obtain satisfactory cosmetic results also are discussed.

DENTAL CERAMICS

The general term ceramics is used to describe porcelain and a variety of materials that are similar in appearance to porcelain but vary in their composition, mode of fabrication, and physical and mechanical properties. Dental ceramics can be classified in a variety of ways based on their composition, processing method, fusing temperature, microstructure, translucency, fracture resistance, and abrasiveness.

GLASS AND NON-GLASS CERAMICS

To simplify the understanding of dental ceramics they will be classified in this chapter into two broad categories according to their composition: glass-based and non–glass-based materials.

- **Glass-based ceramics** have silica as a main component and have a glassy matrix. They include feldspathic porcelains, leucite-reinforced ceramics, and lithium disilicate ceramics. They are more esthetic than the non–glass-based ceramics.
- **Non–glass-based ceramics** are crystalline in nature and composed of simple or complex oxides with no glassy matrix. They include alumina and zirconia. They are the strongest of the ceramics.

ADVANTAGES AND DISADVANTAGES OF CERAMIC RESTORATIONS

Esthetic restorations can be made from composite resin, ceramics with a metal substructure (core), or entirely ceramics.

The primary advantage of **all-ceramic restorations** is their esthetics, because there is no metal substructure to hide. Other advantages over direct-placement restorations such as composite resin, glass ionomer cement, or amalgam include their biocompatibility, wear resistance under function, color stability, stain resistance, and the ability to precisely place contacts and contours of the restorations. All-ceramic restorations are rapidly becoming the restorations of choice for many clinicians.

Disadvantages of all-ceramic restorations compared with direct-placement restorations include their brittleness (can lead to fracture), wear of the opposing enamel or restorations, difficulty or inability to repair them in the mouth, the need for two appointments (except for chairside CAD/CAM restorations), and the difficulty of polishing them in the mouth.

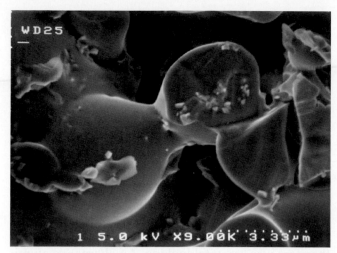

FIG. 9.1 Sintering. In the scanning electron micrograph porcelain particles can be seen that have partly melted at high temperature and fused at their points of contact. This is sintering. (From Rosenstiel SF, Land MF: *Contemporary Fixed Prosthodontics*, ed 5, St Louis, 2016, Elsevier.)

GLASS-BASED CERAMICS

Glass-based ceramics are the most esthetic of the ceramic materials.

PORCELAIN

Porcelain is a term that has been used in dentistry for many years to describe glass-like tooth-colored dental materials. Some people use the term interchangeably with ceramics, but porcelain is actually a subgroup of ceramic materials composed of feldspar, silica or quartz, and kaolin. Ceramic materials that are high in glass content are very esthetic, because their optical properties mimic those of enamel and dentin. However, they are brittle and more prone to fracture than newer low-glass, reinforced glass, or non-glass ceramics. Their flexural strength is no more than 20% of that of the strongest non-glass ceramics.

Feldspathic Porcelain

Until advances in ceramic materials over the past four decades were made, the dental ceramic material most commonly used was feldspathic porcelain manufactured from fine crystalline powders of alumina, feldspar, and silica oxide (or quartz, 44% to 66%) mixed with a flux of sodium or lithium carbonate. As the powder is heated to certain critical temperatures, the porcelain particles fuse together (sinter) at their points of contact to form a type of glass (Fig. 9.1). Examples of feldspathic porcelain include Ceramco 3 (Dentsply), EX-3 (Noritake), Halo (Shofu), and VITA VM13 (Vident/VITA).

Feldspathic porcelain is the oldest of the porcelains used in dentistry (introduced in the early 1900s). It is the most esthetic but the weakest of the ceramic materials in use.

Alumina Porcelain

Alumina porcelain was developed in 1965 by J.W. McLean and T.H. Hughes to enhance (about double) the fracture resistance compared with conventional feldspathic porcelain. It is also a glassy type of porcelain that is about half aluminum oxide by weight in a melted glass (silica) matrix. It is fabricated by first dry-pressing it on a refractory die (die capable of withstanding high temperatures), then sintering it at high temperature.

Uses of Porcelain

Porcelain is manufactured in a variety of colors. The different colors (called shades) are produced by the addition of metal oxides to create the different shades that will match the teeth. The laboratory technician selects powders based on the shade prescription provided by the dentist. These porcelains were initially used for all-porcelain jacket crowns. These jacket crowns were very esthetically pleasing but had a high fracture rate. At present, the feldspathic porcelains have a variety of uses. They are used to cover (or veneer) a metal core to fabricate porcelain-fused-to-metal (PFM) crowns and to veneer high-strength ceramic cores such as zirconia. Zirconia is opaque and lacks the vitality of natural tooth structure, so it is not very esthetic but it is very strong. Veneering it with feldspathic porcelain can produce a more esthetic crown with a strong core. Feldspathic porcelain is also used for very esthetic anterior veneers that can be rather thin, allowing for conservative preparations.

Porcelain veneers are most successful when they are bonded to enamel. Enamel is rigid and provides a firm support for the veneer. A metal or ceramic core also provides rigid support for porcelain. Dentin, however, is not as rigid. If the support for the veneer is mostly dentin, the failure rate with feldspathic porcelain increases. If the dentin flexes slightly under functional loads, either the bond between the veneer and the dentin will fail or the veneer will break. If dentin is the base for the veneer, then a stronger esthetic material should be selected.

Fusing Temperatures

Porcelains can be classified according to their fusing temperature as high fusing (1294 °C to 1371 °C, or 2360 °F to 2500 °F), medium fusing (1093 °C to 1260 °C, or 2000 °F to 2300 °F), and low fusing (871 °C to 1066 °C, or 1600 °F to 1950 °F). High-fusing porcelains are used most often for the manufacture of denture teeth (see Chapter 17 Polymers for Prosthetic Dentistry, Fig. 17.17). Medium-fusing porcelains are used for some all-ceramic restorations. Low-fusing porcelains are used for veneering metal in PFM crowns and to fabricate some all-ceramic restorations.

REINFORCED GLASS-BASED CERAMICS

Because porcelains were prone to fracture, stronger ceramic materials were developed. The most common of these stronger glass-based ceramics are leucite-reinforced ceramics (IPS Empress; Ivoclar Vivadent) and **lithium disilicate ceramics** (IPS e.max and IPS Empress II; Ivoclar Vivadent). Reinforcing the material with leucite crystals or lithium oxide has more than tripled their fracture resistance. The reinforced ceramics require a bit more thickness in order to achieve the desired esthetics.

Lithium Disilicate

Lithium disilicate ceramic is composed of quartz, lithium dioxide, alumina, phosphor oxide, potassium oxide, and small amounts of other components. The resulting glass ceramic has high strength, good marginal integrity, and biocompatibility and, unlike porcelain, can be used in both the anterior and posterior parts of the mouth. It is a very esthetic material because of its high translucency caused by the low refractive index of the lithium disilicate crystals (the crystals let light pass through rather than dispersing it). Because of its favorable properties lithium disilicate ceramic has become very popular for veneers and esthetic anterior and posterior crowns. It also can be used for short-span fixed bridges if not subjected to excessive forces, as with people who grind their teeth (bruxers). It has high flexural strength (approximately 300 MPa), and heat-pressing (pressing a molten ingot into a mold) makes it more resistant to crack propagation. It is manufactured in a variety of shades and comes as ingots for the heat-pressed (890 to 920 °C, or 1634 °F to 1688 °F) technique (e.g., IPS Empress 2 or IPS e.maxPress, Ivoclar Vivadent) or ceramic blocks for CAD/CAM milling (IPS e.max CAD).

Cementation. As with the other glass-based materials, restorations made from lithium disilicate should be bonded to the tooth with resin cement for maximum strength. They are first etched with hydrofluoric acid gel and then coated with silane before applying a resin bonding agent or a self-adhesive resin cement. The length of time for etching is dependent on the type of glass-based material and the concentration of the hydrofluoric acid. Overetching may produce a friable surface that is difficult to bond to. Check the manufacturer recommendations.

SURVIVAL RATES FOR GLASS-BASED CERAMICS

Glass-based ceramic inlays, onlays, and veneers have a 5-year survival rate of 93-98% and 64-95% at 10 years. When used for full crowns limited to the anterior part of the mouth, the survival rate is also high for the reinforced glass materials. These materials owe their high success rate to the fact that they can be bonded to enamel and dentin for support.

NON–GLASS-BASED CERAMICS

Non–glass-based ceramics are crystalline-based with no glass matrix and are composed of oxides of alumina and/or zirconia with minor amounts of other components to improve their properties.

ALUMINA

A non-glass material with a crystalline matrix (composed of alumina) was developed as an alternative to the PFM crown and the first product was In-Ceram Alumina (Vident/VITA). It was the first all-ceramic material that could be used for both anterior and posterior crowns and anterior short-span bridges. While it had higher strength, it was less translucent, and therefore was less vital looking. An alternative alumina material is solid sintered alumina (Procera; Nobel Biocare). The resulting ceramic material has very high flexural strength, about three times that of the glass-based materials.

To provide increased translucency a new material was developed with an alumina/magnesia matrix called *spinel*. In-Ceram Spinell (VITA North America) gives up some of the flexural strength of alumina ceramic but is more esthetic for anterior crowns.

Alumina ceramic systems have been replaced for the most part by zirconia and lithium disilicate because of their higher failure rate when used for molar crowns.

ZIRCONIA

Zirconia (zirconium oxide) ceramics are the strongest ceramic materials currently used in dentistry. They have the highest **flexural strength** (Table 9.1) and **fracture toughness**, at least twice as strong as the alumina-based ceramics. Like lithium disilicate they can be heat-pressed or machined. Common brand names include Lava (3M ESPE), Cercon (Dentsply), and VITA YZ (Vident/VITA). Zirconia can be used in the anterior and posterior parts of the mouth for single-unit crowns or as cores for three-unit bridges.

Cementation

Because of their high strength, zirconia crowns can be cemented with conventional cements or bonded with resin cements. Zirconia restorations are not etched or silanated before cementation. They do not respond to acid etchants like the glass-based ceramics, and attempts at etching might produce a powdery residue on the interior of the crown that is difficult to remove and may interfere with bonding. Several manufacturers have developed primers for preparing the interior of the crown for use with resin cements. Zirconia primers include Metal/Zirconia Primer (Ivoclar Vivadent), Z-PRIME Plus (BISCO), and Clearfil Ceramic Primer (Kuraray America). Some clinicians have reduced the protocol for bonding zirconia to three steps: 1. Sandblasting the interior; 2. Applying primer; and 3. Bonding with adhesive resin cement.

Table 9.1	Strength of Various Types of All-Ceramics				
CERAMIC TYPE	**COMMON BRANDS**	**ESTHETICS**	**FLEXURAL STRENGTH (MPa)***	**FRACTURE TOUGHNESS (MPa · m$^{0.6}$)**	
Feldspathic porcelain	Ceramco VITA VMK Duceram LFC	Very high	120-130	0.78	
Leucite-reinforced glass ceramic	IPS Empress	High	104-160	1.2-2.4	
Lithium disilicate glass ceramic	Empress II IPS e.max	Moderately high	262-306	3.0	
Glass-infiltrated alumina	Procera Alumina In-Ceram (alumina)	Moderate-to-low	340-700	3.2-4.4	
Zirconia	Lava Cercon VITA YZ Procera Zirconia IPS e.max ZirCAD	Moderate-to-low unless veneered with more esthetic material	800-1300	4.0-6.3	

*Approximate, depending on processing.

Improving the Esthetics of Zirconia

Zirconia is a much more opaque ceramic than lithium disilicate ceramic. To achieve better esthetics, a layer of veneering porcelain can be added to the zirconium core. If the crown fractures, it is usually caused by a fracture of the porcelain veneer or a separation of the porcelain from the zirconia. The porcelain veneers chip at the rate of 6-10% for crowns at 5 years and 3-36% for fixed bridges at 5 years.

An alternative to layering porcelain is to heat-press a fluorapatite glass-ceramic material onto the zirconia core. A more recent development is high-translucency zirconia that can be used as an all-zirconia crown without the need for porcelain layering in many posterior applications. Examples of these more translucent zirconia materials include BruxZir (Glidewell Laboratories) and Lava Plus (3M ESPE).

> Glass-based ceramics are the most esthetic and mimic the optical properties of enamel and dentin. However, they have low values for flexural strength. The higher the crystalline component added to the glass matrix, the greater is the strength, i.e., lithium disilicate (IPS e-Max, Ivoclar Vivadent).
>
> Non-glass (crystalline) ceramics have the highest flexural strength but are not as esthetic and are more opaque. The strongest of these materials is zirconia, but it is commonly veneered with porcelain to use where esthetics is important.

PHYSICAL AND MECHANICAL PROPERTIES

FLEXURAL STRENGTH

Ceramic materials are stiff and brittle, and these properties contributed to the fracture of weak feldspathic porcelains in early clinical applications. Newer ceramic materials are much stronger. Although ceramic materials are generally stronger when compressive forces are applied, it is their flexural strength that is more important for resisting fracture. Glass-based ceramic materials such as the porcelains have relatively low flexural strength. Lithium disilicate has the highest flexural strength of these glassy materials. The non–glass-based ceramic materials have very high flexural strengths. Zirconia has the highest flexural strength of the crystalline materials and also has the highest fracture toughness. See Table 9.1 for a comparison of material strengths.

THERMAL PROPERTIES

Ceramic materials act as insulators in that they do not conduct heat or cold readily, as do metallic restorations. They will, however, expand or contract when subjected to temperature changes. The degree to which they expand or contract is called the *coefficient of thermal expansion* (CTE). The higher the CTE, the more the ceramic expands or contracts with temperature changes. This change in dimension is not critically important with a restoration made from a single material. However, when two ceramic materials are used jointly in a restoration, as with porcelain veneer of a zirconia core or porcelain bonded to a metal core (as with a PFM crown), the two materials must have compatible CTEs. Otherwise, the veneering ceramic material may fracture. The laboratory technician must carefully select materials for their compatibility because not all ceramics have the same CTE.

OPTICAL PROPERTIES

Transparency

Transparent materials allow light to pass through in an unaltered path, i.e., window glass (see Fig. 9.2). Since transparent materials do not resemble tooth structure there is little need for them in dentistry.

Translucency

Translucent materials allow light to pass through the surface and into the body of the material; some of the light is reflected back out, unlike a transparent material that allows light to pass all the way through it.

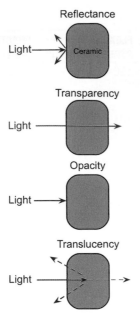

Reflectance

Light → Ceramic

Transparency

Light →

Opacity

Light →

Translucency

Light →

FIG. 9.2 Optical properties (From Powers JM, Wataha JC: *Dental Materials: Properties and Manipulation*, ed 11, St. Louis, 2017, Elsevier.)

Glass-based ceramic materials are more translucent than non-glass ceramics and as a result mimic enamel better.

Reflectance

The surface of a ceramic material may reflect light that hits it. How much light is reflected is influenced by the surface texture and polish and the basic structure of the ceramic material. The portion of the light that is not reflected passes into the ceramic and is either absorbed or passes through it.

Opacity

Opaque ceramic materials do not allow light to pass through them. The light is absorbed or reflected. Non-glass ceramic materials are the most opaque. These materials are the least esthetic of the ceramic materials and must be veneered with more translucent, glassy materials to be used for anterior restorations.

Vitality

Glass-based ceramic crowns have a more lifelike appearance (sometimes called *vitality*) than PFM crowns. They appear vital (similar to natural teeth) because they are fluorescent, that is, they emit light in the visible wave spectrum when ultraviolet light hits them. They are also opalescent because they take on a bluish tinge when light reflects off of them, and an orange-yellow tinge when light passes through them.

BIOCOMPATIBILITY

Ceramic materials are considered to be among the most biocompatible of the restorative dental materials. Clinical studies have not shown an adverse tissue response to these materials. Glass-based ceramic materials will leach some components in minute amounts over time; much less so than alloys or resins. Lithium disilicate shows some initial toxicity in cell cultures that fades with time. Non-glass ceramics have shown no toxicity to date, and zirconia has been successfully used as implant fixtures.

CERAMIC PROCESSING TECHNIQUES

A variety of techniques may be used to fabricate all-ceramic restorations, depending on the type of ceramic material that will be used. Ceramic restorations can be made by sintering, slip-casting, heat-pressing, or computer-aided machining.

SINTERING

Sintering occurs when ceramic particles are heated to the point that they melt and fuse to adjacent particles at their borders (see Fig. 9.1). Methods such as firing the ceramic in a vacuum are needed to reduce porosity and in turn produce a stronger material. To achieve the desired match to the natural tooth, other ceramic materials called *stains* and *glazes* are added and fired to join with the previous layer of ceramic. Alumina-based ceramic and feldspathic porcelain that has been reinforced with leucite are the most commonly used materials for the sintering process. Both of these materials have higher flexural and compressive strength compared with traditional feldspathic porcelain. As ceramic processing techniques advance, sintered all-ceramics are being used less, in favor of heat-pressed or computer-aided machined ceramics.

SLIP-CASTING

Slip-casting is a processing technique whereby the ceramic powder is mixed with a water-based liquid to form a stable suspension called the slip and pressed onto a porous refractory die that soaks up much of the water. The slip is then fired at high temperature (1150 °C, or 2102 °F) to create a porous ceramic core. This core is then infiltrated with molten glass by capillary action to make a dense strong core to which conventional porcelains can be added to develop the desired color and degree of translucency or opacity.

The slip-casting technique can be used with zirconia-based, spinel-based (magnesium aluminum oxide), or alumina-based ceramic materials. Zirconia-based ceramics have the highest flexural strength of these materials and are several times stronger than the ceramic cores made from aluminum oxide that were introduced in the 1960s. They also have fewer defects from processing. Ingots of this glass-infiltrated material can be processed with CAD/CAM units making for a simpler technique.

HEAT-PRESSING

Heat-pressing uses the lost wax technique, similar to that used to cast gold crowns into an investment mold developed from a wax pattern that was burned out in an oven (the lost wax technique is discussed in Chapter 16

Gypsum and Wax Products). Pressable ceramic ingots are made of crystalline particles in a glass matrix. An ingot of the desired shade is heated until it becomes a thick liquid. Then, it is pressed into the mold at high temperature (about 1160 °C, or 2120 °F) and pressure (0.4 MPa), making a denser restoration. To complete the restoration, it can be color-stained and glazed. If the material is used as a core or framework, conventional feldspathic porcelain can be added to complete the color and contour, and surface stains can be added.

A leucite-based ceramic has been used for this process since the 1990s. Commonly known brands are IPS Empress (Ivoclar Vivadent) and Finesse (Dentsply Sirona). An improvement in strength was made with the introduction of a lithium disilicate–based ceramic (IPS Empress II and later versions called IPS e.max; Ivoclar Vivadent). These materials have been used for inlays, onlays, crowns, veneers, and short-span fixed bridges in low stress areas.

COMPUTER-AIDED MACHINING

Various pre-processed ceramic materials are available in blocks for use with CAD/CAM technology. An optical impression of the prepared tooth is made and either used in the dental office or transmitted to the dental laboratory. A computer software program is used to design the restoration to establish the contours, proximal contacts, occlusal contacts, and margins. A block of the ceramic material in the appropriate shade is selected and placed into a milling machine. A computer, using the design created, instructs the milling device to cut out the restoration. Depending on the material selected, heat processing may be required to complete the firing of the ceramic material. Custom staining and glazing of the restoration may be done to achieve maximal esthetics.

CAD/CAM TECHNOLOGY

Advances in technology over the past three decades have led to the development of sophisticated computer-aided design and computer-aided machining (**CAD/CAM**) for general industry and for dental applications. The technology now has widespread acceptance. Initially, CAD/CAM technology in dentistry was used solely for crown and bridge restorations. Preformed ceramics or resin ceramic blocks or disks are used to fabricate a variety of restorations including inlays, onlays, veneers, crowns, and bridges. As the technology has advanced and full arch scanners have become available, many other applications have emerged including surgical guides, custom implant abutments, orthodontic aligners, custom braces, orthodontic appliances, and complete and partial dentures.

In 1986 the CEREC (Chairside Economical Restoration of Esthetic Ceramic) system was the first to be introduced to dentistry. The manufacturer (originally Sirona Dental Systems, Long Island City, NY, and now Dentsply Sirona) has continually improved the system. Presently, there are several manufacturers for CAD/CAM systems for the dental office and the dental laboratory. The two most popular chairside systems in the USA are CEREC 3D (Dentsply Sirona) and E4D (D4D Technologies).

BASIC COMPONENTS OF CAD/CAM SYSTEMS

CAD/CAM systems have three basic components: (1) an optical scanner, (2) a computer with design software, and (3) a milling device (Fig. 9.3). The optical scanner can make "impressions" (digital images) of tooth preparations, opposing teeth and the occlusal relationship that are integrated with computer software (for details on digital impressions see Chapter 15). The computer software then designs the restoration to fit the preparation, establishes proper contours and contacts, and shapes the restoration to fit the opposing occlusion. Improvements in the software permit the operator to view the designed restoration in three dimensions and rotate it in all directions so that each aspect can be inspected. The dentist, hygienist, or assistant can modify the design as needed, using the design tools provided. The design is fed into a computer-controlled machine that uses diamond instruments to mill an all-ceramic restoration from a block of ceramic material (Fig. 9.4).

INCORPORATING CAD/CAM TECHNOLOGY INTO PRIVATE PRACTICE

Benefits of Chairside CAD/CAM Systems

There are a number of benefits that dental practices can derive from using the chairside CAD/CAM systems:

- A three-dimensional image of the tooth preparation can be viewed on the computer monitor from several different angles. The dentist or auxiliary can then modify the preparation as needed before processing the restoration, so potential errors can be eliminated.
- The opposing teeth can be viewed in occlusion with the designed restoration and measurements of the restoration thickness can be made before milling, Thickness of the ceramic can be increased or decreased as needed and contours can be modified with the design software.
- The impression procedure is simplified because no cord packing or impression material is needed. Many potential sources of error are eliminated.
- The completed design of the restoration can be viewed and approved before milling is started.
- Machining eliminates the human error sometimes seen with processing steps done by a laboratory technician.
- Perhaps the most attractive feature is that dental offices that have these systems can prepare and deliver the restoration in the same visit. Patients like this convenience, and this can be a practice-building feature. This improves office efficiency and greatly speeds up the process. The patient needs to be given anesthesia for only one visit; digital scanning of the preparation speeds the "impression" process and no impression materials are needed; no die needs to be poured; no temporary crown is needed; and

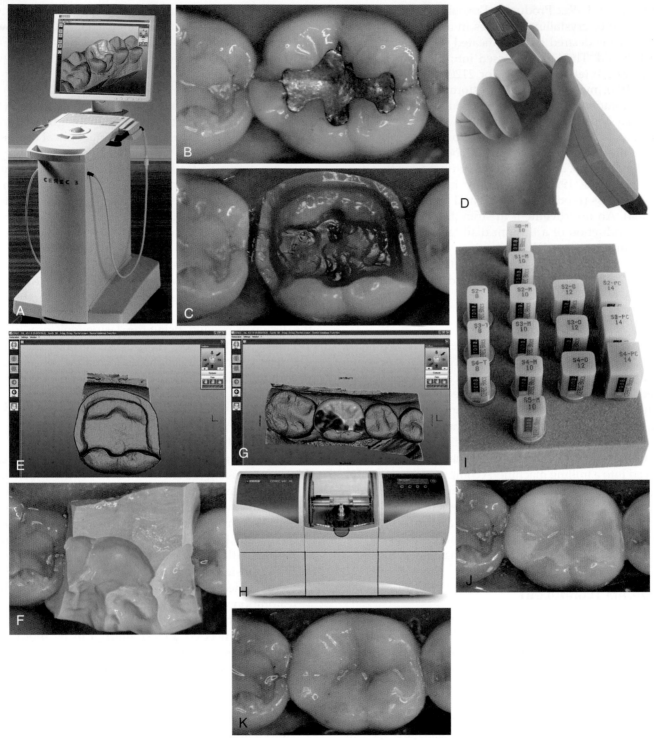

FIG. 9.3 CAD/CAM in-office system for making all-ceramic restorations. **A,** CAD/CAM in-office control unit with attached camera captures and stores images of the prepared teeth and bite relationship. Software designs the restoration and directs the milling unit on how to sculpt the restoration. **B,** Cracked lower first molar needing restoration. **C,** Cracked molar prepared for a ceramic onlay. **D,** Camera captures images of the prepared molar. **E,** The image of the molar and the margins marked in blue. **F,** Bite registration placed over the prepared molar. Its image will be captured, and computer software will configure the occlusal relationship with the ceramic onlay. **G,** Computer-generated occlusal contacts *(blue)* made from the bite registration. **H,** Milling unit that will sculpt the ceramic onlay from a ceramic block of the selected shade. **I,** Ceramic blocks in a variety of shades and sizes. **J,** Unpolished ceramic onlay tried on the molar to confirm its fit. **K,** Ceramic onlay after it has been polished and cemented. (Courtesy of Dentsply Sirona and Todd Ehrlich [private practice in Bee Cave, TX] for clinical photographs.)

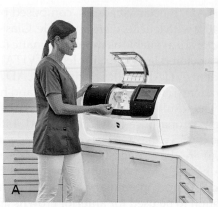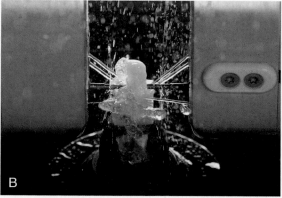

FIG. 9.4 Milling the restoration. **A,** Ceramic block is placed in the milling machine. **B,** Diamond instruments mill the restoration from the ceramic block according to the design feed from the computer software. (CEREC MC XL, Courtesy Dentsply Sirona.)

one cycle of breakdown and setup of the operatory with disposable supplies is eliminated. There is no laboratory fee, so with all of the areas of cost savings the system eventually pays for itself.

The very basics for operating a CAD/CAM system can be learned in a 2-day hands-on course. However, to become proficient and apply all of the features the systems offer, additional training and practice will be needed. Scheduling for restorative procedures that will use the system will need to be altered to accommodate the one-appointment mode. Initially longer appointments will be needed until the dentist and the staff becomes proficient with the system. Consideration will need to be made that at the same visit both preparation and cementation will take place as well as the steps needed to finish, polish, stain, and glaze the restoration.

ROLE OF THE ASSISTANT/HYGIENIST

Many of the steps can be delegated by the dentist to her/his team members who also have undergone training. Training courses are available that are geared specifically for assistants or hygienists. Appropriately trained assistants or hygienists are capable of using the optical scanner to capture images of the prepared and adjacent teeth and the opposing occlusion. They can mark the location of the margins and design the restoration. They can initiate milling of the restoration, polish it, stain and glaze it if necessary, and prepare the restoration for bonding or conventional cementation as dictated by the material selected.

WORKING WITH THE LABORATORY

Sirona has reported approximately 18% of dentists in the United States use chairside CAD/CAM technology. The utilization of CAD/CAM technology by dental laboratories has exceeded chairside use. Dentists who have optical scanners but do not have milling machines in their offices can electronically transmit digital images to a commercial laboratory using the CAD/CAM equipment to have a ceramic restoration made. For those offices without a scanner or milling device, a conventional impression is made of the prepared teeth and sent to the laboratory, where the technician scans a die made from the impression (or scans the impression itself), designs the restoration, and feeds the information to the milling machine. The technician can apply custom stain, and then polish or glaze the restoration and, if needed, stack or press porcelain to high-strength cores.

Drawbacks of Introducing Chairside CAD/CAM into the Practice

Introducing a new technology to the practice is not without certain drawbacks:

- There is the initial expense of the system, periodic software updates, and routine maintenance. The dentist must determine how many esthetic restorations are typically done in the practice or will be done once the new equipment is installed. Is this going to be a cost-effective purchase or will it sit in a corner and collect dust?
- There is a significant learning curve that must be accommodated in the practice schedule. As a result there may be an initial loss of production. Patients may have extended time in the office waiting for new learners to use the system and process the restorations in a single visit. When things do not go as planned both the staff and the patient can get frustrated. So, the patient should be informed ahead of time that the appointment may be a long one.
- To provide good color matching of the restoration to the dentition, custom staining may be needed. This will require additional training and the purchase of a glazing oven.
- There are certain clinical scenarios in which an optical scanner will not be effective, such as preparations with deep subgingival margins. These situations may need cord placement or soft tissue modification with a laser or electrosurgery to expose the margins.

CAD/CAM RESTORATIONS

CAD/CAM technology can be used to produce monolithic (all the same material) single-unit inlays, onlays, crowns, and veneers. In addition, it can be used to make ceramic cores for crowns and bridges that are subsequently veneered with porcelain or other ceramic material. A few manufacturers have developed multi-colored blocks with layers that mimic enamel and dentin. Provisional (temporary) restorations can be fabricated from acrylic blocks. Implant abutments and metal partial denture frameworks can also be milled. Properly designed restorations made with the use of CAD/CAM technology require fewer remakes; shorter seating time and adjustments; and better contours, contacts, and occlusion. Restorations have good marginal integrity which falls within the 50-micron (μm) parameter established by the American Dental Association.

CERAMIC CAD/CAM MATERIALS

Ceramic blocks made for CAD/CAM use have been produced under well-controlled conditions so that they are uniformly dense with no porosity. Porosities are weak points in the material that lead to the development of small cracks that propagate and eventually cause fracture of the restoration. Pre-produced blocks eliminate the variations and errors that can occur with conventional laboratory procedures. Blocks contain bar codes that indicate the density of each block so calculations can be made by the computer software to allow for shrinkage that occurs when the restoration is given its final oven firing.

Blocks of the appropriate materials can be used to generate inlays, onlays, crowns, fixed bridges, veneers and implant abutments. In general, monolithic restorations are stronger than veneered restorations (a core of one material and a veneer of another material). Veneered restorations have the potential to chip or separate at the junction of the veneer material and the core material (called *delamination*).

Glass-Based CAD/CAM Materials

Machinable blocks of glass-based ceramic materials are available for fabrication of inlays, onlays, crowns, and veneers. The first and only ceramic CAD/CAM material available until 1997 was glassy feldspathic porcelain (VITABLOCS Mark II, Vident/VITA). Later, blocks of ProCAD (Ivoclar Vivadent), composed of glass infiltrated 40% with leucite, were available. Glass-based ceramic blocks are available as monochromatic (all one color) or multicolored layers (examples are VITABLOCS TriLuxe [Vident/VITA] or IPS Empress CAD Multi [Ivoclar Vivadent]) and are available in low and high translucency. The resulting restorations are very esthetic and relatively strong once they are bonded. Lithium disilicate blocks (IPS e.max CAD; Ivoclar Vivadent, introduced in 2006) are the strongest of the glass-based ceramics and can be used for posterior crowns and three-unit fixed bridges (from premolars to anterior) and are esthetic enough to be used for anterior crowns and veneers.

Non-Glass Ceramic CAD/CAM Materials

Non-glass ceramics are used mostly as machinable blocks. Aluminum oxide–based ceramics includes Procera AllCeram (Nobel Biocare), In-Ceram AL Block (Vident/VITA), and inCoris AL (Sirona). Zirconia-based ceramics include Lava (3M ESPE), In-Ceram YZ (Vident/VITA), and IPS e.max ZirCAD (Ivoclar Vivadent). They have very high flexural strength (750 to 1200 MPa) and high fracture toughness. They are not very esthetic and must be veneered with more esthetic ceramics to be used in the anterior or visible areas in the posterior part of the mouth. They serve well as high-strength cores for crowns and bridges (Fig. 9.5). To overcome the opacity of zirconia restorations 3M ESPE has developed a high-translucency zirconia material (Lava Plus) that is matched to the VITA shade guides. This should reduce the need for veneering to achieve esthetics in many applications.

Processing the Material

Milling the Blocks Blocks of hard, fully sintered, high-strength materials consisting of lithium disilicate, alumina, and zirconia are difficult and time-consuming to machine (called hard machining) to their final processed form. Milling them can quickly wear out the milling tools and create residual flaws at the surface. To make them easier to machine they are not processed (sintered) completely until after they are milled (called soft or green machining). Some milling units can cut out a full crown in

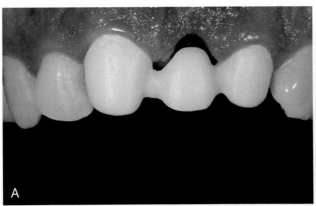
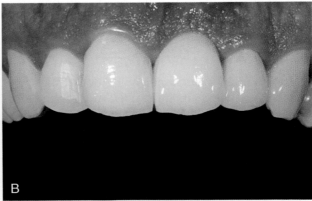

FIG. 9.5 Ceramic bridge teeth #8-#10 (Lava, 3M ESPE). **A,** Zirconia substructure. **B,** Veneered with more translucent ceramic for esthetics. (Courtesy of 3M ESPE and V. Bonatz.)

approximately five minutes. IPS e.max CAD blocks, for example, are only partially sintered and the blocks appear blue or purple (Fig. 9.6). The CAD blocks have a bar code that tells the computer software how large the milled restoration should be based upon the shrinkage that will occur during final sintering and allows for it during milling.

Some milling units can cut the blocks dry, but many units use constant water spray as a coolant. After milling the fit is verified and the restoration is finished and polished. Abrasive rubber wheels and points can be used and a high gloss achieved with diamond paste on bristle brushes. Instead of polishing, some clinicians prefer to apply a spray-on glaze which is fused to the restoration in a ceramic oven.

Firing the blocks. Once milling is complete, the restorations are fired in a ceramic oven to fully sinter them and transform them to the selected color. Materials such as zirconia once took as long as two hours to sinter making them impractical for same-appointment delivery. However, advances in ovens have made firing of zirconia restorations possible in as little as 30 minutes depending on their size and thickness (Fig. 9.7).

Stains and glazes. Color modifiers called stains contain metal oxides and are used on the surface to characterize a restoration by mimicking discolorations, white spots, fine crack lines in enamel, stains in grooves or other imperfections needed to match the natural dentition. They are also used to improve the color of the restoration when a preformed block does not provide an exact color match. A glaze provides a glossy, enamel-like surface. Stains and glazes are applied in thin layers on the surface of the restoration and fired at the time of final sintering. They are heated in a ceramic oven to a point that allows them to fuse with the ceramic restoration.

Sometimes the fusion is not complete and the stain or glaze can wear off. It wears off faster on occlusal surfaces than facial surfaces. If the stain wears off, the result will be a mismatch in color or if the glaze wears off, the result is a rough restoration. Polishing the restoration to a high shine instead of applying a glaze would solve the issue of a rough restoration caused by loss of the glaze.

Resin Hybrid Ceramics

Hybrid resin nanoceramic materials (Lava Ultimate [3M ESPE] (Fig. 9.8); VITA Enamic [Vident/VITA], Shofu Block HC [Shofu] and GC Cerasmart [GC America])

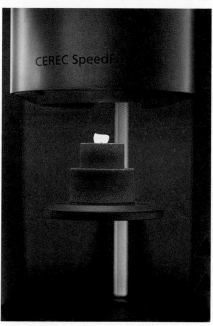

FIG. 9.7 Firing and glazing oven. (CEREC SpeedFire, Courtesy Dentsply Sirona.)

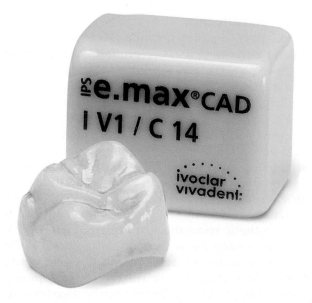

FIG. 9.6 (Top to bottom) Partially sintered block (purple) of lithium disilicate ceramic, and glazed crown (IPS e.max CAD, Ivoclar Vivadent)

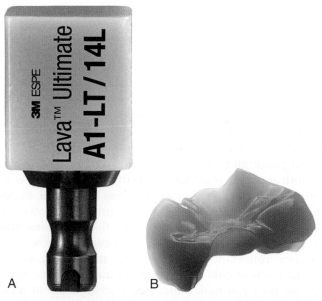

A   B

FIG. 9.8 Hybrid resin nanoceramic. **A,** CAD/CAM block, and **B,** completed onlay. (Lava Ultimate; images courtesy 3M ESPE.)

have been developed that combine desirable properties of both composite resin and nanosized ceramic filler particles. They are easy to mill and polish to a high shine and do not need to be oven fired. Hybrid resin nanoceramic materials produce tough, durable restorations that are not abrasive to the opposing teeth. They are available in several common Vita Classic shades consisting of high and low translucency options. They are stain and wear resistant and color stable. They are indicated for single-unit anterior and posterior crowns, inlays, onlays, and veneers. Because they are relatively new, long-term clinical studies are not yet available on their clinical performance.

SUMMARY OF CAD/CAM STEPS FOR PRODUCING A RESTORATION

- Complete the preparation using principles for all-ceramic restorations
- Use the optical scanner to obtain an image of the preparation lined up with the path of insertion of the restoration. Some scanners require coating the preparation with a powder to enhance scanning accuracy
- Use the computer software to design the restoration: mark margins and establish restoration contours on the computer screen
- Use the software to simulate occlusal excursions
- Select block of the correct shade of the ceramic material and place it in the milling machine
- Program the milling machine for the material being used and activate the machine
- If the milled restoration was in the green (or soft) state, it will need to be fired to complete the sintering process
- Characterization with surface stains can be accomplished while applying the overglaze
- Try in the completed restoration
- Cement the restoration after etching internally and applying silane (zirconia should not be etched or silanated. It has special primers)
- Check and adjust the occlusion as needed after cementation

CLINICAL APPLICATIONS FOR CERAMIC MATERIALS

Many of the newer ceramic materials such as lithium disilicate and zirconium are much stronger than porcelain and have replaced its use in many clinical applications. They are finding wider applications and are strong enough to be used in the posterior part of the mouth in many (but not all) individuals. People who grind their teeth apply greater stress to ceramic materials and are at greater risk of fracturing it. However, some patients are willing to accept the risk of fracture to achieve the high esthetics of all-ceramic crowns. It is very important that patients be made fully aware of the fracture risks of using porcelain or other ceramics, so they can make informed decisions about their care. When the patient has multiple ceramic restorations, use of an occlusal guard is recommended. Many offices use informed consent forms that patients must

sign before esthetic treatments are started. Although the dentist has the final responsibility, the dental assistant or dental hygienist may be called on to inform the patient about the pros and cons of various dental materials.

RATIONALE FOR SELECTION OF CERAMIC MATERIALS

Porcelain

Porcelains (powder/liquid application) are used more for anterior teeth. They (Ceramco 3, EX-3, VITA VM13, and Halo) are used to make porcelain veneers and serve well once they are bonded to the enamel and used in low-stress areas. The risk for fracture and debonding is higher if they are bonded to dentin. They are used as veneers on cores made from stronger but less esthetic materials such as alumina, zirconia, or metal. They are prone to fracture if used in posterior teeth for inlays or onlays or for anterior crowns.

Leucite-Reinforced Ceramics

Leucite-reinforced ceramics (IPS Empress) are esthetic and are available as machinable blocks (VITABLOCS Mark II, IPS Empress CAD) or pressable ingots. They work well for inlays, onlays, thicker veneers, and anterior crowns if they are bonded. They are not strong enough to hold up as posterior crowns.

Lithium Disilicate

Lithium disilicate (IPS e.max and e.max CAD) has twice the strength and fracture toughness of IPS Empress and has enough translucency that it can be used in the anterior or posterior part of the mouth for any solitary restoration. It can be used for three-unit bridges from the premolars to the anteriors. The manufacturer says it can be cemented with conventional luting agents, but for maximal strength it should be bonded.

Alumina and Zirconia.

The non-glass ceramics, alumina (Procera and In-Ceram) and zirconia (Lava, Cercon, In-Ceram Zirconia, IPS e.max ZirCAD, and Procera AllZirkon), are very strong materials but being somewhat opaque are not esthetic for use in the anterior part of the mouth. The alumina materials show an increased risk of fracture when used for molar crowns, and therefore their use should be limited to anteriors and premolars, serving well as inlays and onlays. Their opacity can be useful in hiding the discoloration of endodontically treated teeth. Zirconia is a suitable alternative for PFM crowns. All-zirconia crowns, inlays, and onlays can be used to provide esthetic restorations for bruxers who would otherwise destroy the weaker ceramic materials. Zirconia crowns can be made more esthetic by veneering with porcelain. There is some risk (>5%) of chipping of the veneering porcelains. Zirconia can be used for cores for three-unit bridges and for implant abutments in the anterior smile zone. See Table 9.2 for a summary of indications and contraindications for dental ceramics.

Table 9.2	Indications and Contraindications for Use of Various Types of Ceramics			
CERAMIC TYPE	**COMMON BRANDS**	**MAIN USES**	**OTHER USES**	**CONTRAINDICATIONS**
Feldspathic porcelain	Ceramco VITA VMK Duceram LFC	PFM ceramics Anterior veneers	Single surface inlays in low-stress sites	Inlays, onlays, crowns, bridges (except as metal ceramic veneers)
Leucite-reinforced glass ceramic	IPS Empress	Anterior use for single crowns or veneers	Low-stress inlays and crowns in premolars	Bridges High stress: Bruxers
Lithium disilicate glass ceramic	Empress II IPS e.max	Anterior and premolar crowns Anterior bridges	Anterior veneers Bridges no farther back than premolars	High stress: Bruxers Bridges involving molars
Glass-infiltrated alumina or zirconia	Procera Alumina In-Ceram (alumina, zirconia)	Posterior crowns Bridge substructure to 3 units	Anterior bridge substructure to 3 units	Translucent anterior applications: Veneers and crowns
Zirconia with or without veneering ceramic	Lava Cercon VITA YZ Procera Zirconia IPS e.max ZirCAD BruxZir Solid Zirconia	Posterior crowns and bridges Posterior bridge substructure	Implant abutments in the smile zone	Where high translucency is needed: Anterior veneers, crowns, or bridges Bruxers

PFM, porcelain-fused-to-metal.
Adapted from Anusavice KJ, Shen C, Rawls HR: Dental Ceramics (Table 18-3). In: *Phillips' Science of Dental Materials*, ed 12, St. Louis, 2013, Saunders.

VENEERS

Veneers are thin layers (like press-on nails) of esthetic materials that are used to improve the appearance of the teeth. They are bonded to the fronts of the teeth, most often anterior teeth and premolars. They can be used to lighten the color of teeth, cover stains, repair chips or other defects, lengthen worn teeth, increase the size of small teeth, close spaces (diastemas), or reshape crooked teeth so that they look as though they are in proper alignment.

The most commonly used materials are directly placed composite resins or indirect (made in the laboratory) glass-based ceramics. Indirect ceramic veneers are made in the laboratory of traditional feldspathic porcelains (called *porcelain laminate veneers* or simply *porcelain veneers*), pressed ceramics, or computer-assisted machined ceramics, such as IPS e.maxCAD. Ceramic veneers are more durable than composite veneers: their surface does not discolor over time, they are more wear resistant, and they are stronger.

The first porcelain veneers were used in the 1930s, mostly for Hollywood movie stars. Because bonding to tooth structure by acid-etch techniques did not become commercially available until the 1960s, these Hollywood veneers were just stuck on the teeth with the available denture adhesives. Embarrassing situation could occur if the veneers became dislodged!

Clinical Consideration for Veneers

Until the advent of the newer ceramic materials, porcelain veneers were the most widely used veneers. They can be made relatively thin and require a minimal reduction of the enamel by 0.5 mm on the facial and, if the incisal edge is involved, at least 1.0 mm at the incisal edge. Esthetic demands might require greater reduction to correct overlapping teeth or to hide dark teeth or discolorations. Pressed ceramic veneers are thicker than feldspathic porcelain veneers and therefore require a deeper preparation of the tooth. They are very esthetic for covering mild discolorations but are too translucent for very dark teeth. CAD/CAM-produced veneers of lithium disilicate (IPS e.max) are strong and can be made thinner than pressed ceramics.

Ultrathin porcelain veneers that require no preparation of the teeth are heavily marketed by their manufacturers. Although no preparation may be needed in select cases, in many cases patients might end up with bulky, overcontoured veneers, if adequate space is not created for the veneering material. With an ultrathin material, it is also more difficult to mask dark underlying tooth structure.

Porcelain veneers can be made to be slightly translucent to let the color of the underlying tooth come through, or more opaque to hide the color of a darker natural tooth. Dark teeth are more challenging to cover with veneers and still achieve an esthetic result. Use of some opaque porcelain (up to approximately 15%) helps to hide the darkness, but too much opaqueness will cause a loss of the vitality produced by translucency that mimics natural enamel. Because of their thinness, veneers may not be the best mode of treatment to esthetically improve the appearance of very dark teeth. On occasion, whitening of the dark teeth may be attempted first, to reduce the darkness before veneers are placed. Otherwise, all-ceramic crowns might be a better option for improving the appearance of very dark teeth and still achieving an optimal esthetic effect.

Try-in of veneers. Veneers are tried on the teeth, using water or a try-in gel on the surfaces that contact the teeth. The gel is a water-soluble material that occupies the air space between the veneer and the tooth surface. Without the water or gel, light transmitted through the veneer will be scattered by the air space, altering the appearance of the veneer. The gels can be clear or slightly shaded to correspond to shades of bonding resins. Before they are bonded to the teeth, the ceramic veneers are somewhat fragile, because they are very thin. They must be handled with care when they are tried on the teeth to confirm the fit or to adjust the contact areas. They might crack if too much pressure is applied to them. Once they are bonded, they gain support from the underlying tooth structure and greatly increase in strength.

 Caution

Handle veneers carefully! They are very fragile until bonded!

Cementation of veneers. Veneers are bonded to the teeth with resin cements, using the acid-etch technique, and a resin bonding agent (Fig. 9.9). The resin cements come in a variety of colors, including a clear resin. If needed, a resin color can be selected to slightly alter the final appearance of the veneer to help mask the color of the underlying tooth. To get the resin to stick to the porcelain, the internal surface of the veneer is roughened by etching it with hydrofluoric acid. A coupling agent, called *silane,* is added to the etched porcelain surface to enhance the bond and form a chemical union between the porcelain and the resin cement (see Chapter 5, Procedure 5.2).

Once the tooth surface and the internal veneer surface have been properly prepared, the resin cement is placed on the veneer and is carefully seated while an attempt is made to avoid trapping air. The veneer is lightly vibrated with an instrument or finger to fully seat it and dislodge any entrapped air bubbles. Excess cement can be removed from the margins at this stage with small brushes, or the curing light can be waved over the surface for 3 or 4 seconds to cause the resin to slightly gel but not fully cure. The gelled excess resin can then easily be removed with an explorer or #12 surgical blade. Some additional finishing and polishing might be required. Various techniques are available for this last step, using combinations of finishing strips and disks, carbide and diamond finishing rotary instruments, and rubber polishing points or diamond polishing pastes.

PORCELAIN-METAL RESTORATIONS

Before strong, esthetic ceramics were developed, the most commonly used restorations in fixed (crown and bridge) prosthodontics were combinations of porcelain and metal (**porcelain-metal restorations**). Before the development of the porcelain-fused-to-metal technique in

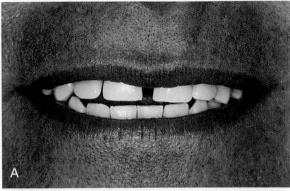
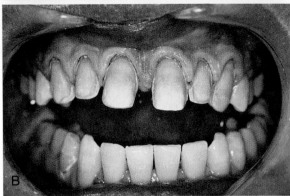
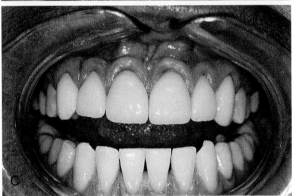

FIG. 9.9 Placement of porcelain veneers to correct a large diastema. **A,** Pretreatment photograph showing large midline diastema. **B,** Maxillary anterior teeth prepared for veneers. Retraction cord is in place. **C,** After cementation of veneers with a resin cement. (Courtesy of Dentsply International [York, PA].)

the 1950s, all-porcelain jacket crowns or metal crowns with acrylic or porcelain facings were used most often in the esthetic zone of the mouth. Acrylic facings stained and wore down over time. Cemented porcelain facings often fractured or became uncemented (bonding was not available at the time). The main advantages of the combination of porcelain and metal are the strength and durability given to the restoration by the bond between a metal internal core and the esthetic external porcelain covering. The restorations are strong enough to be used in the posterior part of the mouth, where biting forces are greater than in the anterior part, and can be provided as single crowns or multi-unit bridges. The survival rate at 5 years for porcelain-metal restorations is about 94%. Trying to hide the metal core with porcelain can present some esthetic challenges. Additionally, a small

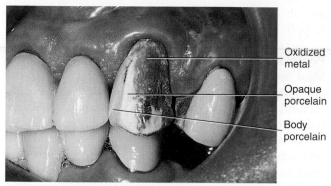

Oxidized metal

Opaque porcelain

Body porcelain

FIG. 9.10 Porcelain failure with porcelain-bonded-to-metal (PBM) crown. The metal is exposed, as is a portion of the opaque layer of porcelain used to prevent metal from showing through the more translucent outer layers of porcelain. (Courtesy of Dr. Steve Eakle, University of California, San Francisco.)

Diagram of longitudinal section through
(A) All-ceramic crown
(B) Porcelain-bonded-to-metal crown

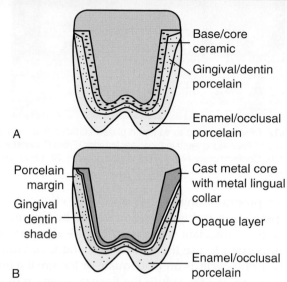

Base/core ceramic

Gingival/dentin porcelain

Enamel/occlusal porcelain

Porcelain margin

Gingival dentin shade

Cast metal core with metal lingual collar

Opaque layer

Enamel/occlusal porcelain

FIG. 9.11 Section through **A,** an all-ceramic crown and **B,** a porcelain-bonded-to-metal crown, showing the layers of porcelain and the metal substructure of the crown.

percentage of patients may have allergies to some of the metals used for the core.

Application of Porcelain to the Metal Core

The method for layering porcelain on a metal core is similar to that for a ceramic core or for building up porcelain on a die. Low-fusing porcelain (i.e., Ceramco 3, Dentsply Sirona) is used for the bonding of porcelain to metal. These restorations are referred to as porcelain-fused-to-metal (PFM) or porcelain-bonded-to-metal (PBM) restorations. The metals that are used as the core for PBM/PFM crowns are alloys of specific metals that will form an oxide layer as the metal is heated. When porcelain is applied to the metal and the two materials are heated together, the porcelain chemically fuses to the oxides on the metal, forming a durable bond. The metal alloys are classified as high noble (precious), noble (semiprecious), or base (nonprecious) metal alloys, based on the presence and amount of gold, palladium, and other precious metals (see Chapter 11 Casting Metals, Solders, and Wrought Metal Alloys). The metal in the area where the porcelain is to be bonded is usually relatively thin, approximately 0.3 to 0.5 mm thick.

A color of porcelain is selected that corresponds to the color or shade that matches the patient's dentition. The first layer of porcelain applied to the metal is opaque porcelain that keeps the metal oxide color from showing through the porcelain and is the main color used for the crown (Fig. 9.10). Base metals often form darker oxides that are more difficult to hide with opaque porcelain.

The porcelain comes as a powder that is mixed into a paste with de-ionized water or a water-based liquid, or may be in a paste form already. The porcelain paste is applied (or stacked) on the metal and shaped. Then it is vibrated with an instrument to reduce porosity and blotted to remove excess moisture. The oxidized metal and porcelain are heated under a vacuum to remove air and increase density at temperatures ranging from 870 °C to 1370 °C (1598 °F to 2498 °F), depending on whether the porcelain

to be used fuses at low, medium, or high temperature. The porcelain particles melt at their borders and fuse together (sintering) and also wet the metal oxides. The oxides and porcelain chemically fuse together and mechanically interlock. Sintering results in shrinkage of the porcelain mass by about 25% to 40%. Then additional layers of porcelain called *body and incisal porcelains* are built up or stacked to simulate dentin and enamel colors and translucency and condensed with a stacking instrument to help eliminate porosity (Fig. 9.11). The incisal porcelain is more translucent, so the body color shows through readily and has a greater influence on the final appearance. The layers of porcelain are fired in the oven until they fuse to each other and to the underlying opaque porcelain.

Firing Porcelain

After completion of the layering of colors, the condensed porcelain on the metal coping is heated to a few hundred degrees to remove residual water. This process is called the drying stage and is done before final firing. A programmable porcelain oven is used to gradually raise the temperature. If the temperature is increased too quickly the water vapor (steam) can cause the condensed mass to blow apart.

Next, the porcelain is fired at high temperature and vacuum. The temperature at which the porcelain is fired is determined by the type of porcelain being used and its components (see manufacturer specifications). The porcelain is low fusing and is first heated to approximately 900 °C to partially fuse (sinter) the particles (see Fig. 9.1). As the glass matrix softens, it flows and reduces porosities. If it is held at firing temperature too long, the glass will slump and the restoration will lose its shape.

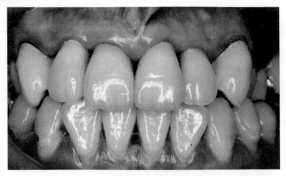

FIG. 9.12 PFM crowns #6 to #11 with glazed surfaces that resemble the luster of the natural teeth in the lower anterior. (From Rosenstiel SF, Land MF: *Contemporary Fixed Prosthodontics*, ed 5, St. Louis, 2016, Elsevier.)

Proper programming of the oven will eliminate the slumping issue, but not all porosity will be eliminated. Typically, a porcelain restoration has 10-30% porosity. It is important to use the correct time and temperature for the firing cycle as an inadequate or too great a temperature can greatly reduce the flexural strength of the restoration. Additionally, the development of translucency occurs only after firing at the proper temperature and time. After firing has been completed, the resulting restoration will have shrunk about 25% because of the fusion of the porcelain particles.

Glazing

After final contouring of the crown, another firing maintaining the temperature at the fusing temperature for a while will produce a surface glaze. The surface layer of porcelain will heat first allowing it to melt and run together producing a dense, shiny, smooth surface (Fig. 9.12). Firing must be stopped at this point to prevent the interior from heating up too much and causing the whole restoration to shump. Some technicians use a layer of special translucent porcelain that fuses at relatively low temperatures to form the glazed surface. This is called *overglazing*.

Color Modification

Stains are used with veneering porcelain for the same purposes as for all-ceramic restorations, that is, they can characterize the restoration and improve color matching.

Re-polishing

The porcelain surface, once it has been fused under temperature, is very hard and smooth. When porcelain or PBM restorations are delivered, the proximal contacts or occlusal surfaces often must be adjusted. These restorations could be returned to the laboratory to be reglazed (refired at porcelain-fusing temperatures to form a glassy surface) before cementing. Because this is seldom practical, various abrasives have been developed for polishing the porcelain surface after adjustment (see Chapter 13 Abrasion, Finishing, and Polishing). Low-fusing porcelains are less abrasive to opposing tooth structure and can be re-polished more easily after adjustments.

Porcelain Failures

Most porcelain failures result from small cracks in the porcelain that develop when the porcelain is put under occlusal loading, and they propagate (spread) over time until the porcelain gives way. Other modes of failure are caused by problems related to the chemical bond between the porcelain and the metal oxides. The oxide layer may be too thick or inadequate in quantity and quality, leading to failure at the interface of the porcelain and metal. It is important that the coefficients of thermal expansion of the porcelain and the metal be compatible. The best arrangement is for the porcelain to have slightly less thermal expansion than the metal. This will keep it from cracking at the metal-porcelain interface and will reduce the chance of failure (see Fig. 9.10).

When porcelain failures occur in non–stress-bearing areas, repairs may be possible using composite resin and bonding techniques, but the repairs are not as strong as the original bonded porcelain (see Chapter 5) and may fail if put under too much biting pressure. The alternative is to do expensive replacements of the entire crown or bridge.

CERAMIC INLAYS, ONLAYS, AND FIXED PARTIAL DENTURES (BRIDGES)

Ceramic inlays, onlays, and fixed bridges are placed in the functional areas of the mouth, and therefore strength is an important factor. Feldspathic porcelains are not the materials of choice, because they are weaker than leucite- or zirconium-based ceramics. Heat-pressed materials are commonly used, but CAD/CAM-produced zirconium materials are gaining in popularity because of their high strength. Ceramic materials with a more opaque core (such as Procera Zirconia [Nobel Biocare] or In-Ceram [Vident/VITA]) may be selected to hide discolorations from root canal therapy or tetracycline stains.

It is important for the clinician to identify the junction of the tooth and the margins of any of these ceramic restorations when removing excess cement or when doing scaling or root-planing procedures. The hand scaler or ultrasonic tip used at high settings may cause chipping of the margins if the clinician is not careful. However, properly fabricated and adjusted ceramic restorations should present minimal problems for the clinician who is doing these procedures. If significant overhang or catching of the margins is noted, the assistant or hygienist should alert the dentist, who may correct them or prescribe replacements.

 Clinical Tip

Ultrasonic scalers, if improperly applied, can chip and craze margins of esthetic materials.

FINISHING AND POLISHING CERAMIC RESTORATIONS

Two important factors in wear of the opposing dentition by ceramic restorations are the crystalline grain (particle) size of the ceramic material and the smoothness of the ceramic surface (Fig. 9.13, *A* and *B*). Modern ceramic materials such as lithium disilicate and zirconia ceramics have smaller grain size than porcelains, are less abrasive, and can be polished smoother. Zirconia that has been glazed will cause more wear of opposing enamel surfaces than highly polished zirconia, because the glaze is thin and will wear away with time leaving a rough, unpolished surface. Once the occlusal surface of a restoration has been adjusted with a diamond bur the roughness of the surface can be very abrasive to the opposing enamel or restorative material. It is imperative to re-establish the surface smoothness through careful finishing and polishing techniques.

Adjustment of ceramic materials with coarse diamond burs can create surface and subsurface damage that can lead to propagation of cracks and future chipping or fracture of the restoration over time from repeated occlusal loading (i.e., eating or bruxing). Coarse diamond burs should not be used to adjust the surface because the larger diamond particles leave a rougher surface that is more difficult to re-polish, and they tend to generate heat that can damage the ceramic. Fine diamond burs are recommended. Zirconia has a unique property (called *transformation strengthening*) due to its crystalline arrangement that allows it to deflect cracks that are forming so they do not propagate through the material. However, if too much heat is generated in finishing and polishing, a shift occurs in the material that negates this "crack-healing" property.

Principles of Finishing and Polishing Ceramics

Some basic principles of finishing and polishing dental ceramic materials should be followed. First, heavy pressure should be avoided; use a light touch. Second, low speed should be used with water spray. Following both of these principles will minimize the generation of heat and surface and subsurface damage.

Sequential finishing and polishing. When trying to achieve a smooth surface it is important to follow a proper sequence progressing to fine and yet finer abrasive finishing and polishing instruments. Steps cannot be skipped. Larger scratches must be sequentially reduced to smaller and smaller scratches until they are no longer perceptible. Several manufacturers have developed special finishing and polishing instruments designed for use with porcelains, lithium disilicate, or zirconia (e.g., Dialite, Dialite LD, and Dialite ZR; Brasseler USA).

Use of polishing pastes. Polishing pastes contain fine abrasives to create a very smooth surface after use of polishing instruments. Pastes containing aluminum

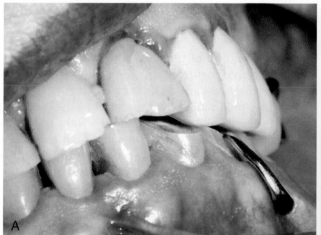
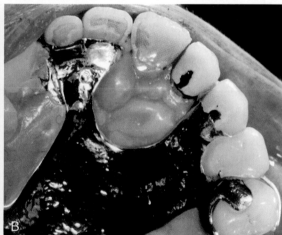
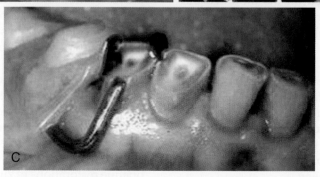

FIG. 9.13 Wear of opposing teeth by porcelain. **A,** Teeth #10 and #11 have PBM crowns; **B,** the porcelain on the PBM crowns extends onto the lingual surfaces of #10 and #11; **C,** the patient is a bruxer and displays excessive abrasion of the teeth opposite the porcelain. Adjacent teeth show moderate incisal attrition. (Courtesy of Steve Eakle, University of California, San Francisco.)

oxide are safe to use on porcelain. If the objective is to produce a high shine or luster, a diamond polishing paste with very fine particles should be used. As with most products, follow the manufacturer's recommendations for which pastes to use on the various ceramic materials.

 Clinical Tip

Generation of heat during adjustment, finishing, and polishing of ceramics can cause damage that may progress to fracture of the restoration. Use rotary instruments at low speed with water spray and light pressure.

CEMENTATION OF ALL-CERAMIC RESTORATIONS

All of the glass-based ceramic materials (porcelain, leucite-reinforced ceramic, and lithium disilicate ceramic) should be bonded to the teeth with resin cement. They all can be etched with acid (usually hydrofluoric) to facilitate bonding them to tooth structure. Bonding them to a rigid substrate greatly enhances their resistance to fracture.

Try-in of Restoration

The delivery of ceramic restorations begins with good isolation. Use of the rubber dam is ideal but not always practical, so alternatives such as the Isolite (Isolite Systems) or absorbent pads and cotton rolls may be used. Next, the provisional restoration is removed, bits of adherent cement are picked off with an explorer or other instrument and the prepared tooth surfaces are cleaned with pumice and water on rubber cups or brushes, then rinsed and dried. The restoration is tried in and interproximal contacts are adjusted. For veneers and other translucent restorations, a water-soluble try-in paste, glycerin, or K-Y Jelly is used to verify the color and to determine the color of resin cement to use. The underlying tooth color can affect the color of the bonded restoration. For zirconia and alumina restorations, their opaqueness hides the color of the underlying tooth. For weaker materials such as porcelain or leucite-reinforced ceramics, the occlusion should not be checked until after cementation because it might crack. The occlusion is checked on the mounted dies before cementation (unless processed by CAD/CAM for which there are no physical dies).

Preparing the Restoration

Glass-based ceramics. If the laboratory has not already etched the internal surface (intaglio) of the restoration, then apply hydrofluoric acid for 5 minutes (leucite-reinforced materials require only 1 minute), and then rinse and dry. After etching, silane coupling agent is applied to the intaglio of the restoration for 60 seconds, and then air dried.

Non-glass ceramics. Non-glass materials (alumina and zirconia) do not etch well with hydrofluoric acid.

These materials can be sandblasted internally with 50-μm alumina at a pressure of 20 to 30 psi (pounds per square inch) (too much pressure can cause damage to the ceramic) to provide a roughened surface to mechanically interlock with the cement. (Glass-based ceramics should not be sandblasted, because it will cause microscopic cracks in the surface.) Zirconia and alumina ceramic materials do not need silane treatment, but may be treated with special primers with acidic adhesive monomers to improve the bond with resin cement.

Preparing the Tooth

The prepared tooth surfaces are wiped with a wet cotton pellet to remove any remnants of try-in materials. If any bleeding has occurred, the tissue can be infiltrated with local anesthetic with epinephrine to constrict the capillaries, or a hemostatic agent can be used. Ferric sulfate hemostatic (e.g., Astringedent; Ultradent) should be avoided because it will interfere with resin bonding and may cause discoloration under the ceramic restoration. Next, the tooth surface (enamel, dentin, or both) is conditioned according to the manufacturer's instructions for the bonding materials being used. A bonding agent is applied to seal open dentinal tubules and to establish a hybrid layer for bonding with the resin cement. An alternative to the etch-and-rinse bonding agent is a self-etch bonding agent that eliminates the need for phosphoric acid etching (see Chapter 5). A self-adhesive resin cement (e.g., Maxcem Elite [Kerr Dental]; RelyX Unicem [3M ESPE]) eliminates the need for a separate bonding agent.

Cementation of the Restoration

The resin cement systems commonly used with ceramic restorations are dual-cured, so if the light from the curing unit is unable to reach all of the cement, it will cure chemically on its own. Many light-cured bonding agents are not compatible with dual-cured resin cements; make sure a compatible bonding agent is used (see the manufacturer's recommendations).

The resin cement is mixed (most are supplied in automixing cartridges) and applied to the internal part of the restoration. Use enough to coat all of the walls of the restoration and the margins. Do not overfill a crown because the hydraulic pressure created in trying to displace the cement when seating the crown may prevent the restoration from seating completely. Wipe away excess cement with a small brush. Use the curing light for about 3 seconds over the area of the margins to cause the resin to gel but not set completely. This is called *tack curing* and will facilitate easy removal of any remaining excess cement. After the excess is removed, a 60-second cure (halogen light) or less with high-intensity lights (laser or plasma arc light) is used to accelerate the set. With opaque restorations of zirconia or alumina the light may be ineffective for reaching cement under the restoration, but the chemical-cure component of the cement will allow it to set in a couple of minutes.

Zirconia and alumina have such high strength that they do not have to be bonded. They can be cemented with conventional cements such as resin-modified glass ionomer cement. This cement is often used because it bonds to the tooth, releases fluoride, is moderately strong, has thermal expansion similar to the tooth, and cleans up easily. However, if the tooth preparation is not very retentive (short walls or over-tapered), then resin cement should be used with bonding to the tooth and internal sandblasting of the crown to aid retention. It has been suggested that lithium disilicate crowns do not need bonding because of their strength, but they are not as strong as zirconia. Therefore, to minimize the risk of fracture it is prudent to bond them.

MAINTENANCE OF ALL-CERAMIC RESTORATIONS

The patient should be given home care instructions for proper brushing and flossing around ceramic restorations. For bridges additional hygiene aids such as floss threaders, interproximal brushes, or Oral-B Superfloss (Procter & Gamble) may be recommended. Patients should be advised against biting on hard objects or food with the ceramic restorations. As previously discussed, some ceramic materials are more fragile than others. At periodic recall appointments recheck the occlusion, review the gingival health, and make sure no excess cement remains.

Care should be taken when working around ceramic crowns. When providing in-office fluoride treatments to adults with ceramic restorations, the hygienist needs to select a fluoride product that is not acidic. Acidulated fluoride products can etch ceramic surfaces. Likewise, when doing bonding procedures on adjacent teeth avoid allowing etching gels to touch the ceramics because they will roughen the surface. Ultrasonic scalers should be used with care around ceramic restorations so as not to induce heat damage or initiate microcracks at the margins. Patients who grind their teeth or have edge-to-edge bites should be provided with occlusal guards to help protect the anterior ceramic crowns and veneers. Restorations made entirely from zirconia (called *monolithic*) may be the exception because of their remarkable strength. However, if the restoration has a zirconia core and is veneered with porcelain for esthetics, then the overlying porcelain could chip or break.

 Caution

Avoid acid etchants and acidic fluorides on ceramic restorations. They will roughen the surface of the ceramic.

REMOVAL OF ALL-CERAMIC RESTORATIONS

The average life span of a crown is about 10 to 15 years, and some fail sooner for a variety of reasons (such as recurrent caries or fracture of the ceramic material).

Clinicians are faced with the task of removing the failing restoration. Gold crowns can readily be removed by sectioning them with a carbide bur. Nonprecious metal crowns can present a problem because of their hardness, and special metal-cutting burs have been developed to address this.

Porcelain restorations can be removed by sectioning with a coarse diamond bur. PFM crowns can be removed by using a combination of coarse diamond burs and metal-cutting burs. First, a pathway through the porcelain to the metal is created with the diamond bur. The pathway should be wide enough so that the metal cutting bur can be used without touching the adjacent porcelain. (The porcelain will dull the carbide bur quickly.) Then, the metal-cutting bur cuts through the metal until the crown is in two segments. The segments are pried apart with a thick instrument (a large spoon, small screwdriver, or crown removal instrument).

The high-strength ceramic materials (lithium disilicate and zirconia) are very difficult to remove with conventional diamond burs. Some manufacturers have developed diamond burs specifically for cutting lithium disilicate and zirconia (e.g., ZR-Diamonds; Komet USA). These diamonds reduce the time needed to remove these high-strength crowns by about half.

SHADE TAKING

The dental assistant or hygienist may be asked to assist the dentist in obtaining the appropriate shade for a restorative procedure. An inappropriate shade selection will result in a mismatch to the patient's dentition. Usually, the restoration will need to be returned to the dental laboratory for a remake or for reapplication of porcelain. This is disappointing for all involved and usually results in an additional laboratory fee and the in-office expense of an additional appointment. Therefore, it is important for all clinical members of the dental team to have an understanding of what goes into the perception of color, how to accurately match the variety of shades within a single tooth, and how to communicate this to the dental technician.

Patients tend to notice differences in value more than differences in hue or chroma when they assess how well a restoration matches their own teeth. So, if a restoration is the same brightness as the natural dentition but is slightly off in its color or color intensity, it will be better accepted by the patient than if the restoration is too dark or too light. Teeth with different colors could have the same value (or brightness), yet have different intensity of color. Likewise, teeth with the same color can vary in brightness. For example, in the classic VITA shade guide, A3 and D3 are similar in color, but A3 is brighter than D3. As teeth darken with age, patients who were once in the A shade range may transition into the D shades.

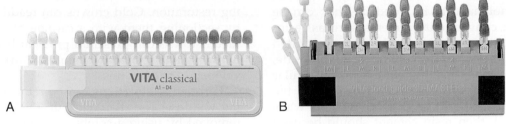

FIG. 9.14 Two popular commercial shade guides that use different methods for selecting the shade: **A,** VITA Classical A1-D4 with whitening shades. **B,** VITA Toothguide 3D Master. (Courtesy of VITA North America, Yorba Linda, CA.)

INVOLVING THE DENTAL ASSISTANT/HYGIENIST AND THE PATIENT

The dentist often relies on the chairside assistant or hygienist to help in shade taking. Having the doctor, assistant, and patient working together to determine the shade often gets a result all can be happy with.

The dental assistant can get the dental office environment ready for taking the shade by:
- Having the patient remove lipstick and colorful makeup
- Covering bright, colorful clothing with a neutral colored bib such as pastel blue
- Placing the patient in a neutral colored room
- Removing debris and surface stain from the teeth
- Keeping the teeth moist; not isolating the teeth until ready to begin preparation
- Turning off or moving the dental unit light away from the mouth
- Headlamps should also be turned off.

The most popular shade guides are the VITA Lumin system (VITAPAN Classical or VITA 3D-Master; VITA North America) (Fig. 9.14) and Chromascop (Ivoclar Vivadent). With the VITA guides shades in the A range are reddish brown, B shades are reddish yellow, C shades are grey, and D shades are reddish grey. In general, the shade should be taken before the tooth is isolated or prepared. Some clinicians arrange the tabs by value from highest to lowest. A typical shade tab is composed of several colors arranged to simulate a natural tooth. An opaque color is used as a backing on the tab for the color of the body of the tooth crown and the color of the root (also called the neck) but does not include the incisal portion that is typically translucent (Fig. 9.15).

STEPS FOR SHADE TAKING

The following steps should be used when taking the shade of the teeth:
- Use natural light when possible
- Use cheek retractors for an unobstructed view of the teeth
- Raise the patient to view the teeth at eye level to use the color-sensitive part of the retina
- Wet the shade tab and the teeth to remove surface texture differences

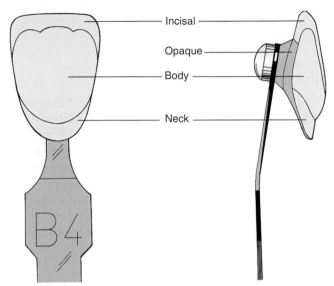

FIG. 9.15 Color arrangements in a typical porcelain shade tab. (From Rosenstiel SF, Land MF: Contemporary Fixed Prosthodontics, ed 5, St Louis, 2016, Elsevier).

- Place the shade tab in the same plane as the teeth, not in front or behind
- View the teeth and tab for no more than 5 seconds at a time
- Rest the eyes between viewings by staring at a neutral gray color
- Pick the best 3 shade tabs quickly
- With the input of patient, doctor, and assistant, select the best of the 3
- If possible, use photography to aid the lab technician. Place the shade tab next to the teeth in the photo.
- Note tooth factors the lab will need to characterize (see Characterizing the Shade below)

The patient, dentist, and assistant should view the tabs and rank them as to the closest match for color intensity and lightness or darkness. It is often necessary to take separate shades for the cervical portion of the tooth, for the occlusal surfaces of posterior teeth, and for the incisal edges of anterior teeth (Fig. 9.16).

Characterizing the Shade

In addition to the shade, the surface luster and texture should be noted. As a person ages, the slight convexities and concavities on the surface of the teeth become smoother from wear and reflect light differently than

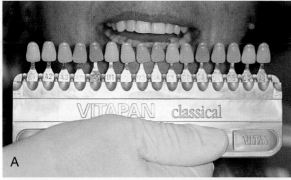

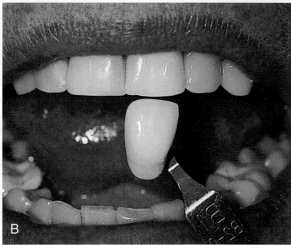

FIG. 9.16 Shade taking for porcelain restorations. A neutral gray is considered a good color to look at to refresh the retina while shade taking. **A,** Shade guide placed near the mouth to select the basic color (hue). **B,** The shade tab in the right color is compared with the teeth to be matched; select the color with the proper value (darkness or brightness) and chroma (intensity of color).

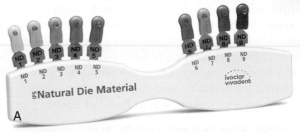

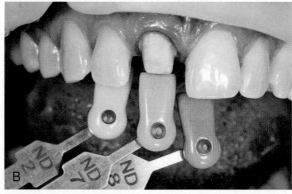

Fig. 9.17 Shade guide for taking dentin shades. **A,** Dentin shade guide and **B,** dentin shade tabs used to match dentin from the prepared tooth. (From Rosenstiel SF, Land MF: *Contemporary Fixed Prosthodontics*, ed 5, St. Louis, 2016, Elsevier.)

highly textured teeth. Textured teeth tend to scatter light. Luster is the degree to which the surface appears shiny and reflects light. The laboratory technician can add surface glazes to ceramic to create a shiny surface and can add texture to scatter light.

The amount of translucency of the enamel and its location (e.g., incisal edge) should also be communicated to the laboratory. The laboratory technician may need to place layers of opaque porcelain to mask darkly colored dentin when fabricating all-ceramic restorations. The opacity will cause of loss of vitality in the restoration. The technician may need to produce the perception of translucency by using color modifiers to tint the porcelain (e.g., blue tints may produce a hint of translucency).

Teeth may have opaque white spots or lines, stained cracks, wear facets, and other characteristics that should be conveyed to the laboratory if the patient is trying to match existing teeth. The process of incorporating into the restoration texture, translucency, opacity, and the many other tooth features is called *characterization*.

A written description and drawing of the shade distribution (called *shade mapping*) and location of translucency and any special characterizations, surface texture, and luster should be sent to the laboratory to help guide the technician. Often it is helpful to the

technician if a digital photograph of the teeth is transmitted. If photography is used, the shade tab should be included in the picture, because some photographs will be a little more red or blue than the actual color. The bright operatory light should not be used to illuminate the patient's mouth, as this will cause the recorded image to appear lighter. The shade tab should be in the same plane as the tooth to be matched, so that it will be in the same focus as the teeth, that is, it should not be in front of the teeth or outside of the mouth and will have the same illumination as the teeth when flash photography is used. The flash used should be rated for a good color rendering (index above 93).

On occasion, some teeth are not a close match to the shade tabs. This requires that the technician see the teeth, so that he or she can custom blend different shades of porcelain or use surface stains to match the color. The patient may be sent to the laboratory, or the technician may come to the operatory for this "custom" shade taking. This is particularly true for whitened teeth. Whitening of teeth has become very popular, and the whitened colors of teeth may not match existing shade guides. So, shade guides with whitening shades that are extra light (low chroma and high value) should be used. Even with these whitening shades, it may be difficult to match the color of whitened teeth.

Dentin Shade Matching for All-Ceramic Restorations

Some of the all-ceramic restorations are relatively translucent. A special shade guide for dentin color is used to help the technician in the fabrication of a crown (Fig. 9.17). Cosmetically, it might be important to hide dark dentin with opaque ceramic colors to achieve a lighter color in the restoration. The final shade of the all-ceramic restoration is influenced by the shade of the ceramic coping (substructure for a crown) or framework (for a bridge), the veneering porcelain or ceramic, the prepared tooth shade, and the shade of the luting material (conventional cement or bonded resin).

DEVICES FOR TAKING THE SHADE

Because of the complexity involved in achieving a good shade match of a ceramic material to the natural tooth, a number of devices have been introduced that help in obtaining an accurate reading of the shade of the teeth. These devices use optical readers (spectrophotometers) to determine the correct shade (Fig. 9.18). Having the information captured by an optical device removes the subjectivity of the individual trying to interpret the shade and trying to describe the shade to the dental laboratory technician. This eliminates the extraneous light sources and conflicting colors in the room or on the patient that confuse the human eye's perception of color. One such device, the VITA Easyshade V (Vident/VITA), can match the shade it records with the company's popular brand of VITA porcelains. These devices can provide a map or layout of the subtle variations in shade within a given tooth.

With proper training, the dental assistant or hygienist can operate the device and acquire the shade. This increases office efficiency and consistency of shade matching. The accuracy of the shade taken by these devices can potentially save time and expense associated with sending the crown back to the laboratory; this can make for a more satisfied patient. Advances in technology are making communication with the laboratory simpler and more accurate.

SUMMARY

A wide variety of tooth-colored esthetic materials are available to the dental team to use to restore a patient's dentition. Patients demand high-quality restorations with a close match to their existing teeth, or in some cases, they demand restorations that produce a lighter, youthful smile. Newer ceramic materials have broadened the choices the clinician has for esthetic restorations. CAD/CAM technology is providing new avenues for the dental team to provide esthetic dentistry with the potential for making many procedures faster and easier on patients.

It is important that all members of the dental team understand the handling characteristics, physical

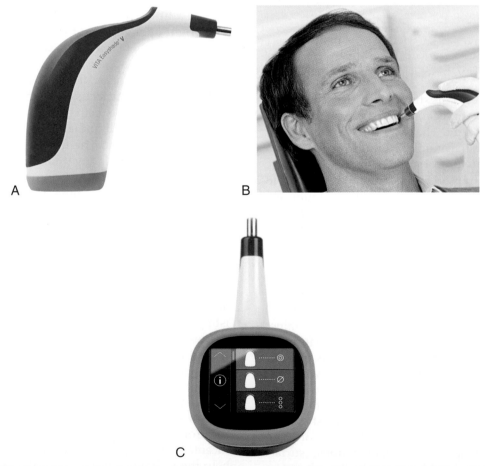

A B

C

FIG. 9.18 Shade taking device. **A,** Easyshade V device. **B,** Device used to take the shade. **C,** Digital display of the shade captured by the device. (Courtesy of VITA North America, Yorba Linda, CA.)

properties, and potential shortcomings of these materials. Before working in the patient's mouth, it is wise to review the dental charting section of the patient's record or perform a brief oral inspection to detect the presence of esthetic restorations. Drying the teeth with an air syringe can help reveal some of the materials, because they may have a different luster than the enamel, or margins may be more readily visible once the saliva has been removed. The selection and use of proper polishing and scaling devices are an important consideration for the hygienist and the chairside assistant when working around these restorations. Ultrasonic scalers have the potential to chip or craze the margins of all-ceramic or composite restorations. When applying topical fluoride, it is important to keep in mind that the surfaces of these esthetic restorations can be affected by the use of acidulated fluoride solutions and gels. The use of these products can dull the surface of the restoration and change the esthetic effect of the original restoration, making for an unhappy patient. Neutral sodium fluoride products or fluoride varnish can be used as alternatives. Certain abrasives used for coronal polishing can also adversely affect the surface luster of composites and porcelain. The radiographic appearance may be different with each of the various esthetic restorative materials. As new esthetic materials are adopted in the practice, it is important to become familiar with their handling characteristics, physical properties, uses, and precautions.

INSTRUCTIONAL VIDEOS

See the Evolve Resources site for a variety of educational videos that reinforce the material covered in this chapter.

Get Ready for Exams!

Review Questions

Select the one correct response for each of the following multiple-choice questions.

1. Porcelain restorations have
   a. Great stain resistance
   b. Low wear resistance
   c. High strength
   d. Easy reparability
2. Porcelain bonds to metal by which one of the following mechanisms?
   a. Micromechanical retention much like resin bonded to etched enamel
   b. Penetration through the surface of the metal
   c. Fusion with oxides on the surface of the metal
   d. Shrinkage when fired so that it locks onto the metal
3. The main advantage of all-ceramic crowns over porcelain-bonded-to-metal crowns is
   a. Their superior esthetics
   b. Their strength
   c. Their ease of cementation
   d. The ease of taking shades
4. The main drawback of feldspathic porcelain for all-porcelain crowns is
   a. Their tendency to fracture
   b. Their opacity
   c. The difficulty involved in making them
   d. That shrinkage when fired makes them difficult to fit to the prepared tooth

5. An in-office CAD/CAM system for ceramic restorations provides all of the following advantages *except* one? Which one?
   a. The restoration does not have to be fabricated in an outside laboratory.
   b. A provisional crown is not needed.
   c. The procedure can be completed in one visit.
   d. Local anesthesia is not needed.
6. The basic color of the tooth is called the
   a. Base shade
   b. True value
   c. Chroma
   d. Hue
7. All of the following should be avoided when taking the shade of a tooth *except* one. Which one?
   a. Lipstick on the patient
   b. Brightly colored clothing
   c. Dirty teeth (covered with plaque)
   d. Neutral wall colors in the room
8. All of the following materials should be avoided around ceramic restorations *except* one. Which one?
   a. Acidulated topical fluoride products
   b. Alginate impression material
   c. Coarse prophy paste
   d. Acid etchant
9. The impression for a CAD/CAM crown typically is
   a. Done with alginate
   b. Done with polyvinylsiloxane impression material
   c. Done with polyether impression material
   d. Done by capturing an image of the prepared tooth with an optical scanner

Continued

Get Ready for Exams!—cont'd

10. When preparing a porcelain-fused-to-metal crown, the technician applies feldspathic porcelain in layers to the metal coping. The initial layer is
    a. Translucent porcelain to mimic enamel
    b. Body porcelain to mimic dentin
    c. Opaque porcelain to hide the oxidized metal

11. On occasion, special porcelain stains are used on the surface of the porcelain. These stains contain metal oxides and are used to
    a. Create a shiny, smooth surface
    b. Mimic white spots or fine crack lines to resemble adjacent teeth
    c. Hide flaws created in the porcelain by firing it at high temperatures

12. Which one of the following statements about porcelain veneers is *false?*
    a. Porcelain veneers are more durable than composite veneers.
    b. Porcelain veneers must be handled carefully when one is trying them on, because they are very fragile until bonded to the tooth.
    c. It is difficult to mask a darkly colored tooth with a porcelain veneer.
    d. Porcelain veneers are usually cemented with zinc phosphate or glass ionomer cement.

13. When assisting the dentist with taking the shade of a tooth, the dental assistant should
    a. Dry the teeth thoroughly
    b. Shine the operatory light directly on the teeth
    c. Cover brightly colored clothing with a pastel, neutral-colored bib
    d. Stare at the tooth and shade guide intensely for at least 30 seconds to let the eyes adjust to the colors

14. Which one of the following ceramic materials is the strongest and most fracture resistant?
    a. Leucite-reinforced porcelain
    b. Zirconia
    c. Feldspathic porcelain
    d. Lithium disilicate

15. Which one of the following ceramic materials is the most opaque and, therefore, the least esthetic?
    a. Feldspathic porcelain
    b. Lithium disilicate
    c. Zirconia
    d. Leucite-reinforced porcelain

16. For anterior ceramic restorations the ceramic material used at the incisal edge tends to be which one of the following?
    a. Opaque
    b. Highly reflectant
    c. Translucent
    d. Transparent

17. The lightness or darkness of a color is referred to as which one of the following?
    a. Chroma
    b. Value
    c. Hue
    d. Radiance

18. Which of the following ceramic materials is not etched by hydrofluoric acid in preparation for cementation but may be sandblasted internally instead?
    a. Zirconia
    b. Lithium disilicate
    c. Feldspathic porcelain
    d. Leucite-reinforced porcelain

19. Porcelain veneers are bonded to the tooth with resin cement. This provides the opportunity to do all of the following *except* one. Which one?
    a. Increase the strength of the restoration
    b. Increase the retention of the restoration
    c. Slightly modify the shade of the cemented restoration with a colored resin cement
    d. Whiten the tooth with the acid etchant

20. All of the following considerations should be applied when finishing or polishing a ceramic material *except* one. Which one?
    a. Use slow speed
    b. Use a coarse diamond bur for adjustments
    c. Use light pressure
    d. Progress from medium abrasives to finer ones

21. All of the following are processing methods for ceramic materials *except* one. Which one?
    a. Sintering
    b. Heat pressing
    c. Cold curing
    d. CAD/CAM

22. When one is taking photographs of the teeth to send to the dental laboratory to help convey the correct shade, what is the proper location for the shade tab in the photograph?
    a. Outside of the mouth
    b. Inside the mouth and in front of the teeth
    c. In the same plane as the tooth being matched
    d. None of the above (the shade tab does not have to be included in the photograph)

For answers to Review Questions, see the Appendix.

Case-Based Discussion Topics

1. A 57-year-old secretary comes to the dental office for a periodic examination and prophylaxis. She has maxillary anterior composite veneers and all-ceramic crowns on her mandibular incisors.
Describe the factors that might contribute to fracture of the porcelain restorations. What must the dental hygienist and dental assistant be concerned about when treating patients who have esthetic composite and porcelain restorations present in their mouths?

2. An active 80-year-old woman comes to the dental office for preparation of her maxillary anterior and premolar teeth for porcelain veneers. She wants to lighten her teeth but wants to keep the same color (hue). She is wearing brightly colored clothing and lipstick.
What steps can the dental assistant or hygienist perform to help in the initial shade taking? Under what lighting conditions should the shade be taken?

Get Ready for Exams!—cont'd

3. A 60-year-old male postal worker was hit in the mouth by a falling package in the warehouse. The mesio-incisal edge of a porcelain-fused-to-metal crown on tooth #8 was fractured. He would like to have it fixed.

What are his treatment options? If he desires that it be fixed at today's visit, what materials could be used? What must he be told regarding the long-term prognosis of a repair?

4. A 30-year-old business executive has several large occlusal amalgam restorations on her lower molars and premolars that are visible when she speaks. She frequently gives presentations to small groups and would like to eliminate the dark restorations. She grinds her teeth in her sleep and clenches during the day.

What materials could be used to satisfy her esthetic needs? Of the ceramic materials, which would be most likely to fracture in her mouth and which would be most likely to survive her bruxing?

5. A 25-year-old fashion model has large mesial and distal class III composites on tooth #8, which have turned brown; the composites are visible when she smiles. She wants to get rid of the composites and the discoloration. The dentist has recommended a porcelain-fused-to-metal crown. The fashion model wants an all-porcelain crown to maximize the esthetics.

What are the pros and cons of each type of crown for this application? If an all-ceramic crown is done, what type of ceramic material is best for this application? Should the crown be bonded or just cemented? Why?

BIBLIOGRAPHY

Al Dehailan L: *Review of the Current Status of All-Ceramic Restorations.* Indiana University School of Dentistry. Available at: https://www.dentistry.iu.edu/files/3713/7597/9182/ceramic_lit_review.pdf

Anusavice KJ, Shen C, Rawls HR: Dental ceramics. In *Phillips' Science of Dental Materials*, ed 12, St. Louis, 2013, Saunders.

Baum L, Phillips R, Lund M: *The Metal-Ceramic Restoration. Textbook of Operative Dentistry*, ed 3, Philadelphia, 1995, Saunders.

Ferracane JL: *Materials for Inlays, Onlays, Crowns and Bridges. Materials in Dentistry*, ed 2, Baltimore, 2001, Lippincott Williams & Wilkins.

Giordano R: Materials for chairside CAD/CAM-produced restorations, *J Am Dent Assoc* 137:14S–21S, 2006.

Heyman HO, Swift EJ, Ritter AV: Additional conservative esthetic procedures. In *Sturdevant's Art and Science of Operative Dentistry*, ed 6, St. Louis, 2013, Mosby.

Kois JC, Chaiyabutr Y: Intraoral occlusal adjustment and polishing for modern ceramic materials, *Inside Dentistry* 11(3), 2015.

McLean JW, Hughes TH: The reinforcement of dental porcelain with ceramic oxides, *Br Dent J* 119:251–267, 1965.

McLaren EA: CAD/CAM dental technology: a perspective on its evolution and status, *Compendium* 32(4), 2011.

McLaren EA, Whiteman YY: Ceramics: rationale for material selection, *Inside Dentistry* 38–50, 2012.

Phillips RW, Moore KB: *Dental Ceramics. Elements of Dental Materials for Dental Hygienists and Dental Assistants*, ed 5, Philadelphia, 1994, Saunders.

Poticny DJ, Klim J: CAD/CAM in-office technology: innovations after 25 years of predictable, esthetic outcomes, *JADA* 141(Suppl 6):5S–9S, 2010.

Powers JM, Farah JW, O'Keefe KL, et al.: Guide to all-ceramic bonding, *The Dental Advisor*, 29(4), 2012.

Powers JM, Wataha JC: Dental ceramics. In *Dental Materials: Foundations and Applications*, ed 11, St. Louis, 2017, Elsevier.

Rosenstiel SF, Land MF, Fujimoto J: All-ceramic restorations. In *Contemporary Fixed Prosthodontics*, ed 4, St. Louis, 2006, Mosby.

Sakaguchi RL, Powers JM: Ceramics. In *Craig's Restorative Dental Materials*, ed 13, St. Louis, 2012, Mosby.

Santos MJ, Costa MD, Rubo JH, et. al.: Current all-ceramic systems in dentistry: a review. *Compend Contin Educ Dent.* 36(1):31–7, 2015.

Sorensen JA: Finishing and polishing with modern ceramic systems, *Inside Dentistry* 9:10–16, 2013.

Trost L, Stines S, Burt L: Making informed decisions about incorporating a CAD/CAM system into dental practice, *J Am Dent Assoc* 137:32S–36S, 2006.

10 Dental Amalgam

Chapter Objectives

Upon completion of this chapter, the student should be able to:

1. List the main components in dental amalgam.
2. Describe the advantages of high-copper amalgams over low-copper amalgams.
3. Explain the role of the gamma-2 phase in corrosion of amalgam.
4. Describe the particle shapes in lathe-cut, admix, and spherical alloys, and discuss their effects on the condensation resistance of freshly mixed amalgam.
5. Define creep, corrosion, and tarnish.
6. Compare the strength of amalgam with that of composite resin or glass ionomer cement.
7. Discuss the effect of mixing time on the strength and manipulation of amalgam.
8. Discuss the advantages and disadvantages of amalgam as a restorative material.
9. Discuss the safety of amalgam as a restorative material.
10. Perform safe mercury hygiene practices in the dental office.
11. Collect and process amalgam scrap for recycling.
12. Select an appropriate size of matrix band for a class II amalgam preparation.
13. Assemble a Tofflemire band in its retainer.
14. Evaluate a class II amalgam matrix setup for meeting proper placement criteria.
15. Assist with or place (as allowed by state law) amalgam in a class II cavity preparation.

Key Terms

Alloy a mixture of two or more metals

Amalgamation reaction that occurs when silver-based alloy is mixed with mercury to form an amalgam

Dental Amalgam metallic restorative material composed of silver-based alloy mixed with mercury

Lathe-Cut Alloy irregularly shaped particles formed by shaving fine particles from an alloy ingot

Spherical Alloy small spheres of alloy particles produced by spraying a fine mist of liquid alloy into an inert gas environment

Admixed Alloy mixture of lathe-cut and spherical alloys

Gamma-2 Phase a chemical reaction between tin in the silver-based alloy and mercury that causes corrosion in the amalgam

Delayed Expansion expansion of amalgam containing zinc when it is contaminated with moisture (e.g., saliva) during condensation. Inside the amalgam hydrogen gas develops from the interaction of water and zinc, and it creates an outward pressure that causes creep to occur

Creep gradual change in the shape of a restoration usually caused by compression from occlusion or adjacent

teeth and can cause amalgam to bulge out of the cavity preparation

Tarnish oxidation affecting a thin layer of a metal at its surface that does not change the metal's mechanical properties

Corrosion breakdown of a metal by chemical or electrochemical reaction with substances in the environment such as water or air. It negatively impacts the properties of amalgam

Triturator or Amalgamator mechanical device used to mix silver-based alloy particles with mercury to produce amalgam

Condensation the act of pressing amalgam mix into a cavity preparation with instruments to produce a dense mass

Burnishing after the amalgam mix is placed an instrument is used to further condense and smooth the amalgam surface

Amalgam separator a device that collects amalgam particles and mercury from evacuation systems that might otherwise escape into the wastewater and therefore enter the environment

Dental amalgam has been in use for more than 180 years and has been used for hundreds of millions of restorations. Dental amalgam is an amalgamation or combination of metals, mostly silver alloy powders and mercury. It is easy to manipulate, has good clinical durability, and is low-cost. However, its use has been gradually diminishing in many countries as patients demand more esthetic materials such as composite resin and ceramic restorations which have continually improved in their physical properties and handling characteristics. In addition, health and environmental concerns have been raised due to the mercury content of the amalgam causing some countries to move away from the use of amalgam.

It is essential that oral health practitioners have an understanding of the characteristics of the various amalgam alloys, so they can correctly select, mix, place, and carve them. In addition, knowledge of safe mercury hygiene measures is important for health and safety reasons. Dental assistants and hygienists will be asked questions by patients regarding the mercury content of amalgams and the health risks. Patients need to be provided with accurate information about this issue. Some states mandate patients be provided with a dental materials fact sheet listing pros and cons of the materials. This chapter covers the properties and handling of amalgam and mercury hygiene.

DENTAL AMALGAM

Millions of amalgam restorations are placed each year. Amalgam has been studied and tested more than any other restorative material. Although composite resins are being requested by patients with increasing frequency for posterior restorations, amalgam is still a widely used direct-placement material for the posterior region of the mouth and accounts for about 30% of the direct restorations placed in this region. No other direct restorative material has the durability, ease of handling, and good physical characteristics of amalgam. Its wear resistance and compressive strength are superior to composite resin and glass ionomer cement. Clinical studies indicate a typical life expectancy of about 15 years for conservative class I and II amalgams. Many can last much longer, with a few amalgams documented as lasting 40 to 50 years. The safety of amalgam has been called into question in recent years, but a study conducted by the National Institutes of Health (NIH) from 1991 to 1993 concluded that amalgam is safe for human use. In addition, the U.S. Public Health Service, the U.S. Food and Drug Administration (FDA), the American Dental Association, the Centers for Disease Control and Prevention, and the World Health Organization all consider amalgam to be a safe material. Less than 0.01% of people have an adverse reaction to the components of amalgam. However, a combination of concerns by patients about its safety and its lack of esthetics has prompted many patients to request tooth-colored restorative materials. Insurance carriers have seen a reduction in the use of amalgam for posterior restorations by approximately 45% in the past 20 years. Health and safety concerns will be discussed in detail later in the chapter.

ALLOYS USED IN DENTAL AMALGAM

An **alloy** is a mixture of two or more metals. The alloy used to produce dental amalgam is composed predominantly of silver but also contains copper and tin. A variety of other metals, such as palladium, indium, or zinc, may be added in much smaller quantities to produce specific properties in the alloy. When the silver-based alloy particles are mixed with mercury the reaction that occurs is called **amalgamation** and the material that is produced is a strong, hard, durable material called **dental amalgam**.

SILVER-BASED AMALGAM ALLOY PARTICLES

Silver-based amalgam alloys are classified as irregular, spherical or admixed according to the shape of the particles in the powder (Fig. 10.1). Each of these particle shapes contributes certain handling characteristics to the amalgam, and to some degree the amalgam type is selected by the dentist according to these characteristics.

Lathe-cut alloy

Irregularly shaped particles are formed by shaving fine particles (10-70 μm in width and 60-120 μm in length) off a heat-treated ingot of the alloy with a cutting machine called a lathe (thus, **lathe-cut alloy**). The particles are sifted to separate them into fine and ultrafine particles.

Spherical alloy

Spherical particles are produced by spraying (atomizing) a mist of molten alloy into an inert gas. Small spherical particles (2-43 μm) are formed as the atomized droplets cool (thus producing **spherical alloy**). The spherical particles are heat-treated and washed in acid to remove surface contaminants.

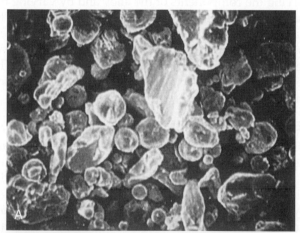
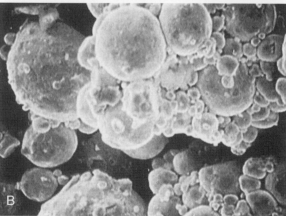

FIG. 10.1 A, Scanning electron micrograph (SEM) of admixed alloy showing a mixture of irregularly shaped particles and spherical particles. **B,** SEM of spherical alloy with spherical particles of various sizes. (Courtesy of Grayson W. Marshall, University of California School of Dentistry [San Francisco, CA].)

Admixed alloy

Admixed particles consist of a mixture of lathe-cut and spherical particles (**admixed alloy**).

Composition of Amalgam Alloys

Dental alloys for amalgam are composed mainly of silver and tin. Copper is added to replace some of the silver to lessen the brittleness. Alloys can be grouped or classified by their copper content. Modern dental alloys are considered to be high in copper content (13% to 30%) compared with their predecessors, which had 4% to 6% copper by weight (Table 10.1). They generally contain 40% to 70% silver and 12% to 30% tin. They are mixed with mercury 42% to 52% by weight (wt. %). Spherical alloys require less mercury to wet the particles, because the surface area of spheres is less than that of lathe-cut particles. Spherical alloys require about 42 to 45 wt. % of mercury whereas lathe-cut and admix alloys require 50 to 52 wt. %. Spherical amalgam generally sets faster than lathe-cut amalgam. Manufacturers may also add indium (1% to 4%), palladium (0.5%), and zinc (0.01% to 2%). Zinc may inhibit corrosion by reducing the oxidation of the other metals in the amalgam.

The manufacturer can affect how amalgam handles by varying the components of the alloy and by varying the shape, size, and distribution of the sizes of particles. The manufacturer, too, can control how fast the amalgam sets by various treatments of the alloy particles, such as heat-treating them or removing oxides from their surface. The dentist, then, can select alloys with slower or faster setting times depending on the intended application.

SETTING TRANSFORMATION (AMALGAMATION)

When the alloy in powder form is mixed with liquid mercury, a chemical reaction occurs. The reaction starts at the surface of the alloy, so the size and shape of the alloy particles will affect the setting process. The alloy particles dissolve into the mercury. When no more metal can dissolve into the mercury, a mixture of metallic compounds begins to crystallize in the mercury (a process called *amalgamation*) and continues until the liquid mercury is used up. Not all of the alloy particles are dissolved before the mercury is used up, so they remain in the core of the amalgam, held together by compounds of mercury with silver and tin (acting as a matrix), and make up about half of the amalgam volume. These particles contribute to the strength and corrosion resistance of the amalgam. The freshly mixed amalgam has a putty-like consistency that can be packed into the cavity preparation. Over the next several minutes, the free mercury is used up in the crystal formation and the mix gradually becomes firmer. During the first part of this firming phase, the amalgam can be carved (during the working time or time available to manipulate the amalgam) to the anatomic shape of the tooth. Once it reaches its initial set, it can no longer be carved and is firm but is not fully reacted. It is relatively brittle at this point, and the patient is advised not to bite on it for several hours. Many of the high-copper spherical amalgams gain approximately 50% of their compressive strength in the first hour, but it takes up to 24 hours for most amalgams to gain their maximum strength. Once fully set, they are hard, strong, durable restorations.

Setting Reactions

The chemical reaction that occurs when the alloy and mercury are mixed has three phases. The first phase, called the *gamma phase* (γ), is the silver alloy phase. It is the strongest phase and has the least corrosion. The second phase is the *gamma-1 phase* (γ_1), consisting of mercury reacting with the silver. It is strong and corrosion resistant, although not as resistant as the gamma phase. The third phase, the **gamma-2 phase** (γ_2), consists of the reaction of mercury with tin. Gamma-2 is weak and corrodes readily. Tin is used to control the rate of set of the amalgam. Both silver and tin dissolve into the liquid mercury until the solution becomes saturated with them, and they also absorb mercury. Newly formed particles begin to precipitate (crystallize) out of the mercury until there is no more mercury left to react. This process may take up to 24 hours to go to completion. Low-copper amalgams had much more corrosion because of the chemical reaction of tin and

Table 10.1	Main Components of Amalgam Alloy				
COMPONENT	**FUNCTION**	**OTHER EFFECTS**	**HIGH-COPPER ALLOY, %**	**LOW-COPPER ALLOY, %**
Silver (Ag)	Increases strength Increases durability Decreases creep	Decreases setting time Tarnishes easily	40–70	68–72
Tin (Sn)	Improves physical properties when compounded with silver	Reduces setting expansion Increases setting time	12–30	28–36
Copper (Cu)	Increases strength Increases hardness Reduces corrosion	Increases setting expansion Decreases creep	13–30	4–6
Zinc (Zn)	Reduces oxidation of other metals	Causes delayed expansion with moisture contamination	0–1	0–2

mercury (gamma-2 phase). Copper reacts with the tin to keep it from being available for the gamma-2 phase. High-copper amalgams do not have a gamma-2 phase and are superior in their clinical performance, displaying reduced corrosion and tarnish, higher compressive strength, less dimensional change, and better integrity of margins than low-copper amalgams.

PROPERTIES OF AMALGAM

Strength

Amalgam is among the strongest of the directly placed restorative materials. Its compressive strength is similar to tooth structure. It has the ability to resist the strong forces of the bite repeatedly over many years when properly placed. Amalgams are stronger in compression (approximately 400 to 450 megapascals [MPa]) than composites (300-350 MPa) or glass ionomers (50-150 MPa). However, they are relatively weak in tension (about 12% of compressive strength) and shear. All amalgams are considered to be brittle. Therefore, they require adequate bulk to resist breaking. If the cavity preparation is too shallow or the occlusal morphology of the restoration is carved too deeply, the restoration is more likely to fracture. Thin excesses of amalgam left over the cavosurface margins lack strength and chip away over time, creating an irregular margin that tends to collect plaque and contribute to recurrent caries. Additionally, cavosurface margins of the cavity preparation should be at 90 degrees to follow the direction of the enamel rods and to prevent forming thin edges of amalgam that may fracture. Excessive forces from bruxing, chewing on ice or biting on a popcorn kernel can cause fracture of the amalgam.

The strength of the amalgam can be affected by the speed and duration of trituration. Under or over triturating the amalgam mix amd a mix that is too wet or dry can decrease the strength of the amalgam. Likewise, the amount of mercury used in the mix can affect strength. A mix that is poorly condensed into the cavity preparation can result in voids that weaken the final restoration. In general, spherical alloys require less condensation pressure than admix alloys and they develop a degree of strength more quickly.

In general, high-copper amalgams have a higher early compressive strength (1 hour) than low-copper amalgams. This is advantageous because it helps resist breakage if the patient inadvertently bites on a newly placed amalgam. Some high-copper amalgams gain approximately 80% of their strength in the first 8 hours. Low- and high-copper amalgams are comparable in compressive strength once they have completely set at about 24 hours. See Table 10.2 for some of the properties of high-copper amalgam.

The American National Standards Institute/American Dental Association (ANSI/ADA) Standard No. 1 for Amalgam has set maximum values for dimensional change and creep and minimum values for

Table 10.2	Properties of High-Copper Amalgam	
	ADMIX	SPHERICAL
Compressive Strength (MPa)		
1 hour	110–220	260–315
1 day	400–440	450–500
Tensile Strength (MPa)1 day	43–50	49–64
Dimensional Change at 24 hours (µm/cm)	−1.9 to −3	−5 to −8.8
Creep (%)	0.25–0.45	0.05–0.15

(approximate – values vary with each product)

Table 10.3	ANSI/ADA Standard No. 1 for Amalgam
PROPERTY	VALUE
Dimensional change	Maximum of 20 µm/cm
Creep	Maximum of 1%
Compressive strength	Minimum at 1 hr: 80 MPa Minimum at 24 hr: 300 MPa

ANSI/ADA, American National Standards Institute/American Dental Association; MPa (megapascals).

compressive strength as a measure of amalgam quality. See Table 10.3.

Dimensional Change

Ideally, the dimensions of a newly placed amalgam should not change. If amalgam contracts excessively, it will open gaps at the margins, contributing to leakage of fluids and bacteria and causing sensitivity. If it expands excessively, it can put pressure on the cusps and cause pain with biting pressure or may result in fracture of the cusps. Some expansion and contraction occur during the setting reaction of the amalgam. It is the net effect of these two processes that is important. The composition of the alloy particles, the ratio of the mercury to alloy powder by weight, and salivary/moisture contamination are other factors that contribute to dimensional changes. Low-copper amalgams containing zinc are prone to expansion over time if they are exposed to moisture during placement. This gradual expansion after placement is called **delayed expansion** (Fig. 10.2). It is caused by the formation of hydrogen gas resulting from a reaction of zinc and water that causes an outward pressure on the amalgam, causing it to creep. Delayed expansion can cause the restoration to expand beyond the cavity walls, causing cracking in the adjacent enamel. Most high-copper amalgams do not contain zinc or have very small amounts, and therefore delayed expansion is less common. In fact, most present-day amalgams have contracted slightly by the time they set because of smaller alloy particle size and the use of less mercury (see negative numbers for dimensional change in Table 10.2 indicating shrinkage).

Creep

Creep in dental amalgams refers to the gradual change in shape of the restoration from compression by the opposing dentition during chewing or by pressure from

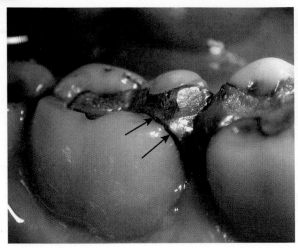

FIG. 10.2 Delayed expansion of amalgam. Margins of the restoration stand up from the tooth. (Courtesy of Dr. Steve Eakle, University of California, San Francisco.)

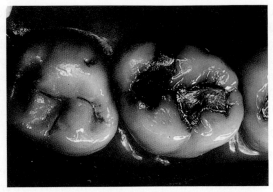

FIG. 10.3 Low-copper amalgam restoration showing surface tarnish, margin deterioration, and corrosion. Tooth has darkened as corrosion products from the amalgam have penetrated the dentinal tubules. (From Bird, DL, Robinson DS: *Modern Dental Assisting*, ed. 11, St. Louis, 2015, Saunders.)

adjacent teeth. It is a phenomenon associated with the gamma-2 phase seen with low-copper alloys (about 6%) and results in deterioration of the margins. High-copper alloys exhibit far less creep (less than 0.5%) and have superior marginal integrity.

Tarnish

Tarnish is an oxidation that attacks the surface of the amalgam and extends slightly below the surface. It results from contact with oxygen, chlorides, and sulfides in the mouth. It causes a dark, dull appearance, but it is not very destructive to the amalgam (Fig. 10.3). The rougher the surface, the more it tends to tarnish. Metals such as palladium are sometimes added to help reduce tarnish. Polishing of the restoration can also reduce tarnish. Polishing of amalgams is best done after the restoration has set for a period of 24 hours or longer. Some clinicians have advocated polishing fast-set amalgams in as little as 20 minutes after placement. However, amalgams polished this soon after placement usually do not achieve a high shine. High-copper amalgams have a smoother surface after carving than low-copper amalgams and tend to tarnish less. Polishing is not as critical to their longevity as with low-copper amalgams. Because of this fact, controversy exists among dental educators and clinicians as to whether high-copper amalgams need polishing if they are well carved and contoured at the time of placement. Generation of excessive heat during polishing can cause a release of mercury from the silver-mercury phase resulting in a mercury-rich surface that will corrode more readily and deteriorate at the margins.

Corrosion

Corrosion can occur from a chemical reaction between the amalgam and substances in saliva or food, resulting in oxidation of the amalgam. It can also occur when two dissimilar metals interact in a solution containing electrolytes (saliva is such a solution). An electrical current is generated between the metals (much like a battery) in a process called *galvanism*. The result of the galvanic reaction is oxidation of one of the metals. This oxidation is responsible for corrosion of the amalgam. Corrosion also takes place within the amalgam through interaction of its metal components. It weakens the amalgam over time, can stain surrounding tooth structure as corrosion products enter the dentinal tubules, and can lead to deterioration of the margins (see Fig. 10.3). The high copper content of newer alloys eliminates the formation of the gamma-2 reaction product that caused weakening of the amalgam. High-copper alloys have virtually replaced low-copper alloys, because high-copper amalgams are more durable, with less deterioration at the margins (better marginal integrity), less corrosion (with less staining of surrounding tooth structure), and higher strength.

Clinically, a galvanic reaction may occur when a newly placed amalgam contacts another metal restoration such as a gold crown. The patient feels a mild electrical shock and may experience a metallic taste. This problem may persist until the amalgam completes its setting reactions, until enough oxides build up on one of the metals to stop the electrical current, or until the offending restoration is replaced with a non-conducting restoration such as composite or with a restoration of a metal similar to the one next to it. Corrosion, however, can occur within an amalgam without the patient ever being aware of the process.

Thermal Conductivity

Amalgam, being a mix of metals, is a good conductor of heat and cold. In shallow cavity preparations the thickness of the dentin remaining over the pulp is usually adequate to dissipate the heat or cold. However, in deeper cavity preparations or in teeth that were sensitive before the placement of the amalgam restoration, a base or liner should be used for the comfort of the patient. Hot coffee or ice cream can produce quite a painful shock to the patient when thermal insulation is not used in these deeper preparations.

APPLICATIONS FOR DENTAL AMALGAM

Amalgam is useful for small to moderate intracoronal restorations in posterior teeth where esthetics is not a concern. These cavity preparations include Class I, II, V, and VI. Amalgams do well in stress-bearing areas. Amalgams are used in large cavity preparations and to replace missing cusps when patients cannot afford crowns and onlays. They are used for foundations (build-ups) for crowns. They are sometimes used to seal a root apex after apical surgery. They are often the material of choice when restoring a cavity where control of saliva and blood is difficult. Amalgams are the least technique sensitive of the direct placement restorative materials.

MATRIX SYSTEMS

A **matrix** for amalgam restorations usually consists of three components: (1) a flexible metal band that is placed around all or part of the tooth to temporarily form a wall that helps contain and shape the amalgam during placement, (2) a device that helps to retain or hold the band in place, and (3) a wooden or plastic wedge that secures the band against the tooth and produces some separation of the two adjacent teeth.

USE OF MATRIX BANDS

A matrix band is used to help contain the amalgam during condensation in a class II preparation and helps to form the proximal contours and contacts of the restoration. Matrix bands are thin strips of material that encompass all (circumferential bands) or part (sectional bands) of the tooth. For amalgam the bands are typically composed of stainless steel. Metal bands are available in thicknesses of 0.001, 0.0015, and 0.002 inch with 0.001 being the thinnest. The bands are made in various heights occlusogingivally (narrow and wide) to accommodate shorter or taller teeth (premolars, adult molars, and primary molars). The universal matrix band will adapt to most posterior teeth, but occasionally on taller teeth or teeth with deep gingival box forms the universal band will be too short to cover the entire cavity preparation. A band with extensions to cover deep mesial and distal box forms (called an extension band or a mesiooccluso-distal [MOD] band) is then selected (Fig. 10.4).

If the metal band is flat as the conventional bands often are, then it must be shaped to form the proper contours of the final restoration. Using a flat band will produce a contact area that does not have full contour. To shape the band place it on a soft paper pad and at the location of the contact area begin rubbing a burnisher against the inner portion of the band until a

smooth convexity is formed on the outside of the band (Fig. 10.5).

This will form the contact area when the amalgam is condensed into the box form of the Class II cavity preparation. Bands that are 0.002 inch in thickness are easier to contour and hold their shape better when placed in the retainer. Bands are also available that are already contoured and need little or no adjustment (Fig. 10.6).

Matrix Band Retainers

Some bands require a retainer to hold the band in place around the tooth which enables the operator to tighten the band around the tooth. The Tofflemire-type retainer (developed by Ben Tofflemire, a graduate of UCSF School of Dentistry) is the most widely used (and has been used for about a century). It comes in two designs, straight or contra-angled. A smaller version is available for use on primary teeth. The contra-angled retainer is useful when the retainer is placed on the lingual side of the teeth instead of the typical buccal placement and on posterior teeth where the straight retainer does not fit well. The retainer has four parts: a U-shaped head that has three slots for positioning the band, a locking vise with a sliding component that holds the band, a long knurled knob that is turned to tighten the diameter of the band, and a short knob that locks the band within the sliding component (Fig. 10.7).

Placing the Band in the Retainer

The band is slightly curved so that when it is folded to form a loop, there will be a larger circumference on one edge and a smaller circumference on the other edge. (See Fig. 10.5) The edge with the smaller circumference is placed toward the gingiva, because most teeth constrict toward the cervical. The edge with the wider

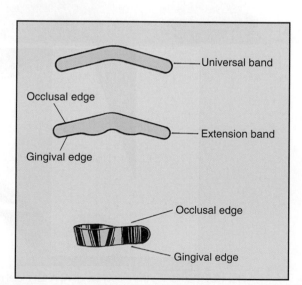

FIG. 10.4 Common types of posterior metal matrix bands for Tofflemire-type retainer. (From Bird DL, Robinson DS: *Modern Dental Assisting*, ed 11, St. Louis, 2015, Elsevier.)

circumference is oriented toward the occlusal side and is placed into the retainer. The ends of the band are placed into the slot of the locking vise, and then the loop of the band is positioned into the slot of the retainer head that orients it toward the tooth with the retainer on the buccal side of the tooth. The small locking knob is turned clockwise to secure the band in the retainer.

Placing the Band on the Tooth

If the band loop has been constricted when putting the band in the retainer, use a mirror handle inside the loop to open it and round it out (Fig. 10.8).

If the diameter of the loop is larger than needed to go around the tooth, then adjust the diameter by tightening the inner knob. Slide the matrix band around the tooth. If it cannot pass through a tight contact area, try placing a wedge to slightly separate the teeth. The gingival edge of the band should be properly oriented and the open end of the retainer head should be positioned toward the gingiva (to allow ease of removal in an occlusal direction). Fully seat the band so that the gingival edge extends at least 0.5

mm beyond the gingival floor of the preparation and the occlusal edge extends approximately 1 mm above the marginal ridge of the adjacent tooth (assuming both teeth had marginal ridges at the same height before the preparation).

If the universal band is short of the gingival floor of the proximal box, then the MOD extension band should be used. If the preparation involves only one proximal surface or only one proximal box is deep, then with scissors cut away the extension of the band that is not needed (i.e., if the distal box is deep but not the mesial, then cut away the mesial extension level with the rest of the band), otherwise that unneeded extension may not let the band seat fully (Fig. 10.9).

While holding the band from the occlusal surface with a finger, tighten the band to the tooth by turning the long knob clockwise until the band is snug to the tooth. Check with an explorer to see that there is no gap at the gingival margin with the band. Next, use a plastic instrument or an interproximal burnisher to burnish the band against the adjacent tooth.

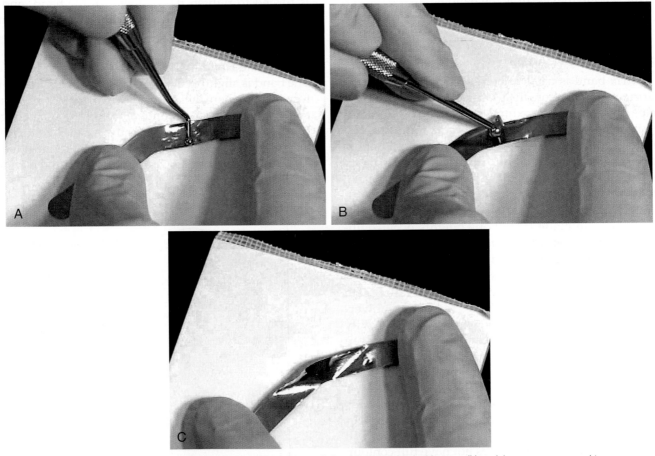

FIG. 10.5 Burnishing the matrix band. **A,** A flat metal matrix band is burnished with a small burnisher on a paper pad to provide proper contours for the contact area. **B,** A football burnisher forms the contours for mesial and distal contact areas. **C,** The band is burnished and ready to use. (Courtesy Aldridge Wilder, DDS from Heymann H, Swift E, Ritter A: *Sturdevant's Art & Science of Operative Dentistry*, ed 6, St. Louis, 2013, Elsevier.)

Criteria for Matrix Band Placement for Class II Preparation

CRITERIA	REASON
1. Band approximately 1 mm above level of the marginal ridge	1. If band is higher, amalgam packed too high at the ridge is likely to fracture when removing the band
2. Band should not be lower than marginal ridge level	2. Amalgam packed over the top of the band will fracture when removing the band. Difficult to establish marginal ridge contours.
3. External surface of band should be convex and establish contact with adjacent contact area.	3. Establishes proper proximal contours and contact
4. Band firmly in contact with the gingival margin of box	4. Prevents overhang at gingival margin
5. Band well adapted at buccal and lingual margings of box.	5. Reduces excess amalgam at buccal and lingual margins and makes carving easier.

The Wedge

The function of the wedge is to adapt the matrix tightly against the gingival margin of the proximal box and to produce some separation of the teeth to compensate for the thickness of the matrix band. Otherwise, when the band is removed there would be a gap between the restoration and the adjacent tooth (called an open contact). Commercially made wedges are often triangular-shaped pieces of wood or plastic. Some clinicians prefer to use wedges made from round toothpicks.

Select a wedge that is large enough to fit the gingival embrasure space and will hold the band against the

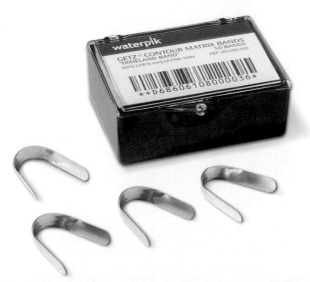

FIG. 10.6 Pre-contoured matrix bands. (Getz Contour Bands, Waterpik.)

gingival margin of the box form without distorting the band (Fig. 10.10).

The wedge is usually inserted firmly into the gingival embrasure from the lingual side, because this is typically the widest of the two embrasures. The wedge must be placed firmly enough to make up

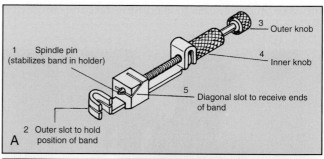

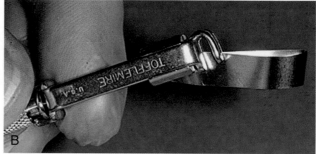

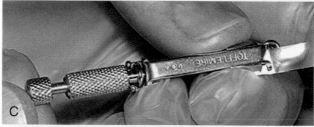

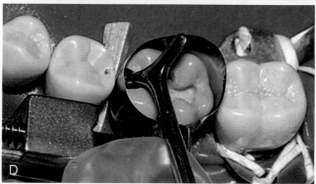

FIG. 10.7 Use of the Tofflemire-type retainer. **A,** Components of the retainer. **B,** Metal band placed in guide slot and diagonal slot. The closed end of the guide slots is oriented toward the occlusal surface of the teeth, and the occlusal edge of the band is inserted first toward the closed end. **C,** Tighten locking nut to secure band in the retainer. **D,** Note that band has been angled through the left guide slot to be positioned on the buccal surface of the tooth. The band is tightened around the tooth by turning the inner knob clockwise. A wedge is inserted firmly into the lingual embrasure to create separation of the teeth and hold the band against the tooth gingivally. (**A,** From Bird DL, Robinson DS: *Modern Dental Assisting,* ed. 11, St. Louis, 2015, Elsevier. **B,** From Darby ML, Walsh MM: *Dental Hygiene: Theory and Practice,* ed. 4, St. Louis, 2015, Elsevier. **C,** From Darby ML, Walsh MM: *Dental Hygiene: Theory and Practice,* ed. 3, St. Louis, 2010, Elsevier.)

for the thickness of the matrix band. If a circumferential band (encircles the tooth) is used, there are two thickness of matrix band (mesial and distal) to compensate for. So, the wedging pressure must be greater than when a sectional band (goes only on one proximal surface) is used (see Chapter 6 for sectional matrix systems). Some manufactured wedges are concave on their sides to accommodate the convexity of the tooth (e.g., Wedge Wands or G-Wedges by Garrison Dental. See Chapter 6, Figure 6.14). If the cavity preparation includes both mesial and distal proximal boxes, then a wedge will be needed for each embrasure.

Once the wedge is in place, loosen the retainer by turning it counterclockwise one quarter turn. This

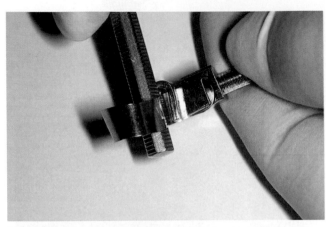

FIG. 10.8 Opening and rounding a constricted matrix band loop. (From Bird DL, Robinson DS: *Modern Dental Assisting*, ed 11, St. Louis, 2015, Elsevier.)

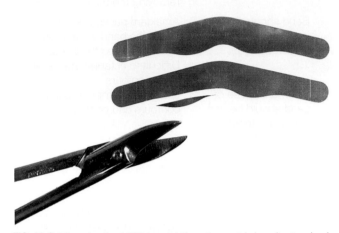

FIG. 10.9 Trimming the MOD band. When the matrix band extension is needed only on one proximal surface, the other extension is removed to allow full seating of the band. (From Heymann H, Swift E, Ritter A: *Sturdevant's Art & Science of Operative Dentistry*, ed 6, St. Louis, 2013, Elsevier.)

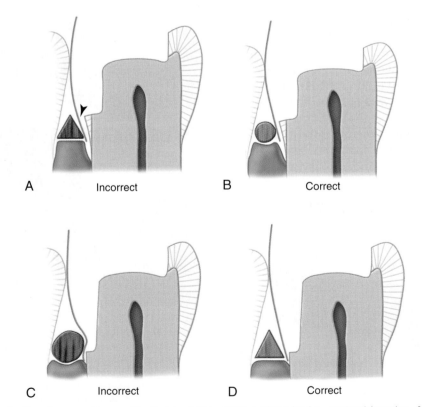

A   Incorrect   B   Correct

C   Incorrect   D   Correct

FIG. 10.10 Indications for use of a round toothpick wedge versus a triangular (i.e., anatomic) wedge. **A,** Often the triangular wedge does not firmly support the matrix band against the gingival margin in conservative Class II preparations *(arrowhead).* **B,** The round toothpick wedge is preferred for these preparations because its wedging action is nearer the gingival margin. **C,** In Class II preparations with deep gingival margins, the round toothpick wedge crimps the matrix band contour if it is placed occlusal to the gingival margin. **D,** The triangular wedge is preferred with these preparations because its greatest width is at its base. (From Heymann H, Swift E, Ritter A: *Sturdevant's Art & Science of Operative Dentistry*, ed 6, St. Louis, 2013, Elsevier.)

will loosen the band slightly so it can be adapted to the adjacent contact area and will allow the condensed amalgam to push the band against the adjacent contact. Once the band is loosened, burnish it against the adjacent tooth with an interproximal burnisher or the back of a large spoon excavator.

Atypical Wedge Placement

The wedge may have to be placed in an unconventional way depending on a number of factors:

1. On occasion, the shape of the wedge is not compatible with the convex shape of the tooth. In this case, the wedge can be custom-shaped by carving it with an amalgam knife or a scalpel.
2. If the wedge sits too high in the embrasure space, it may distort the matrix band, fail to seal the gingival margin, and cause concave proximal contours in the gingival aspect of the restoration (Fig. 10.11).
3. If the embrasure space is very large because the gingival tissue has receded, it will be difficult to secure the band against the gingival margin of the proximal box with a single wedge because it will be apical to the gingival margin. It may be necessary to place a second, smaller wedge on top of the first wedge.
4. If the cavity preparation has resulted in a very wide proximal box (from facial to lingual), it may be necessary to place two wedges, one from the facial and one from the lingual, in order to ensure that the two gingival corners of the proximal box are sealed.

The presence of a rubber dam may make wedge insertion more difficult as it tends to push the wedge back out. To lessen this problem, stretch the interseptal rubber dam in the opposite direction of wedge placement while inserting the wedge. After the wedge is fully seated, gently release the dam.

Criteria for Wedge Placement for Class II Preparation

CRITERIA	REASON
1. Wedge firmly seated	1. To separate teeth enough to make up for thickness of band
2. Wedge holds matrix band against gingival margin of proximal box	2. Prevents amalgam overhang
3. Wedge is not located coronal to the gingival margin of proximal box	3. Prevents amalgam from escaping under the band to create an overhang
4. Wedge is not located too far apical to gingival margin of proximal box	4. Prevents overhang
5. Wedge does not deform the band contours	5. Allows proper anatomic proximal contours

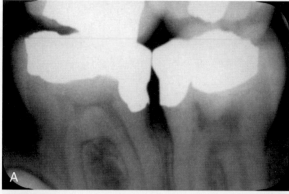

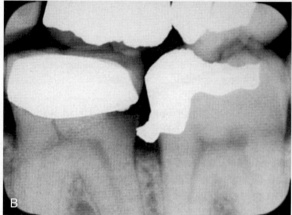

FIG. 10.11 Radiographs depicting poor proximal contours of the amalgams: **A,** caused by a wedge place too far coronal to the gingival margin of the cavity preparation that distorted the matrix band; **B,** overhang of amalgam caused by a wedge that was not firmly placed, was placed slightly above the gingival margin, or the band did not cover the deep gingival margin. (Courtesy Dentaljuce CPD Providers Ltd, https://www.dentaljuce.com/direct-restorations-wedges.)

Pre-Wedging

Some clinicians prefer to place a wedge interproximally before starting to cut the proximal box of a Class II cavity preparation. The wedge separates the approximating teeth slightly to allow preparation of the box form with less risk of damaging the adjacent proximal surface. It also provides some protection of the interseptal gingiva. There is a commercially available product called the Fender Wedge (Garrison Dental Solutions) that has a protective metal sheet that extends from the wedge occlusally to protect the adjacent tooth during preparation of the proximal box (Fig. 10.12).

Final Evaluation of the Matrix before Condensation

Once the matrix band has been placed around the prepared tooth, the retainer appropriately tightened and the wedge snugly pressed into place, a final check is made of the matrix assembly before the preparation is filled with amalgam. Check for the following features (see Fig. 10.13):

1. The matrix band extends apical to the gingival margin of the proximal box by about 1 mm.

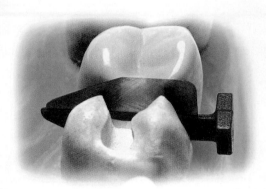

Fig. 10.12 Wedge with a metal shield attached that acts to protect the proximal surface of the adjacent tooth during cavity preparation. (Fender Wedge, courtesy of Garrison Dental Solutions.)

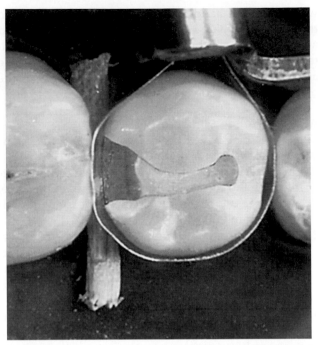

FIG. 10.13 Properly placed and wedged matrix band for Class II cavity preparation. The gingival margin is sealed with the band and wedge and the band is adapted to the adjacent tooth. (From Heymann H, Swift E, Ritter A: *Sturdevant's Art & Science of Operative Dentistry*, ed 6, St. Louis, 2013, Elsevier.)

2. There is no gap between the band and the gingival margin of the box form.
3. There is no gingival tissue or rubber dam caught between the band and the tooth.
4. The top edge of the band extends beyond the adjacent marginal ridge by approximately 1 mm.
5. The wedge is firmly in place, so that it will produce some separation of the teeth.
6. The band is well adapted to the buccal and lingual walls of the proximal box.
7. The band is adapted to the adjacent tooth.
8. The wedge has not distorted the convexity of the band in the cervical area.
9. The band is stable so that it will not move around during placement and condensation of the amalgam.

See Procedure 10.1 at chapter end for placement and carving of Class II amalgam.

Retainerless Matrix Systems

Some matrix systems do not require a retainer. The AutoMatrix (Dentsply) and ReelMatrix (Garrison Dental) have a band formed into a circle with a coil-like loop at the end. A special tool is used to wind the coil and tighten the band (Fig. 10.14). Other bands include the copper T-band (Fig. 10.15) used in pediatric dentistry and custom spot welded bands that are formed to the teeth, then removed and spot welded to retain the loop.

SECTIONAL MATRIX SYSTEMS

Some systems use bands that do not go entirely around the tooth. These are called *sectional bands*. They are typically used with composite resin restorations but can be used for class II or III (distal of canines) amalgam preparations, particularly where only one proximal surface has been prepared (mesio-occlusal or distocclusal). A wedge is placed just as with all of the other matrix systems. A pressure ring is applied that holds the band in place and produces

some separation of the teeth to make up for the thickness of the matrix band to ensure a snug contact (see Figure 6.15, Chapter 6 [Composites, Glass Ionomers, and Compomers]). When using a sectional band with a pressure ring, be sure to check the contact with floss right after removing the matrix band. If the contact is too tight, insert a wedge snugly and pass floss through the contact several times to loosen the tight contact.

HANDLING CHARACTERISTICS OF HIGH-COPPER ALLOYS

High-copper alloys are mostly admix or spherical types (see Table 10.4 for a comparison of admix and spherical alloys). Spherical particles have a smaller surface area with which the mercury can react. Therefore they need approximately 10% less mercury for the amalgamation process. Freshly mixed spherical amalgam has very little resistance to condensation into the cavity preparation and feels soft compared with an admixed amalgam. Spherical amalgams do not displace a matrix band and force it into contact with the adjacent tooth in class II preparations as well as admixed amalgams. Therefore spherical amalgams may require a bit more physical separation of the teeth with the wedge in order to establish a good proximal contact after the matrix band has been removed. Spherical amalgams have higher 1-hour and 24-hour compressive strengths than admixed amalgams. Newly placed spherical amalgams have slightly more shrinkage than admixed amalgams. At 24 hours, both

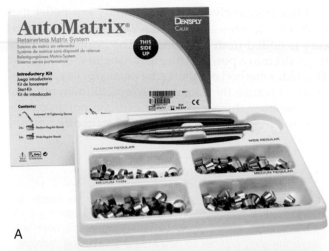

A

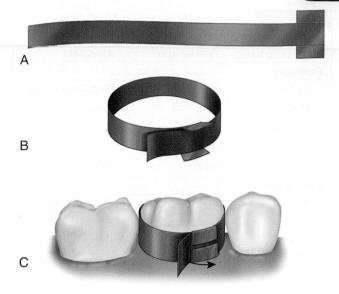

A

B

C

FIG. 10.15 Copper T-band used for primary molars. **A,** T-band **B,** T-band prepared for placement. **C,** T-band positioned around the tooth and tightened by folding the flaps. (Copyright Elsevier Collection.)

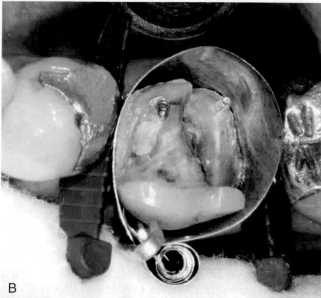

B

FIG. 10.14 Retainerless matrix systems use a tool to tighten the matrix band into a coil. **A,** Automatrix Kit (Courtesy of Dentsply Caulk). **B,** Coil is tightened with tool to tighten it against the tooth (Automatrix band). (**B,** Courtesy Dentaljuce CPD Providers Ltd, https://www.dentaljuce.com/direct-restorations-wedges.)

Table **10.4**	High-Copper Amalgams: Admix and Spherical	
ADMIX	**SPHERICAL**
Needs greater condensation pressure	Needs less condensation pressure
Adapts readily to cavity preparation	Requires both vertical and lateral condensation
Establishes contact readily	Requires heavier wedging to establish contact
Medium early strength	High early strength
Needs more mercury	Needs 10% less mercury
Longer working time	Faster set

MANIPULATION OF AMALGAM

(See Procedure 10.1.)

Selection of Alloy

Because most of the modern dental alloys are high-copper, the dentist selects the dental alloy based on personal preference for its handling characteristics (see Table 10.5 for commercially available alloys and their particle types). There are variations among the commercially available alloys in working and setting times, resistance to condensation pressures, and resistance to carving pressures. Admix amalgam generally has a longer working time than spherical amalgam. So, if the clinician is doing a large multi-surface amalgam and needs more time to place and carve the amalgam, an admix alloy may be selected. Some alloys are specifically manufactured to be fast setting, and these alloys may be selected when the clinician needs early strength in the restoration. High-copper alloys are selected because they have superior properties.

DISPENSING OF ALLOY AND MERCURY

Amalgam must be handled properly from the start through the entire placement process if a restoration is to be successful. The preferred dispensing of alloy powder and mercury is done in commercially prepared capsules that contain factory-measured amounts of alloy and mercury separated from each other by a plastic membrane. The manufacturers determine the optimal ratio of alloy and mercury for their products based on testing of materials for their best properties.

admixed and spherical high-copper amalgams shrink slightly.

Table 10.5	Common High-Copper Amalgams	
MANUFACTURER AND BRAND NAME	**TYPE OF ALLOY**	**SET SPEEDS AVAILABLE**
Dentsply		
Dispersalloy	Admix	Regular and Fast
Megalloy EZ	Spherical	Regular
Ivoclar Vivadent		
Valiant	Spherical	Regular
Valiant Ph.D.	Admix	Regular
Kerr Dental		
Contour	Admix	Regular and Fast
Tytin	Spherical	Slow and Regular
Tytin FC	Spherical	Regular and Fast

Usually capsules are available with different quantities of materials depending on the size of the restoration. They are offered as single mix (also called *one spill*, containing 400 mg of alloy), double mix (two spill, 600 mg), triple mix (three spill, 800 mg) or more, depending on the manufacturer, and capsules are color-coded to indicate the quantity. With large preparations, several capsules may be needed.

MATRIX APPLICATION

Some cavity preparations will require the use of a matrix system to contain and shape the amalgam, particularly when all or a part of one or more walls of the tooth are missing. The operator will select a matrix system (with retainer or retainerless) well suited for the clinical situation. A sectional or circumferential matrix band will be adapted to the tooth and wedges will be placed as needed to seal the cervical area and create separation of the teeth. If a matrix is needed, it should be applied prior to triturating the amalgam.

TRITURATION

(See Procedure 10.1). The powder and mercury are mixed together in a mechanical device called a **triturator** (or **amalgamator**). The triturator has settings that allow adjustment in the speed and time of the mixing process. The manufacturer's recommendations for the selected material should be followed. Some capsules require activation before trituration to break the membrane and allow the powder and mercury to mix. Other capsules are self-activating meaning the membrane ruptures with the forces created by rapid movement of the triturator. Some capsules have a small plastic or metal rod called a *pestle* inside to aid in the mixing. A capsule is placed in the retaining arms of the triturator (see Procedure 10.1, Fig. 10.24), the proper settings of time and speed are made, and the device is activated. The retaining arms move back and forth rapidly to mix the powder and mercury, much like an automatic paint mixer.

A less frequently used form of alloy is a pellet that is placed into a reusable capsule with a pestle and mercury is added from a dispenser. The pestle pulverizes the pellet into a powder during mixing in the triturator. This older method of mixing the amalgam has declined in use, because the capsules often leak mercury into the operatory during mixing, mixes are not as consistent, and the dispenser is a potential source of mercury spills.

> ### 💡 Clinical Tip
>
> Do not activate the capsule before you are ready to begin mixing it. Activating the capsule and placing it in the triturator before completing the cavity preparation will allow the alloy powder to be partially wet by the mercury. When the mix is actually triturated a few minutes later, some of the reaction will have already started. The resulting amalgam will not have optimal properties and may have reduced working time. Self-activating capsules avoid this potential problem.

Expansion, contraction, creep, and corrosion can be caused by improper manipulation, moisture contamination, overtrituration, and undertrituration. Undertriturated alloy has a dry, crumbly appearance, sets too quickly, and does not condense well. It results in a weaker restoration, because the components have not totally mixed, leaving a higher level of unreacted mercury and alloy particles. On the other hand, overtriturated alloy is too wet and has low resistance to condensation. It also results in an amalgam that sets too quickly because of the heat produced by prolonged mixing. It results in a weaker restoration that will corrode more readily, because it forms too many reaction products (silver-mercury and copper-tin). Properly triturated alloy has a satin appearance (Fig. 10.16) and produces the desired physical properties and resistance to condensation.

WORKING AND SETTING TIMES

After the amalgam has been mixed a certain amount of time is needed to place, condense, and carve the amalgam before it begins to harden. This time is called the working time. After the working time has been exceeded the amalgam cannot be condensed or carved without causing problems in the material. Alloys are commercially available in fast, regular, and slow set forms. The amount of working time selected is by operator preference. A slower set material may be desired if a very large restoration needs to be done and more time is needed to place and condense the material.

The setting time has two components: the initial setting time and the final setting time. The initial setting time is the time at which the amalgam reaches a predefined firmness in the setting process. Usually, this is

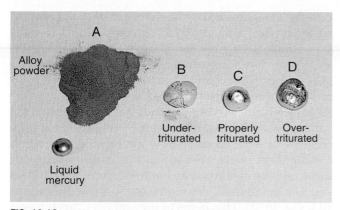

FIG. 10.16 **A,** Alloy powder and mercury. **B,** Undertriturated amalgam is dry and crumbly. **C,** Properly triturated amalgam has a satin-like appearance. **D,** Overtriturated amalgam appears too wet.

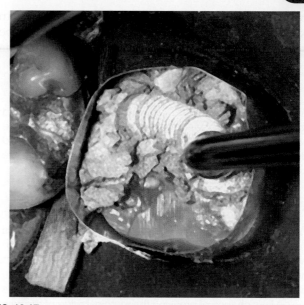

FIG. 10.17 Amalgam is condensed with overlapping steps of the condenser to avoid voids within the amalgam that might weaken it. (Courtesy of David Graham, University of California School of Dentistry [San Francisco, CA].)

the time when the restoration can no longer be carved and the occlusion can be checked and adjusted without damaging the amalgam. The final setting time is the time when the setting reaction has been completed. The final set usually occurs 12 to 24 hours after trituration depending on the type of alloy used.

PLACEMENT AND CONDENSATION
(See Procedure 10.1.)

Amalgam Placement
After mixing, the amalgam is removed from the capsule and placed into an amalgam well or the small end of a Dappen dish. The pestle (if one is present) and the plastic membrane are removed from the mixed amalgam. The amalgam is picked up in increments from the well by an amalgam carrier and is placed by the assistant into the cavity preparation (see Procedure 10.1, Figs. 10.25 and 10.26).

Condensation
The main objectives of **condensation** are to reduce the porosity in the amalgam and to adapt the amalgam to the walls of the cavity preparation. Amalgam condensers are used to carefully work the amalgam into all of the corners and retentive areas of the preparation, using vertical and lateral condensation. Condensers should be carefully stepped around the preparation in vertical overlapping steps to prevent voids in the material (Fig. 10.17), and lateral condensation is used to adapt the material closely to the walls of the preparation. Voids in the amalgam will produce a weaker restoration. Amalgam that is poorly adapted to the walls of the preparation may allow microleakage and cause post-placement sensitivity.

Condensation should occur in a well-isolated, clean, dry preparation. A well placed rubber dam is the ideal method of isolation. Amalgam is the most forgiving of the direct restorative materials in the presence of saliva and blood, but will have its properties diminished none-the-less.

Spherical amalgams have less resistance to condensation pressures and require the use of larger condensers, whereas admix amalgams require more pressure to condense and typically condensation is started with smaller condensers progressing to larger ones. The cavity preparation is slightly overfilled to allow enough material to carve to contours and to remove excess mercury that has been forced to the surface during the condensation process. If excess mercury is left, physical and mechanical properties will be poorer.

 Clinical Tip

When filling a large, complex cavity preparation or crown buildup with amalgam, the slower, novice operator should choose an amalgam alloy that will provide additional working time (such as an admix alloy like Dispersalloy [Dentsply]). If the earlier increments of amalgam begin to set before the large restoration or buildup is completed, the later increments may not adequately join to them and parts of the amalgam may fall away as the matrix band is removed.

 Caution

Ultrasonic condensation devices used on amalgam can produce unsafe mercury vapor levels in the dental office.

When a large cavity preparation is restored, several capsules of the mixed amalgam might be needed. If placement of the newly mixed amalgam is too slow and the material placed in the cavity preparation starts to get firm, then additional mixes of the material added on top might not join with the firm material. This could result in a weak restoration that will separate under chewing forces at that non-joined interface. Careful coordination and timing of mixing and placement between the dental assistant and the operator are crucial to a successful restoration.

Clinical Tip

Amalgam should be placed as soon as it is mixed. If allowed to stand for a couple of minutes, the amalgam will be weaker because crystals that are forming will be disrupted during condensation. The amalgam will feel drier and more crumbly. Discard this mix and make a new one.

Clinical Tip

When removing the matrix band from a newly placed class II amalgam, hold the marginal ridge of the amalgam down with a large condenser to prevent the amalgam ridge from breaking. If the wedge is left in place while removing the band, some separation of the teeth will remain and there will be less chance of breaking the marginal ridge of the new amalgam when the band is removed.

BURNISHING AND CARVING

(See Procedure 10.1.)

Burnishing

Burnishing is a controversial procedure for amalgam. Some feel that burnishing brings excess to mercury to the surface where it can be carved away. Others do not burnish, because they feel that burnishing may damage the amalgam at the margins. Of those clinicians who burnish their amalgams, some burnish just before carving and others burnish gently after carving to produce a smooth, dense surface.

When clinicians burnish the amalgam before they begin carving, they use a large burnisher to further condense the amalgam with pressure in the faciolingual and mesiodistal directions (see Procedure 10.1, Fig. 10.27). Burnishing before carving produces a much smoother and denser surface.

Carving

After the amalgam has been burnished, a carver (the cleoid end of a discoid/cleoid carver is useful) is used with a light touch to remove the gross excess of amalgam on the occlusal surface without touching the cavosurface margins. As the amalgam gradually becomes firmer, begin carving the occlusal anatomy and shaping the proximal surfaces. Remove all excess at the margins on the proximal surface with a suitable carver (such as a half-Hollenback) before completing the occlusal anatomy. Access to the proximal surfaces is more difficult, so these areas should be completed before the amalgam sets. Once the amalgam is hard, attempts at carving may damage the amalgam margins or cause fracture of portions of the amalgam mass. The time the amalgam takes to harden can vary depending on the type of amalgam and its composition. In general, admix amalgams set more slowly than spherical amalgams, but some amalgams are formulated to be fast-setting and can set in 2 to 3 minutes versus 5 to 10 minutes for regular set amalgams.

A variety of carving instruments can be used for various parts of the restoration—occlusal, proximal, and cervical—based on operator preference. In general, carving instruments are used so that part of the instrument rests on the adjacent tooth structure for support and as a guide to follow tooth contours (see Procedure 10.1, Fig. 10.31). This helps to prevent over carving and exposure of the cavosurface margin of the preparation. After carving the amalgam surface can be smoothed further by gently rubbing the surface with a damp cotton pellet.

CHECKING THE OCCLUSION

After the restoration is carved to restore tooth contours, the occlusion should be checked. If the amalgam forming the a marginal ridge is too high, then the patient could bite too hard and break the amalgam. To avoid this mishap, first check to see that the marginal ridge of the amalgam is about the same height as the marginal ridge of the adjacent tooth and then instruct the patient to close very lightly at first on the articulating paper. After the amalgam has been completed, the patient should be instructed to avoid chewing on the newly placed amalgam until the next day (most amalgams will gain about 80% of their strength by 8 hours). The ADA Standard No. 1 requires a minimum compressive strength of 80 MPa at 1 hour (see Table 10.3).

Caution

In general, the height of the marginal ridge of the newly placed class II amalgam should be at the level of the adjacent marginal ridge. If it is much higher, it should be reduced *before* the occlusion is checked. Otherwise, the ridge might fracture when the patient bites down on the articulating paper. Remember, the patient might still be numb and cannot tell how hard he/she is biting.

FINISHING AND POLISHING

Finishing and polishing (see Chapter 13 [Abrasion, Finishing, and Polishing]) is best done 24 hours or more after the initial placement to allow crystallization within the amalgam to go to completion. The purpose of finishing is to make the amalgam flush with the cavosurface margins of the tooth, adjust the contours, and eliminate roughness. It is usually accomplished with multi-fluted finishing burs or fine abrasive disks. Polishing further smoothes the surface and creates a high shine (see Procedure 10.1, Fig. 10.32, tooth #29). Many clinicians do not finish and polish their amalgam restorations, because (1) it requires a second visit,

(2) modern amalgams are smoother after carving, and (3) high-copper amalgams have low tarnish and corrosion. Although not ideal, some clinicians choose to finish and polish at the time of placement. With their high early strength, spherical amalgams can be lightly polished after their initial set. Polishing should be done using a water coolant and a light touch to avoid generating heat that can potentially irritate the pulp and bring mercury to the surface. Typically, polishing agents such as silex or a slurry mix of fine pumice or abrasive-impregnated rubber polishers are used. When amalgam is polished early (after the initial set) a smooth satin surface is produced but a high shine cannot be achieved.

Advantages and Disadvantages of Amalgam

ADVANTAGES	DISADVANTAGES
Can withstand high chewing forces	Not an esthetic material
Biocompatible	May require more tooth structure removal to retain the restoration
Useful when isolation is difficult	Cannot chew on it immediately after placement
Easy to manipulate	Possible temperature sensitivity after placement
Very durable and wear resistant	Possible galvanic reaction with other metals in the mouth
Relatively inexpensive	Requires mercury hygiene measures with scrap material
Alternative for cusp replacement when patient cannot afford a crown	Fills the cavity preparation but does not support the surrounding walls like a bonded composite or ceramic restoration
Strongest direct placement material for crown buildups (cores)	Cannot be used for buildup with all-ceramic restorations (gray color shows through)

> **💡 Clinical Tip**
>
> Care should be taken when polishing amalgam to avoid generating heat. Heat greater than 60 °C (140 °F) causes mercury to come to the surface of the restoration, weakening the surface and margins; and pulpal irritation can occur. Do not polish dry. Use low speed and a light touch, particularly with abrasive rubber points and cups.

USE OF A CAVITY SEALER

For many years a copal resin varnish (e.g., Copalite, Temrex Corporation) was routinely placed in the cavity preparation before the amalgam was inserted (Fig. 10.18). The purpose of the varnish was to prevent microleakage at the amalgam margins and thereby, reduce sensitivity. The copal resin tended to wash out with time. Corrosion products at the

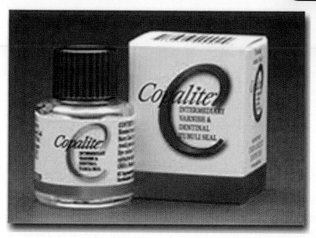

FIG. 10.18 Copal resin varnish for cavity sealing (Copalite, Temrex Corporation.)

interface of the amalgam and the preparation over time greatly reduced the microleakage. With low-copper amalgams corrosion occurred relatively quickly as the varnish began to disappear. However, with the introduction of high-copper amalgam, corrosion was greatly reduced and the amalgam shrank as it set. So, as the copal resin washed out, microleakage and resulting post-operative sensitivity was often seen. Some clinicians lined the dentin with calcium hydroxide (a popular commercial preparation was Dycal by Dentsply Sirona) to cover exposed dentin and act as a thermal insulator under the amalgam. Studies showed that calcium hydroxide also washed out over time (Fig. 10.19). Currently, many clinicians use bonding agents as sealers at the margins and over exposed dentin. These materials tend to hold up better over time than cavity varnish, and they can actually seal the dentinal tubules while cavity varnish merely placed a temporary cover over the tubules.

Bases and liners are used less frequently under amalgam then in the past, because the need for their use on a routine basis has not been established. They are applied mostly in deeper cavity preparations for thermal insulation and pulpal protection.

LONGEVITY OF AMALGAMS

High-copper amalgams in use today last longer than low-copper amalgams due to their superior physical and mechanical properties. High-copper amalgams are stronger, corrode less, creep less, and have better marginal integrity. Although there are many factors that go into how long amalgams last, the typical survival rate ranges from 7 to 15 years. However, some amalgams have been documented to last as long as 40 to 50 years, whereas some fail in just a few years. Amalgams in conservative cavity preparations last

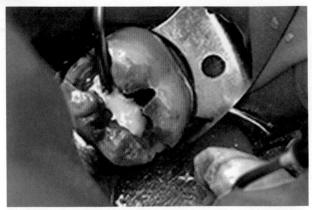

FIG. 10.19 Calcium hydroxide cavity liner for pulpal protection (Dycal, Dentsply Sirona) (From Dentistry Today: New Options for Restoring a Deep Carious Lesion. Category: Dental Materials Created: Monday, 18 March 2013 13:56 Written by Robert E. Rada, DDS, MBA.)

Why Amalgams Fail

Reasons for Amalgam Failure

Poor Case Selection	Not a good place to use amalgam
Improper Cavity Design	Too deep, too shallow, inadequate extensions of the preparation, improper isthmus width, inadequate retention, cavosurface margins not 90 degrees
Improper Manipulation	Overtrituration or undertrituration
Poor Placement	Improper condensation leaving voids or porosity, using a mix that is too dry or wet
Improper Carving	Too deep or too shallow, poor carving or finishing of margins leaving gross overhangs
Inadequate Isolation	Contamination of the cavity preparation by blood and saliva
Improper Use of Matrix	Poor matrix selection, careless matrix placement and removal, poor contouring and wedging
Other Factors	Too much force placed on the new restoration before it has gained full strength causing fracture, a restoration that is too high in occlusion, poor oral hygiene leading to recurrent caries

longer than those in larger preparations. Conservative Class I amalgams last about 15-18 years and conservative Class II amalgams last about 12-15 years. The accompanying box lists some of the reasons that amalgams fail.

Clinically, an amalgam restoration needs to be replaced when it is no longer functional. Meaning, you can no longer chew on it, it is loose, part of it has fallen out, or part of the tooth has fractured away from the amalgam. Other reasons include defective margins, recurrent caries, voids or cracks in the amalgam, gross overhangs causing damage to the periodontium, or poor contours or contacts causing food impaction.

Many of the reasons for failure of the amalgam are caused by operator error such as poor case selection (not a good place to use amalgam), improper cavity design (too deep, too shallow, inadequate extensions of the preparation, improper isthmus width, inadequate retention) or improper manipulation (over- or undertrituration), placement (improper condensation or using a mix that is too dry or wet), and carving (too deep or too shallow) of the amalgam. Contamination of the cavity preparation by blood and saliva by inadequate isolation is another factor in failure of the restoration. Poor matrix selection, careless placement or removal, poor contouring, and wedging can all contribute to amalgam failure. Other factors are too much force placed on the new restoration before it has gained its full strength or a restoration that is too high in the occlusion.

Occasionally after placement a new amalgam may have post-operative sensitivity or pain. Some of the reasons for this are: inadequate cooling of the tooth during preparation, leaking margins, incomplete caries removal, hyperocclusion, cracked tooth, or galvanism.

REPAIR OF AMALGAM
Using Amalgam

At times part of a large amalgam may fracture or have a relatively minor defect. A decision involving the patient's informed consent may be made to repair the existing amalgam rather than replace it. To repair the amalgam a retentive preparation (possibly using mechanical interlocks, undercuts, grooves, and troughs) needs to be made in the existing amalgam and possibly the surrounding tooth structure. The prepared surfaces need to be rough but free of any cutting debris, blood, or saliva. Fresh amalgam is then condensed into the preparation against the roughened amalgam walls. The repair will not have the strength of unrepaired amalgam but if not under excessive occlusal loading may serve the patient well for a number of years.

Using Flowable Composite

On occasion, a gap might form in an amalgam at an accessible margin but the amalgam is otherwise serviceable. To close the gap and extend the life of the amalgam the margin could be repaired by the use of bonded flowable composite. Any debris is removed from the gap and the absence of decay is confirmed. Acid etchant is placed on the gap between the amalgam and tooth for 10 to 20 seconds, rinsed, and dried. A bonding agent is applied and cured followed by the application of flowable composite to the gap. An explorer or fine brush is used to work the composite into the gap and displace entrapped air; then the composite is light cured. This process reseals the margin to prevent leakage and recurrent caries at that site. Although repairing the amalgam is not ideal, it can often extend the life of the existing amalgam, conserving tooth structure and reducing expense to the patient.

BONDING AMALGAM

Amalgam is retained in the cavity preparation by parallel walls or undercut walls and by its adaptation to irregularities in the tooth created during preparation. Amalgam placed in this manner simply occupies the space of the cavity preparation; it is not bonded to and does not support the surrounding walls. Low-copper amalgam expands slightly as it sets and forms corrosion products at the tooth-amalgam interface as it ages. The expansion and corrosion help to reduce microleakage at the tooth-amalgam interface. High-copper amalgams shrink slightly during setting and form corrosion products more slowly and to a lesser degree. They tend to have more microleakage initially, which in some cases can result in transient tooth sensitivity.

Bonding of amalgam was popular in the 1990s, but mixed research results have cast a shadow on its usefulness. This technique uses bonding methods similar to those used with composite resin. After etching and application of bonding agent, a dual-cure bonding resin is applied to the cavity preparation and while it is still wet the amalgam is placed. The wet resin mechanically intermixes with the amalgam during condensation, and when the resin sets, it mechanically locks the amalgam in place and the resin bonds to the tooth. The resin along the margins of the restoration creates a seal, reducing microleakage. There is some concern that the resin bond will hydrolyze over time and lose its effectiveness.

ALLERGY TO AMALGAM

Allergy to components of amalgam is very uncommon occurring in less than 1% of patients. A local hypersensitivity reaction is most typically encountered; more severe reactions with swelling, difficulty breathing, and anaphylaxis are extremely rare. Local contact dermatitis is usually seen as red or combined red and white lesions (resembling lichen planus and thus called lichenoid lesions) of the buccal mucosa (Fig. 10.20) or lateral border of the tongue in close proximity to the amalgam. On occasion, the gingiva surrounding a cervical amalgam may be affected as well. Usually, replacement of the amalgam restoration with an alternative material (such as composite, ceramic, or gold) will usually resolve the problem.

MERCURY SAFETY PROCEDURES

Mercury is a toxic metal, but the elemental mercury used in amalgam is less toxic than organic mercury (methylmercury) that can end up in the food chain, especially in seafood and can be absorbed through the digestive tract.

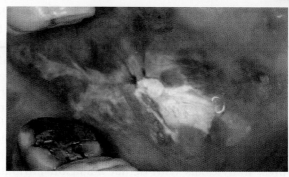

FIG. 10.20 Inflammatory response of the buccal mucosa (lichenoid lesion) to contact with an amalgam restoration in a sensitive patient. (From https://www.proprofs.com/flashcards/cardshowall.php?title=oral-path-exam-3).

Mercury is the only metal that is in a liquid state at room temperature. Elemental mercury can pass through the gastrointestinal tract without being absorbed. It is mercury vapor that is of greatest health concern as it is absorbed by the lungs. Exposure to mercury vapor occurs during placement or removal. Low levels of mercury vapor are released from the set amalgam under function (eating) or bruxing. Mercury can accumulate over time in certain body tissues such as the brain and kidneys. Low level exposure creates no demonstrable problems. However, higher levels such as those experienced by workers who are exposed to the vapors at their jobs may experience signs and symptoms. These include headaches, irritability, fatigue, memory loss, or neurological signs.

Concerns about the safety of amalgam and the mercury it contains should be considered from three aspects:

a. Safety of the patient
b. Safety of the dental staff
c. Safety of the environment

ADA STANCE ON DENTAL AMALGAM SAFETY

The amount of mercury that is released from a set amalgam is very small and has not been shown to be dangerous to patients. The amount of mercury released in vapor form from amalgam is about 1 to 2 micrograms (µg)/day, but the total exposure to the patient will depend on a number of factors, including the number and type of amalgam restorations and their size, frequency of chewing, and whether or not the patient grinds their teeth. The ADA has addressed health concerns about mercury in amalgam (see the ADA Council on Scientific Affairs [CSA] Statement on Dental Amalgam and the CSA Amalgam Safety Update, both of which can be accessed at the ADA website, www.ada.org), as has the FDA (see their Update/Review of Potential Adverse Health Risks Associated with Exposure to Mercury in Dental Amalgam, which can be accessed at www.fda.gov).

In 2004 a review of the scientific literature was conducted by the Life Sciences Research Office and funded by the National Institute of Dental and Craniofacial Research (National Institutes of Health) and the Center for Devices and Radiological Health (a branch of the FDA). Their report states that "The current data are insufficient to support an association between mercury release from dental amalgam and the various complaints that have been attributed to this restoration material. These complaints are broad and nonspecific compared to the well-defined set of effects that have been documented for occupational and accidental elemental mercury exposures. Individuals with dental amalgam–attributed complaints had neither elevated urinary mercury nor increased prevalence of hypersensitivity to dental amalgam or mercury when compared with controls."

CONCERNS ABOUT THE SAFETY OF AMALGAM

Safety for patients

Prudent oral health providers should limit the exposure of patients to mercury. Mercury can enter the body through ingestion, through direct contact with the skin, and by inhalation of the vapor. Care should be taken when placing or removing amalgam restorations to prevent swallowing of amalgam particles or inhalation of mercury vapor. However, the mercury in swallowed particles is not absorbed well and typically excreted. Use of the rubber dam and high-volume evacuation will aid in minimizing both.

Mercury in the bloodstream of pregnant mothers can pass through the placental barrier to reach the developing fetus. It can also be passed in breast milk to nursing infants. The developing nervous system may be more sensitive to the mercury vapor. There is very little research or clinical data on the long-term effects of mercury exposure to developing fetuses or young children. Therefore, in order to be prudent many countries throughout the world have banned the use of amalgam in pregnant women or young children.

Safety for office staff

In some dental offices, dentists and their staff have been found to have higher levels of mercury than the population in general. Precautions should be taken in the dental office to limit the exposure to the dental team. The Occupational Safety and Health Administration (OSHA) has set an acceptable level of exposure to mercury at 0.05 mg/m^3 for a 40-hour workweek. Because excessive exposure to mercury can cause it to build up in the body faster than it is eliminated, it is essential to practice good mercury hygiene. Most dental offices comply with mercury hygiene standards, as demonstrated by studies that have shown mercury levels in most dental offices to be far below OSHA's recommended minimum.

Several measures can be taken by the office staff to minimize mercury exposure. Free mercury vapor is released if amalgam is heated above 800° C (1472° F). Instruments contaminated with amalgam should never be heated to this temperature in the operatory. Sterilization rooms must have adequate ventilation to disperse any mercury vapor that may come from the sterilizer during the sterilization process. Staff members should stand an arm's length away from the sterilizer when opening the door to avoid inhaling any vapors that might be released. Operatory floors should have surfaces that are nonporous and easy to clean. Carpets and tiled floors with seams tend to trap amalgam particles and mercury droplets and therefore are not recommended. Gloves, masks, and eye protection should be worn when working around amalgam and mercury. Use of factory encapsulated alloy and mercury will minimize handling of mercury and reduce the risk of mercury spills. Keep a variety of capsules with various portions (spills) of amalgam on hand to minimize amalgam waste. Amalgam scrap should be stored in airtight containers. Operatories should be well ventilated. If staff members have concerns about mercury exposure, offices can be monitored for mercury vapor (available through private companies). Individual staff members could also wear monitors and have periodic blood and urine analyses.

Safety for the Environment

Although dental offices do not contribute as much mercury to the environment as large companies, their contribution is not insignificant. In 2003 dental offices were estimated to be responsible for 50% of the mercury contamination from waste water entering publicly owned treatment works (POTWs). In 2008 the Environmental Protection Agency (EPA) estimated that the approximately 162,000 dentists who use or remove amalgam discharged 3.7 tons of mercury annually into POTWs. The POTWs typically remove about 90% of the amalgam, so the remaining 10% goes into streams, rivers, lakes, and oceans. Therefore, it is vitally important to our environment that the dental profession do all it can to manage amalgam waste.

Special collection devices called **amalgam separator**s are available to collect amalgam particles and mercury that might escape into the wastewater. The Environmental Protection Agency mandated under the Clean Water Act that in July 2017 dental practices must control amalgam waste through the use of amalgam separators certified by the International Organization for Standardization (ISO). The ISO standard 11143 for amalgam separators requires they collect at least 95% of the mercury waste. Practices that place and remove amalgam are also subject to two best practices: (1) they must collect and recycle scrap amalgam and (2) they must clean waterline traps with cleaners not containing bleach or chlorine so that mercury is not released. Amalgam scrap that is collected from used capsules, remnants from the amalgam well, and amalgam debris from high-volume evacuation traps and vacuum pump filters should be appropriately recycled. Do not dispose of the waste in biohazard bags, infectious waste (red) bags, or discard it in the trash that ends up in landfills. Some recyclers want the amalgam scrap separated into contact

TABLE 10.6	Best Practices for Amalgam Waste	
DO THESE:	**DO *NOT* DO THESE:**
Use factory encapsulated alloy	Do not use bulk mercury
Store in air-tight containers and recycle amalgam scrap, capsules, and extracted teeth with amalgam	Do not dispose of amalgam scrap, capsules, or extracted teeth with amalgam in biohazard bags, infectious waste bags, or regular trash
Use chairside amalgam traps, vacuum pump filters, and amalgam separators. Recycle scrap	Do not clean traps, filters, or separators over the sink
Use line cleaners that do not dissolve amalgam	Avoid cleaners that contain bleach or chlorine
Train all staff in safe handling procedures and review state regulations	Avoid direct contact with amalgam and its scrap

mercury. Provisions of the treaty included a global ban on the import and export of mercury-containing products by 2020. However, dental amalgam was exempted from an outright ban. Instead, countries still using it were encouraged to find alternatives to amalgam, phase out amalgam over time, and promote best environmental practices.

Sources of Office Staff Exposure to Mercury

1. Placing or removing amalgam
2. Leaking amalgam capsules (less frequent with factory-sealed capsules)
3. Mercury droplets collecting on triturator surfaces
4. Sterilizing instruments contaminated with amalgam
5. Improper disposal of amalgam capsules and waste
6. Improper storage of amalgam scrap
7. Amalgam particles in traps within high-volume evacuation system
8. Carpeted operatories or floors with tile or linoleum seams that can collect spilled mercury

Methods for Mercury Vapor Reduction

Use factory-sealed amalgam capsules, not bulk alloy and mercury that could spill.
Use an amalgamator with a completely enclosed mixing arm to prevent spread of mercury during mixing.
Store amalgam scrap in a sealed container. Do not use x-ray fixer for amalgam scrap storage because the fixer is another environmental hazard.
Recap used amalgam capsules and dispose of them in a sealed container.
Use copious water and high-volume evacuation when removing old amalgam to prevent release of mercury vapor into the air.
Use a rubber dam whenever possible to prevent patients from swallowing scrap or breathing mercury vapors.
Use facemask and shield to avoid splatter and vapors.
Use traps or filters (or both) in evacuation systems. Check and clean regularly.
Avoid the use of mechanical or ultrasonic condensers. They increase mercury vapor release.
Clean up spilled mercury promptly with a commercial spill kit. Avoid handling with bare skin. Dispose of it in a sealed container (one comes with the kit).
Clean instruments of any adherent amalgam before sterilization.
Avoid carpeted operatories. Use floor coverings that are nonabsorbent, seamless, and easy to clean.
Remove professional protective clothing before leaving the workplace.

Handling of Mercury Spills

1. Do not use a vacuum cleaner to removed spilled mercury.
2. Do not use cleaning products, especially those that contain bleach, chlorine, or ammonia.
3. Do not use a broom or brush to collect the mercury.
4. Do not dispose of the mercury in the drain.
5. If clothing or shoes have been contaminated with mercury, remove them and leave them at the spill site.
6. Use a commercially available clean-up kit to safely contain and remove mercury.

and noncontact containers. Noncontact amalgam scrap is that which is left over in the amalgam well or other sources that have not touched the patient and, obviously, contact amalgam scrap is that collected after touching the patient which includes extracted teeth (Table 10.6).

RESTRICTIONS ON AMALGAM USE

The stance taken in the USA on amalgam safety has been largely retrospective, meaning that no studies so far have shown a harmful effect from the use of amalgam in the general population or in specific groups such as pregnant women or children. So, amalgam can be used until studies show a harmful effect. However, in Europe and some other countries a more precautionary approach is used. They conclude that because mercury is a known toxin, it is prudent to restrict the use in pregnant women and young children unless it is proven safe.

In 1956 Japan experienced a public health disaster from mercury poisoning in the city of Minamata that killed thousands and sickened many others. Seafood contaminated with mercury from industrial waste was the culprit. In the 1980s, primarily to reduce mercury in the environment, Japan became one of the first nations to restrict dental amalgam use. Since then, many countries have taken steps to reduce the use of amalgam both for environmental reasons and patient safety, especially in pregnant women and children under 6 years of age. These countries include members of the European Union (United Kingdom, Germany, Netherlands, Hungary, Switzerland, and Austria) as well as Finland, Canada, New Zealand, and Singapore. The use of amalgam has been banned in Norway, Sweden, and Denmark.

In October 2013 an international meeting called the Minamata Convention was held in Minamata, Japan, to address health and environmental concerns involving mercury pollution. By November of that year 93 countries had signed a treaty to reduce the risks to human health and to the environment from the use and release of

SUMMARY

Dental amalgam is a widely used restorative material. Amalgam is an economical, durable, and useful restorative material, although composite resins have surpassed amalgam in popularity. Dental auxiliaries play an important role in the delivery of amalgam restorations to patients by assisting the dentist or, in some states when properly licensed, the placement, carving, and finishing and polishing of the amalgams. Knowledge of the physical properties, mixing and placement techniques, and finishing and polishing methods is important for the proper handling of amalgam and ultimately the longevity of restorations. Safe mercury hygiene practices in the workplace are essential to the health and well-being of patients, office staff, and to the environment in general.

Patient education is an essential role of the dental auxiliary in the dental practice. The ability to describe the pros and cons of the various materials used in practice to the patient and the ability to aid in the treatment process depends on your knowledge of these materials. As new materials are introduced into dental practice, it is important to stay current about their indications, contraindications, and application techniques. Manufacturers' instructions for their care and use should also be followed. Many manufacturers have websites on which they post information relative to their materials.

INSTRUCTIONAL VIDEOS

See the Evolve Resources site for a variety of educational videos that reinforce the material covered in this chapter.

Procedure 10.1 Placing and Carving Class II Amalgam

See Evolve site for Competency Sheet.

EQUIPMENT/SUPPLIES (Fig. 10.21)

a. Local anesthesia setup
b. Operative dentistry setup: Assorted burs, excavators, hand-cutting instruments
c. Amalgam placement setup: Amalgam carrier and well, large and small condensers, ball burnisher; coronal and interproximal carvers; matrix retainer, pre-burnished bands, wedges; articulating paper and holder and dental floss
d. Encapsulated amalgam alloy and mercury
e. Dental dam setup
f. Disposables: Gauze, cotton pellets, high-volume evacuation (HVE) tip, air-water syringe tip

PROCEDURE STEPS

1. After the administration of local anesthetic, application of the dental dam, and preparation of the cavity, place the preassembled Tofflemire matrix band and retainer on the tooth and firmly insert the wedge in the interproximal space from the lingual side (Fig. 10.22).

NOTE: After placement, the band should be burnished against the adjacent tooth with an interproximal burnisher or the blade of a plastic instrument to create the proper contour of the contact area.

The band should:
   (a) be sealed against the tooth at the gingival margin by the wedge
   (b) extend approximately 1 mm coronal to the level of the marginal ridge
   (c) be in contact with the proximal surface of the adjacent tooth

The wedge should:
   (a) press the band against the tooth to seal the gingival margin
   (b) create a separation of the teeth to make up for the thickness of the matrix band so an open contact is not formed when the band is removed

2. Place a base, liner, or cavity varnish, as needed.

NOTE: Copal resin is seldom used as a cavity varnish, because it quickly washes out of the preparation. Some offices have replaced it with dentin sealers or bonding agents that occlude the dentinal tubules. At present, bases and liners are used less frequently and are applied mostly in deeper cavity preparations,

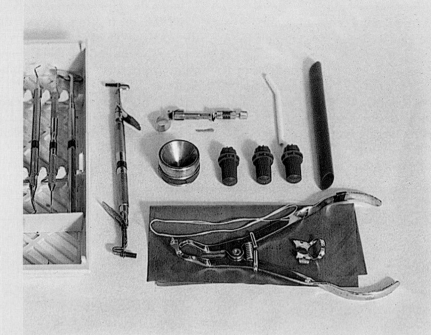

FIG. 10.21

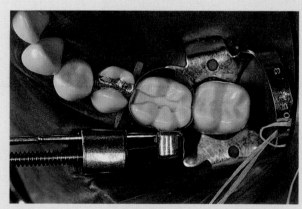

FIG. 10.22

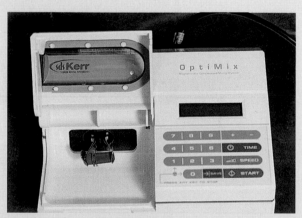

FIG. 10.23

because the need for their use has not been established on a routine basis. Deeper preparations may need a base or liner for thermal insulation.

3. After the base or liner has set, activate the amalgam capsule (unless it is self-activating), place it into the arms of the triturator, and set for the recommended time and speed (Fig. 10.23).

4. Mix the amalgam, open the capsule, and place the mixed amalgam in the amalgam well (Fig. 10.24).

5. Fill both ends of the amalgam carrier and place the amalgam in the proximal box from the small end first (Fig. 10.25).

NOTE: Some clinicians who use spherical alloy prefer to place the amalgam in large increments and quickly condense it into the cavity preparation.

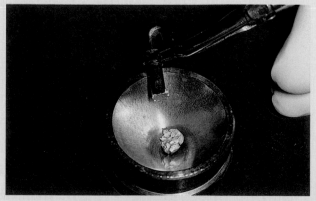

FIG. 10.24

Continued

Procedure 10.1   Placing and Carving Class II Amalgam—cont'd

Spherical amalgam requires much less condensation pressure and displaces easily into the preparation as compared with an admixed amalgam.

6. Continue to fill the preparation with amalgam. Mix additional amalgam as needed to complete the restoration.

NOTE:. Usually, the smaller end of the condenser is used first to condense amalgam onto the gingival floor of the box and against the facial and lingual walls. Both vertical and lateral condensation forces should be used to adapt the amalgam to the preparation.

7. After the preparation has been slightly overfilled, the amalgam is burnished with the ball burnisher over its surface and margins (Fig. 10.26). Some clinicians use an anatomic burnisher (e.g., acorn burnisher) to begin the initial contour of the occlusal morphology.

NOTE: Burnishing creates a denser surface, adapts the amalgam closely to the margins, and brings excess mercury to the surface that is then carved away. Not all clinicians burnish their amalgams.

8. An explorer tip is used to carve excess amalgam away from the band and to begin shaping the marginal ridge (Fig. 10.27). A discoid carver is used to remove large excesses of amalgam from the occlusal surface.

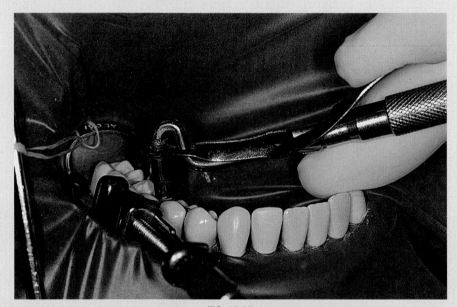

FIG. 10.25

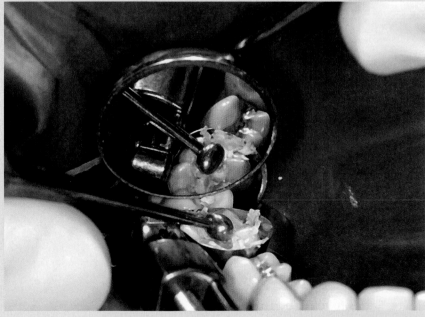

FIG. 10.26

Procedure 10.1   Placing and Carving Class II Amalgam—cont'd

NOTE: Removing excess amalgam adjacent to the band helps prevent fracture of the amalgam during removal of the band.

9. Remove the matrix retainer. While holding the marginal ridge of the amalgam restoration down with a large condenser, remove the matrix band in an occlusal direction with a gentle rocking motion (Fig. 10.28).

NOTE: Some clinicians prefer to leave the wedge in place while removing the band to maintain some separation of the teeth. This helps to minimize risk of fracture of the marginal ridge. If the marginal ridge is not held down during removal of the band, the unset amalgam is at risk of fracture, requiring its removal and placement of fresh amalgam.

10. An interproximal carver (e.g., 1/2 Hollenbeck) is used to carve first the gingival margin, then facial and lingual margins to remove any excess material (Fig. 10.29). Next, a discoid/cleoid or similar carver is used to carve the occlusal surface (Fig. 10.30). The blade of the carver is held partially on the adjacent enamel to act as a guide so that the amalgam margins are not overcarved.

11. After the amalgam is firm, pass dental floss through the contact to clear the embrasure of excess carving debris and to test the adequacy of the contact relationship (Fig. 10.31).

NOTE: A weak, open, or poorly contoured contact relationship with the adjacent tooth can lead to food impaction into the gingival tissues and periodontal pocket formation.

12. Remove the dental dam and mark the occlusal contacts with articulating paper (Fig. 10.32). High spots as indicated by heavy marks from the articulating paper are carefully carved away. Repeat the process until contact is no longer heavy and the patient indicates that the restoration does not feel high. As a last step, some clinicians smooth the surface of the amalgam with a wet cotton pellet.

NOTE: Before checking the occlusal contacts make sure the marginal ridges of the amalgam are at the same level as the ridges of the adjacent teeth. The patient should be instructed to close very lightly and then open again. If the patient closes too firmly and the amalgam is high, especially at the marginal ridge, it might fracture. When patients are still numb from the local anesthetic, they often cannot judge how hard they are biting. Some clinicians prefer to wait a couple of minutes after completing the carving before

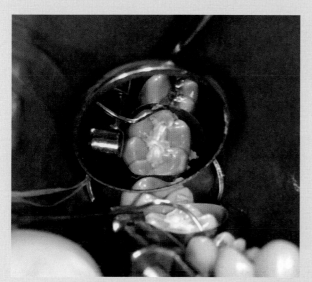

FIG. 10.27

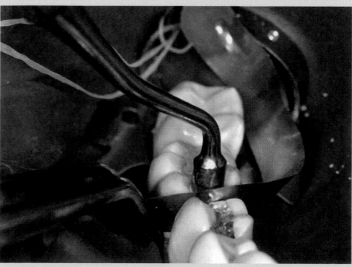

FIG. 10.28

Continued

Procedure 10.1 Placing and Carving Class II Amalgam—cont'd

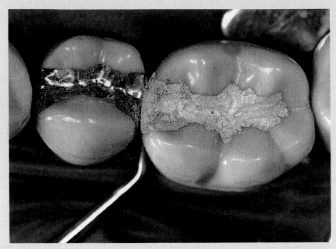

FIG. 10.29

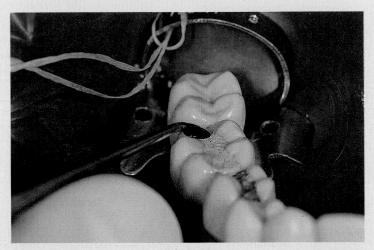

FIG. 10.30

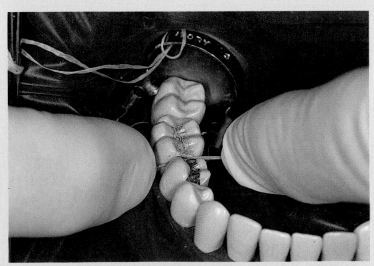

FIG. 10.31

Procedure 10.1   Placing and Carving Class II Amalgam—cont'd

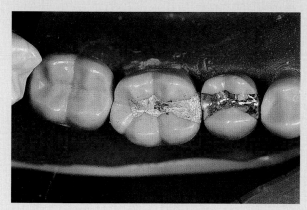

FIG. 10.32

checking the occlusal contacts to allow the amalgam to gain some firmness, especially for very large amalgams.

In some states, dental hygienists and assistants licensed in expanded functions can place, condense, and carve the amalgam.

13. Instruct the patient to avoid chewing on the new amalgam restoration until the next day. Advise the patient to take care while they are still numb from the anesthetic when chewing or consuming hot foods or beverages due to the risk of biting the lip or tongue or burning the oral tissues or throat.

NOTE: High-copper amalgams, especially spherical ones, have a high early strength and gain about 80% of their compressive strength in the first 8 hours. The set is usually complete within 24 hours.

Get Ready for Exams!

Review Questions

Select the one correct response for each of the following *multiple-choice questions.*

1. In an amalgam restoration, which of the following elements has the greatest effect on reduction of corrosion?
   a. Silver (Ag)
   b. Mercury (Hg)
   c. Copper (Cu)
   d. Indium

2. In the amalgam restoration, the two main components are
   a. Silver and copper
   b. Copper and tin
   c. Silver and mercury
   d. Mercury and zinc

3. Why should all remnants of amalgam be removed from the placement instruments before they are autoclaved?
   a. The steam causes the amalgam to fuse to the stainless steel.
   b. Amalgam corrosion products produced by the steam are toxic.
   c. The heat causes mercury vapor to be released from the amalgam.
   d. The heat melts the silver component, and it will clog the drain of the autoclave.

4. The strength of the amalgam restoration can be affected by
   a. Overtrituration
   b. Undertrituration
   c. Corrosion
   d. All of the above

5. A properly mixed amalgam should appear
   a. Dry and crumbly
   b. Soupy and shiny
   c. As a homogeneous mass with a slight shine
   d. Liquid-like and should pour easily out of the capsule

6. Scrap amalgam should be
   a. Autoclaved before it is sent to the recycler
   b. Thrown into the incinerator
   c. Stored in a sealed container
   d. Put into the general nonmedical waste

7. With high-copper alloys, which metal reacts with copper to reduce gamma-2 phase corrosion?
   a. Tin
   b. Zinc
   c. Silver
   d. Palladium

8. The fact that mercury makes up almost half of amalgam has caused concerns about
   a. Its safety for patient use
   b. Risks to the office staff
   c. Environmental effects of improper disposal of amalgam waste
   d. All of the above

9. Amalgam has been popular for the restoration of carious teeth because
   a. It is economical
   b. It has excellent physical properties
   c. It is easy to manipulate
   d. All of the above

10. For best mercury hygiene practices, which type of flooring is preferred for the dental operatory?
    a. Hardwood plank flooring
    b. Ceramic tile
    c. Seamless vinyl
    d. Tight-knit carpet

11. How does tarnish differ from corrosion?
    a. Tarnish occurs only on the surface.
    b. Tarnish is more harmful to the restoration than is corrosion.
    c. Tarnish contributes to the destructive effects seen in the gamma-2 phase.
    d. Tarnish cannot be removed by polishing, whereas corrosion can.

12. Which one of the following amalgam mixes has the least resistance to condensation pressure?
    a. Lathe-cut low-copper
    b. Spherical high-copper
    c. Admix high-copper
    d. Lathe-cut high-copper

13. Delayed expansion of amalgam is caused by contact of water with which component of amalgam?
    a. Mercury
    b. Copper
    c. Tin
    d. Zinc

14. Polishing of amalgam should be done
    a. With light pressure, using water as a coolant
    b. With rubber abrasive points without water
    c. Immediately after carving
    d. With heavy pressure, using pumice in a rubber cup

15. Amalgam is strongest in which one of the following?
    a. Tension
    b. Shear
    c. Compression
    d. Torsion

16. All of the following features meet the criteria for a well placed matrix assembly **except** one. Which one?
    a. The narrow portion of the band is oriented toward the gingival margin.
    b. Matrix band extends apical to gingival margin of proximal box by at least 1 mm.
    c. No gap is present between the band and the gingival margin of the proximal box.
    d. Top edge of the band extends 3 mm above the adjacent marginal ridge.

17. Which one of the following statements does **NO**T fit the criteria of a well placed wedge for a Class II cavity preparation matrix assembly?
    a. The wedge is located just coronal to the gingival margin of the proximal box.
    b. The wedge does not deform the contours of the matrix band.
    c. The wedge is seated firmly to produce separation of the teeth.

d. The wedge holds the band against the gingival margin of the proximal box.

18. The dental staff is most at risk for mercury overexposure from which one of the following sources?
   a. Inhaling mercury vapor
   b. Handling amalgam with gloved hands
   c. Triturating commerically prepared capsules of amalgam
   d. Polishing amalgam under water spray

For answers to Review Questions, see the Appendix.

Case-Based Discussion Topics

1. A healthy 23-year-old college student reports to the dental office for a routine examination. It is discovered that she has several class II carious lesions in her molars that require restoration. She does not have a lot of money and wants a durable restoration. She is not concerned about whether the restorations show when she speaks.

Discuss the advantages and disadvantages of amalgam and composite resin for her situation. Which would you choose for yourself? Why?

2. A 43-year-old housewife comes to the dental office and reports that another dentist has told her that all of her old amalgams must be removed because they contain mercury. She asks you about the safety of amalgam fillings.

Discuss the safety issues related to amalgam, its mercury content, and the risks involved in removing the restorations.

3. You have just triturated a double mix capsule of amalgam, and mercury has leaked while the capsule was being shaken and can be seen in small puddles on the outer surface of the triturator.

Discuss appropriate ways to capture the spilled mercury and dispose of it. What risks does the spill present to the office staff?

4. While removing the matrix band from a newly placed MOD amalgam on tooth #19, the mesial marginal ridge of the amalgam fractured off.

Can this fracture be fixed by replacing the matrix band and adding more amalgam from a fresh mix? Why or why not? What steps can be taken to avoid the marginal ridge fracture when removing the band?

5. A 36-year-old nurse had an MO amalgam placed on a moderately deep cavity preparation in tooth #3. When she drinks hot coffee or eats ice cream she gets a sudden sharp pain in the tooth that lasts 2 to 3 seconds.

What is the likely cause of the pain? How could this problem have been prevented?

BIBLIOGRAPHY

ADA Council on Scientific Affairs: Dental mercury hygiene recommendations, *J Am Dent Assoc*, 134:1498–1499, 2003.

American Dental Association (ADA): *Amalgam Waste Best Management*, Available at ada.org/-/media/ADA/Member%20Center/Files/topics_amalgamwaste_brochure.ashx, 2007.

Anusavice KJ, Shen C, Rawls HR: Dental amalgams. In *Phillips' Science of Dental Materials*, ed 12, Philadelphia, 2013, Saunders, p 2013.

Bird DL, Robinson DS: Restorative and esthetic dental materials. In *Modern Dental Assisting*, ed 12, Philadelphia, 2018, Saunders.

DermNet NZ: *Lichenoid Amalgam Reaction*, Available at: http://dermnetnz.org/reactions/amalgam-lichenoid.html, 2010.

Eakle WS, Staninec M, Lacy AM: Effect of bonded amalgam on the fracture resistance of teeth, *J Pros Dent*, 69(2):257–260, 1992.

European Commission, Department of Health and Food Safety: *Final Opinion on Dental Amalgam*, https://ec.europa.eu/health/scientific_committees/consultations/public_consultations/scenihr_consultation_24_en, 2014.

Heyman HO, Swift EJ, Ritter AV: *Class I, II and VI Amalgam Restorations in Sturdevant's Art and Science of Operative Dentistry*, ed 6, St. Louis, 2013, Mosby.

Life Sciences Research Office: *Executive Summary: Review and Analysis of the Literature on the Health Effects of Dental Amalgam*, Available at: http://www.lsro.org/presentation_files/amalgam/amalgam_execsum.pdf.

Mackey TM, Contreras JT, Liang BA: The Minamata Convention on Mercury: attempting to address the global controversy of dental amalgam use and mercury waste disposal, *Science of the Total Environment*, 472:125–129, 2014.

Marshall GW, Marshall SJ, Bayne SC: Restorative dental materials: Scanning electron microscopy and x-ray microanalysis, *Scanning Microsc*, 2:2007–2028, 1988.

Office of Environmental Health Hazard Assessment: *Mercury in Dental Amalgam Fillings. State of California*, March 2016. Oehha.ca.gov/media/downloads/proposition-65/chemicals/mercurydentalamalgamfactsheet.pdf.

Powers JM, Wataha JC: *Dental amalgam*. In *Dental Materials: Foundations and Applications*, ed 11, St. Louis, 2017, Elsevier.

Sakaguchi RL, Powers JM: Restorative materials – metals. In *Craig's Restorative Dental Materials*, ed 13, Philadelphia, 2012, Mosby.

Stafford G: *The Environmentally Responsible Dentist—Dental Amalgam Recycling: Principles, Pathways and Practice*, July 2011. Available at: https://www.researchgate.net/publication/263370547_The_Environmentally_Responsible_Dentist_-_Dental_Amalgam_Recycling_Principles_Pathways_and_Practice.

U.S. Department of Health and Human Services: Public Health Service (DHHS/PHS): *Dental Amalgam: A Scientific Review and Recommended Public Health Service Strategy for Research, Education and Regulation*, Washington DC: DHHS/PHS, 1993. https://health.gov/environment/amalgam1/ct.htm

U.S. Department of Labor, Occupational Safety and Health Administration. *Permissible Exposure Limits. Annotated OSHA Z-2 Table*, December 19, 2016. https://www.osha.gov/dsg/annotated-pels/tablez-2.html

U.S. Food and Drug Administration. *About Dental Amalgam Fillings*, Updated 1/27/2015. Fda.gov/MedicalDevices/ProductsandMedicalProcedures/DentalProducts/DentalAmalgam/ucm171094.htm.

Xu HH, Eichmiller FC, Giuseppetti AA, et al.: Three-body wear of a hand-consolidated silver alternative to amalgam, *J Dent Res*, 78:1560–1567, 1999.

Chapter Objectives

Upon completion of this chapter, the student should be able to:

1. Describe the differences among the types of gold alloy used for dental restorations.
2. Differentiate between high-noble, noble, and base-metal alloys.
3. Describe the properties needed for porcelain bonding alloys.
4. Describe the properties of metals used for casting partial denture frameworks.
5. Explain the biocompatibility issues associated with some alloys.
6. Explain how solders are used.
7. List metals used for solders.
8. Describe how wrought metal alloys differ from casting alloys.
9. Describe the uses of wrought wire.
10. Explain the use of the different types of metal for orthodontic arch wire.
11. Explain the purpose of an endodontic post.
12. Describe the types of materials used for preformed endodontic posts.

Key Terms

Alloy a solid compound made up of two or more elements of which at least one is a metal

High-Noble Alloy alloy containing at least 60% noble metals, 40% of which must be gold

Base-Metal Alloy alloy composed of non-noble metals which corrode more readily

Noble Alloy alloy composed of metals that do not corrode readily; at least 25% must be noble metals

Precious Metal classification of metal based on its high cost

Elastic Modulus a measure of the stiffness of a material. A high modulus indicates a stiff material and a low modulus a more flexible one

Porcelain Bonding Alloys special casting alloys manufactured for their compatibility with porcelain that is bonded to them at high temperature

Coping a thin covering like a thimble that serves as a substructure for a porcelain-bonded-to-metal crown (in this case, the coping is metal)

Firing a process of heating porcelain powders at high temperature until they fuse

Glazing firing porcelain at high temperature to achieve a smooth, shiny surface

Sintering a process whereby particles are heated to the point that they fuse together at their borders but do not clump into one solid mass

Yield Strength amount of stress at which a substance deforms

Solder an alloy used to join two metals together or to repair cast metal restorations

Wrought Metal Alloy an alloy that has been mechanically changed into another form to improve its properties (including ductility and malleability)

Anneal to modify physical properties of a metal by heating it

Nitinol an alloy of nickel and titanium often used for orthodontic wires

Gauge a measure of the thickness of a wire; the lower the gauge, the thicker the wire (e.g., 8 gauge is thicker than 16 gauge)

Endodontic Post a metal or nonmetal dowel placed within the root canal to retain a core buildup

---

Historically, the most widely used material in restorative and corrective dentistry has been metal. Because a pure metal may not possess the physical and mechanical properties desired for a restoration, it may be combined with one or more other elements to form an alloy with the properties desired. Metal alloys generally have high strength and consequently make durable dental restorations. They melt at high temperatures, conduct temperature and electricity, can be polished to a high shine (luster), and have varying degrees of ductility (ability to be pulled or drawn into a wire). Gold is malleable and ductile and the margins of gold restorations can be burnished for better adaptation to the tooth preparation margins. As esthetic nonmetal materials improve in their physical properties, they are gradually replacing metals in many applications.

The dental health care worker (clinical or laboratory) is in contact with and involved in the manipulation of metal dental materials in various ways every day. Grinding dust from certain metal alloys can present the dental health care worker with health hazards, so personal protective

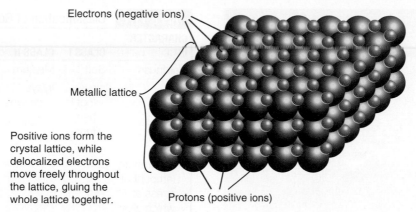

Electrons (negative ions)

Metallic lattice

Positive ions form the
crystal lattice, while
delocalized electrons
move freely throughout
the lattice, gluing the
whole lattice together.

Protons (positive ions)

FIG. 11.1 Representation of a crystal lattice structure of a metal. A sea of free electrons in the outer shell are shared among all of atoms. (Modified from HSC Physics, Dux College.)

equipment must be used. It is essential that the dental auxiliary have an understanding of the properties of various metal materials in order to correctly manipulate and care for them and to be able to answer questions by patients relative to a particular material that will be used for their treatment.

STRUCTURE OF METALS AND ALLOYS

PURE METALS

Pure metals are composed of multiple small interlocking crystals (also called grains) arranged in a highly ordered, three dimensional structure called a lattice (Fig. 11.1). There are fourteen types of lattice arrangements found in metals. Each crystal is composed of multiple, closely packed metal ions surrounded by a sea of free electrons in the outer shell that are shared among all of the atoms. The force of attraction between the metal ions and the electrons circulating among them forms the metallic bond. The metallic bond is very strong, helps the metal to maintain a regular shape, and is responsible for the physical properties of the metal. These physical properties include high melting and boiling points, high strength, ductility, malleability, thermal and electrical conductivity, high density, hardness, opacity, and luster.

ALLOYS

Since most pure metals lack the properties desired for dental uses, they are combined with other metals or nonmetal elements to form an **alloy**. Alloys are formed by melting the metal and added elements, mixing them together and then cooling them back into a solid. Alloys typically have higher strength and hardness than pure metals. Instead of a melting point like pure metals, alloys have a melting range determined by its different components.

Both pure metals and their alloys are crystalline solids. The properties that are desired for dental uses can be controlled by the changes to the crystalline structure that occur when they are processed or heated, for example,

the manner in which steel is heated and cooled can increase its hardness but can also make it more brittle.

All-Metal Casting Alloys

In the early 1900s, W.H. Taggart developed a technique for making dental restorations from metal that was melted and cast into a mold, using the lost wax technique (see Chapter 16 Gypsum and Wax Products). A variation of this technique with improved equipment is still used today for casting metal dental restorations.

Pure metals are seldom used in dentistry, because they lack properties that make them useful in the oral cavity. Therefore, they are usually combined with other metals or nonmetal materials in portions that achieve desirable physical and mechanical properties. Alloys used with the lost wax technique are called *dental casting alloys*. Unlike amalgam, restorations made from these alloys are not placed directly into the preparation but are made outside the mouth by an indirect technique, and then are cemented in place (see Chapter 6 Composites, Glass Ionomers, and Compomers and Chapter 14 Dental Cement). Cast metal restorations can be classified as intracoronal (preparation is made within the crown of the tooth) or extracoronal (preparation is made primarily on the outside of the crown of the tooth). An inlay is an intracoronal restoration, whereas an onlay has both intracoronal and extracoronal components in that it has an inlay preparation and also covers the outer surface of one or more cusps (Fig. 11.2). Other extracoronal cast restorations include partial coverage (¾ and ⅞ crowns) and full coverage crowns (Fig. 11.3). Cast metal alloys can also be used to make fixed partial dentures (bridges) and removable partial dentures for replacement of missing teeth.

The International Organization for Standardization (ISO) sets specifications for casting alloys; these can be found at its website (www.iso.org). Dental casting alloys can also be classified by their use:

- All-metal alloys for crown and bridge
- Ceramo-metal alloys (porcelain fused to metal) for crown and bridge
- All-metal alloys for removable partial dentures

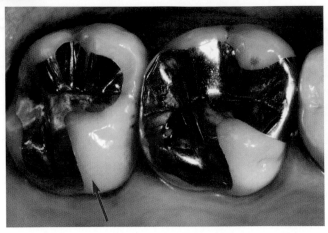

FIG. 11.2 Inlay (blue arrow) and onlay using high-noble metal (gold alloy). (Courtesy of Richard V. Tucker, Department of Restorative Dentistry, University of Washington [Seattle, WA].)

TABLE 11.1   Classification of Gold Alloys

CHARACTERISTIC	CLASS I	CLASS II	CLASS III	CLASS IV
Hardness	Soft	Medium	Hard	Extra hard
Use	Inlays (not in heavy function)	Inlays, crowns	Inlays, crowns, bridges	Partial denture framework, bridges
Yield strength (amount of stress at which alloy deforms)	Low	Medium	High	High
Wear resistance	Low	Medium	High	High

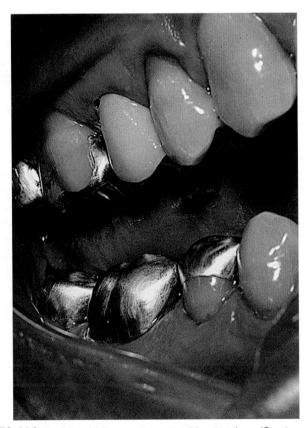

FIG. 11.3 Partial and full coverage cast gold restorations. (Courtesy of David Graham, University of California, San Francisco [San Francisco, CA].)

Noble Metal Dental Casting Alloys

A noble alloy is one that does not tarnish or corrode very readily in the oral environment. Gold (chemical symbol, Au) is the most corrosion resistant noble metal and has been used in dentistry for centuries. However, its use in dentistry is declining because of its high cost, and it is not considered esthetic in Western cultures. Gold alloy is classified as karats, percentage, or fineness (obtained by multiplying percentage of gold by 10) according to its gold content.

As an example, pure gold is 24 karat, 100%, or 1000 fine, and half gold is 12 karat, 50%, or 500 fine. The term *karat* is used more to signify the gold content of jewelry than dental alloys. Pure gold has limited use in dentistry today but is used in the form of gold foil by a small number of dentists for direct-placement restorations. Pure gold is too soft to use for dental castings; however, gold alloys have excellent properties and handling characteristics.

The American Dental Association classifies dental casting alloys according to their noble metal content and divides them into three categories: high-noble, noble, and base-metal alloys. To be considered a **high-noble alloy**, they must contain at least 60% noble elements (gold, palladium, and platinum), of which 40% must be gold. Base metals (usually copper, silver, or gallium) make up the remaining 40%. **Noble alloys** contain at least 25% noble elements with no requirement for gold, and the remaining 75% consists of base metals. **Base-metal alloys** have no requirement for gold and require less than 25% by weight of noble metals.

Dental gold casting alloys can also be classified (Table 11.1) by their

- Hardness (resistance to penetration)
- Malleability (ability to be shaped, as by tapping or pounding)
- Ductility (ability to be elongated, as by stretching or pulling)

The more ductile the alloy, the more the margins can be burnished (pushing or pulling the metal at the margins to close small gaps between the restoration and the tooth). Dental casting alloys should possess the following properties: strength, resistance to corrosion and tarnish, melting temperature compatible with investment materials (gypsum materials used in the lost wax technique of casting to encase the wax pattern, see Chapter 16), thermal expansion compatible with porcelains (for porcelain-fused-to-metal restorations), and biocompatibility.

Other Noble Metals for Casting Alloys. Other noble metals include platinum (Pt) and palladium (Pd). Platinum is not used much because of its expense, high melting point, and difficulty mixing with gold. Palladium is used widely, because it has good corrosion resistance, increases hardness of the alloy, and is less expensive than gold (however, palladium alloys have greatly increased in price because of shortages in the supply of palladium). These noble metals are sometimes referred to as **precious metals** because of their high monetary value. Although silver (Ag) is considered to be a precious metal, it is not considered noble because of its tarnish and corrosion in the oral cavity.

Gold, palladium, and platinum are the noble metals most widely used in dentistry. The remaining four of the seven noble metals (rhodium, iridium, ruthenium, and osmium) are used in very small amounts to enhance the physical properties of a dental alloy. Other metals that may be added to noble metals to enhance their properties and handling characteristics include copper, silver, zinc, tin, indium, gallium, and nickel (Table 11.2).

Base-Metal Dental Casting Alloys

Base-metal dental casting alloys consists of less than 25% noble metals. The most common base-metal alloys are chrome-cobalt and nickel-chrome. It is the chromium content that gives these metals their corrosion resistance. Other base metals used in casting alloys are copper (Cu), nickel (Ni), silver (Ag), zinc (Zn), tin (Sn), and titanium (Ti). Copper and silver are often added to gold alloys to increase their hardness. Zinc is added to reduce oxidation when the alloy is cast.

Because of their low cost, base metals have also been called *nonprecious metals.* They are inexpensive alternatives to noble metals for all-metal crowns and porcelain-to-metal crowns. Base metal alloys have about half the density of gold alloys, making them much lighter. Although they are not considered to be as good as the noble metals, the base metals are essential for many applications in dentistry. The stiffness (modulus of elasticity) of base alloys is twice as great as that of gold-based alloys which makes them useful for removable partial denture frameworks.

Drawbacks of base metals include their higher casting temperatures that require different equipment and investing materials than the gold-based alloys and their potential biocompatibility problems. They are much harder than noble metals, making them difficult to cut and finish. Other base metals used for casting removable prostheses are discussed later in this chapter (see Removable Prosthetic Casting Alloys).

PROPERTIES OF CASTING ALLOYS

Color of Casting Alloys

Most dental casting alloys are either yellow or silver ("white") in color. Often an assumption is made that yellow casting alloys have a higher gold content than

TABLE 11.2   Function of Metals Added to Gold Alloys

METAL (SYMBOL)	FUNCTION	MELTING POINT (°C)	COLOR
Palladium (Pd)	Reduces corrosion and tarnish Improves mechanical properties	1554	White
Platinum (Pt)	Raises melting temperature Improves hardness and elasticity	1772	Blue-white
Copper (Cu)	Hardens and strengthens the alloy Allows heat-treatment properties	1083.4	Reddish
Silver (Ag)	Hardens gold alloy Counters copper's redness	961.9	Silver
Zinc (Zn)	Acts as oxygen scavenger during casting process	419.6	Blue-white
Indium (In)	Used as a replacement for zinc	156.6	Gray-white
Nickel (Ni)	Seldom used. Increases hardness and strength	1453	White
Tin (Sn)	Acts with palladium and platinum to harden the alloy	232	White
Gallium (Ga)	Forms oxides for bonding ceramic to metal	29.8	Gray-white
Iridium (Ir)	Improves yield strength by creating smaller grains	2410	Silver-white
Ruthenium (Ru)	Improves yield strength by creating smaller grains	2310	White

silver-colored alloys. However, this may not be true. It is possible for a yellow casting alloy to have absolutely no gold at all! On the other hand, a silver casting alloy may have a high gold content. Because beauty is in the eye of the beholder, some patients may prefer the yellow color, whereas others prefer the silver color, and others still prefer no metal showing at all.

Melting Range

A dental casting alloy, being composed of more than one metal, will have a temperature range at which it melts rather than a single melting point. The temperature at the start of the range is when the alloy shows an initial shift toward melting and the temperature at the end of the range represents the point at which the entire alloy is liquid. So, an alloy with a range of 1100 °C to 1300 °C has the first signs of melting at 1100 °C and will be totally melted (called *liquidus*) at 1300 °C. When cooling a melted metal the temperature at which it becomes a solid is called *solidus.*

Elastic Modulus

The **elastic modulus** is a measure of stiffness of the alloy. The higher the elastic modulus of the alloy, the stiffer the alloy will be. Alloys used for fixed bridge restorations need to be stiff to avoid bending or distorting. If the crown or bridge has porcelain fused to it, bending would cause the brittle porcelain to fracture. Likewise, alloys used for removable partial dentures need to be stiff so that the framework does not flex too much and stress the abutment teeth when the patient chews. Wires used for orthodontic purposes must have a low elastic modulus to allow them to be bent without breaking.

Thermal Expansion

When a metal is heated, atoms within the metal increase in vibration. The result is a small increase in its length, width, and volume known as thermal expansion. How much expansion occurs depends on the particular metal. In the case where the metal will be heated to high temperature in order to bake porcelain on it for a porcelain-fused-to-metal crown, the expansion of the metal must be compatible with the expansion of the porcelain when they are heated. Otherwise, the brittle porcelain will crack.

Thermal and Electrical Conductivity

Metals are good conductors of heat and electricity. Thermal and electrical conductivity is determined mainly by the movement of free electrons throughout the lattice structure of the metal. Heat excites the tightly packed particles in the metal so that their vibrations quickly pass from one to the next. Electricity causes electrically charged particles—the free electrons—to flow through the lattice structure of the metal.

Density

Gold and platinum are among the densest (and heaviest) of the metals used in dental casting alloys. On the other hand, titanium is less dense and is lighter in weight. Gold alloys are easier to cast than chrome-cobalt alloys because their weight drives the molten metal into the investment better under casting forces than the lighter alloys.

Strength

Dental casting alloys must be strong enough to resist fracture or distortion. Typically, they are strong in both compression and tension. When the strength of alloys is compared, it is their yield strength that is considered. The yield strength is the stress or force needed to cause permanent distortion of the alloy. Typically, base-metal alloys have greater yield strength than gold alloys.

Hardness

Alloys that have low yield strength (like gold alloys) will be softer than those with higher yield strength (like base-metal alloys). A hard alloy will be more

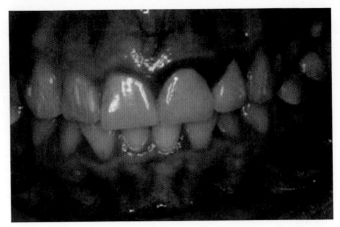

FIG. 11.4 Chronic gingival inflammation due to allergic reaction to a metal substructure of the porcelain-fused–to-metal crown. (Courtesy of Dr. Nicole Vane, Encinitas, CA.)

resistant to denting or scratching and will be more difficult to polish. Gold restorations, being softer, will also be kinder to the opposing enamel.

Crystal Formation (Grains)

After casting alloys have been melted and cast into the mold, they cool and form crystals (also called *grains*). Small crystals produce more desirable properties (especially improved yield strength) in the metal alloy than large crystals. Some elements such as iridium or ruthenium are added to gold-based alloys to keep the crystals from growing too large. Reheating gold-based alloys (called *annealing*) can improve some of the properties. After heating, slow cooling produces a harder metal and rapid cooling keeps the metal soft. However, with base-metal alloys, reheating will degrade the physical properties.

Resistance to Tarnish and Corrosion

It is important that dental casting alloys be composed of materials that resist tarnish and corrosion in the oral environment. The noble metal alloys naturally resist tarnish and corrosion. Base metal alloys are more likely to corrode in the mouth, so they are blended with other metals such as chromium that make them more corrosion resistant.

BIOCOMPATIBILITY

Noble metals are more biocompatible with the oral tissues, because they tend to corrode less than base metals. As metals corrode, they release metal corrosion products into the oral cavity. Some of these products are responsible for allergic responses (Fig. 11.4). Of the base metals, nickel has the highest incidence of allergic response. Women have a higher rate of allergy to nickel than do men, by a ratio of 10 to 1. A prior exposure to nickel in jewelry is thought to be the likely source of the exposure that sensitizes women to nickel. The overall allergy rate to nickel for the general population is about 9% to 12%. The allergic response is sometimes seen around the free gingival tissues, especially at the margins of base-metal crowns. This is less common for removable partial dentures because the metal often is not in direct contact with the tissues, and they are not worn constantly as fixed partial dentures or single crowns are worn. Some responses to nickel cause a skin reaction rather than a response in the mouth, even though the oral cavity is the source of the nickel.

Beryllium is a base metal added to nickel-chrome alloys to reduce the fusion temperature for easier casting and to improve physical properties by creating smaller metal crystals when the molten metal cools after casting. Beryllium is toxic and can cause chronic lung scarring with difficulty breathing. It can also cause allergic reactions with skin rashes. Once exposed the individual is at risk for disease for her lifetime even if exposure is stopped. Laboratory technicians are at risk for nickel and beryllium exposure when casting (metal vapors), grinding, and polishing these metals. In the laboratory an exhaust hood should be used for grinding procedures and the room should have good ventilation. When grinding in the mouth, high-volume evacuation should be used as well as isolation with a rubber dam where applicable. In addition, dental personnel should wear personal protective equipment (PPE) when working with these materials.

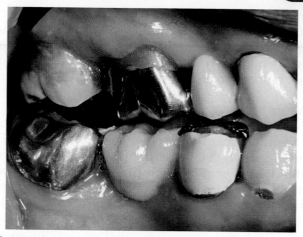

FIG. 11.5 Variety of metal alloys used to restore the teeth. Shown are gold and base metal alloys and alloys used for porcelain-fused-to-metal crowns. (Courtesy of Steve Eakle, University of California, San Francisco [San Francisco, CA].)

 Caution

Inhalation of beryllium is known to contribute to a lung disease called *berylliosis*. All dental personnel should wear PPE when grinding these alloys to prevent inhalation of small particles and to prevent fine particles from getting into the eyes. They should follow Occupational Safety and Health Administration (OSHA) guidelines for occupational hazards.

PORCELAIN BONDING ALLOYS

Porcelain bonding alloys were developed in the late 1950s. They are similar to the other casting alloys with similar physical properties. They are also classified as high-noble, noble, and base-metal alloys (Fig. 11.5). However, they have minor changes in their composition that make them compatible with dental ceramic materials. The most common ceramic materials used with these metals are conventional feldspar-based porcelains (see Chapter 9 Dental Ceramics). The metals in porcelain bonding alloys are selected and blended so that they have the ability to withstand the high temperatures at which porcelain is fired without melting or distorting. They also have a lower thermal expansion than gold alloys used for all-metal crowns, so they will not expand too greatly and crack the brittle porcelain that lies over top. In addition, small amounts of metals such as indium, iron, tin, or gallium are added to form oxides on the metal surface to which porcelain will bond (or fuse) at high temperature. Alloys that contain silver and copper may cause green staining (called *greening*) of the porcelain when fired at high

temperatures, and therefore they are usually avoided for use with ceramic materials. Most of the alloys are silver ("white") in color, but alloys that are gold colored (yellow) contain mostly gold with platinum and palladium added to increase the melting temperature.

PORCELAIN-BONDED-TO-METAL RESTORATIONS

Preparing the Metal

Porcelain-bonded-to-metal (also called *porcelain-fused-to-metal*, or *PFM*) crowns have a metal substructure (typically 0.3 to 0.5 mm thick) that is covered with layers of porcelain. The metal substructure (also called a **coping**) must be at least 0.3 mm thick to prevent distortion at high temperatures and must be convex in shape with no sharp angles. Sharp angles would create stress areas in the overlying porcelain that would be subject to fracture. To make room for a thin metal substructure and layers of porcelain that are at least 1.5 mm thick in areas under function, these crowns require a greater reduction of the tooth than all-metal crowns. For porcelain to bond to the metal, after the substructure is cast it is heated at high temperature to form oxides on the surface of the metal, a process called *degassing* (oxidizing would be a more accurate term).

Fusing Porcelain to Metal

The first layer of porcelain applied to the metal is opaque porcelain that keeps the metal oxide color from showing through and is the main color used for the crown (see Chapter 9, Fig. 9.11). Base metals often form darker oxides that are more difficult to hide with opaque porcelain. The oxidized metal and porcelain are heated (**fired**) at temperatures ranging from 870 °C to 1370 °C, depending on whether the porcelain fuses at low, medium, or high temperature. The oxides and porcelain chemically fuse together and mechanically interlock. Then additional layers of porcelain called *body and incisal porcelains* are built up or stacked to simulate dentin and enamel colors and translucency. After final contouring of the crown, another **firing** that maintains the temperature at the fusing temperature for a while will produce a surface glaze (a smooth, shiny surface created by the **glazing** process).

Failure Modes

The metal and porcelain must have compatible rates of thermal expansion or the porcelain will crack as it and the metal cool. Porcelain manufacturers will indicate the type of alloy needed for compatibility. Problems seen clinically with ceramic-alloy crowns are usually associated with fracture within the porcelain, where a piece of porcelain breaks off (called *debonding*) at the metal-porcelain interface, leaving metal exposed (see Chapter 9, Fig. 9.10). Failure can also result from formation on the metal surface of an inadequate oxide layer, an oxide layer that is too thick, or contamination of the oxide layer. The American National Standards Institute/American Dental Association (ANSI/ADA) Specification #38 sets the standard for testing the porcelain-metal bond. On occasion, composite resin bonding techniques can repair porcelain failures, but the repairs are prone to failure of the bond to porcelain or metal if they are subjected to chewing pressures. Often the crown needs to be replaced if the fracture causes an esthetic or functional issue. In addition to potential fracture problems, PFM crowns can cause accelerated wear of the opposing enamel, where it contacts the porcelain. Low-fusing porcelains are used more frequently, because they produce less wear of opposing enamel than is produced by medium- or high-fusing porcelains. Once the glaze on the surface of the porcelain is disrupted (e.g., adjusting the bite and not adequately repolishing the porcelain) it is rough and very abrasive to the opposing teeth.

Crown Design

Ceramic-metal crowns can have several different designs based on the esthetic demands of the patient and the need for maximal strength. In highly esthetic zones, patients usually do not want any metal to show, so the metal must be covered with porcelain. In parts of the mouth where esthetics is secondary to the need for maximal strength (as with a maxillary molar or premolar), the occlusal surface might be kept in metal and the buccal surface covered with porcelain to look like a tooth when the patient smiles. Patients who grind their teeth are at greater risk of chipping or breaking the porcelain, so they are good candidates for metal occlusal surfaces when possible.

The margins of the crowns can also have different configurations. The most esthetic margin is a porcelain facial margin. This is achieved by not extending the metal substructure all the way to the margin and leaving room to place porcelain to complete the margin. These porcelain margins are technically more difficult to produce, and therefore the laboratories charge more for this service. Another margin configuration is the disappearing metal margin. The metal at this margin has been ground to a thin, knife-edge where it extends to the edge of the preparation margin. Porcelain is applied over the metal (most of the metal disappears from view), but a thin dark line of metal may be visible. Therefore, to hide this metal line, the preparation of the tooth usually extends below the crest of the marginal gingiva. Over time, the gingiva may recede and expose the dark line of metal. Patients do not like the appearance of this dark line and may mistake it for dental caries. The dental auxiliary may be asked by the patient what is causing that dark line, so it is important to be able to provide an accurate explanation. A third configuration of the margin of the crown is an all-metal margin or collar. The all-metal collar is used, because it usually provides the best marginal fit, but it is used only in a non-esthetic zone (Fig. 11.6).

TITANIUM AND ITS ALLOYS

Titanium and its alloys can be used for implant fixtures, partial denture frameworks, and all-metal and metal-ceramic crowns and bridges. Titanium and its alloys have very high melting temperatures (approximately 1670 °C) and require special equipment in order to melt and cast them. They have low density and therefore, are very lightweight and harder to cast into the investment mold. Casting is done under pressure and vacuum or centrifuge and vacuum. Because of the difficulties in casting titanium, some crowns and partial denture frameworks are fabricated from metal blocks using CAD/CAM techniques.

Titanium and its alloys have a low coefficient of thermal expansion, so they need special low-expansion porcelains when being used for metal-ceramic restorations. The most widely used titanium alloy is Ti-6Al-4V (6% aluminum and 4% vanadium). It has high hardness, high strength, and more fatigue resistance than other titanium alloys. However, there are potential health concerns, because it contains aluminum and vanadium that slowly leach from the alloy by way of electrochemical corrosion. The concentration of the metal ions will affect how much toxicity results. Small amounts may cause no discernible problems. Aluminum ions are known to be more toxic than vanadium ions. Pure titanium is less toxic than aluminum and vanadium as well as nickel, chromium, and cobalt.

Although titanium alloys have good physical and mechanical properties to serve as partial denture frameworks, their high melting temperature and difficulty in casting them make them harder to work with than chrome-cobalt alloys. Surface oxides resulting from casting are more tedious to remove and internal porosities from casting can make the clasps more susceptible to fracture.

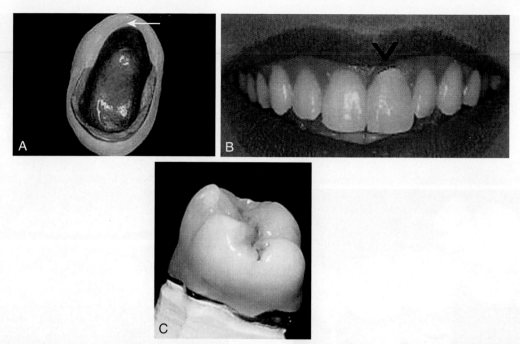

FIG. 11.6 Margin configurations for porcelain-fused-to-metal crowns. **A,** Porcelain facial margin. **B,** Disappearing metal margin seen as a dark line at the margin after gingival recession exposes it. **C,** All-metal margin (metal collar). (**A,** Courtesy of Dr. George Freedman. **B,** Courtesy of Infodentis. **C,** Courtesy of Marotta Dental Studio.)

SINTERED COMPOSITE ALLOYS

Alloys in this class differ from the casting metal alloys, because they are formed under high temperature through a process called **sintering**. In this process, powdered metal is heated and pressed into shapes with uniform content. Particles of metal alloy, in this case gold-palladium-platinum, are distributed in casting wax. The mixture is placed in an oven and the wax is burned off. The alloy particles are heated to the point that they fuse or sinter together at their points of contact but do not melt into one solid mass. This leaves a mass with lots of spaces between the particles—a meshwork. This material is hand-pressed onto a refractory die (a die made from special gypsum material that can withstand high temperatures) to form the first layer of a metal coping (the metal substructure to which porcelain is added) for a crown. Next, a wax containing gold-silver alloy particles is put on the first sintered alloy mass and is heated to the point that the gold-silver alloy melts but the gold-palladium-platinum alloy does not (it has a higher melting point). The second alloy melts, flows into, and fills by capillary action the spaces of the first meshwork. This produces a composite of the two alloys that serves as the coping or substructure for a porcelain-to-metal crown or bridge. To get the porcelain to bond to the alloy, it is necessary to apply yet another alloy to the composite alloy to allow the development of a ceramic-alloy fusion zone rather than an oxide-porcelain fusion. The fusion zone allows porcelain to melt and mechanically bond to the metal surface rather than undergo chemical fusion to an oxide layer as with traditional alloys (Fig. 11.7). A commercially available product is the *Captek* coping (Argen Corporation). It contains 88.2% gold, 9% platinum-group metals, and 2.8% silver. The Captek coping can be as thin as 50 microns (μm) at the margins and therefore requires less tooth reduction compared with conventional metal-ceramic crowns. Combined coping and porcelain thickness for anterior crowns can be as thin as 0.7 to 1.0 mm and 1.2 mm for posterior crowns.

REMOVABLE PROSTHETIC CASTING ALLOYS

At one time, type IV gold alloys were the predominate metals used for partial denture frameworks. However, they became quite expensive as the price of gold increased after deregulation of gold prices in 1971. The metals used today are mostly base metal alloys with or without minor amounts of noble elements (Fig. 11.8). Because the base metals are less dense than gold, they are lighter in weight. These base metals include nickel, titanium, chromium, aluminum, cobalt, vanadium, iron, beryllium, molybdenum, gallium, and carbon. In addition to corrosion resistance, hardness and resistance to deformation under function (**yield strength**) are important properties for these metals. Hardness indicates their resistance to scratching and denting and the increased effort needed to polish them. Their resistance to deformation is especially important for use in partial denture frameworks, where flexing of the framework would put undue stress on abutment teeth. Base metal alloys used for partial denture frameworks should also be resistant to fatigue, so that repeated flexing of the clasp arms as the partial denture is seated and removed does not cause them to break off. Cobalt-chromium

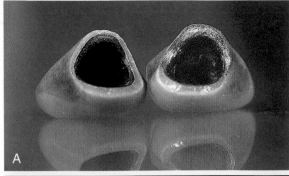

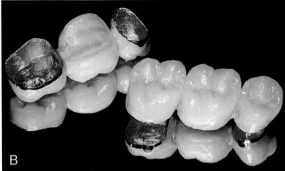

FIG. 11.7 Sintered alloy composite. **A,** A traditional porcelain-fused-to-metal crown on the *left* includes dark oxidized metal that must be covered with opaque porcelain. The Captek crown on the *right* with the sintered alloy has a gold color that does not require the opaquing needed for the traditional crown. **B,** Fixed partial denture (bridge) made with a sintered alloy substructure. (Courtesy of Argen Corporation, San Diego, CA.)

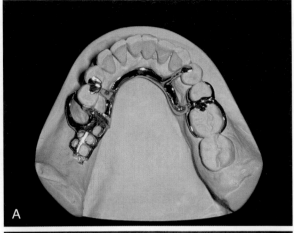

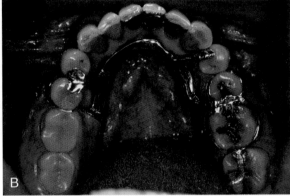

FIG. 11.8 Chrome-cobalt metal framework for a removable partial denture. **A,** Framework on the cast. **B,** The completed partial denture in the mouth after processing of acrylic and teeth over the retentive area. (Courtesy of Mark Dellinges, University of California School of Dentistry [San Francisco, CA].)

alloys are the most resistant to this type of fatigue and most commonly used for partial denture frameworks.

Because these metals are among the hardest of the alloys and are quite difficult to cast, they require special casting machines and are cast by commercial dental laboratories. Other metals may be used for attachments for prostheses, such as attachment bars between tooth abutments (see Chapter 12 Dental Implants, Fig. 12.15), overdenture attachments, and precision and nonprecision attachments for partial dentures. These attachments are made from high-noble, noble, or base metals. Attachments are used more frequently with the increasing use of combinations of implants and removable partial or complete denture combinations.

! Caution

Patients should be advised not to soak their appliances with metal components in household bleach. It will attack and corrode the metal.

IDENTALLOY PROGRAM

Manufacturers of dental alloys have developed a program that certifies the content of the alloys they produce. A certificate (IdentAlloy) is provided for each alloy (Fig. 11.9). It lists the manufacturer, name of the alloy, composition, and the ADA classification and is color-coded based on the noble metal content. The certificate is provided with a duplicate, so that both the

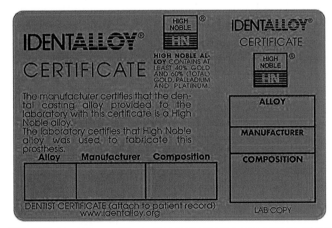

FIG. 11.9 IdentAlloy certificate that indicates the components of the metals used. (Courtesy of the IdentAlloy/IdentCeram Council.)

laboratory and the dentist can have a copy. Benefits of this program include the following: assurance the alloy meets the ADA classification criteria; provision of a record for the laboratory in case the U.S. Food and Drug Administration (FDA) has a recall, the dentist has questions, or future repairs are needed; insurance claims documentation and documentation in the patient's record concerning what was used in case the patient has an allergic reaction to the alloy.

SOLDERS

Metals are joined by three processes:
1. Soldering
2. Brazing
3. Welding

Soldering and brazing are similar and use a molten filler metal to join two other metals together. The difference between soldering and brazing is the temperature at which the procedure is completed. Soldering is performed at temperatures below 450 °C and brazing is done at temperatures above 450 °C. Because the term *soldering* is the one most commonly used, we use it here to discuss both soldering and brazing. Welding, on the other hand, is a process that uses high heat to fuse two metals together where they contact each other without the use of a filler metal. At one time custom matrix bands were made by spot welding two ends of a strip of matrix band material together by a device using electrical resistance.

GOLD SOLDERS

Solders are used to join metals together or repair cast restorations. Solders used for crown and bridgework are generally gold-based alloys, because they are used with gold alloys that make up the crowns. They generally contain gold, silver, and copper with small portions of zinc and tin. Gold-based solders are used to join together units of a bridge, add contacts, close holes ground in the occlusal surface by adjusting the bite, or correct small marginal deficiencies on onlays and crowns when they are found to be deficient at the try-in appointment. Gold-based solder is often categorized according to its fineness. The higher the fineness number, the higher the gold content and the lower the melting point of the solder.

Gold solders are available with different melting ranges (690 °C to 870 °C), depending on their composition, to accommodate the melting ranges of the gold alloys to which they will be soldered. This is important when two gold castings are soldered together or when a contact is added to a gold crown, because the solder must melt before the casting. Tin is often added to the solders to lower the melting range. To solder two units of a bridge together, they first must be invested in a special gypsum soldering investment in the proper relationship to each other (see Chapter 16). A flux is applied to the alloy surfaces to be soldered. The flux removes surface oxides so that the solder will flow freely and will wet the alloy surfaces as it melts. Flux for gold alloys usually contains borax. The alloys are heated with a torch until they turn red. The solder is added and heated until it melts and flows over the exposed surfaces of the bridge units. Often a contact can be added to a single crown without investing it by holding it over a Bunsen burner. Graphite from a pencil "lead" can be used to outline the limits of the contact area to be soldered. It acts as an antiflux to prevent the solder from flowing too far over the surface.

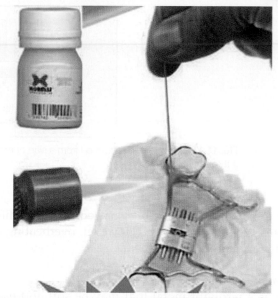

FIG. 11.10 An arch expander unit is attached to a metal orthodontic band with silver solder. (Courtesy of Royal Dent.)

Soldering of units of porcelain-fused-to-metal is much more challenging, because the ceramic and the metal alloy have different melting temperatures, and uneven heating of the unit can cause the porcelain to crack. Often soldering of PFM units is done in a special furnace where the temperature can be better controlled than with a torch.

SILVER SOLDERS

Silver-based solders are used more often in orthodontics and pediatric dentistry to solder fixed-space maintainer components (e.g., wire loop soldered to an orthodontic band) and to solder wire components to removable and fixed orthodontic appliances (Fig. 11.10). These solders contain varying amounts of silver, copper, and zinc and small amounts of tin which lowers the melting temperature and improves the flow of the molten metal. Silver solder is selected because it melts at a lower temperature (620 °C to 700 °C) than gold solder. The higher heat required to melt gold solder, which is greater than that for silver solder, sometimes will degrade the wire adjacent to the solder joint and weaken it. Flux for nongold alloys usually is a potassium fluoride flux.

WROUGHT METAL ALLOYS

Wrought metal alloys are different from casting alloys in that they are formed after the metal is cast. Usually the metal is drawn or extruded through a die or formed in a press to the desired shape, such as a flat plate or a wire or a knife or other instrument shape (Fig. 11.11). So, wrought alloys are alloys that have been mechanically changed into another form. The result is an alloy that is harder and has greater yield strength (the point at which a force can create permanent deformation of the metal). Wrought metal has the characteristic of being

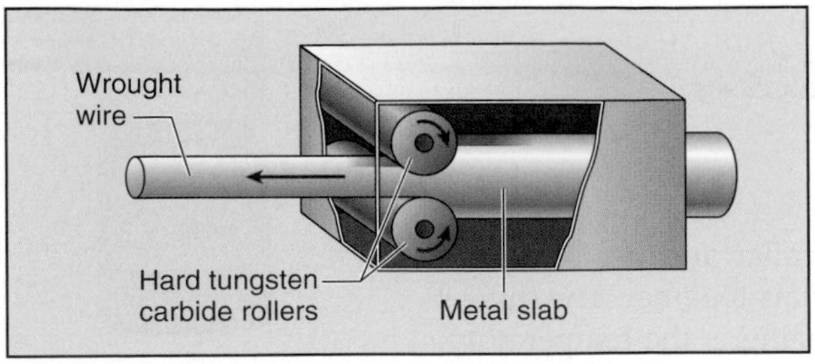

FIG. 11.11 Wrought wire is formed from a slab or thick rod of metal (A) by pulling it through a hard metal die or (B) forcing it through rollers.

able to be heat-modified, or **annealed**, to create differing resistance to deformity. However, overheating can degrade the properties of the metal.

Wire

Wire is a wrought metal that may be soft and easily shaped or may resist bending as does a spring. Various degrees of resistance to bending can be created by annealing. Wrought metal is used in removable prosthetic appliances, primarily for clasps. It can be a base metal such as stainless steel or a high-noble alloy composed of platinum-gold-palladium (called *PGP wire*). Additional examples of wrought wire used in dentistry include archwires and ligature (tie) wires used in orthodontics and arch bars and ligature wires used in oral surgery for stabilization of a jaw fracture.

Stainless Alloys

Steel is made from iron to which a small amount of carbon has been added. Stainless steel is steel to which chromium (12% or more) has been added to reduce tarnish and corrosion. Chromium acts by forming a very thin and transparent protective layer of oxides on the steel when it is in contact with oxygen. If this protective layer is scraped off inadvertently, corrosion can occur. In the oral cavity, this usually is not an issue, because the applications for stainless steel are often limited in the length of time they are used (e.g., use of endodontic files or archwires for orthodontics). Other metals such as molybdenum and nickel may also be added to stainless steel to improve its physical and mechanical properties. Because of their low cost, good mechanical properties, and corrosion resistance, stainless steel alloys have the following applications in dentistry: endodontic files; wires, brackets, and bands used in orthodontics; and fixed-space maintainers and stainless steel crowns used in pediatric dentistry.

PREFORMED PROVISIONAL CROWNS

Wrought alloys of stainless steel are used for the fabrication of preformed provisional crowns. They are the most durable of the preformed crowns and can last for months or even years. They come in a variety of sizes that fit most molars and premolars (see Chapter 18 Provisional Restorations, Figs. 18.4 and 18.5). Because

more esthetic alternatives are available, they are no longer used much for anterior teeth. These crowns are thin and flexible to fit over minimally prepared teeth. They have applications in pediatric dentistry when trying to protect a primary tooth until it exfoliates or on an abutment for a fixed space maintainer. Applications for these durable stainless steel crowns also include primary teeth following pulpotomy or pulpectomy, caries involving multiple surfaces where amalgam would not hold up, or fractured teeth. They are also used for adults to protect a tooth when the patient cannot afford a cast metal crown.

METALS USED IN ORTHODONTICS

WIRES

Orthodontic wires are composed mostly of base metals. They are also wrought metal alloys commonly made of stainless steel, cobalt-chrome-nickel, titanium, or an alloy of nickel and titanium. Of these metal alloys, stainless steel is the most commonly used in orthodontics and is easily bent by the dentist.

Special characteristics are manufactured into these archwires to create the desired amount of resistance to deformity. Resistance to deformity creates "memory" in the wire so that it tries to reassume its original shape. It is the "memory" that exerts the forces that move the teeth.

Nickel-titanium (NiTi) alloy was developed in 1963 by Buehler who was a space program metallurgist. It is called **nitinol** as an acronym for nickel titanium Naval Ordinance Laboratory where it was developed. It was introduced to orthodontics around 1970 and has become very popular. Nitinol now encompasses a group of alloys with variations in the ratios of nickel to titanium. Nitinol wires are resilient and springy and maintain their shape. Nitinol wire has the most springback or memory to return to its original shape compared with the other alloy wires, so it more readily facilitates tooth movement with lower force. Because they cannot be bent easily at chairside, they are usually used as preformed archwires. If bent sharply, they are prone to fracture. Another limitation of nitinol is that it cannot be soldered or welded because heating changes its microstructure.

The orthodontist will order wires either preformed or straight wires in various lengths and diameters. The diameter of wire is sometimes referred to as its gauge. The thicker the wire, the smaller its gauge; thus 8-gauge wire is thicker than 16-gauge wire. The diameter of wire is more commonly described in hundredths of an inch (e.g., 0.36 inch). Most orthodontic wires are supplied using the inch diameter classification, although some manufacturers, particularly in Europe, use millimeters as the unit of measure. Wire is strong but can be made to fracture by repeatedly bending it back and forth. Repeated bending reduces the wire's ductility and strain hardens it, eventually causing it to break. Some archwires are preformed to the approximate shape of a dental arch.

BRACKETS AND BANDS

Orthodontic brackets and bands are bonded or cemented on the teeth, and they retain the archwire that the orthodontist has shaped. The archwire is shaped into a form that will guide the teeth into their new position. When the wire is tied to the brackets of the teeth, the wire tries to assume its ideal form, and as a result, exerts a force on the teeth that gradually moves them in the desired direction. The archwire is held to the bracket or band by ligature wire or elastics. Metal orthodontic brackets are cut and shaped from stainless steel alloy and are attached to a stainless mesh backing (see Chapter 5 Principles of Bonding, Fig. 5.33). They are bonded to the tooth with bonding resin or other appropriate luting cement that locks into the mesh backing (see Chapter 5, Procedure 5.3). The edgewise bracket, which is the most common, has a horizontal slot between four wings. The slot is where the archwire is placed, and the wings are used to hold the elastics or ligature wire that secures the archwire. Orthodontic bands are formed from a stainless steel alloy and are preformed or formed at chairside by the dentist. Stainless steel brackets, tubes, and hooks are welded onto the bands or brackets for the purpose of attaching intraoral wires, elastics, or extraoral headgear (Fig. 11.12).

RETAINERS AND REMOVABLE ORTHODONTIC APPLIANCES

A retainer is often placed to help maintain the position of the teeth after orthodontic treatment. It provides long-term stabilization of the anterior teeth. Retainers can be fixed or removable and often use a round wire to help hold the teeth in position. A fixed lingual retainer is simply a wire adapted to the lingual surfaces of the mandibular anterior teeth and bonded in place with composite resin (Fig. 11.13). On occasion, a similar fixed retainer is used on the lingual surfaces of the maxillary anterior teeth. It may be shortened to include only the maxillary central incisors if its purpose is merely to prevent a midline diastema from reforming after orthodontic closure. A removable retainer often uses a wire embedded in acrylic. The wire engages the facial surfaces of the teeth and holds them in

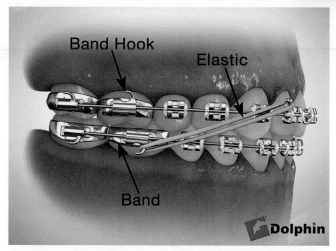

FIG. 11.12 Orthodontic bands with tubes and hooks, edgewise brackets, archwires, and elastics used for tooth movement. (Courtesy of North Coast Orthodontics.)

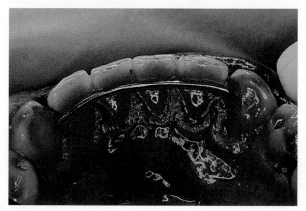

FIG. 11.13 Orthodontic bonded wire lingual retainer. (Courtesy of Steve Eakle, University of California, San Francisco [San Francisco, CA].)

position. Some removable appliances used for minor tooth movement also use a wire embedded in acrylic. In this case, the wire is activated to put pressure on the teeth to be moved (Fig. 11.14). After the teeth have moved into their desired position, the appliance can be used as a retainer by keeping the wire resting passively against the facial surfaces of the teeth.

SPACE MAINTAINERS

When teeth are lost prematurely, it is desirable to prevent adjacent teeth from drifting into the space. If the space of a primary tooth is lost, the permanent tooth may not have room to erupt into its proper position. If a drifting neighbor takes up the space of a lost permanent tooth, there may not be adequate room for a bridge or implant and the drifting tooth may tip into the space, altering its proper alignment. Fixed and removable space maintainers are often used temporarily to hold the space. Common fixed space maintainers consist of a wire loop that is attached to a stainless steel crown or an orthodontic band. The loop rests against the adjacent tooth and holds it in position (Fig. 11.15).

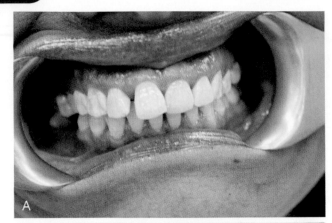

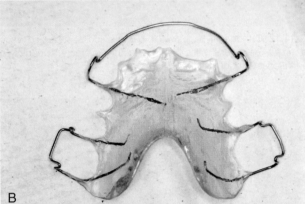

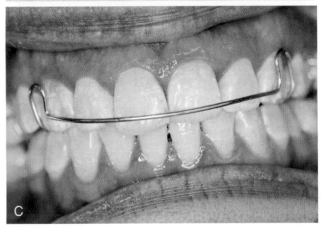

FIG. 11.14 Removable orthodontic appliance to retract tooth #8. It can serve as a retainer after tooth movement has been accomplished. **A,** Protruding maxillary central incisor. **B,** Hawley appliance with adjustable labial wire bow to move tooth lingually. **C,** Tooth has been repositioned. (Courtesy of Dr. Scott Rooker, Bend, OR.)

METALS USED IN ENDODONTICS

ENDODONTIC FILES AND REAMERS

Endodontic files and reamers are other examples of wrought metal used in dentistry. They are made of wrought wire that has been twisted to produce multiple cutting edges (Fig. 11.16). Files are made of stainless steel or nickel-titanium and are used within the root canal to clean and shape it for final filling. Stainless steel files become stiffer as the diameter of the file increases. This stiffness is not desirable when curved canals are instrumented, because the files tend to remove more dentin at

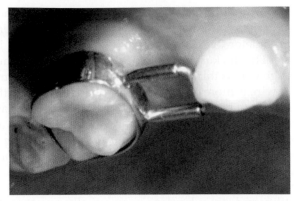

FIG. 11.15 Fixed band and loop space maintainer. (Courtesy of Brent Lin, Pediatric Dentistry, University of California, San Francisco.)

the point of the curvature. Nickel-titanium (nitinol) files are far more flexible than stainless steel files. They have an enhanced elastic characteristic that allows them to return to their original shape after they have had a load or force put on them. When used for instrumenting curved canals, they will regain their shape, unlike stainless steel files.

Some files are used to instrument root canals by hand, and some are used in slow-speed dental handpieces at low speeds and are called *rotary instruments*. Rotary instruments are usually composed of nickel and titanium alloys. Rotary instruments are very popular and allow root canal therapy to proceed much faster and more efficiently. Their flexibility is highly desirable in a curved canal, because they can follow the curvature of the canal more easily and remove less dentin than stainless steel files.

Both hand files and rotary files are subject to metal fatigue that can cause fracture of the file after repeated use. If the file fractures within the root canal, it might not be able to be removed. This could result in failure of the root canal treatment. The dentist and the assistant should determine how many times a file can be used, and then should discard the file when it has reached that limit. A tracking system must be developed to document how many times each file has been used.

Reamers are similar to files except that they have fewer twists in the metal and cut faster. Reamers are made by twisting a tapered triangular or square rod so that its cutting edge is parallel to its long axis. It is used for cutting canal walls to enlarge and shape them. A reamer will remove debris more efficiently than a file.

ENDODONTIC POSTS

Teeth in which the pulpal tissues are infected or die often receive root canal therapy (endodontic treatment). Conventional root canal therapy generally entails making an access preparation through the crown of the tooth to the pulp chamber, removing the diseased pulpal tissue from within the root canal with a series of fine files, and sealing the root canal space with a special sealing material (gutta percha) and a sealing cement so that bacteria cannot grow in the space.

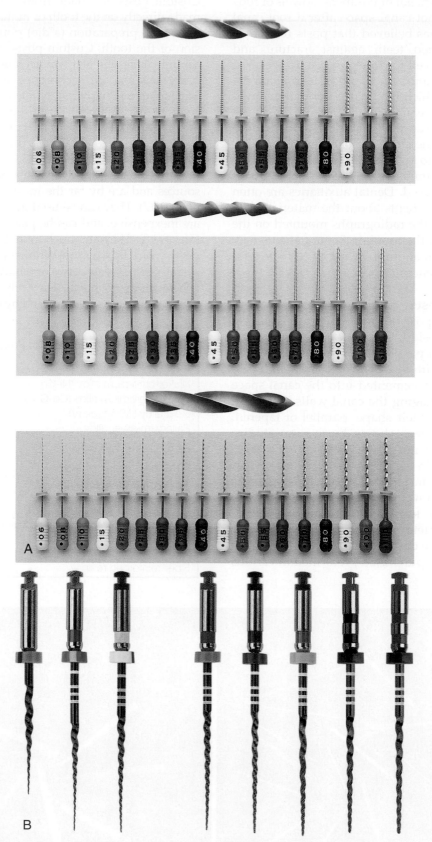

FIG. 11.16 A variety of endodontic files. **A,** Types of hand files. **B,** Rotary files. (**A,** From Robinson DS, Bird DL: Endodontics. In *Essentials of Dental Assisting,* ed 6. St. Louis, 2017, Elsevier. **B,** Courtesy of Dentsply Sirona.)

Purpose of the Post

Endodontic posts are metal or nonmetal dowels or rods placed within the root canal space after a root canal treatment. It once was believed that posts reinforced endodontically treated teeth against fracture, and many posts were placed for this purpose. However, it is now clear that the purpose of a post is to retain the core buildup over which the final restoration (crown) is placed. If there is adequate tooth structure remaining to hold the core buildup without a post, a post should not be used. While the choice of using posts or other retaining designs is up to the dentist, it is important for all clinicians to be familiar with the various types of posts that might be used. Dental auxiliaries are often asked questions by patients about the materials they see in their teeth on the radiographs mounted on the view box or seen on the monitor. Some patients may confuse the post with an implant and need to be educated as to the differences.

Classification of Posts

It is beyond the purpose of this section to discuss retention and post design, but basically posts can be classified as active or passive. Active posts engage the root canal surface with threads like a screw, and passive posts are simply cemented into the canal space without actively engaging the canal walls. Posts can also be classified by their shape: parallel or tapered. Parallel posts have been shown by in vitro studies (meaning they were not conducted in living creatures but were done in the laboratory) to transmit less stress to the root than tapered posts. Tapered posts when loaded place a wedging force on the root, with a higher risk of root fracture. Posts can be made of metal or can be nonmetal such as resin-fiber posts (Table 11.3). Posts can be custom-made in the laboratory (cast posts) or can be purchased preformed in various sizes and materials.

Custom Posts

Custom posts are made from a wax or resin pattern made directly on the tooth or in the laboratory on a replica of the preparation (a die) poured from an impression of the tooth. Custom posts are cast into metal or ceramic using the lost wax technique, or can be milled using CAD/CAM techniques (see Computer-Aided Machining in Chapter 9). Noble or base-metal alloys or ceramic-fired materials are used. Cast posts generally are made as one unit with the core already attached.

Preformed Posts

Preformed posts are available from many commercial sources and are by far the most commonly used posts (Fig. 11.17). They can be used in most clinical situations, are inexpensive, and can be placed in one appointment (Fig. 11.18). They are much more time efficient than cast posts, which take two appointments. The designs of these preformed posts are active or passive, parallel or tapered, and metal or nonmetal. They rely on retention by their length, diameter, and shape and by the use of a cementing

TABLE **11.3**   Composition of Posts
CUSTOM CAST POSTS
Nickel-chromium alloy (Ni-Cr)   Cobalt-chromium alloy (Co-Cr)   Gold alloy (ADA type IV)   Palladium-silver alloy
PREFORMED POSTS
A. Metal
Titanium (99% pure)   Stainless steel (Fe-Ni-Cr)   Titanium-aluminum-vanadium alloy (Ti-Al-V)
B. Nonmetal
Ceramic (zirconia)   Fiber-reinforced resin

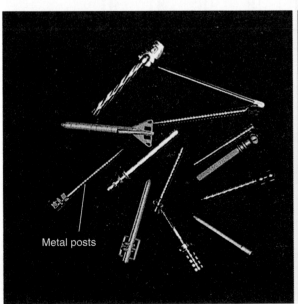
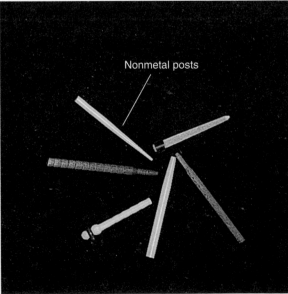

Metal posts

Nonmetal posts

FIG. 11.17 A variety of preformed metal and nonmetal posts.

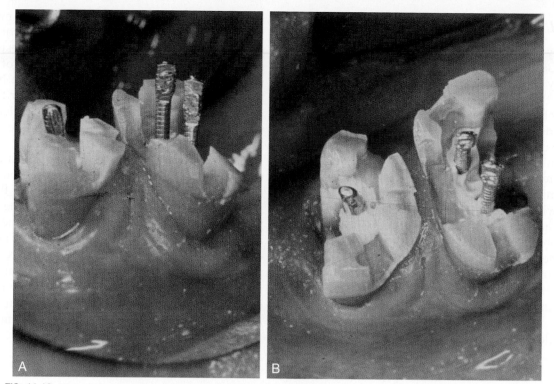

FIG. 11.18 Clinical photographs of preformed metal posts. **A and B** show two views of preformed metal posts that will be used to retain a composite resin core. Supplemental retention boxes have been cut to lock in the core material. (Courtesy Dr. Dennis J. Weir, Novato, California.)

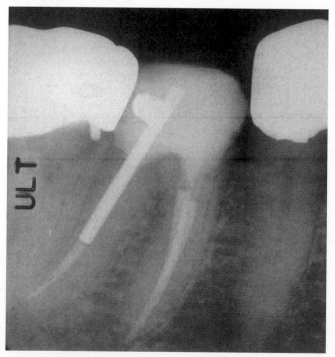

FIG. 11.19 Radiograph of lower first molar with endodontic gutta percha filling and metal preformed post in the distal canal. A composite core has been added. The post retains the core. (Courtesy of Dr. Steve Eakle.)

or bonding medium (see Chapters 5 and 14 for discussions of bonding and cementing materials). Preformed posts come in kits with drills specific to the size and style of the post. Preformed metal posts (Fig. 11.17) are made of stainless steel, titanium, or titanium alloy. Preformed nonmetal posts are made of fiber-reinforced resin or ceramic materials. Preformed posts generally do not have a core attached by the manufacturer, so one must be added (Fig. 11.19). The core can be made of amalgam, composite resin, or resin-modified glass ionomer cement.

SUMMARY

Metals play a major role in restorative and corrective dentistry. Gold and alloys of gold are some of the most biologically compatible materials and have many uses, even with the shift toward cosmetic dentistry. Noble and non-noble metals have a significant role in modern prosthetic dentistry. They are the main support for removable partial dentures, fixed bridges, and prostheses used in combination with implants. Orthodontic treatment relies heavily on the use of metal. Brackets are predominantly metal, although some are ceramic. Wrought wire, with its "memory," exerts predictable forces and has made the job of the orthodontic clinician easier, improved comfort for the patient, and reduced the time needed for treatment. Titanium is a lightweight metal and has good characteristics of strength and elasticity. Titanium alloy is the main alloy used for dental implant fixtures (see Chapter 12). It is used as an alloy with nickel for archwires in orthodontics and for endodontic hand files and rotary instruments.

Endodontic treatment has moved into the modern era with the use of rotary files and the controlled speed of the electrical handpiece. Likewise, the restoration of endodontically treated teeth and the use of post and core materials have changed dramatically. Now, both metal and nonmetal posts are available for the dentist to select for the process of restoring endodontically treated teeth. The indications for each are important for the clinician to understand.

Patient education is an important aspect of the role of the dental auxiliary in dental practice. Your ability to describe to the patient the pros and cons of the various materials used in practice and to aid in the treatment process depends on your knowledge of these materials. As new metal-based materials are introduced into dental practice, it is important to stay current on their properties, indications, contraindications, and application techniques. Manufacturers' instructions for their care and use should be followed. Many manufacturers have websites on which they post information relative to their materials.

Get Ready for Exams!

Review Questions

Select the one correct response for each of the following multiple-choice questions.

1. The ADA recognizes which three major categories of alloys?
   a. High noble, noble, and low noble
   b. High noble, noble, and base metal
   c. Precious, semiprecious, and nonprecious
   d. Class I, II, and III

2. High-noble metal classification must contain what percent by weight of gold?
   a. 40%
   b. 60%
   c. 75%
   d. 90%

3. Noble metal elements include all of the following *except*
   a. Silver
   b. Gold
   c. Palladium
   d. Platinum

4. How does porcelain bond to metal alloys?
   a. By fusing to oxides formed on the surface of the metal
   b. By sandblasting the metal surface to roughen it
   c. By the use of metal bonding adhesive systems
   d. By melting the surface of the metal and embedding the porcelain in it

5. When bonding porcelain to metal for a crown, the metal must have which one of the following properties to prevent cracking of the porcelain?
   a. high hardness
   b. high density
   c. low melting range
   d. low thermal expansion

6. Metal that is formed by casting into an ingot or bar and then is altered in its form by extruding or pressing it is known as
   a. Stainless steel
   b. Wrought metal
   c. Milled metal
   d. Brazed metal

7. High-noble alloys usually have which metals added to increase their hardness?
   a. Silver or copper
   b. Nickel or beryllium
   c. Iron or aluminum
   d. Chromium or cobalt

8. Which type of orthodontic wire has the most springiness and tendency to maintain its original shape?
   a. Stainless steel
   b. Cobalt-chrome nickel
   c. Gold
   d. Nickel-titanium (nitinol)

9. Allergy to nickel
   a. Occurs in less than 3% of the population
   b. Is seen only in the oral cavity
   c. Occurs 10 times more often in women than in men
   d. Is associated more often with orthodontic wire than with crowns

10. Solder has all of the following uses *except* one. Which one?
    a. Adding a contact to a crown
    b. Joining a pontic to a bridge retainer
    c. Repairing a hole in the occlusal surface of a crown discovered in a patient's mouth
    d. Joining a wire loop to a band to make a space retainer

Get Ready for Exams!—cont'd

11. The purpose of a flux used during soldering is to
    a. Lower the melting point of the solder
    b. Make the solder harden quickly
    c. Prevent the solder from flowing to areas where the solder is not needed
    d. Remove oxides from the surfaces of the metals so the solder can flow and wet the surfaces better

12. Preformed metal posts are available in all of the following materials ***except*** one. Which one?
    a. Pure gold
    b. Stainless steel
    c. Titanium
    d. Titanium alloy

13. The purpose of a post is to
    a. Strengthen the root
    b. Put a permanent seal over the root canal filling material
    c. Strengthen the core material
    d. Retain the core material

14. An all-metal crown that is yellow in color has which one of the following?
    a. A high gold content
    b. A high copper content
    c. A high palladium content
    d. Can't tell the composition from the color

15. All of the following statements about cast posts are true ***except*** one. Which one?
    a. They may be formed from a wax or acrylic resin pattern.
    b. They can be cast using high-noble, noble, or base-metal alloys.
    c. They usually have the core already attached to the post.
    d. They are used in practice far more often than preformed posts.

16. The alloy most used for partial denture frameworks and most resistant to fatigue failure of the clasps is which one of the following?
    a. cobalt-chromium alloy
    b. stainless steel
    c. gold alloy
    d. titanium alloy

For answers to Review Questions, see the Appendix.

Case-Based Discussion Topics

1. A 33-year-old schoolteacher comes to the dental office to have a crown placed on tooth #18. The dentist has told the patient that she should have a gold crown. After the dentist has left the room, the patient asks you if there are any cheaper metals that could be used. She says that she has no insurance and is short of money at this time.

What can you tell her about the general types of metals used for cast crowns and what the pros and cons are for each?

2. A 65-year-old retired accountant comes to the dental office with a gold crown for tooth #19 in his hand. It came off last night while he was eating sticky candy. The patient complains that since the crown was placed last year, he has been packing food between the crown and tooth #20, which has a disto-occlusal amalgam. The crown has an acceptable fit to the tooth and no dental caries are present. The amalgam is also acceptable.

What procedures can you suggest to solve the food impaction problem without remaking the crown or the amalgam? What materials should be used? Describe the correct sequence for the procedure(s).

3. A 46-year-old businesswoman at her annual oral examination complains that as her gum has receded on tooth #12, a dark line can be seen at the margin of a porcelain-bonded-to-metal crown that was placed 5 years ago. She is unhappy with the appearance and is concerned that it might be "decay."

What is the likely cause of the dark line she is referring to? How might the dentist have prevented this from occurring?

4. A 34-year-old female schoolteacher presents to your dental office complaining that she broke off a cusp on her lower left first molar. Visual inspection reveals that tooth #19 is missing the distolingual cusp down to the gingival crest, and a large MOD amalgam is present. The patient is a heavy bruxer and she admits that she wakes up sometimes grinding her teeth. The dentist recommends a crown to restore the tooth.

From a strictly functional perspective, what type of crown would be the most trouble free and durable? If the patient selects a porcelain-fused-to-metal (PFM) crown with porcelain on the occlusal surface, what should the patient be told regarding the risks and benefits of this type of crown?

5. As you are preparing for a cementation appointment for a porcelain-bonded-to-metal crown for tooth #12, you notice several small cracks in the porcelain. The crown has just come from the lab and has not been in the patient's mouth.

If the crown was not dropped or otherwise mishandled, why did these cracks appear? Discuss compatibility problems as they relate to the physical properties of the porcelain and the porcelain-bonded alloy. Should the dentist proceed with the cementation of the crown?

6. A 58-year-old female mail carrier presents for her annual periodic examination. She says she has noticed some inflammation in the gum around tooth #14 that started 2 weeks after a base-metal crown was placed last year. She says she has been brushing and flossing carefully but the inflammation does not go away.

What are some possible causes for the inflammation? If a prophylaxis and application of antibiotics to the sulcus have no effect, what now becomes a greater suspect for the cause? If the dental laboratory uses IdentAlloy labels, what information can you glean that might help in determining the likely cause?

BIBLIOGRAPHY

American Dental Association (ADA): *Council on Scientific Affairs: Products of Excellence: ADA Seal Program*, Chicago, 1999, ADA.

Anusavice KJ, Shen C, Rawls HR (eds): Dental casting alloys and metal joining, wrought metals. In *Phillips' Science of Dental Materials*, ed 12, Philadelphia, 2013, Saunders.

Department of Health and Human Services, Agency for Toxic Substances and Disease Registry: *Beryllium Toxicity: Patient Education Care Instruction Sheet*. Updated May 2008. Accessible at https://www.atsdr.cdc.gov/csem/csem.asp?csem=5&po=15.

Leinfelder KF: An evaluation of casting alloys used for restorative procedures, *J Am Dent Assoc* 128:37–45, 1997.

Powers JM, Wataha JC: Casting alloys, wrought alloys and solders. In Yen-Wei Chen, editor: *Dental Materials: Foundations and Applications*, ed 11, St. Louis, 2017, Elsevier.

Roach M: Base metal alloys used for dental restorations and implants, *Dent Clin N Am,* 51:(3):603–627, 2007.

Robinson DS, Bird DL: Endodontics. In *Essentials of Dental Assisting*, ed 6, St. Louis, 2017, Elsevier.

Rosenstiel SF, Land MF, Fujimoto J (eds): *Laboratory Procedures. Contemporary Fixed Prosthodontics*, ed 5, St. Louis, 2016, Elsevier.

Sakaguchi RL, Powers JM (eds): Restorative materials—metals. In *Craig's Restorative Dental Materials*, ed 13, Philadelphia, 2012, Mosby.

Sansone V, Pagani D, Melato M: The effects on bone cells of metal ions released from orthopaedic implants. A review, *Clin Cases Miner Bone Metab*, 10(1):34–40, 2013.

Van Noort R: Structure of metals and alloys. In Michele Barbour, editor: *Introduction to Dental Materials*, ed 4, St. Louis, 2013, Mosby.

Dental Implants

http://evolve.elsevier.com/Eakle/materials/

Chapter Objectives

Upon completion of this chapter, the student should be able to:

1. Describe the components of an implant used for a crown.
2. Describe the most common materials used for dental implants.
3. Explain osseointegration of an implant.
4. Discuss the indications and contraindications for dental implants.
5. Explain the advantages of image-guided implant surgery.
6. Identify risks to the patient for implant surgery.
7. Describe the sequence of the one-stage surgical procedure.
8. Present postsurgical instructions to a patient.
9. Compare the one-stage, two-stage, and immediate surgical procedures.
10. Discuss the pros and cons of immediate loading of an implant.
11. Explain the process of taking an implant impression.
12. Compare the open-tray and closed-tray impression procedures.
13. Make an impression for an implant, using the open- or closed-tray procedure (as permitted by state law).
14. Identify the uses for mini-implants.
15. Define the types of bone grafting.
16. Describe the purpose of the sinus lift procedure.
17. Identify when sutures would be utilized in a dental procedure.
18. List the different types of sutures.
19. Describe the types of needles used to place sutures.
20. Demonstrate the removal of sutures.
21. Describe the assessments that should be done for dental implants at the hygiene visit.
22. Demonstrate to a patient the use of home care aids for dental implants.
23. Explain the rationale for the selection of instruments for cleaning titanium implants.
24. Perform periodontal maintenance around an implant (hygienists) using appropriate probes, scalers, curettes, and ultrasonic tips.

Key Terms

Endosseous Implant implant placed into the bone

Implant Fixture metal or ceramic component placed into bone to support a crown or prosthesis

Implant Abutment metal or ceramic component that connects the implant crown to the implant fixture

Healing Abutment a component placed temporarily on the implant fixture during the healing phase to allow the gingiva to adapt to it and form a cuff that will function around the implant

Osseointegration bone growing into intimate contact with an implant fixture after placement (a microscopic space exists between the bone and the implant surface)

Biointegration a total integration of the implant fixture with the bone (without a microscopic space) that occurs with ceramic implant materials

Mini-Implant a very small–diameter implant that can be placed with minimal surgery involved

Cone Beam Computed Tomography (CBCT) type of digital tomographic radiography used to produce three-dimensional images of the jaws; useful for analyzing the structures before surgery

Cover Screw component placed in the top of the implant fixture to prevent tissue from growing into the screw hole when the fixture is covered with the flap in a two-stage surgical procedure

Impression Abutment component used in the implant impression to align the implant analog in the same way as the implant fixture was in the mouth

Implant Analog a substitute for the implant fixture used during the laboratory fabrication of the implant crown

Open-Tray Impression impression for implants that uses a tray with a hole over the impression abutments to be able to remove the abutments with the impression

Closed-Tray Impression impression for implant that removes the impression with the impression abutment still attached to the implant fixture; the abutment is later removed and placed in the impression

Temporary Anchor Devices (TADs) small, tack-like mini-implants used on a temporary basis as anchors for orthodontic tooth movement

Autograft graft tissue harvested from the patient's own body

Allograft tissue taken from a donor (usually deceased) for grafting in another human

Xenograft graft tissue taken from an animal (usually bovine) for use in a human

Alloplast synthetic graft material

Barrier Membrane protective membrane that prevents the in-growth of fibrous connective tissue into a graft site and also holds the graft material in place

Sinus Lift a surgical procedure that lifts up the floor of the maxillary sinus to allow placement of a bone graft. It is used to provide adequate bone for an implant when there was not enough available over the maxillary sinus

Peri-Implantitis an infection around an implant that can cause gingival inflammation and loss of bone around the implant

Sutures natural or synthetic material with the appearance of thread used to hold tissues together or to reposition tissues after trauma or surgical procedures

Absorbable Sutures sutures broken down naturally by the body's enzymes and absorbed

Non-Absorbable Sutures sutures made of materials that are not broken down by the body and require removal by a dental professional

For centuries people have attempted to replace missing teeth with some form of implant. The first evidence of attempted implants was bamboo pegs placed in a jawbone in ancient China 4000 years ago. Then 3000 years ago in ancient Egypt, a copper stud had been nailed into a jawbone. The Mayans, in about 600 C.E., tried implanting carved shells into the anterior mandible. Centuries later, in 1905, C.R. Scholl introduced a porcelain root-form implant to the modern world. Over the next 60+ years many materials and implant designs were used with limited success. The major breakthrough came in 1969 when P.-I. Brånemark and co-workers using medical implants reported their finding of integration of bone with an implant surface. The Brånemark dental implant system was introduced into the United States in 1982. The development of endosseous root-form implant treatment has rapidly progressed over the last 40+ years with high success rates. Advances in technology with cone beam computed tomography (CBCT) and computer-aided design software have helped dentists more accurately plan for and place dental implants. Bone grafting and guided tissue regeneration have helped to improve bone in sites for implant placement where previously the patient would have not been considered a candidate for implants. The introduction of narrow-diameter implants has also broadened the applications of dental implants. The use of implants in modern dentistry has accelerated rapidly, with sales of implant components exceeding 3.5 billion dollars worldwide.

This chapter emphasizes endosseous implants, because they are the most widely used. The materials used for implants and the indications, contraindications, placement, restoration, integration with bone, components, and maintenance are discussed. It is essential that the dental hygienist have an understanding of the characteristics of the various implant materials to correctly manipulate and care for them. The dental assistant and hygienist must be able to answer questions by patients relative to the material and techniques that will be used for their treatment. In addition, they must have an understanding of the process of restoring implant fixtures so they can ably assist the dentist. Where allowed by state law, hygienists and assistants trained in expanded functions can make impressions for implant restorations and play an important role in implant maintenance.

DENTAL IMPLANTS

Dental implants are of three main types: subperiosteal, transosteal, and endosseous (Fig. 12.1). With

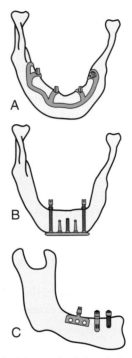

FIG. 12.1 Older implant types. **A,** Subperiosteal. **B,** Transosteal. **C,** Older variety of endosseous implants. (From Phillips RW, Moore BK: *Elements of Dental Materials for Dental Hygienists and Dental Assistants.* Philadelphia, 1994, WB Saunders.)

subperiosteal implants a surgical excision exposes the bony ridge and an impression is made. A metal framework is fabricated and placed over the bony ridge (and beneath the periosteum) with metal struts protruding through the soft tissues to support a prosthesis. The transosteal implant (also called a *mandibular staple*) is placed from under the chin and has a flat plate from which two to four threaded posts projected through the anterior mandible into the oral cavity. The posts are used to support a complete denture. Subperiosteal and transosteal implants are rarely done because of the high success rate of endosseous implants. Endosseous implants are the most commonly used implants in dentistry today and are the focus of this chapter.

ENDOSSEOUS IMPLANTS

Endosseous implants are surgically placed into the bone and act like a root substitute for missing teeth to support a crown or prosthesis (Fig. 12.2). Implants can be used to replace one or more single units as

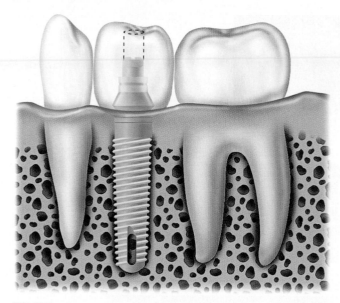

FIG. 12.2 Contemporary endosseous dental implant. (From Rosenstiel SF, Land MF, Fujimoto J: *Contemporary Fixed Prosthodontics*, ed 4, St. Louis, 2006, Mosby.)

individual crowns or as fixed bridges, or they can support a partial or full denture. Their use is expanding as implant materials and techniques continue to improve, and their success rate remains high with careful case selection. Clinical studies have shown these implants to be very successful, with long-term survival (greater than 10 years) of approximately 90% in the maxilla and 95% in the mandible. The difference in success rates between the two jaws is related to the quality of the bone in each jaw. The bone in the mandible is generally much denser.

INDICATIONS FOR IMPLANTS

Implants are indicated for a variety of clinical situations. Because of the excellent survival rate of implants, they are often the treatment of choice in place of a partial denture or a fixed bridge when a single tooth has been lost, particularly when the potential abutment teeth are unrestored. When most of the posterior teeth have been lost in an arch, implants are often preferred to a distal extension partial denture. When a patient has a problem stabilizing a denture because of extreme ridge resorption, implants can be used to anchor the denture. Implants may also be indicated to improve function and esthetics.

CONTRAINDICATIONS FOR IMPLANTS

Implants are contraindicated in patients who have medical conditions (such as advanced cardiovascular or respiratory disease) that make them poor candidates for surgery. Patients with conditions that can affect their ability to fight infections or heal properly (such as diabetes) are not good candidates for implants. Patients who have recently taken bisphosphonates (such as Boniva and Zometa) to prevent osteoporosis or that have had radiation therapy affecting the implant site are not candidates for implants because of the risk of delayed bone healing and bone infection (osteonecrosis). Patients with compromised immune systems are also not candidates for implants. Smokers are not good candidates because their healing may be compromised. In addition, patients who are mentally or physically not able to maintain good oral hygiene or those with unrealistic expectations are not candidates for implants.

BENEFITS OF IMPLANTS

Dental implants have several benefits that make them a desirable means for restoring the dentition. When implants are used in place of a fixed bridge, tooth structure is preserved because abutments do not have to be prepared. The individual implant units are easier to keep clean than a fixed bridge, so the gingiva stays healthier and the caries incidence of adjacent teeth is lowered. When teeth are extracted the bone at the site begins to resorb fairly rapidly soon afterward and then continues more slowly over time. When an implant is placed it helps to preserve the bone both in ridge height and width.

Patients with complete dentures can bite and chew with only a small fraction of the force they could with their natural teeth. The muscles of mastication weaken and show signs of atrophy and the ridges resorb. With an implant-supported denture, biting, chewing, and speaking are improved. Muscle tone is regained and the implants help preserve bone. The patient is more comfortable, especially when chewing hard foods, and does not have the discomfort associated with shifting of the denture and pressure on the soft tissues. The esthetic result often is improved because the teeth can be set where most attractive rather than being limited to placement over the center of a ridge that has resorbed.

IMPLANT COMPONENTS

Numerous components are used for restoration with an implant. Some components are permanent parts of the implant, and others are used temporarily for healing phases, impression making, or crown construction. Different terms may be used to describe them, depending on the manufacturer. Conventional dental implants used to support crowns and bridges have three basic components: the implant fixture, abutment, and crown (or bridge) (Fig. 12.3).

Implant fixture: The **implant fixture** is that portion of the implant that is placed in the bone and remains there to support the crown (or other prosthesis).

Implant abutment: The **implant abutment** is an attachment to the implant fixture that protrudes through the gingiva and acts like a tooth preparation on which the crown attaches or the prosthesis rests. The abutment is usually attached to the fixture with a screw. Another type of abutment is the **healing abutment.** The healing abutment is attached to the fixture and is

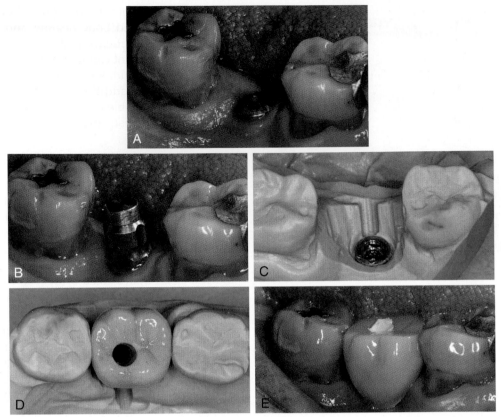

FIG. 12.3 Implant components. **A,** Healing abutment placed after the surgeon uncovers the top of the implant fixture to allow the soft tissue to adapt. **B,** Impression abutment facilitates orientation of an implant analog to the cast in the same way the implant fixture was oriented in the mouth. **C,** Implant analog is used in the laboratory as a substitute for the implant fixture, so the implant crown can be made. **D,** Screw-retained implant crown with occlusal screw-access hole. **E,** Implant crown in the mouth with the access hole filled. (Courtesy of Fritz Finzen, University of California School of Dentistry [San Francisco, CA].)

placed temporarily to allow the gingiva to heal around it and form a gingival cuff and sulcus. Both the abutment for a crown and the healing abutment may be prefabricated or custom made. Prefabricated abutments are generally round, so the gingiva conforms to the round shape. However, teeth are rarely round in shape. Custom abutments are shaped more like the root form of the teeth they are replacing. The custom abutment may be made by a laboratory technician or milled by a CAD/CAM (computer-aided design/computer-aided machining) unit.

Implant crown or *prosthesis:* When a single tooth is being replaced, a crown is made to fit to the abutment much like a crown is made to fit to a prepared tooth. When multiple teeth are being replaced, an implant supported fixed bridge, removable complete denture, or partial denture is used.

Other Components

Additional components are needed in the implant procedure. Titanium alloy screws are used to attach the abutment to the implant fixture and in some cases will attach the crown to the abutment. Of course, a screwdriver is also needed. The **cover screw** is the component that is placed in the top of the implant fixture in the two-stage surgery; it prevents bone and tissue

growth into the top of the implant while it is covered with the surgical flap during the healing phase. The healing abutment replaces the cover screw after the top of the implant is uncovered during the second stage of the two-stage surgery procedure (see Fig. 12.3, *A*). A torque wrench is used to tighten various components of the implant to very specific amounts of force (expressed in newtons [N]). Impression and laboratory components are discussed in the section "Implant Impression and Laboratory Components."

IMPLANT MATERIALS

Various materials have been used for implant fixtures over the years, but metal and ceramics are the materials currently used. The metals of choice are titanium and titanium alloy.

Titanium

Titanium (Ti) and titanium alloys are the metals most commonly used because of their favorable biocompatibility with the oral tissues. Their elastic modulus is the closest to bone of the materials used for implants. As a result, forces placed on the implant will be more evenly distributed between the implant and the bone. Those implant materials with an elastic modulus much greater than bone will concentrate stress within the implant.

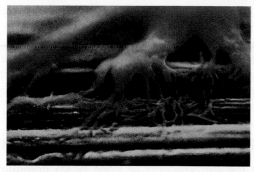

FIG. 12.4 Osseointegration - bone cells growing in contact with a titanium implant (Courtesy Professor Per-Ingvar Branemark, Institute for Applied Biotechnology, Gothenburg, Sweden.)

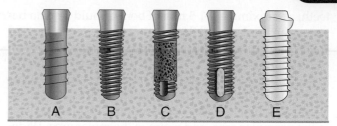

FIG. 12.5 Implant designs. From left to right: **A,** Cylinder. **B,** Tapered. **C,** Textured. **D,** Vented. **E,** Ceramic cylinder.

Titanium is a lightweight, corrosion-resistant, biocompatible material that is 99% titanium with oxygen and trace elements. Bone will grow around and closely adapt to titanium and titanium alloy implants (a process called **osseointegration**) when they are placed intimately in contact with the bone (Fig. 12.4). There should be no fibrous connective tissue formed at the interface, but there will be a microscopic space present between the fixture surface and the bone. There will be no mobility of the implant.

Titanium is not as rigid or strong as titanium alloy, and this property can occasionally lead to failure of an implant if it is placed under heavy loading forces (such as with patients who grind their teeth frequently). Titanium quickly forms a thin surface layer of oxides that will integrate with the bone. Titanium alloys contain small amounts of vanadium (decreases corrosion) and aluminum (increases strength, decreases density) to improve their mechanical properties, particularly their tensile strength. Ti-6Al-4V is a commonly used titanium alloy containing 6% aluminum and 4% vanadium. Because of the favorable mechanical properties of titanium alloys, they are also used for the screws that hold the implant components together.

Ceramics and Other Implant Materials

Other materials that have been used for dental implant fixtures are ceramics, composites, vitreous carbon, polymers, and a variety of metals including gold. These materials have been used with limited success. Composite, vitreous carbon, and polymer implant fixtures did not integrate with the bone. Negative aspects of the early ceramic materials were their brittleness and lack of flexibility, causing them to transmit greater stress to the implant site; these implant fixtures were at greater risk of fracture from functional forces.

Newer ceramics such as zirconia (see Chapter 9 Dental Ceramics) are much stronger and hold up better than older ceramics that were brittle and ran the risk of fracture. Ceramic implants will integrate with the bone more intimately than titanium implants. It is thought that they integrate chemically with the bone so that that there is continuity between the ceramic surface and the bone (with no microscopic space as seen with osseointegration); this is called **biointegration**.

Ceramics are also used for implant abutments in the esthetic zone, particularly where all-ceramic crowns are used to restore the implants. Metal abutments tend to show through and cause a gray coloration in the cervical area of the crowns, due to the partial translucency of the ceramic crowns. Zirconia and titanium are equally biocompatible implant fixtures.

IMPLANT FIXTURE DESIGNS

Over the years, various endosseous implant designs have been used. Today, the most commonly used implant fixtures are the threaded type with a cylindrical or tapered shape. The threads vary in their spacing and angulation. Some designs include the use of very small threads at the coronal aspect of the implant to aid in directing forces away from the implant top. This helps to prevent loss of bone at the crest with resultant gingival recession and compromised esthetics.

Some threads are sharp and will cut into the bone. An initial pilot hole is made slightly smaller than the implant, which is screwed into place, making for a very close adaptation to the bone. Nobel Biocare makes an implant with self-cutting threads. Other manufacturers produce implants with non-cutting threads (Straumann, for example). Some designs have a hollow core with or without holes in the apical portion. The holes were placed to allow bone to grow into them and mechanically lock the implant in place. The expectation is that these surface designs will help the integration of bone with the implant (Fig. 12.5).

Early implant fixtures were flat on top, allowing bacterial contamination of the internal portion of the implant with an ensuing inflammatory response from the tissue. Current implants use a conical connection that provides a seal against bacteria and as a result a healthier periodontium.

Implant Dimensions

The dimensions of implant fixtures can vary in diameter and length to fit the implant site and amount of available bone. The size of the tooth being replaced is a factor in determining the diameter and length of the implant fixture used. A wider diameter implant fixture provides more surface area for support of the crown or prosthesis. When an implant is placed between two adjacent teeth, approximately 1.5 mm of bone should remain between the implant and the adjacent tooth root to prevent compromising the bone. Likewise, there should be 1.5 mm of bone on the facial and lingual surfaces to prevent bone remodeling and gingival recession. When the patient is partially or totally edentulous, implant size in the mandibular anterior may be 3 mm or smaller, 4 mm in the premolar area, and 6 mm in the molar area. Wide-bodied implants have diameters ranging from 8 to 10 mm. They are often used when a shorter length of implant is needed; their larger diameter provides additional surface area for support to make up for the lack of length. Very small–diameter implants (**mini-implants**) are growing in popularity for mandibular complete denture support (they are discussed in the section "Retention of the Removable Prosthesis").

Surface Treatment

Titanium and its alloys are very reactive and will readily form oxides on their surfaces. Manufacturers will create these oxides in a controlled environment to prevent contamination of the oxide layer. To further protect from contaminants, after their manufacture the implant fixtures are sealed in containers and are protected until they are ready to be placed in bone. The oxide layer is very thin but is essential to integration with bone. Special care must be used when cleaning implants in the mouth to prevent scratching the implant surface. Scratching will disrupt the oxide layer and allow contaminants to form on the damaged surface.

Manufacturers may roughen the surfaces of the implant fixtures to increase the surface area available for integration with bone. Roughening has been accomplished by sandblasting, etching with acid, or coating with titanium plasma spray. Some studies show faster healing and greater integration with the bone with rough-surface implants. Bone apposition of 80% or more occurs when surface roughening is used as opposed to only 40% bone-to-implant contact with implants that were not roughened.

Ceramic coatings have been used on titanium alloys to promote more rapid integration with the bone. The ceramic materials are applied in thin layers by a plasma spraying process. The bond of the ceramic coating may break down with time, and therefore use of this process is controversial.

Epithelial Seal

Epithelial cells will adapt to and adhere to the surface of the implant to provide a seal to prevent the ingress of bacteria along the implant interface with the bone. This seal is important to the longevity of the implant.

ADA Seal of Acceptance

Of the many companies that manufacture implants, only a few (including Nobel Biocare, Astra, and Straumann) have obtained the American Dental Association (ADA) Seal of Acceptance. The ADA requires companies to submit information about the materials used, research, and 5 years of clinical testing. The U.S. Food and Drug Administration (FDA) does not require clinical testing. Although the ADA seal is not required to sell implants, it demonstrates a commitment by the companies to produce a reliable product.

IMAGE-GUIDED IMPLANT PLANNING AND SURGERY

Before the introduction of **cone beam computed tomography (CBCT)**, most surgeons relied on their clinical examination and two-dimensional radiographs. Panoramic radiographs magnify dental structures by about 25%, and thus the risk of introducing errors is increased. The use of CBCT provides the dentist with very accurate three-dimensional images of the dental structures. With CBCT the density of the bone, the thickness and height of the ridge at the planned implant site, the location of nerves and major blood vessels, and the size and configuration of the maxillary sinuses can all be assessed. Therefore, the surgeon can have an image of the anatomy of the patient's jaw with all of its concavities and irregularities prior to the surgery.

IMPLANT PLANNING SOFTWARE

Treatment planning software can import CBCT images, allowing the surgeon and restorative dentist to plan for the implant placement surgery. They can virtually extract teeth and determine precisely where the implant should be placed. They can plan for the type of implant; the proper diameter and length of the implant; and the proper position in the buccolingual, mesiodistal, and apicocoronal dimensions. Bone density can be determined, and the surgeon can simulate placement of the implant. The CAD simulation can determine the angulation and position of the implant for ideal esthetics and gingival contours. Once the proper placement is determined, then CAD/CAM technology can be used to create accurate acrylic models of the patient's jaws, if needed, and make precision surgical guides for placement of the implants (Fig. 12.6). Three-dimensional (3D) design software creates a digital image of the surgical guide. The guide can be fabricated by milling or 3D printing. If printing the guide, the design information is fed to a 3D printer. Instead of cutting away material as milling does, 3D printing builds up the surgical guide as it sprays the material in successive layers to make the desired form.

ADVANTAGES OF GUIDED IMPLANT SURGERY

Implant surgery that is precision guided by this technology affords several distinct advantages. Among these advantages are the following:
- The option to place the implant without laying a flap; this leads to less postoperative discomfort and faster healing

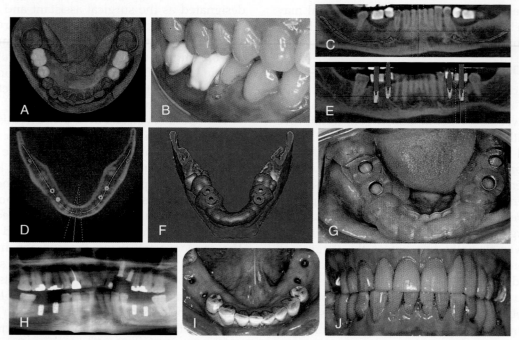

FIG. 12.6 Image-guided implant planning and surgery combines cone beam computed tomography (CBCT) and implant planning computer software. **A,** Plastic guide with barium-filled teeth marks positions in the CBCT scan. **B,** Scan guide in the mouth. **C,** Barium-filled teeth show up in the scan (white opaque). **D,** Scan lines (orange) orient position of transverse cross-section of the mandible. **E,** Software allows simulation of implant placement. **F,** Software designed surgical guide for correct position of implants. **G,** Surgical guide positioned in the mouth. **H,** Implant fixtures seen in panoramic radiograph. **I,** Implant fixture heads seen in the mouth. **J,** Restored implants in the mouth (From Rosenstiel SF, Land MF, Fujimoto J: *Contemporary Fixed Prosthodontics,* ed 4, St. Louis, 2006, Elsevier.)

- Fewer perforations of bone by a misaligned drill
- Improved prosthetic outcomes of treatment and enhanced esthetics because of better implant placement
- Increased survival rates for the implants

Minimally invasive surgical techniques are greatly facilitated by image-guided surgery.

CAD/CAM TECHNOLOGY

In Chapter 9, Ceramics, CAD/CAM technology was discussed regarding fabrication of ceramic restorations. The same technology can be applied to fabrication of custom implant abutments and crowns. Additionally, when implants are placed in the socket immediately after extraction of the tooth, a provisional restoration can be fabricated to support the gingival tissues and help maintain their contours during healing. A digital impression could be made prior to the extraction to fabricate a provisional restoration shell that can be relined with acrylic to fit the newly placed implant and support the gingival tissues. Otherwise, the provisional restoration can be made immediately after the extraction and placement of the implant. Milling or 3D printing can be used to fabricate the provisional restoration to fit the implant. After the soft tissues and bone have healed, a custom abutment and crown can be made from a new digital scan. A new scan is made because the gingival tissues will likely have shrunk some during healing and the contours of the crown will be made to accommodate for that change.

IMPLANT PLACEMENT AND RESTORATION

Variations are seen in the surgical approaches to implant placement and in healing times before the crown or other prosthesis is placed. Decisions underlying these variations depend on whether there is already a healed edentulous space with adequate bone or whether a tooth needs to be extracted first. The surgery for implant placement is often done by an oral surgeon or a periodontist. However, many well-trained general dentists are now placing implants in the more straightforward cases—those patients who are healthy and have adequate bone. Implants are restored by general practitioners and prosthodontists.

INFORMED CONSENT

Before the surgical procedure the patient must be fully informed of the risks, benefits, and alternatives to implants. The patient must be given the opportunity to ask questions and have things explained in terms they can understand. Many times the patient will ask the dental assistant or hygienist questions about implants or the surgery, so it is important to be knowledgeable about the entire implant process.

SURGICAL RISKS

Risks from the implant surgery include the usual surgical risks of excessive bleeding and swelling, infection, and necrosis of the gingival flap. In addition, there are risks of perforation of the bone or the maxillary sinus, puncture of major blood vessels, and damage to nerves. Also, bone grafting material may not develop a blood supply and new bone, and the implant fixture may not integrate with the bone.

PREPARATION OF THE PATIENT FOR SURGERY

Several steps can be taken to enhance the success of the surgery. An oral hygiene appointment should be scheduled a week or so before the surgery to improve gingival health and remove any calculus that could break off and fall into a surgical site. Prior to the surgery, postoperative instructions should be reviewed with the patient while they are still capable of listening to and understanding the instructions. The patient should also be given written instructions as many patients will forget or misunderstand portions of the instructions given verbally. Just before the surgery all removable prostheses should be removed and the mouth rinsed with an antibacterial rinse such as chlorhexidine (e.g., Peridex or PerioGard) to reduce bacterial levels in the mouth. Some clinicians like to administer an antibiotic and an anti-inflammatory medication (e.g., ibuprofen) to minimize the risk of infection and reduce swelling. The surgery can be done under a local anesthetic, but some patients prefer oral or intravenous sedation. Sedated patients may be kept in recovery for an hour or more and should have someone drive them home after the surgery.

POSTSURGICAL INSTRUCTIONS

First, provide the patient with a cold pack to place on the face in the area of the surgery to help minimize swelling. The patient can apply an ice pack at home—10 minutes on, 10 minutes off—for a couple of hours. Postsurgical instructions should be reviewed again or reviewed with a companion who will be with the patient at home. A pack of sterile gauze should be provided to use with pressure for an hour or two on the surgical site to control bleeding. The patient should rest and limit physical activity, eat soft foods, drink plenty of fluids but not through a straw (to avoid disrupting any clots), avoid smoking, and avoid vigorous rinsing. All medications should be taken as prescribed. Warm salt water rinses three or four times a day can be started the day after the surgery and continued for about 4 days (unless the patient has high or uncontrolled blood pressure which would limit sodium intake). The surgical site should not be brushed but can be cleaned gently with a cotton swab or gently wiped with a piece of gauze during the first week. Heavy or prolonged bleeding, abnormal swelling, intense pain, and allergic reactions should be reported to the surgeon at once. For any adverse reactions perceived to be life-threatening, the patient or companion should call 911.

PREPARING THE OPERATORY FOR SURGERY

A team approach is important for implant surgery. Team members should know the role they will play and their responsibilities. One assistant should be designated as the surgical assistant and a second assistant should be a roving assistant to retrieve supplies. The responsibility of the surgical assistant is to set up the operatory; transfer instruments; retract cheeks, tongue, or the flap; evacuate saliva from the mouth and blood from the surgical site; and carefully monitor the patient during the procedure.

The operatory needs to be properly disinfected and clean zones with barriers established for placement of sterile instruments and supplies. A sterile field must be maintained during the surgery. Implant kits are available that are prepackaged and sterile. The kits contain many small parts and drills. A system should be established to keep all of the parts organized. Many kits contain labeled holders for the drills and components. The sequence for using the components of the kit should be rehearsed. Members of the surgical team should know the terminology of the parts so that communication during the surgery is clear. In addition, a throat drape or barrier should be used to prevent aspiration or the swallowing of small parts if they are dropped in the mouth. A common safeguard is to tie a long piece of floss around the handle of small screwdrivers to quickly retrieve them. Sterile saline is used for irrigation and as a coolant because city water supplies will have bacterial contaminants.

IMPLANT PLACEMENT SURGERIES

Presently there are three modes of implant placement surgery:
- two-stage
- one-stage
- immediate placement

TWO-STAGE SURGICAL PROCEDURE

The surgical procedures are done in two stages.

First Stage

The first stage involves exposing the bone at the chosen placement site with a surgical flap. Next, a hole (called an *osteotomy*) is drilled in the bone at low speed and with sterile saline irrigation to prevent overheating the bone. A series of burs will be used, starting with a small-diameter bur and increasing to the size of the implant fixture being used. The hole is the shape and length of the implant fixture and a size that is just slightly smaller than the fixture. Depending on the implant fixture design, the implant is either lightly tapped into place to have a frictional fit with the bone, or it is screwed into place. Often an acrylic resin surgical guide (called a *stent*) is made ahead of time with holes drilled through it at the same angulation at which the implant should be positioned. The surgeon places it over the ridge at the time of surgery and inserts a bone-cutting bur through the predetermined holes to cut the hole for the implant at the correct angulation. The stent is particularly helpful when the surgeon must place several implants that need to be parallel to each other for purposes of the restoration that will be placed on the implants. It is important that excessive heat not be generated during drilling of the bone. The bone can be damaged easily and then will not integrate with the implant fixture.

After the implant fixture is placed in the bone, a cover screw is placed into the opening at the top of the fixture (Fig. 12.7). The cover screw prevents tissue from growing into the screw hole to which the future abutment will be attached. The surgical flap is repositioned and sutured closed over the implant.

Second Stage

Approximately 3 months later, the surgeon uncovers the top of the implant fixture, removes the cover screw, and places a smooth, prefabricated or custom healing abutment (Fig. 12.3, A) that screws onto the top of the fixture. Next, the soft tissue (gingiva) is positioned around the healing abutment, leaving it exposed to the oral cavity while the gingiva heals around it. This process allows the gingiva to form a cuff around the implant, which will adapt to the crown when it is placed. After a few weeks, the crown impression procedure can begin.

ONE-STAGE SURGICAL PROCEDURE

With the one-stage procedure, surgery for placement of the implant fixture is performed just as with the two-stage procedure. The difference is that with the one-stage procedure, a cover screw is not placed at the top of the fixture and it is not covered with the gingival flap. Instead, the healing abutment is placed and the gingiva is positioned around the healing abutment and sutured (Fig. 12.8). The one-stage procedure is increasing in popularity, because it saves the patient from having to go through a second surgery. It is best used when the patient's restorative needs are not complicated. Occasionally, a provisional crown is placed that is out of occlusion while healing takes place.

The two-stage surgery was popular when osseointegration was first introduced to dentistry in the 1980s, because it was thought that covering the implant during healing was needed to ensure success. Research has shown that there is no difference in survival of the implant between the one-stage and the two-stage surgery.

IMMEDIATE-PLACEMENT SURGICAL PROCEDURE

When the implant procedure involves the extraction of a tooth, some clinicians place the implant fixture at the time of extraction directly into the new socket. This is called an *immediate-placement implant,* and this procedure is growing in popularity. A soft tissue flap is used to cover the extraction site until bone fills in and integrates with the fixture. Often an artificial bone material is also placed in the socket to aid the growth of new bone into the socket and to help stabilize the fixture.

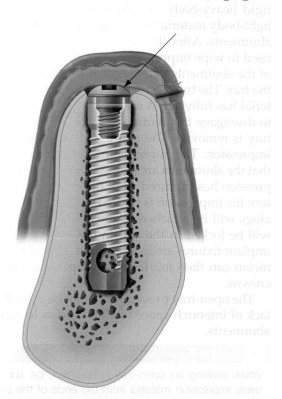

FIG. 12.7 Cover screw (also called healing screw) used in a two-stage surgical procedure. It prevents tissue from growing into the screw hole after the implant fixture is covered with the surgical flap. (From Rosenstiel SF, Land MF, Fujimoto J: *Contemporary Fixed Prosthodontics,* ed 4, St. Louis, 2006, Mosby.)

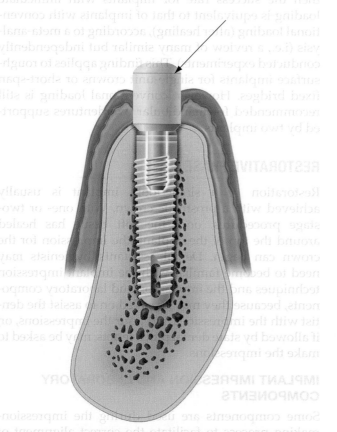

FIG. 12.8 Healing abutment used immediately in a one-stage surgical procedure or in a two-stage procedure after initial healing of 2 to 3 months. The healing abutment is placed to allow the gingiva to form a cuff around it. (From Rosenstiel SF, Land MF, Fujimoto J: *Contemporary Fixed Prosthodontics,* ed 4, St. Louis, 2006, Mosby.)

There is a slightly higher rate of failure of the implant after initial placement with this procedure compared with the one- or two-stage surgical approaches.

IMMEDIATE LOADING

Initially, it was thought that 3 to 6 months of healing was needed so that osseointegration could occur before the implant could be loaded. Loading, it was thought, would cause movement of the fixture that would result in failure to integrate with the bone and loss of the implant. However, more recent findings suggest that it is the stability of the implant in bone that is important for loading rather than osseointegration. Therefore, many clinicians are placing the abutment and a provisional crown at the same visit as the placement of the implant fixture. Usually, this is done when the implant is long and wide enough to engage sufficient bone in the socket and beyond to have a stable fixture. If needed, bone grafting material is packed around the fixture to provide additional stability. Loading of the implant under chewing forces, then, occurs before integration of the fixture with the surrounding bone. However, forces still need to be controlled, distributed, and directed along the long axis of the implant.

If the surgical procedure is performed in accordance with a careful protocol and the fixture is very stable, then the success rate for implants with immediate loading is equivalent to that of implants with conventional loading (after healing), according to a meta-analysis (i.e., a review of many similar but independently conducted experiments). This finding applies to rough-surface implants for single-unit crowns or short-span fixed bridges. However, conventional loading is still recommended for mandibular overdentures supported by two implants.

RESTORATIVE PHASE

Restoration of a single-tooth implant is usually achieved with a prosthetic crown. With one- or two-stage procedures, once the soft tissue has healed around the top of the implant, the impression for the crown can begin. Dental assistants/hygienists may need to become familiar with the implant impression techniques and the impression and laboratory components, because they may be called on to assist the dentist with the impressions and pour the impressions, or, if allowed by state dental practice acts, may be asked to make the impressions.

IMPLANT IMPRESSION AND LABORATORY COMPONENTS

Some components are used during the impression-making process to facilitate the correct alignment of the implant to the cast. An **impression abutment** (also referred to as the *impression post, transfer post,* or *impression coping*) is attached to the implant fixture (see Fig. 12.3, *B*), and an imprint of it is captured in the impression. The abutment is transferred from the mouth to the impression, and when the impression is poured, it becomes part of the cast. The **implant analog** is the component used during laboratory construction of the implant crown. It attaches to the impression abutment and is used to replicate the implant fixture for the laboratory cast (see Fig. 12.3, *C*); the impression abutment orients the analog in the cast in the same way that the implant fixture is oriented in the mouth.

IMPRESSION PROCEDURES

There are two conventional impression techniques used for dental implants:
- open-tray impression
- closed-tray impression

Open-tray impression. The **open-tray impression** (also called a *pick-up impression* because it picks up the abutments in the impression) is the easiest for the inexperienced clinician (Fig. 12.9). With this procedure a plastic impression tray is tried in for fit to the arch. Then, the impression abutments are attached to the implant fixtures. The plastic tray is reinserted into the mouth, and the location of the abutments is marked on the tray. An acrylic bur in the straight handpiece is used to cut a window in the tray over the abutments, so the ends of the abutments can be accessed when the tray is in place. Next, the impression is made. Usually, polyether or polyvinyl siloxane impression materials are used. A rigid heavy-body material is used in the tray and a light-body material is syringed around the impression abutments. After the tray is seated, a gloved finger is used to wipe impression material away from the ends of the abutments that are accessed through the hole in the tray. The tray is stabilized until the impression material has fully set. A screwdriver (hex driver) is used to disengage the abutments from the fixtures, and the tray is removed. The abutments will come out in the impression. The impression is inspected to determine that the abutments are properly seated and that the impression has captured all of the structures needed. Before the impression is poured in die stone, implant analogs will be attached to the abutments. The analogs will be locked in the cast in the same position as the implant fixtures are in the mouth. The laboratory technician can then fabricate the implant abutments and crowns.

The open-tray procedure cannot be used if there is a lack of interarch space to allow access to unscrew the abutments.

 Clinical Tip

When making an open-tray impression, be sure to wipe away impression material from the ends of the abutments after the tray is fully seated. Otherwise, you will be frantically searching for the abutments in set material! Don't forget to fully loosen the abutments fully before removing the tray!

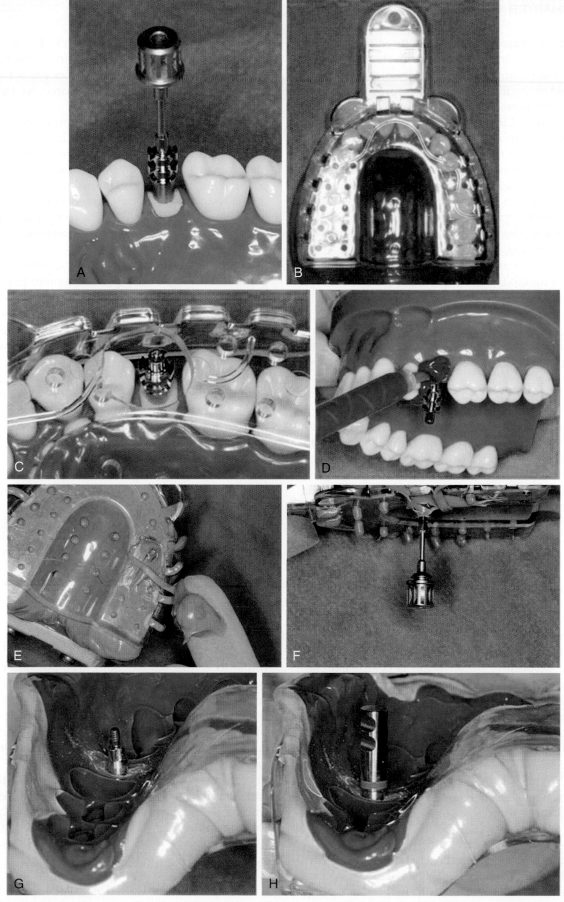

FIG. 12.9 Open-tray impression procedure. **A,** Screw impression abutment into the implant fixture. **B,** Select a plastic impression tray to fit the arch. **C,** Cut a hole in the tray over the top of the impression abutment to allow access to it after the impression material is placed. **D,** Monophase or light-bodied impression is syringed around the abutment and heavy-bodied impression material is placed in the tray, and then the tray is seated. **E,** Impression material is wiped away from the abutment through the hole in the tray. **F,** After the impression material has set, unscrew the impression abutment before removing the impression. **G,** Impression with impression abutment in place. **H,** Carefully attach the implant analog to the end of the impression abutment, making sure it does not shift position within the impression. When poured in stone, the analog will represent the implant fixture (see Fig. 12.3, C). (Courtesy of Arun Sharma, University of California San Francisco School of Dentistry.)

Closed-tray impression. With the closed-tray impression (also called a *transfer impression*), there is no hole cut in the impression tray. The impression abutments are screwed to the fixtures and the impression is made using the same types of materials as with the open-tray procedure (Fig. 12.10). When the set impression is removed from the mouth, the abutments remain in the mouth, attached to the fixtures. The abutments are removed from the fixtures, and then the implant analogs are attached to them. The abutments are reinserted into the impression in their proper orientation. Some clinicians like to syringe some soft tissue-simulating material around the neck of the analog before pouring the impression (Fig. 12.10, panels E-H). (This material will act as gingiva around the analog and is more easily trimmed for laboratory procedures than stone.) The impression is poured in stone and the cast will look the same as with the open-tray procedure.

The biggest drawback of the closed-tray procedure is the potential source of error if the abutments are not placed back into the impression fully or in their proper orientation.

Digital impressions. Digital impression techniques will be discussed in detail in Chapter 15, Impression Materials. Intraoral scanners that can take digital images of the oral structures have been available for over a quarter of a century. This technology can be applied to capturing images of implant components for purposes of fabricating custom implant abutments and crowns. The precise location of the implant can be captured as well as the internal details of the head of the fixture that has anti-rotation and seating orientation features for the abutment.

For the digital impression, a scannable impression coping is placed into the implant fixture and its seating verified with a radiograph. The scan is made and checked to see that all necessary components have been captured: opposing teeth, bite registration, contact areas of adjacent teeth, and gingival contours (Fig. 12.11). The laboratory prescription is completed containing the tooth shade and abutment and crown materials. The scan and prescription can be transmitted by way of the internet allowing the laboratory to start work immediately without having to produce models for the abutment or crown.

RETENTION OF THE IMPLANT CROWN.

Implant crowns can be retained by screws or by cementing. There are pros and cons with each type of retention.

Screw-retained implant crowns. The implant crown can be attached to the implant fixture core by a small screw often made of titanium alloy or gold alloy (Fig. 12.12). Screw-retained crowns are retrievable so that the implant fixture or abutment can be evaluated or the crown replaced or repaired. However, if screws are used and are not tightened properly, they may come

out. If they are tightened too much, the metal of the screw might be strained to the point of breaking. Special wrenches called *torque wrenches* are set to deliver the recommended amount of force to tighten the screws (typically about 35 N).

Screw-retained crowns require an access hole in the crown (see Fig. 12.3, *D* and Fig. 12.12, *A*) for placement or removal of the screw. After the screw is tightened, a soft material such as cotton, gutta percha, or Teflon tape is placed over the screw head (to make retrieval easier), and then a restorative material, usually composite, is placed into the hole (see Fig. 12.3, *E*). The composite may wear or stain with time and may need replacement.

Cement-retained implant crowns. Cementing the implant crown (Fig. 12.13) is a much more popular technique, particularly for anterior crowns. If the crown is cemented with permanent cement, it will not likely be retrievable. But if it is cemented with provisional cement, then retrievability is possible. The downside is that the crowns may come off unexpectedly. It is very important to ensure that no cement remains under the tissue. Cement remnants could cause peri-implantitis and loss of the implant (Fig. 12.14).

If an implant is not aligned properly, it is easier to use a cemented crown to correct the misalignment than a screw-retained crown. With the screw-retained crown the access hole may end up in an undesirable location such as on the facial surface in order to make up for the misalignment.

 Caution

After cementing an implant crown, it is critically important to ensure that all cement has been removed from the gingival sulcus. Cement retained under the gingiva can lead to infection and loss of the implant!

RETENTION OF THE REMOVABLE PROSTHESIS

Implants can be used to support a partial or full denture. In the mandible, atrophy (loss of bone through resorption) of the alveolar ridge is common in patients who have lost teeth at a relatively young age. A complete denture often has very little retention in this circumstance. Implants are a viable option for support and stability of the prosthesis (Fig. 12.15). They can also be used to anchor a prosthesis used to replace missing facial parts, such as a nose, eye, or ear lost to trauma or cancer surgery (see Chapter 17 Polymers for Prosthetic Dentistry, Fig. 17.22).

MINI-IMPLANTS

Mini-implants (also called *narrow-body implants*) are smaller in diameter than conventional implants and typically range in diameter from 1.8 to 2.9 mm. They can be placed in sites where the available bone would be inadequate for conventional implants. They are

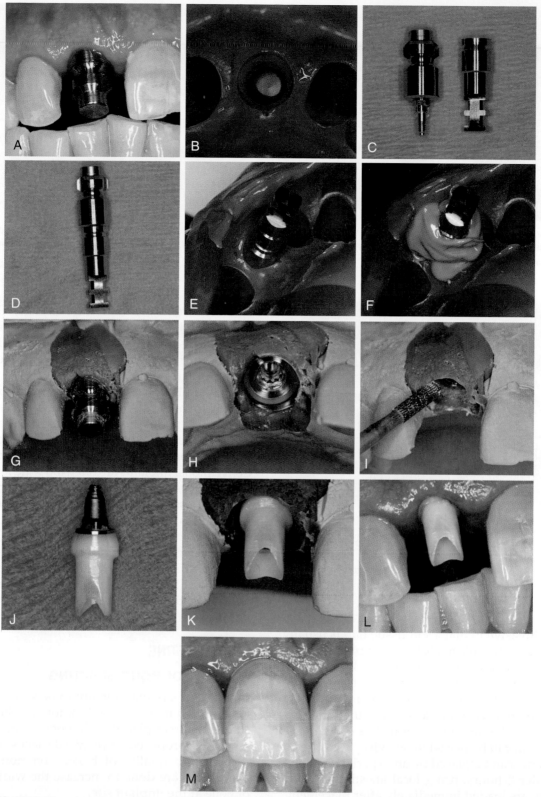

FIG. 12.10 Closed-tray impression technique for a single implant crown. **A,** Impression abutment in place in the implant fixture. **B,** Closed-tray impression showing imprint of the impression abutment. **C,** Impression abutment (on *left*) has been removed from the mouth and is next to the implant analog. **D,** Impression abutment is attached to the implant analog. **E,** Impression abutment is seated into its imprint in the impression. **F,** Soft tissue simulation material is placed around the top of the implant analog before casting in dental stone. **G,** Poured cast with the impression abutment showing. **H,** Implant analog can be seen after the impression abutment has been removed. Impression abutment positions the analog the same way the implant fixture is in the mouth. **I,** Soft tissue material can be shaped to develop the emergence profile of the crown. **J,** Ceramic abutment selected. **K,** Zirconia abutment seated on the cast for crown fabrication. **L,** Zirconia abutment seated in the mouth. **M,** Ceramic crown cemented on the abutment. (From Rosenstiel SF, Land MF: *Contemporary Fixed Prosthodontics,* ed 5, St. Louis, 2016, Elsevier.)

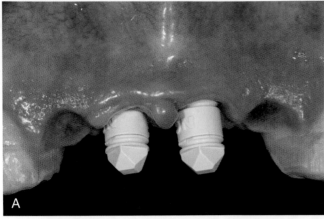
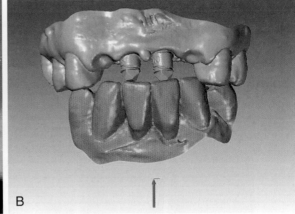

FIG. 12.11 Digital impression for fabrication of implant abutments and cantilevered bridge #7-10. **A,** impression abutments on implant fixtures #8 and 9. **B,** digital impression scan captured the impression abutments, gingival contours, opposing teeth, bite relationship and proximal contact areas of adjacent teeth. (Courtesy Sang J. Lee, DMD, MMSc.)

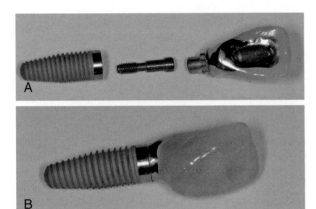

FIG. 12.12 Assembly of implant components. **A,** Screw-retained implant crown with implant fixture and retaining screw. The screw-access hole can be seen on the lingual surface of the crown, and the implant abutment can be seen at the apical end of the crown. **B,** Crown retained on implant fixture by the screw. (Courtesy of Fritz Finzen, University of California School of Dentistry [San Francisco, CA].)

minimally invasive in that a soft tissue flap is usually not needed and the hole made by the implant is much smaller than conventional implants. Healing is faster with less discomfort. The survival rates for mini-implants are similar to conventional implants, ranging from 91% to 96%. They are less costly than conventional implants, because they require less of a surgical procedure and can be placed in one visit. Two to four mini-implants can be placed by an experienced operator in under 2 hours, using local anesthesia. Commonly, they are loaded immediately after placement.

USES FOR MINI-IMPLANTS

One of the main uses for mini-implants is to stabilize a denture. One system (MDI; 3M ESPE) has a ball on the head of the implant that engages an assembly placed in the denture base with a rubber O-ring that snaps over the ball when the denture is fully seated. The denture rests gently on the ridge and gains support and retention from the mini-implant and O-ring (Fig. 12.16). Another system (Locator Overdenture Implant System; Zest Anchors) uses a replaceable retentive head on the implant that engages a retentive cap placed in the denture base instead of an O-ring.

Mini-implants are also used in sites with minimal bone that could not accommodate a conventional implant unless grafting was done. They are used to replace teeth with narrow roots such as lower incisors or upper lateral incisors, and then they are restored with a crown. Conventional implants are often too wide for these sites. A growing use for mini-implants is as **temporary anchor devices (TADs)** in orthodontic treatment when adequate anchorage is not naturally present (Fig. 12.17). They are even smaller than the typical mini-implant, with diameters ranging from 1.2 to 2.0 mm. They can be useful to move molars distally, intrude them, or to help close open bites. The TADs are used short-term (about 6 to 12 months), and then are easily removed.

BONE GRAFTING

PURPOSE OF BONE GRAFTING

In order for a dental implant to be successful it must be anchored in an adequate amount of bone to withstand the forces placed on it. Bone grafting is needed when the proposed implant site lacks an adequate amount and quality of bone. Common bone graft procedures are done to increase the width or height of bone at the implant site.

One type of bone grafting is done before placement of the implant. The alveolar ridge may be deficient in bone, in width or height, or both. Grafting can help to replace the lost bone. The use of three-dimensional imaging, such as cone beam CT, can help the dentist determine which sites are deficient in bone. In addition, in the upper posterior arch the maxillary sinus may be positioned too close to the alveolar ridge so that there is not enough bone to

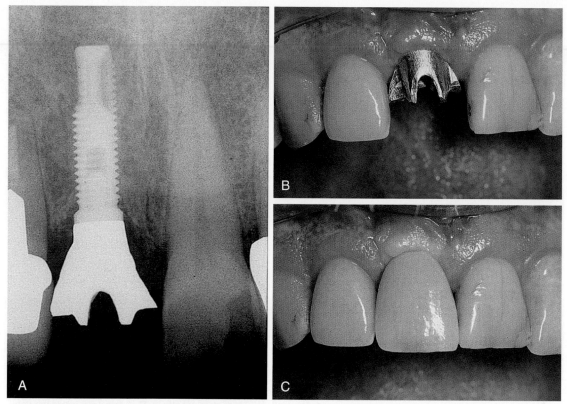

FIG. 12.13 Single-tooth implant with a cemented crown. **A,** Radiograph of fixture in bone and the attached implant abutment. **B,** Abutment is attached to the fixture by a screw. **C,** Crown is cemented onto the abutment. (Courtesy of Mark Dellinges, University of California School of Dentistry, San Francisco, CA.)

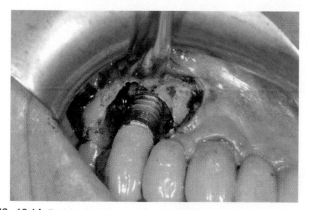

FIG. 12.14 Peri-implantitis resulting in bone loss around the dental implant. (Courtesy of Toronto Implant Institute.)

place an implant. Bone grafting is done to develop adequate bone for placement of the implant.

Another type of bone graft is done at the time of implant placement. It is done when there is generally sufficient bone for implant placement, but some portion of the implant may not be completely covered with bone. Graft material is placed to cover the exposed parts of the implant. Still another use for bone grafting is when an implant is placed in the socket immediately after a tooth is extracted. Bone graft material is placed in the socket around the newly placed implant to help stabilize it and to stimulate new bone to fill in the socket and integrate with the implant.

TYPES OF BONE GRAFTS

Bone graft materials can come from the patient's own body, from a tissue bank with freeze-dried bone from another person, from animal bone components (usually bovine), or from synthetic bone materials. The most effective graft material comes from the patient's own body. Freeze-dried human bone is next in effectiveness followed by animal bone, and then synthetic bone materials. These basic types of bone grafts can be put into four general categories:

* autografts
* allografts
* xenografts
* alloplasts

Autografts. **Autografts** are those harvested from the patient's own body. Typical sites for harvesting this bone are the back of the lower jaw (ramus), chin, hip (iliac crest), or shin (tibia). This grafting material is very effective, because it contains the patient's own bone marrow with cells that can promote bone growth and healing. The negative aspect is that it requires another surgery with a certain amount of discomfort, healing time, and expense.

Allografts. **Allografts** are human bone taken from donors who have donated body parts at the time of their death (cadaver bone). The bone is rigorously washed

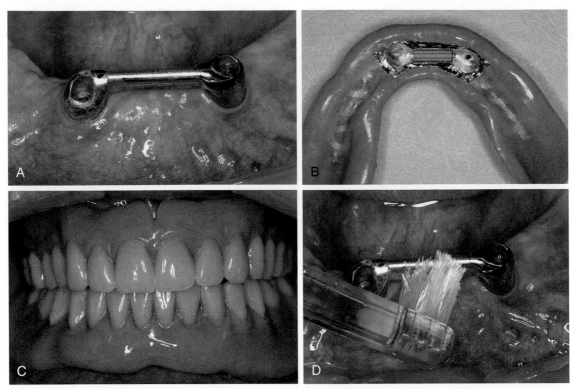

FIG. 12.15 Implant-supported denture. Implants were used because the ridge had resorbed and was inadequate to retain the denture. **A,** Implants supporting a connector bar onto which a lower denture will attach. **B,** A metal clip inside the denture slides over the bar (**A**) to retain the denture. **C,** Lower denture supported by the implants. **D,** The implants and the bar are cleaned with a brush. (Courtesy of Fritz Finzen, University of California School of Dentistry, San Francisco, CA.)

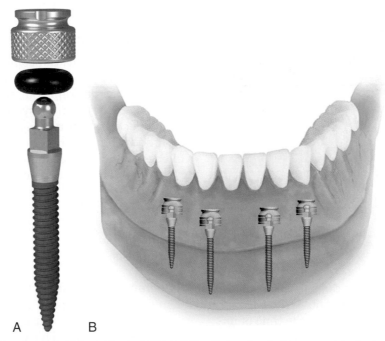

A   B

FIG. 12.16 Mini-implants. **A,** MDI mini-implant (3M ESPE) with housing that is secured to the inside of the denture. The rubber O-ring resides in the housing and snaps over the ball on the head of the implant for retention. **B,** Complete denture is retained by the mini-implants. (Images Courtesy of 3M™ ESPE™ MDI Mini Dental Implants, 2010. All rights reserved.)

and sterilized. It is freeze-dried and stored in a tissue bank. The rigorous processing protocol eliminates concerns of transmitting disease from the donor to the recipient. Allograft materials that are commercially available include Puros (Zimmer Dental) (Fig. 12.18), CreoS (Nobel Biocare), MinerOss (BioHorizons), and DFDB (Biomet).

Xenografts. **Xenograft** material is obtained from animals, usually cows (bovine bone), but occasionally

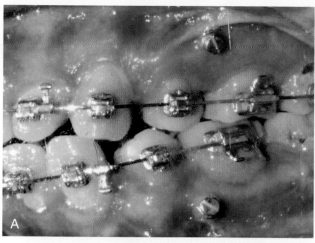
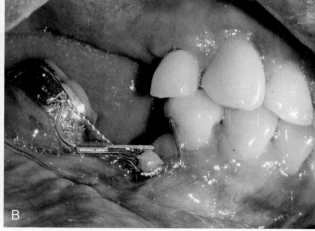

FIG. 12.17 Temporary anchor devices (TADs) are used when there is not enough anchorage in the natural dentition to orthodontically move teeth. They are removed after tooth movement is complete. **A,** TADs for additional anchorage for retraction of teeth. **B,** TAD anchor for molar uprighting. (Courtesy of Jesse Patino, University of California, San Francisco, CA.)

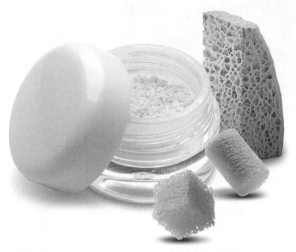

FIG. 12.18 Allograft cadaver bone in granules and large and small pieces. (Puros, Zimmer Dental.)

pigs (porcine bone). The bovine bone is very similar in structure to human bone, so it works well for grafting. The bovine graft material is processed to make it sterile and biocompatible. Only the mineral components are used, and it acts as a matrix or filler around which new bone grows (Fig. 12.19). Xenograft materials include Bio-Oss (Geistlich), PepGen P-15 (Dentsply Sirona), and Endobon Xenograft Granules (Biomet 3i).

Alloplasts. **Alloplasts** are inert, synthetic materials that stimulate new bone growth. They are commonly composed of calcium phosphate or hydroxyapatite, components found in human bone (Fig. 12.20). Often the material is mixed with the patient's bone marrow or with growth factors to stimulate bone activity. It also acts as a matrix or scaffold on which new bone is laid. Some types of alloplastic graft material are resorbed by the body and some types are not resorbed.

Common synthetic graft materials include Bioplant (Kerr Dental), Gem 21S (Osteohealth), and IngeniOs (Zimmer Dental).

Table **12.1**	**Bone Graft Materials**	
TYPE	**MATERIAL**	**SOURCE**
Autograft	Human bone (host)	Iliac crest (hip) Ramus (posterior mandible) Tibia (shin) Mandibular tori
Allograft	Cadaver bone (Fresh, freeze dried, demineralized freeze dried)	CreroS (Nobel BioCare) MinerOss (BioHorizons) Puros (Zimmer Dental)
Xenograft	Mainly bovine bone or porcine	BioOss (Geistlich) Zcore (Osteogenics) MinerOssX (BioHorizons)
Alloplast	Hydroxyapatite Bioactive glass Calcium phosphate Calcium sulfate	Novabone (Novabone Products) PerioGlass (Novabone Products) SynOss (Collagen Matrix)

Potential risks with bone grafting

- Bleeding
- Infection
- Postoperative pain
- Nerve damage causing numbness in lips, gums, and cheek
- Sinus problems with sinus lift or implant encroaching on sinus
- Swelling and bruising
- Inadvertant damage to adjacent teeth or tissues

Newer Additions to Grafting

Bone grafting has been enhanced by the use of human growth factors, such as bone morphogenetic proteins or platelet-derived human growth factor, which can stimulate new bone growth. Bone morphogenetic protein (BMP) can induce rapid bone growth from the body's own

A

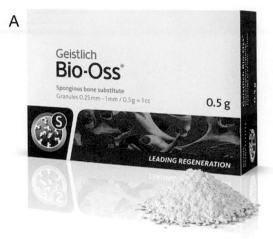

B

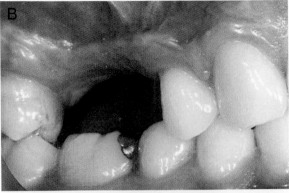

C

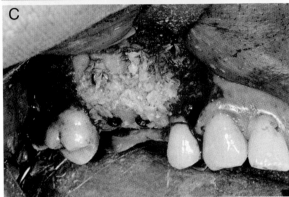

FIG. 12.19 Xenograft mineral granules used for bone graft. **A,** Granular xenograft bone substitute material (also available in blocks). **B,** Edentulous site with inadequate bone for implant. **C,** Xenograft granular bone substitute material packed around newly placed implant fixtures. (**A,** Image used with the courtesy of Geistlich Pharma AG [Wolhusen, Switzerland]. **B** and **C,** Image used with the courtesy of Prof. Dr. M. Chiapasco [Milan, Italy] and Geistlich Pharma AG [Wolhusen, Switzerland].)

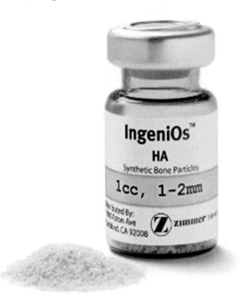

FIG. 12.20 Alloplast synthetic bone made from hydroxyapatite (HA). (Courtesy of Zimmer Dental.)

mesenchymal cells (a process called *osteoinduction*). Some commercial products containing BMP include Regenafil (Exactech), OP-1 (Stryker Biotech), and Infuse (Medtronics). Also, stem cells can be saved in human allograft materials, and they can accelerate the formation of new bone.

For years orthopedic surgeons have used the patient's own blood components, called *platelet-rich fibrin*, to promote bone growth and healing. Some oral surgeons like to use it in their grafting procedures for the same purposes.

Studies are showing that autogenous bone grafts with growth factors are producing the best results compared with other graft materials. The other graft materials lack the live cellular material possessed by autografts.

BARRIER MEMBRANES

At times it is beneficial to cover a bone graft with a protective barrier. The **barrier membrane** is in the form of a thin membrane that prevents fibrous tissue from growing into the site where bone is needed, and it prevents the graft material from being lost from the graft site (Fig. 12.21). The barrier membrane can be made of resorbable or nonresorbable materials. Both types are well tolerated by the tissues.

Resorbable membranes are composed of materials derived from collagen. The ideal situation is to be able to cover the membrane with a soft tissue flap (primary closure), but this is not always possible. Even when not covered by a flap, the collagen-type membrane will stick to and integrate with the surrounding soft tissue. Nonresorbable membranes (such as polytetrafluoroethylene, also known as Teflon) are often chosen when the graft site will be exposed to the mouth. They are removed in approximately 3 weeks.

SINUS LIFT

A **sinus lift** is a surgical procedure that adds bone in the molar and premolar region when the maxillary sinus has extended into that area, bone has resorbed from the alveolar ridge after teeth were lost, or both.

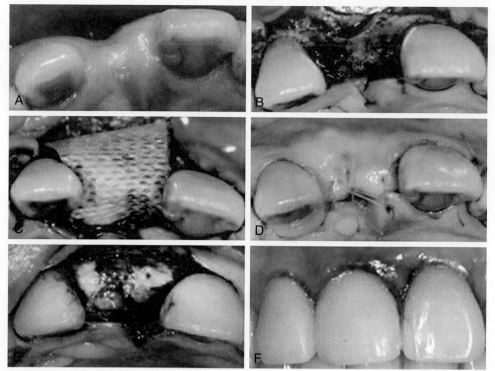

FIG. 12.21 Barrier membrane placed to protect bone graft. **A,** Presurgical edentulous site. **B,** Gingival flap reflected. **C,** Bovine collagen barrier membrane trimmed, hydrated, and placed over graft material. **D,** Gingival flap sutured over bone graft and barrier membrane. **E,** Surgical site 4 months postoperative. **F,** Provisional restoration placed on dental implant. (From Jaypee Journals, Copyright 2013 Jaypee Bros Medical Publishers Article: Comparison of Guided Bone Regeneration using a Bovine Collagen Membrane vs a Calcium Sulfate Barrier, Ghaly M, Kerns DG, Hallman WW, et. al. Jaypee Journals, 2013; 3(3), 138-143.)

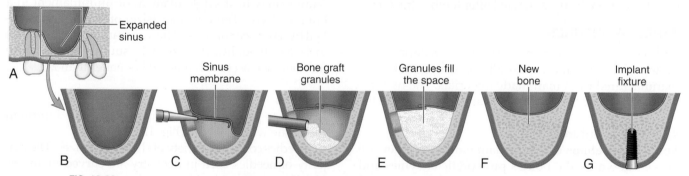

FIG. 12.22 Sinus lift procedure and implant placement. **A,** Maxillary sinus expanded into edentulous space reducing the amount of bone at the ridge. **B,** frontal section through the sinus and ridge. **C,** Entry is made through the lateral sinus wall and an instrument is used to lift the sinus membrane off the sinus floor. **D,** Bone grafting granules are placed on the sinus floor. **E,** Graft material fills the space that was created. **F,** New bone formed around the graft material. **G,** Adequate bone is present and an implant fixture is placed.

An oral surgeon or a periodontist usually does the surgery. For the procedure, a soft tissue flap is raised to expose the bone. The bone is cut to create a window to the floor of the maxillary sinus. An instrument is used to separate the sinus membrane from the bone and lift it up. Bone graft material is placed into the space created by lifting the sinus membrane. The soft tissue flap is repositioned and sutured. New bone will form around the graft material. The area is allowed to heal (typically 4 to 6 months) before an implant is placed in the site (Fig. 12.22). As with any surgery, there can be complications, and the patient needs to be informed of these and give informed consent before the surgery. There can be problems with infection, bleeding, and swelling. The sinus membrane could be perforated or torn and require closure with sutures or a barrier membrane. The patient's bone may fail to integrate with the graft material and the graft may fail to develop a blood supply. These complications may necessitate additional surgery or may preclude placement of an implant in that site.

SUTURES

Extraction of teeth, placement of implant fixtures, bone grafting, and sinus lift procedures often require sutures. The dental assistant or hygienist frequently will assist in placement of sutures and may be asked to remove them (as permitted by state dental practice

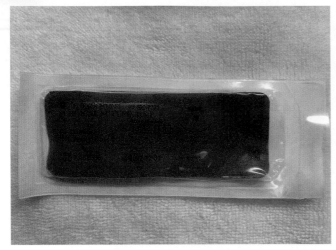

FIG. 12.23 Chromic gut sutures, size 5-0 derived from animal collagen.

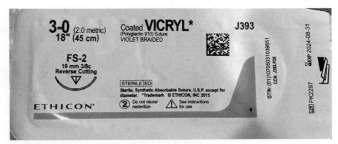

FIG. 12.24 Synthetic polyglycolic acid sutures, size 2-0 (Vicryl, Ethicon Inc.) are made from a biodegradable thermoplastic polymer. (Courtesy of Matt Crimaldi.)

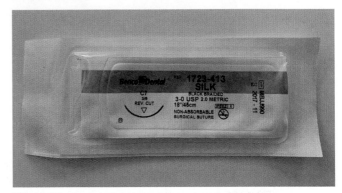

FIG. 12.25 Non-absorbable suture made of braided silk, size 3-0.

acts) after initial healing has occurred. It is important for these dental auxiliaries to know why sutures were needed, which suture materials were used, how long they should remain in place, what to do if sutures come out prematurely, and which suture materials need to be removed or will absorb on their own.

Sutures, also known as stitches, are used to hold tissues together so they can grow together or to reposition tissues after trauma or surgical procedures. Initial healing is considered the point at which sutures are no longer needed, typically 7 to 10 days. Until initial healing has occurred sutures aid in bleeding control and prevent blood clots from being dislodged after tooth extraction.

TYPES OF SUTURES

Sutures can be made from a variety of materials consisting of those that are naturally occurring and those manufactured from man-made materials. The two categories of sutures are absorbable and non-absorbable.

Absorbable Sutures

Absorbable sutures do as the name indicates; they are broken down by the body's proteolytic enzymes and absorbed, thereby eliminating the need for a second removal appointment. Absorbable sutures include synthetic polyglycolic acid and surgical gut in plain or chromic. Surgical gut sutures are composed of purified collagen taken from the serosal or submucosal layer of intestines from cattle, sheep, or goats. With chromic gut sutures the collagen has been treated with chromic acid which almost doubles the length of time over plain gut before they absorb (Fig. 12.23). Synthetic polyglycolic acid (Vicryl) (Fig. 12.24) sutures are made from a biodegradable thermoplastic polymer.

Non-Absorbable Sutures

Non-absorbable sutures are not absorbed by the body's enzymes and must be removed at a later appointment. See Procedure 12.1 for suture removal technique. If not removed the body will see the sutures as a foreign body and initiate the inflammatory process. Non-absorbable sutures

include surgical silk (Fig. 12.25), polyester fiber and nylon.

Characteristics of Sutures

Sutures may be a single filament or multifilament in a braid or twist. The diameter (size) of sutures is identified by a number of zeros. The sizes range from 0 (ought) to 8-0 (eight ought). The size of the suture declines as the number increases such that 8-0 is smaller than 2-0.

Needles

In order to place sutures the filament is pulled through the tissue with a needle (Fig. 12.26).

Needles come in a variety of shapes and sizes. The majority of needles used in dentistry are curved in an arc. Needles are tapered with a round cross-section or cutting with a triangular cross-section. Cutting needles have a sharp triangular apex. Those with the cutting surface on the bottom of the triangle are called reverse cutting.

Needles are predominately composed of stainless steel. Needles can have an opening (eye) that the suture material passes through and a knot is tied to hold the suture to the needle.

The second needle option does not have an eye and is called a swaged needle. The end opposite the sharp tip is a tube that the suture material is inserted and the tube crushed (swaged) onto the suture binding it to the needle. Due to the absence of a knot, swaged needles pass through the tissue more easily and cause less tissue damage.

Suturing Techniques

Interrupted sutures are those placed where each stitch is tied and knotted separately. Examples include

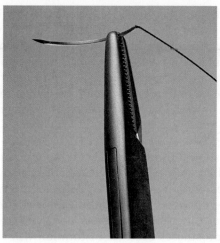

FIG. 12.26 Suture needle attached to suture. (From Hupp JR, Ellis E III, Tucker M: *Contemporary oral and maxillofacial surgery*, ed 6, St Louis, 2014, Mosby.)

single interrupted suture and mattress interrupted suture. The continuous suture is a series of sutures made with one thread that is tied at the beginning and end of the series. Examples include the continuous blanket suture and the simple continuous suture. (Fig. 12.27)

IMPLANT LONGEVITY

IMPLANT FAILURE

Early failure of an implant is usually due to failure of the bone to integrate with the implant. Lack of integration can be due to poor surgical technique, lack of proper infection control, excessive generation of heat when the implant hole is drilled in the bone; infection of the implant site; poor quality of bone; or placement of loading forces too soon on the implant. Failure of the implant that occurs after the initial integration is often caused by bacterial infection extending from the peri-implant tissues into the bone, or overloading of the implant during function, leading to loss of the supporting bone.

Potential Adverse Outcomes from Implant Placement

- Failure of implant to integrate with bone
- Loss of integration
- Infection around the implant
- Systemic infection
- Perforation of maxillary sinus, nasal cavity, inferior alveolar canal, buccal or lingual cortical plate of bone
- Inadequate sterility of implant fixture, leading to infection and implant loss
- Heat damage to bone during drilling for implant site
- Improper angulation of implant that compromises esthetics or function
- Damage to adjacent teeth during implant placement
- Nerve damage
- Lingering numbness or pain

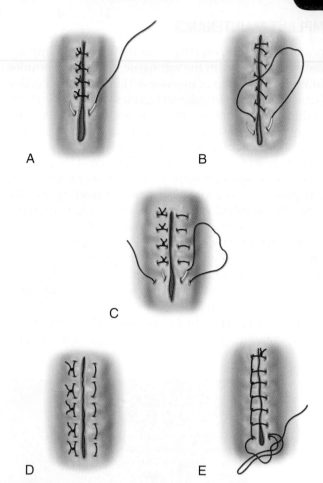

FIG. 12.27 Types of suturing techniques. **A,** Interrupted sutures. **B,** Continuous suture. **C,** Vertical mattress suture. **D,** Horizontal mattress suture. **E,** Continuous box suture. (From Singh PP, Cranin AN: *Atlas of Oral Implantology*, ed 3, St. Louis, 2010, Mosby. In Bird DL, Robinson DS: *Modern Dental Assisting*, ed 11, St. Louis, 2015, Elsevier.)

LONG-TERM SUCCESS

Long-term success is found with implants that have integrated with the bone, and when the implant components are kept clean, the surrounding gingiva is maintained in a healthy state, and forces on the implant are not excessive and are aligned with the implant. Forces on the implant must be properly managed. Because the implant has no periodontal ligament, patients cannot sense how much pressure they are applying to the implants. Therefore, forces must be distributed across the arch to other teeth or prostheses. Excessive force can result in loss of bone around the implant as well as fracture of ceramic crowns, denture bases, denture teeth, and implant components. Bruxers can stress the implant components to the point of fracture, resulting in implant failure. Occlusal guards are often indicated for bruxers.

When the negative factors are well controlled, implants have success rates of 95% or more and the implant crowns may last 10 to 20 years or more. Complete and partial dentures may need replacement as teeth wear or bases break.

IMPLANT MAINTENANCE

In addition to its interface with the bone, the implant has an interface with the soft tissue, where it protrudes through the gingiva or mucosa. Although no connective tissue fibers (i.e., periodontal ligament or junctional epithelium) are connected to the implant surface, as they are to the cementum on the root surface of a natural tooth, close adaptation and attachment of the sulcular epithelium to the implant surface are noted (Fig. 12.28). This close adaptation helps to develop a biological seal that prevents microorganisms from invading the tissues. The implant surface can accumulate bacterial plaque and calculus, just as teeth do. If this occurs, the tissues surrounding the implant (peri-implant tissues) will become inflamed, much like the gingiva around the teeth. If not controlled, this inflammation and bacterial invasion can progress into the bone (**peri-implantitis**) surrounding the implant and can contribute to its loss. It is critically important to the success of the implant that the patient employ meticulous oral hygiene techniques and work with the dentist and dental hygienist to implement an effective tissue management program. The dental hygienist plays an integral role in helping the patient maintain the health of the implants and in reinforcing home care techniques. Likewise, the dental assistant can reinforce oral hygiene techniques when the patient comes in for periodic examinations or treatment.

HOME CARE

Patients should thoroughly clean the implant surfaces no less than once a day. If the patient has an implant-supported complete or partial denture, the prosthesis should be removed to facilitate cleaning of the implant and the prosthesis. The number and type of implants and the prostheses used for restoration will vary from patient to patient. Therefore it is important to customize the home care regimen for each patient. Home care aids that are beneficial to patients with implants include a variety of each of the following:

- Disclosing agents
- Brushes

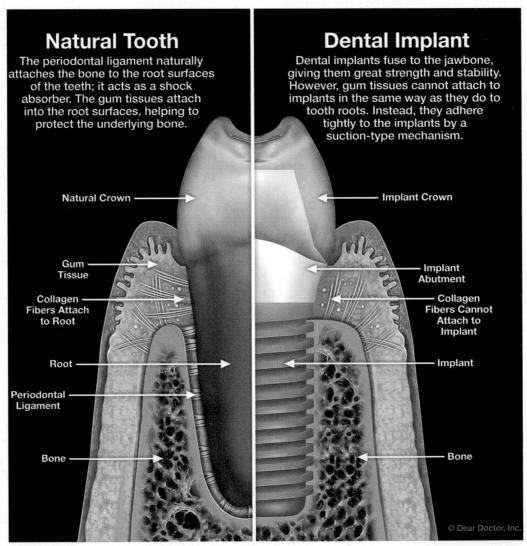

Natural Tooth

The periodontal ligament naturally attaches the bone to the root surfaces of the teeth; it acts as a shock absorber. The gum tissues attach into the root surfaces, helping to protect the underlying bone.

- Natural Crown
- Gum Tissue
- Collagen Fibers Attach to Root
- Root
- Periodontal Ligament
- Bone

Dental Implant

Dental implants fuse to the jawbone, giving them great strength and stability. However, gum tissues cannot attach to implants in the same way as they do to tooth roots. Instead, they adhere tightly to the implants by a suction-type mechanism.

- Implant Crown
- Implant Abutment
- Collagen Fibers Cannot Attach to Implant
- Implant
- Bone

© Dear Doctor, Inc.

FIG. 12.28 Gingival adaptation to titanium dental implant compared to that with a natural tooth. (Courtesy Dear Doctor, Inc., Hopewell Junction, New York.)

- Flosses
- Wooden plaque removers
- Antibacterial agents

Disclosing Agents

Plaque-disclosing agents can help patients visualize the location of plaque in difficult-to-reach areas. These agents should be used daily for the first few weeks until the patient becomes more proficient in keeping the implants clean, and then periodically to check on the effectiveness of hygiene techniques. The patient should be given a disposable mouth mirror to help visualize all areas of the mouth. Adequate lighting is important also.

Brushes. Gentle sulcular brushing is recommended to help maintain peri-implant tissue health. Brushes also need to be positioned at a variety of angles to clean around and under the prosthesis. In many cases conventional toothbrushes can be used, but selection of brushes will depend in part on the number and spacing of the implants. For single-tooth implants, as well as for implant-supported fixed bridges, interproximal brushes are helpful for reaching between the implant and the adjacent tooth or pontic (artificial replacement tooth that is part of a fixed bridge). Interproximal brushes that have a plastic coating on the wire holding the bristles together are recommended to avoid scratching the implant (Fig. 12.29). End-tuft brushes can be helpful when the space between implants is greater than is practical for interproximal brushes (Fig. 12.30). For most brushes with plastic handles, the angulation of the brush head can be altered by heating the handle in hot water and bending it to the desired angle. Patients who have problems with manual dexterity because of arthritis, stroke, or other medical problems can use power brushes. Rotary brushes with bristles forming a point are useful for reaching between implants that are spaced far apart. If a dentifrice is used, one should be selected that is not abrasive. A foam tip (Oral B, Procter & Gamble) is also useful for interproximal cleaning (Fig. 12.31). It can be soaked in chemotherapeutic agents to deliver them to specific sites.

Flosses. Several types of flosses are available. Regular-thickness floss, dental tape, flossing cord, knitting yarn, twill tape (from fabric stores), gauze strips, and fuzzy-type floss with threader (Oral-B Superfloss; Procter & Gamble) all have applications for plaque removal, depending on the nature of the implants and the overlying prosthesis (Fig. 12.32). Floss threaders are helpful for carrying floss under prostheses such as implant-supported complete dentures or fixed bridges, particularly where access is difficult.

Wooden plaque removers. Balsa wood triangular sticks (e.g., Stim-U-Dents [Revive Personal Products]) and toothpicks can be used with care to aid in plaque removal. These items will not scratch implants.

Antibacterial agents. Chlorhexidine gluconate solution (0.12%) (such as Peridex [3M ESPE]) is an effective antibacterial agent. It may be used as a rinse for about a week after implant placement or during the second surgical

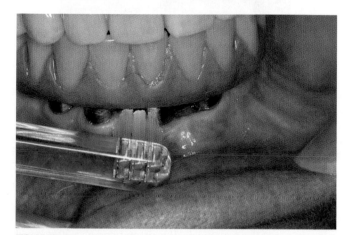

FIG. 12.30 End-tuft brush to clean implant. (Reprinted by permission from *Endosteal Dental Implants*, St. Louis, 1991, Mosby, Figure 31-6, p. 404.)

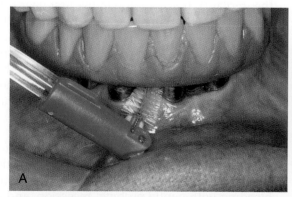

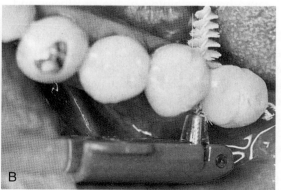

FIG. 12.29 A, Interproximal brush used to clean implant. **B,** Nylon-coated proxy brush to clean between individual implants. (**A,** Reprinted by permission from Endosteal Dental Implants, St. Louis, 1991, Mosby, Figure 31-6, p. 404 **B,** From Darby ML, Walsh MM: *Dental Hygiene: Theory and Practice*, ed 4, St. Louis, 2015, Elsevier.)

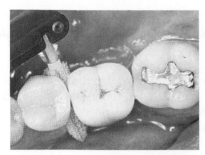

FIG. 12.31 Use of foam tip for cleaning interproximal surfaces of an implant. (Courtesy Procter & Gamble.)

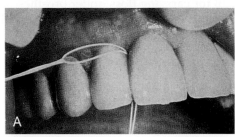

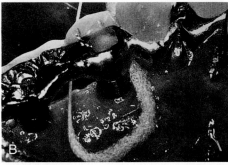

FIG. 12.32 Floss threader used to pass floss under a bridge. **A,** Use of floss threader to go under a bridge pontic **B,** Superfloss used to clean under implant-supported bridge. **A,** Floss passed under the connector between the implant and the pontic **B,** Superfloss used to clean the proximal surfaces of the implant and pontic. (A. From Babbush CA: Dental implants: the art and science, Philadelphia, 2001, Saunders. B. Courtesy Procter & Gamble.)

stage when the implant is uncovered. It is also useful when inflammation is found in peri-implant tissues after placement of the prosthesis. It is often used as a 30-second daily rinse for 1 to 2 weeks. It can also be applied directly to the problem site on an interproximal brush, end-tuft brush, foam tip, or cotton swab. Frequent use of chlorhexidine will cause brown staining of the prosthesis and natural teeth. An alternative antibacterial agent that is beneficial in controlling gingivitis but is not as effective as chlorhexidine is a phenolic compound (e.g., Listerine; Johnson & Johnson) (see Chapter 7 Preventive and Desensitizing Materials). Oral irrigation may be used to deliver antibacterial solutions, but it should be used at low pressure and not directed into the sulcus. If the pressure used is too high, damage to the biological seal between the epithelium and the implant may occur.

When a patient has inflammation around the implant that is not responding to good oral hygiene measures and hygiene visits, then prescription antibacterial agents may be needed. Arestin (OraPharma) is a powder of slow-releasing minocycline that can be placed in the sulcus around the implant to help manage bacteria. Orally administered doxycycline hyclate (Periostat, 20-mg tablets; Galderma Laboratories) taken twice a day may help to manage the inflammation.

Home Care Aids for Implant Patients
Brushes
Regular soft-bristled toothbrush
Interproximal brush with plastic-coated wire
End-tuft brush
Power brushes: Standard or rotary with pointed brush tip
Flosses
Regular floss or tape
Yarn or Superfloss
Cord
Twill tape
Gauze strips
Wooden sticks
Balsa wood sticks (Stim-U-Dents [Revive Personal Products])
Toothpicks
Antibacterial agents
Chlorhexidine solution
Phenolic compound rinse (Listerine; Johnson & Johnson)

HYGIENE VISIT

The patient should return to the dental office 3 to 4 months after implant placement for assessment and maintenance. The interval between subsequent visits should be based on how well the patient is doing with oral hygiene measures, the health of the peri-implant tissues, and how rapidly calculus accumulates. At the maintenance visit, review of the health history and vital signs and examination of extraoral and intraoral structures are conducted in the same manner as for patients without implants. However, questions specific to implants should be asked, such as those involving the presence of implant mobility, soreness, bleeding of peri-implant tissues, pain with chewing, and looseness of the prosthesis.

Radiographic assessment. The dentist may request periodic radiographs to check the bone level surrounding the implants. It is common in the first year for about 1 mm of crestal alveolar bone to be lost around the top of the implant. Conventional bitewings may not extend far enough apically to capture the bone around the crest of the implant, and therefore vertical bitewings should be used. Periapical radiographs alone usually are angled, so the true level of the bone around the top of the implant cannot be determined.

Visual assessment. The hygienist should perform a visual inspection of the peri-implant soft tissues to evaluate for edema (swelling), erythema (redness), bleeding with gentle probing, recession, and other indications of a developing problem. Exudate (pus) may be discovered upon probing or palpation of the area

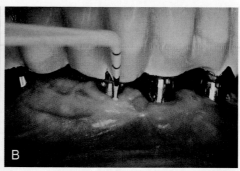

FIG. 12.33 Use of plastic probe around implant. **A,** Plastic probe for measuring sulcus around implant. **B,** Probe measuring sulcus without scratching implant (Sensor Probe, Pro-Dentec, courtesy of J. Kleinman). (From Darby ML, Walsh MM, *Dental Hygiene: Theory and Practice,* ed 4, St. Louis, 2015, Elsevier.)

with a cotton-tip applicator. Usually, when these signs are limited to the tissue around the top of the implant, it is caused by bacterial plaque on the implant. Problem areas can be pointed out to the patient, and a review of oral hygiene techniques should be done. If the patient has a particular problem area, alternative cleaning aids and techniques can be recommended.

Probing. At one time probing was not recommended for fear of damaging the epithelial cuff around the implant and introducing bacteria into these tissues. However, the current consensus is to perform gentle probing at maintenance visits. When probing of the peri-implant sulcus is done to check the status of an implant, it should be done with a light touch and a plastic probe (e.g., Colorvue Probe [Hu-Friedy] or Sensor Probe [DenMat]) so as not to disturb the biological seal and scratch the implant surface (Fig. 12.33). The plastic probe will also allow for proper adaptation to the surface of the implant as some flexibility is needed and the plastic probe provides the appropriate amount of flexibility without damaging the biological seal. Sites with increased probing depths, exudate, and bleeding should be recorded.

Mobility. Implants should be checked for mobility. An implant that has integrated with the bone should not be mobile. Mobility can be tested by using the handles of two dental instruments to try to push the implant back and forth buccolingually. Do not use your fingers because the soft pads of tissue on the finger tips will compress when trying to move the implant. This can be mistaken for mobility of the implant. On occasion, the patient may complain that the implant is loose, but careful examination may determine that a component of the implant such as a retention screw has loosened or broken. If the implant is loose, there should be some radiographic finding of bone loss.

Cleaning the implant surface. The clinically accessible surfaces of the implant should be thoroughly cleaned of plaque and calculus at each maintenance visit. Stainless steel scalers and curettes should not be used on titanium implants because they will scratch them. When titanium is exposed, special scaling instruments should be used to

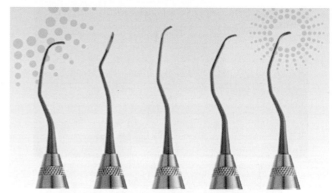

FIG. 12.34 Titanium scalers for titanium implants. (Courtesy of Hu-Friedy Manufacturing Company, Inc., Chicago.)

avoid damage to the surface of the implant. Titanium scalers are preferred because they will not scratch the titanium implant components and the blades are narrower allowing greater access to tight spots (Fig. 12.34). Titanium-coated, gold-coated, or Teflon-coated instruments may lose their coating with time and the underlying metal could scratch the implant. Plastic (e.g., Implacare Implant Scalers; Hu-Friedy) curettes and scalers (Fig. 12.35) or ultrasonic implant tips with plastic or rubber coating or sleeve (e.g., Cavitron SofTip Implant Ultrasonic Insert, Dentsply Sirona; Piezon Implant Cleaner, EMS and TIS-P Implant Scaler, Tony Riso) (Fig. 12.36) should not be used when rough surfaces or implant fixture threads are exposed. Research has shown that tiny bits of the plastic or rubber can become lodged on these rough surfaces, remain subgingival, and act as soft tissue irritants and plaque traps. Some clinicians still use plastic instruments but limit their use to biofilm/plaque removal on smooth surfaces. Implant and abutment-safe tips must be used if an ultrasonic scaler is needed.

Prophylaxis pastes with coarse or medium grit should not be used on titanium. Even very fine paste can produce some surface scratches on the implant. If polishing is deemed necessary, tin oxide or other nonabrasive polishing paste in a rubber cup applied with light pressure may be used.

Air-polishing. Air-polishing devices (also called air-powder polishing devices) were derived from technology developed by Dr. Robert Black in the 1940s. These

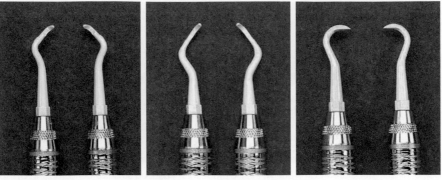

FIG. 12.35 Scaling instruments for implants with replaceable high-grade resin tips. (From Implacare Maintenance Instruments, courtesy of Hu-Friedy Manufacturing Company, Inc., Chicago.)

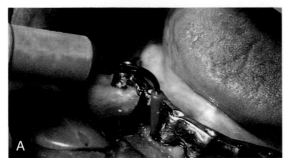

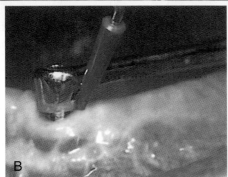

FIG. 12.36 Plastic tips for ultrasonic scalers. **A,** Disposable polysulfone plastic tip (Cavitron SofTip, courtesy of Dentsply International, York, PA.) **B,** Plastic ultrasonic scaler insert for titanium implants. (Courtesy of Tom Riso Company, North Miami Beach, FL.)

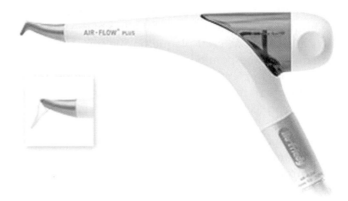

FIG. 12.37 Air-polisher with subgingival nozzle (Air-Flow 3.0 Premium, Hu-Friedy EMS). (Courtesy of Hu-Friedy Manufacturing Company, Inc., Chicago.)

devices spray a stream of compressed air and water containing an abrasive powder through a nozzle onto the implant surface to remove plaque and stain. They are not meant to remove calculus. High volume evacuation should be used with air-polishing to capture as much of the aerosol as possible to minimize the amount the patient inhales and swallows. Air-powder polishers are generally considered safe to use on implants according to in vitro studies. However, these systems must be used with caution. The use of incorrect powders can scratch titanium implant surfaces and can injure surrounding soft tissues. Incorrect use or too much air pressure can result in air being forced into tissue spaces (called tissue emphysema). The risk is greatest if the stream is aimed directly into the gingival sulcus rather than angled toward the implant.

Abrasive particles. Sodium bicarbonate to which flavoring agents have been added is the most common powder used with supragingival air-polishing. The size of the powder particles is kept small, 60-80 μm. Sodium bicarbonate is less than half as abrasive as pumice, which is used in prophylaxis paste. However, some studies have shown sodium bicarbonate to cause some changes to the implant surface. It has also caused some soft tissue abrasions.

Glycine (an amino acid) powder is an alternative to sodium bicarbonate and is a very mild abrasive with a particle size of 20-30 μm. One air-polisher (Air-Flow Perio, Hu-Friedy EMS) uses glycine and with its nozzles designed for subgingival use has been found to be highly effective at removing subgingival biofilm (Fig. 12.37). In one study comparing glycine to sodium bicarbonate, glycine was found to be 80% less abrasive.

Contraindications for air-polishing. Contraindications for air-polishing include patients with respiratory problems such as chronic asthma or pulmonary disease that may be aggravated by inhaling the powder spray. Patients with transmissible diseases that could be spread by the aerosol created and those with compromised immune systems are also not good candidates for air-polishing.

SUMMARY

Dental implants are increasing in use, with more than 2 million placed annually. Screw-type titanium alloy implants are the most commonly used and have a success rate of approximately 95% with proper case selection and careful surgical technique. Image-guided implant planning and surgical procedures have minimized surgical complications. Two-stage surgical procedures were once the norm but are being replaced by the more popular one-stage and immediate-placement procedures. Dental assistants and hygienists can play an integral role in making the impressions for the implant restorations.

When implants were introduced, it was thought that immediate loading should be avoided at all costs. More recent findings indicate that as long as the implant is firmly embedded in bone and is stable, immediate loading can be successful if occlusal forces are properly controlled. Mini-implants have been introduced that are minimally invasive and can be used in sites where conventional implants could not. They are very useful for supporting dentures where there is little remaining alveolar ridge, and variants of them, called TADs, are used as temporary anchorage for orthodontic tooth movement. Bone grafting can improve sites for implants by building bone both in width and height. Bone grafting is also used in sinus lift procedures.

It is not enough to just place and restore implants; they must be routinely maintained to ensure the success of the implants. Patients must be shown how to use the various aids for cleaning implants. In addition, a detailed assessment of the implants should be done at each hygiene visit. Care must be taken when providing periodontal preventive care around titanium fixtures to prevent scratching their surfaces. Hygienists must know which hand instruments and ultrasonic tips can be used with implants to avoid damaging them.

Patient education is an important aspect of the role of the dental assistant and the dental hygienist in dental practice. The ability to describe to the patient the pros and cons of the various materials used in practice and to aid in the treatment process depends on your knowledge of these materials. As new materials are introduced into dental practice, it is important to stay current on their indications, contraindications, and application techniques. Manufacturers' instructions for their care and use should be followed. Many manufacturers have websites on which they post information relative to their materials.

INSTRUCTIONAL VIDEOS

See the Evolve Resources site for a variety of educational videos that reinforce the material covered in this chapter.

Procedure 12.1 Suture Removal

See Evolve Site for Competency Sheet

EQUIPMENT/SUPPLIES (FIG. 12.38)

- Mouth mirror
- Explorer
- Hydrogen peroxide or diluted mouthwash
- Cotton tip applicator
- Suture scissors
- Cotton pliers
- Gauze squares

PROCEDURE STEPS

1. Using a cotton tip applicator swab teeth and tissues with antiseptic agent (hydrogen peroxide or diluted disinfectant mouthwash) to remove bacteria and debris (Fig. 12.39).

   NOTE: Inspect surgical site for closure of the wound, absence of drainage and inflammation.

2. With cotton pliers grasp suture knot.

   NOTE: Be sure not to pinch tissues.

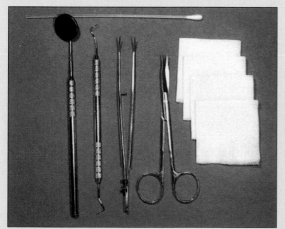

FIG. 12.38   (From Bird DL, Robinson DS: Modern Dental Assisting, ed 12, St. Louis, 2018, Elsevier.)

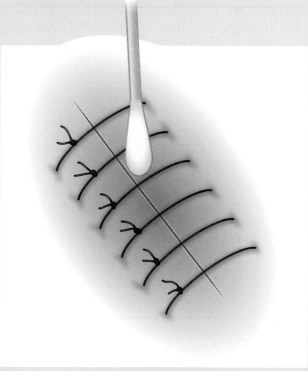

FIG. 12.39

Continued

3. Lift knot gently away from tissues creating a space to insert scissor blade (Fig. 12.40).

NOTE: This will expose a portion of suture that has been under tissue and thought to be free of bacteria.

4. Insert one cutting tip of suture scissors into the space between suture and tissue (Fig. 12.41).

NOTE: If suture scissors have a half moon cut out in one of the blades, this blade should be inserted under the suture.

5. Snip one thread close to tissue taking care not to cut tissue (Fig. 12. 42).

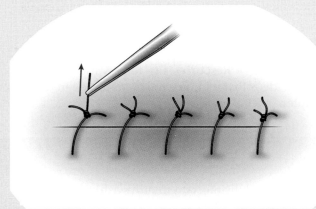

FIG. 12.40

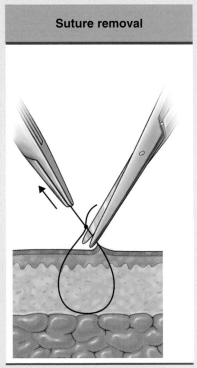

FIG. 12.41 (From Robinson JK et al: Surgery of the Skin, ed 1, St. Louis, 2005, Mosby.)

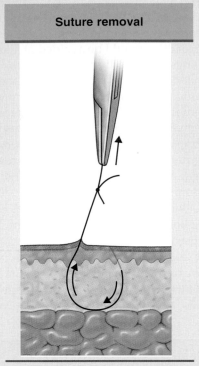

FIG. **12.42** (From Robinson JK et al: *Surgery of the Skin*, ed 1, St. Louis, 2005, Mosby.)

NOTE: Cutting suture material close to knot will allow suture previously exposed in the oral cavity to pass through tissue. This will contaminate sub-epithelial tissues with bacteria.

NOTE: Cutting both ends of suture may result in suture material being left in the tissue.

NOTE: If cutting scissors are used, the blade is inserted in the space with the tip curved away from tissue to prevent laceration/cutting of tissue.

6. Using a smooth continuous action to pull the suture out of the tissue in one piece.

NOTE: Do not pass the knot through the tissue, as this would cause the patient discomfort.

7. Place suture on gauze square.

8. Remove all visible sutures and place them on gauze square.

NOTE: To control bleeding, apply pressure to area with gauze square.

9. When all sutures have been removed, count the number of sutures on the gauze square to confirm the number is equal to the number recorded in the patient chart during the surgical appointment.

10. Record the number of sutures removed in the patient chart and any significant observations about the wound healing.

Get Ready for Exams!

Review Questions

Select the one correct response for each of the following multiple-choice questions.

1. The metal most commonly used for dental implants is
   a. Gold
   b. Silver
   c. Stainless steel
   d. Titanium

2. An implant inserted into a hole drilled into bone is which of the following types?
   a. Subperiosteal
   b. Endosseous
   c. Transosteal
   d. Exosteal

3. Why is the surface of a titanium implant fixture roughened?
   a. To remove oxides
   b. To provide a larger surface area for osseointegration
   c. To remove adherent bacteria
   d. To prevent the implant from rotating under function

4. With a two-stage implant, after the fixture is placed, which one of the following occurs?
   a. The implant crown is placed.
   b. The fixture is covered with bone.
   c. A cover screw is placed and the fixture is covered by the soft tissue flap.
   d. The healing abutment is placed and the soft tissue is allowed to heal around it.

5. Potential adverse outcomes when an implant fixture is surgically placed include
   a. Infection around the implant
   b. Perforation of one of the cortical plates of bone
   c. Improper angulation of the implant
   d. Damage to a nerve or a large blood vessel
   e. All of the above

6. Immediate-placement implants are done
   a. About 3 weeks after the extraction of a tooth
   b. At the time of extraction of the tooth that will be replaced
   c. Only when a bone graft is needed
   d. To plug the hole made when the maxillary sinus is accidentally perforated

7. Implants can be used to support which of the following prostheses?
   a. Single crowns
   b. Fixed bridges
   c. Partial or complete dentures
   d. All of the above

8. Implant crowns are fixed to the implant abutment by which method?
   a. Cemented only
   b. Cemented or held by screws

   c. Held in place by screws only
   d. Welded on

9. The instruments used to remove calculus from implants where titanium is exposed include
   a. Carbon steel curettes
   b. Air polishers
   c. Metal ultrasonic tips
   d. Titanium curettes and scalers

10. The closed-tray impression procedure requires that one of the following components be repositioned in its proper alignment into the set impression after it is removed from the mouth; which one is it?
    a. Impression abutment
    b. Implant analog
    c. Fixture
    d. Healing abutment

11. The purpose of the cover screw is to
    a. Cover the screw hole on top of the fixture to prevent tissue from growing into it
    b. Allow a cuff of gingiva to heal around it after the surgical flap has been repositioned
    c. Hold the abutment to the fixture
    d. Cover the screw hole in the implant crown used to place the retention screw

12. Mini-implants can be used for which of the following purposes?
    a. To support complete dentures
    b. To support crowns for narrow-rooted teeth such as mandibular incisors
    c. To serve as anchors for orthodontic tooth movement
    d. All of the above

13. Which type of bone graft is derived from animal tissue?
    a. Allograft
    b. Autograft
    c. Xenograft
    d. Alloplast

14. Which one of the following statements regarding the gingiva around an implant is *false*?
    a. The gingiva has connective tissue fibers that connect or integrate with the surface of the implant.
    b. When healthy, the gingiva produces a biological seal against the implant that prevents microorganisms from invading the deeper tissues.
    c. The gingiva is closely adapted to the implant but is not attached to the surface.
    d. Chronic inflammation of the gingiva around the implant could lead to peri-implantitis.

15. The consequences of not maintaining good oral hygiene around an implant include all of the following *except* one. Which one?
    a. Inflammation and swelling of the gingiva
    b. Loss of the biological seal

Continued

Get Ready for Exams!—cont'd

c. Bacterial invasion and potential loosening of the implant

d. Increased bone growth due to chronic irritation

16. Biointegration where the bone totally integrates with the implant is seen with which implant material?
    a. ceramics
    b. stainless steel
    c. gold
    d. titanium

17. Which part of the implant is placed in bone?
    a. healing abutment
    b. fixture
    c. analog
    d. impression coping

18. This type of suture will be absorbed naturally by the body's enzymes
    a. Silk
    b. Nylon
    c. Vicryl
    d. Polyester fiber

19. When removing sutures, the suture material should be cut close to the knot to prevent contamination of the sub-epithelial tissues with_____ as the suture is pulled through the tissue.
    a. viruses
    b. bacteria
    c. mucus

For answers to Review Questions, see the Appendix.

Case-Based Discussion Topics

1. The dentist has discussed a treatment plan with a patient who is a candidate for implants to support a mandibular complete denture. The dentist has described to the patient both conventional endosseous implants and mini-implants. After the dentist leaves the operatory, the patient is somewhat confused and asks you to explain the difference.
   In laymen's terms, describe the difference to the patient. If the patient asks you specific details about why the dentist is recommending one type of implant over another, what should you do?

2. A 74-year-old retired grocer comes to the dental office for a maintenance visit. He has several implants supporting two fixed bridges in the posterior part of the maxilla.
   When the patient has his implants cleaned, describe the types of instruments the hygienist will likely use and the instruments that should be avoided if titanium will be scraped. Explain the selection of these instruments.

3. The patient described in the preceding discussion topic is found to have inflammation in the peri-implant tissues around three implants and moderate amounts of calculus and plaque on the proximal surfaces of the implants. He tells you that he had missed his previously scheduled maintenance appointment and that he is just using a regular toothbrush with hard bristles to clean his implants.
   What can you do to reinforce regular maintenance visits? What home care aids can you recommend to help him keep his implants clean? Should an antibacterial agent be suggested? If yes, which one?

4. You are in the room when the dentist reviews the informed consent for implants with a patient. The patient is 78 years old and seems to be confused about what was just said to her. You question whether she has the mental capacity to give informed consent.
   What should you do? What topics should be covered in an informed consent discussion?

BIBLIOGRAPHY

American Dental Association (ADA): *Council on Scientific Affairs. Products of Excellence: ADA Seal Program*, Chicago, 1999, ADA.

Bird DL, Robinson DS: Dental implants. In *Modern Dental Assisting*, ed 12, St. Louis, 2018, Elsevier.

Bird DL, Robinson DS: Oral and maxillofacial surgery. In *Modern Dental Assisting*, ed 12, St. Louis, 2018, Elsevier.

Darby ML, Walsh MM: Dental implant maintenance. In *Dental Hygiene Theory and Practice*, Darby and Walshed 4, St. Louis, 2015, Elsevier/Saunders.

Edel A: *Air Polishing for Implant Maintenance*, CDE World, 2017. Available at https://cdeworld.com/courses/20704-Air_Polishing_for_Implant_Maintenance.

Grisdale J: The clinical applications of synthetic bone alloplast, *J Can Dent Assoc*, 65:559–562, 1999.

Kotick PG, Blumenkopf B: Abutment selection for implant restorations, *Inside Dentistry* 7(7), 2011.

McKinney RV: Oral hygiene protocol for implant patients. In McKinney RV, editor: *Endosteal Dental Implants*, St. Louis, 1991, Mosby.

Moldovan S: Dental implants: a comprehensive review. *Continuing Education Course*. Available at http://www.dentalcare.com/en-US/dental-education/continuing-education/ce420/ce420.aspx.

Perry DA, Beemsterboer PL, Taggart EJ: Dental implants. In *Clinical Periodontics for the Dental Hygienist*, ed 2, Philadelphia, 2001, Saunders.

Powers JM, Wataha JC: Dental implants. In *Dental Materials: Properties and Manipulation*, Yen-Wei Chened 11, St. Louis, 2017.

Rethman MP: *Introduction and Historical Perspectives on Dental Elsevier Implants*. White paper commissioned by Hu-Friedy. Available at http://www.friendsofhu-friedy.com/userfiles/file/Implant Maintenance White Paper/Implant Maintenance White Paper Final.pdf

Robinson DS, Bird DL: Oral and maxillofacial surgery. In *Essentials of Dental Assisting*, Bird and Robinsoned 6, St. Louis, 2017, Elsevier.

Sakaguchi RL, Powers JM: Dental and orofacial implants. In *Craig's Restorative Dental Materials*, Sakaguchi and Powersed 13, St. Louis, 2012, Mosby.

Wilk BL: Intraoral digital impressioning for dental implant restorations versus traditional implant impression techniques, *Compend Contin Educ Dent*, 36(7):529–533, 2015.

Wilkins E: Sutures and dressings. In *Clinical Practice of the Dental Hygienist*, ed 12, Philadephia, 2017, Wolters Kluwer.

Chapter Objectives

Upon completion of this chapter, the student should be able to:

1. Define abrasion, finishing, polishing, and cleaning.
2. Discuss the purpose of finishing, polishing, and cleaning of dental restorations and tooth surfaces.
3. Identify and discuss the factors that affect the rate and efficiency of abrasion.
4. Compare the relative ranking of abrasives on restorations and tooth structures.
5. Describe methods by which dental abrasives are applied.
6. Discuss the contraindications to the use of abrasives on tooth structure and restorations.
7. Describe the clinical decisions made to determine which abrasive to use when finishing, polishing, or cleaning dental restorations or tooth structures.
8. Describe the abrasives and the procedures used for finishing and polishing metals, composite, and porcelain.
9. Describe the abrasives and the procedures used for polishing and cleaning metals, composite, ceramic, and gold alloys as part of oral prophylaxis.
10. Describe the safety and infection control precautions taken by the operator when using abrasives.
11. Relate the instructions given to patients to prevent and remove stain from tooth surfaces and restorations.
12. Finish and polish a preexisting amalgam restoration.
13. Polish a preexisting composite restoration.

Key Terms

Finishing a procedure used to remove excess restorative material to develop appropriate occlusion, contour, and functional form; usually done with rotary cutting instruments. Finishing removes surface blemishes and produces a smooth surface

Polishing a procedure that produces a smooth, shiny surface by eliminating minor surface imperfections, fine scratches, and surface stains using mild abrasives frequently found in the form of pastes or compounds. Polishing produces little change in the surface.

Mohs Hardness a measure of hardness on a scale of 1 to 10 where 1 is a very soft material such as talc and 10 is the hardest material such as diamond

Cleaning a procedure that is primarily meant to remove soft deposits from the surface of restorations and tooth structures. Polishing and cleaning are done to remove surface stains and soft deposits from the clinical crowns and exposed root surfaces of teeth after all hard deposits are removed

Abrasive a material composed of particles of sufficient hardness and sharpness to cut or scratch a softer material when drawn across its surface

Hardness is the ability of a material to resist abrasion

Grit the size of the abrasive particles, typically classified as coarse, medium, fine, and superfine

Margination a procedure for removal of excessive restorative material from the margins of restorations

Flash feather-like excesses of material present at the margins of a restoration typically on occlusal and proximal surfaces

Overhang excessive material present at the cervical cavosurface margin

Supragingival Air Polishing the process of polishing or finishing the clinical crown using fine, soft particles under air pressure to remove biofilm and stain from enamel surfaces and in pits and fissures; an alternative to prophy pastes

Subgingival Air Polishing the process of polishing the anatomical crown and clinical root surface using fine, soft particles under air pressure to remove biofilm subgingivally

Air Abrasion or Microabrasion like air polishing, but using greater air pressure and harder particles. Used to cleanse cast appliances before cementation, repair porcelain and composite restorations, prepare tooth surfaces before bonding, and cut tooth structure for restorative preparations

---

Proper finishing, polishing, and cleaning of tooth structures and restorative materials is clinically relevant because this improves esthetic and tissue health, while increasing the longevity of the restorative material. The demands for improved esthetics through whiter and brighter teeth have *grown dramatically causing a multitude of clinical and over-the-counter products available to provide this benefit to grow. The allied dental professional must carefully evaluate the clinical procedures used for the removal of stains and soft deposits with the use of abrasives. These procedures should be selective procedures, performed after the needs of the individual patient are considered, and the types of stains and restorative materials present are properly identified. The routine polishing of teeth with abrasive prophylactic (prophy) paste after scaling and root planing is not recommended. The clinician must critically evaluate the potential negative effects of the coronal polish procedure against the benefits.*

The goal of finishing and polishing restorations, intraoral appliances, and tooth structure is to remove excess material, smooth roughened surfaces, and produce an esthetically pleasing appearance with minimal trauma to hard and soft tissues. The finishing and polishing of a surface involves removing marginal irregularities, defining anatomic contours and occlusion, removing the surface roughness of the restoration, and producing a mirror-like surface luster. Many benefits are derived from smooth tooth surfaces, restorations, or appliances in the intraoral environment. A smooth surface resists accumulation of soft deposits and stains, is less irritating to the gingival or mucosal tissue, and is esthetically pleasing because it reflects light better. A smooth and polished tooth surface can help to motivate the patient to maintain these positive results with better self-care procedures. A smooth, highly polished restorative surface is more resistant to the effects of corrosion and surface breakdown. A properly finished and polished surface will contribute to the appearance and longevity of the restoration or appliance and the health of the surrounding oral tissues (Fig. 13.1).

Clinicians who perform finishing and polishing procedures must have a clear understanding of the factors that cause and control abrasion. Improper use of abrasives can lead to roughening and over-reduction of tooth and restorative surfaces. The clinician must be able to recognize that different types of tooth structures and restorative surfaces abrade differently and must use the proper protocol for finishing, polishing, or cleaning each surface. It is also the clinician's responsibility to teach the patient how to properly care for the surfaces with home care devices and how to prevent the staining habits that diminish their appearance (see Chapter 2 Oral Environment and Patient Considerations for identification of restorative materials).

FINISHING, POLISHING, CLEANING

The process of finishing and polishing involves using sequentially coarser to finer abrasives on a surface to first contour, then smooth, and finally bring a luster to the surface. Contouring to cut or grind away excessive materials with rotary instruments may be required first to produce the desired anatomic form.

Finishing removes excess material to develop the surface morphology and functional form. Contouring of the restoration is most often done with rotary instruments in high-and low-speed handpieces. Gross finishing is done first to remove large excesses

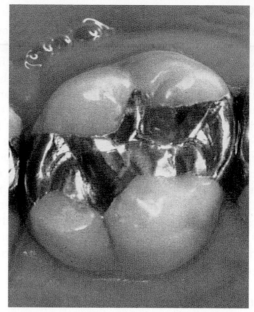

FIG. 13.1 A finished and polished amalgam restoration.

of restorative material using coarse or medium grit diamond burs, carbide finishing burs, and abrasive discs and strips. Fine finishing refines the anatomic morphology, that is, occlusal surfaces and occlusion, embrasure spaces, and marginal ridge form using medium to fine versions of the gross finishing instruments. Fine finishing prepares the surface for polishing.

Polishing is the process of removing scratches from the surface of a restoration with a series of particles, coarse to fine, to produce a smooth, glossy surface that is esthetically pleasing, tolerated well by soft tissues, and resistant to biofilm adhesion. Polishing produces little change in the surface. It may have to be repeated periodically during the life of the restoration if tarnish or stains develop. Polishing requires materials with a **Mohs' hardness** of only 1 to 2 units above the substrate being polished. Finishing and polishing are intended to produce selective and controlled wear of the surface being manipulated.

Cleaning does not produce scratches or wear and is primarily used for the removal of biofilm. Polishing and cleaning are done to remove surface stains and soft deposits from the clinical crowns and exposed root surfaces of teeth after all hard deposits are removed. Aside from abrasives, there are also chemical cleaning products that are primarily used for removable appliances. Cleaning requires materials with Mohs' hardness no greater than equal to the substrate.

There is no single type of abrasive that can be used safely and effectively on all types of dental materials and tooth structures. The effect of abrasion is directly related to the properties of the abrasive and the material (substrate) it is abrading.

FACTORS AFFECTING ABRASION

An understanding of the properties of **abrasives** and the factors that control the rate or efficiency of abrasion will help the clinician make appropriate clinical decisions. The rate of abrasion is determined by the abrasive being used and the surface being abraded (the *substrate*). The abrasiveness of particles is determined by size, irregularity, and hardness; the number of particles contacting the surface; and the pressure and speed at which they are applied. The rate of abrasion is also dependent on the surface being abraded; a hard substrate such as enamel is much more resistant to abrasion than softer cementum. An understanding of these factors will assist the clinician in making appropriate clinical decisions for the indications, contraindications, and control of abrasion.

Size, Irregularity, and Hardness of Abrasive Particles

The size, irregularity, and hardness of the abrasive particle determine the depth of the scratches in the material being abraded and therefore the amount of material being removed. An example is the effect of pumice, which comes in several grades of coarseness, on cementum and amalgam. Coarse pumice, consisting of larger and irregular particles, will remove more surface from the softer cementum than from the harder amalgam. If superfine pumice (also called *flour of pumice*), consisting of much smaller and more regular particles is used, the effect will be to polish the cementum as well as the amalgam. Diamonds are the most abrasive materials used in dentistry. Coarse diamond abrasives, often used for contouring restorations as part of gross finishing, can remove large amounts of tooth structure and restorative material. They can also be used for fine finishing and polishing of restorations, all according to diamond particle size and regularity. Their rate of abrasion will also depend on the material being abraded, the pressure applied, and the speed of the rotating device.

If the surface being abraded is harder than the abrasive, there is little or no effect. If the clinician is using prophy paste with appropriate technique on enamel, it will polish the surface; if the same paste and technique is used on demineralized enamel it will result in enamel loss. It is important that the clinician have an appreciation for the relative hardness of various intraoral natural and restorative materials and abrasives used on these materials. **Hardness** is the ability of a material to resist abrasion. The Mohs scale of hardness ranks materials by their relative abrasion resistance. The Knoop hardness test is based on the ability of materials to resist indentation. In both of these tests the farther apart the substrate and the abrasive are in hardness number, the more effective is the abrasive process. As seen in Table 13.1, diamond

Table 13.1	Mohs and Knoop Hardness Scales	
	MOHS	**KNOOP**
Diamond	10	7,000-10,000
Silicon carbide (carborundum)	9-10	2,500
Tungsten carbide	9	1,900
Aluminum oxide (corundum), emery	7-9	2,100
Sand (quartz)	7	820
Zirconium silicate	6.5-7.5	
Silicon dioxide (Silex)	6-7	
Flour of pumice	6-7	460-560
*CAD/CAM ceramic	6-7	
Porcelain (ceramic)	6-7	560
Tin oxide	6	
Perlite	5.5-7	
Enamel	5.5-6	340-431
Composite	5-7	30-55
Rouge	5-6	
Amalgam	5-6	90
Gold Type IV alloy	3-4	220
Dentin	3-4	70
Cementum	2-3	40
Denture base resin (acrylic)	2-3	20
Calcium carbonate	3	
Aluminum trihydroxide	2.5-4	
Sodium bicarbonate	2.5-3	
Glycine	2	
Potassium and sodium	0.04-0.05	

Tooth structure in shaded rows
*CAD/CAM, computer-assisted design/computer-assisted machining.

has the highest resistance to abrasion and is therefore considered the hardest; flour of pumice rates a 6 to 7 on the Mohs scale and 460 to 560 on the Knoop scale, which is similar to tooth enamel but harder than amalgam and dentin. Therefore, pumice may be used to polish enamel, whereas contact with exposed dentin would be too abrasive. It is important to note that porcelain is harder than enamel and dentin. Abrasive wear of tooth structures in contact with porcelain restorations is a problem for many patients. The greater the difference in hardness between the abrasive and the surface it is abrading, the faster and more effective the abrasive action. To effectively polish, a particle must be harder by 1 to 2 Mohs units than the surface it is polishing. Cleaning, when no abrasion is indicated, requires a substance 1 Mohs unit less than or equal to the surface on which it is directed. Compare Mohs and Knoop hardness rankings for enamel and dentin. You can surmise that exposed dentin is

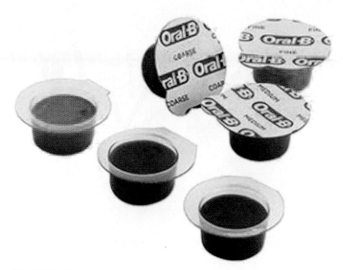

FIG. 13.2 The grit in prophy paste (available as single-dose units in holders) comes in various sizes. (Courtesy of Proctor & Gamble.)

abraded at a much greater rate than enamel during dental polishing procedures. Compare the Mohs and Knoop rankings of composite and gold. If the same polishing agent were used on these as on enamel, the result would be greater loss of the restorative material. As you can also see, denture base materials are very susceptible to abrasion.

> ### Clinical Tip
> It is important that patients be given instructions to use only approved denture cleaners for their home care; even toothpaste may be too abrasive for acrylic intraoral appliances such as dentures.

The size and shape of the particles must be considered in manipulating an abrasive. Particles that are large and irregular, with jagged edges, will cut more efficiently. The sharpness, or efficiency, of the particles is usually lost with use as the jagged edges break down and become rounder and the particles no longer "grab" the surface. Unlike the shape of the particles, the size of the particles does not always change significantly with use. Abrasive particles are classified from coarse to fine, based on their size measured in micrometers (also called *microns* [symbol, μm]). One micrometer is equal to one-thousandth of a millimeter (1 mm = 1000 μm). Abrasives are classified as coarse (particles 100 μm and above), medium (20 to 100 μm), and fine (20 μm to submicron particle sizes). Manufacturers use the term **grit** to refer to the size of abrasive particles. Particles are passed through a standardized sieve that allows a specific size of particles to pass, categorizing them from coarse through superfine. Prophylactic polishing pastes are commonly manufactured in various degrees of coarseness, as are abrasive disks and rotary diamonds (Fig. 13.2).

If too hard an abrasive is used the result will be deep scratches that cannot be finished or polished out. The clinician must make decisions as to the coarseness of the abrasive and the application method needed for each procedure.

Number of Particles That Contact the Surface
The more concentrated the particles that contact the surface, the more quickly the surface will be abraded. If a lubricant is used to dilute the concentration of the particles, the abrasiveness of the material is reduced. Water and saliva are lubricants commonly used to dilute the effect of abrasion. When using an abrasive, the clinician has control of how much lubricant to add to the material, whether this is done before it is placed in the mouth or while it is being used intraorally as it picks up saliva. Pumice (Fig. 13.3) is manufactured as a powder or paste which allows the clinician the opportunity to further dilute this abrasive. Rotary cutting instruments such as abrasive disks and stones will lose effectiveness as particles break away from their surface or debris clogs the surface. Many rotary cutting stones and diamonds use the water from the handpiece or three-way syringe to assist in the movement of debris from the cutting edge and act as a surface coolant, thus allowing the surface to maintain its abrasive action much longer.

Speed and Pressure
Increasing the speed and pressure at which an abrasive is applied will increase the rate of abrasion. Increased speed alone can produce undesired effects if it results in lack of control. Increased pressure will produce deeper scratches, as well as several other possible results:
- Less control of the amount of material being removed
- Decreased clinician's tactile sensitivity, possibly leading to an undesired over-abraded surface
- Reduced cutting efficiency of the abrasive, the result of decreased instrumental torque

Increased speed and pressure also result in frictional heat, which may have a detrimental effect on the tooth structure, the pulp, and on patient comfort. Heat generated from rotary instruments can bring mercury to the surface of an amalgam restoration and degrade its properties. Polishing that is done dry with continuous application produces the highest temperature increase on the surface of the restoration. If polishing needs to be done dry, then intermittent application with light pressure should be used.

> **Caution**
> Care must be taken to control the amount of pressure and speed with which abrasives are applied. For most applications a light intermittent touch is recommended.

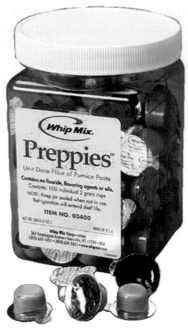

FIG. 13.3 Pumice delivered in a single dose of premixed paste. (Copied from smartpractice.com.)

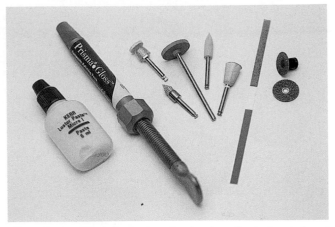

FIG. 13.4 Various delivery designs for abrasives: Paste, bonded, and coated.

When is polishing accomplished? Patients can detect surface roughness on restorations with their tongue: the tongue can sense a surface roughness of less than 1 μm, and roughness greater than 1 μm may lead to breakdown of the restoration surface due to biofilm accumulation and corrosion. Gloss and/or luster are produced when the scratches on the restoration surface are smaller than the wavelength of visible light (<0.5 μm) resulting in a shiny surface that reflects light.

The clinician must be able to determine if the surface of the restoration is smooth in order to properly determine the amount and rate of abrasion needed to polish the surface. When the surface of a restoration is rough, polishing should be completed in order to smooth the surface. The clinician will select the appropriate type of material to polish the surface without causing excessive damage; this is known as selective polishing. Determining the amount and rate of abrasion is an important consideration when clinical decisions are made regarding what type of material to be abraded, how much material is to be removed, and the desired outcome.

MODE OF DELIVERY OF ABRASIVES

Dental abrasives are supplied in a number of forms (Fig. 13.4):
- Two-body abrasives, including:
  - Bonded abrasives
  - Coated abrasives
- Three-body abrasives, including:
  - Paste abrasives
  - Loose abrasives

- Microparticle (or hard-particle) abrasives, delivered by air pressure

Two-body abrasives, also known as *direct contact abrasives*, include abrasive agents that are fixed on an abrasive instrument such as on sandpaper disks, strips, or burs. Tooth-to-tooth contact, known as *attrition*, is an example of two-body abrasion. Three-body abrasives are those that are free to rotate between the delivery device and the surface being polished. Prophy paste in a rubber cup is an example of a three-body abrasive. Toothpaste is a three-body abrasive, as are abrasive foods or materials that might be introduced during mastication. Microparticle abrasives are those that are forced against the substrate by air pressure. This technique, called *air polishing* (with a ProphyJet, Dentsply) or *air abrasion* depending on the particles and air pressure used, is an example of the use of hard-particle abrasives.

Bonded Abrasives (Two-Body, Direct Contact Abrasives)

Bonded abrasives are attached to rotary instruments; the abrasive particles are uniformly incorporated in a binder and bonded to the device. The devices vary in the available shape, such as points, disks, cups, brushes, and wheels. These devices are frequently used for intermediate finishing and initial polishing of restorations (Fig. 13.5).

Coated Abrasives (Two-Body, Direct Contact Abrasives)

Coated abrasives are supplied on rotary disks and handheld finishing strips. The abrasive particles are secured to one side of a flexible backing with an adhesive. Devices with coating on only one side protect the adjacent tooth from the abrasive and are referred to as *safe-sided*. Flexible backing such as paper or plastic gives such devices the advantage of flexibility but eliminates their ability to be sterilized. Abrasive coated rotary devices are typically attached to a

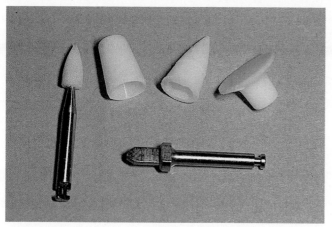

FIG. 13.5 Bonded abrasives: Reusable point on mandrel, and disposable cup, point, and disk with sterilizable mandrel.

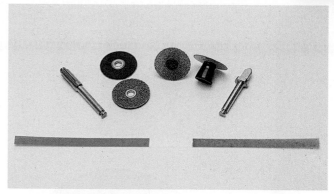

FIG. 13.6 Coated abrasives: Various designs of sandpaper disk and mandrels and sandpaper strip.

autoclavable shaft or mandrel, for convenience and cost-effectiveness (Fig. 13.6). Sof-Lex spiral finishing and polishing wheels (3M ESPE) (Fig. 13.7).

Paste Abrasives (Three-Body Abrasives)

Paste abrasives are found in the form of prophy paste and toothpaste. A more complete discussion of both follows in the section "Preparations Used for Abrasion" (below).

Loose Abrasives (Three-Body Abrasives)

Loose abrasives are manufactured as powders and pastes and are classified by their grit or particle size. Grits of coarse, medium, fine, and superfine are available for finishing, polishing, and cleaning surfaces. These may be applied with wheels, brushes, cups, or soft pads. The concentration of particles that contact the surface is clinically controlled. If the clinician uses a coarse, thick paste, rapid removal of surface material will result, along with possible pulpal damage due to excessive frictional heat. However, if a superfine, highly diluted paste is used, little or no material may be removed. The proper grit and dilution of the loose abrasive must be considered to obtain the best results in finishing and polishing a given surface.

Abrasives are manufactured for use at chairside and in the laboratory. Some may be used for either purpose. Regardless of how the abrasive material is supplied, the clinician must control the rate of abrasion.

MATERIALS USED IN ABRASION

Many types of natural and synthetic (human-made) materials are available for use in dentistry. The following materials are listed from most to least abrasive.

Diamond

Diamond is the hardest known substance rating a 10 on the Mohs hardness scale. It will efficiently abrade any substance. Rotary diamonds are expensive and

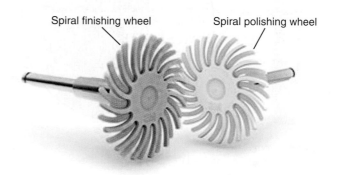

Spiral finishing wheel   Spiral polishing wheel

FIG. 13.7 A Sof-Lex spiral finishing and polishing wheel. Its shape adapts to all tooth surfaces, making it an alternative to traditional points, cups, disks, and brushes. (Courtesy of 3M ESPE [St. Paul, MN].)

usually are not disposable, so they are found most often bonded in varying degrees of coarseness to rotary cutting shanks or disks (Fig. 13.8). They are sterilizable and can be reused several times before they wear out. Coarse and medium grit diamond burs are used cut crown and bridge preparations and fine and ultrafine diamond burs are used to finish and polish composite restorations. Fine particle diamonds come in a paste for polishing composite and porcelain restorations.

Silicon Carbide

Rare in nature, silicon carbide is typically synthesized as an extremely hard and efficient abrasive material (9 to 10 on the Mohs scale). Silicon carbide–coated disks and bonded rotary devices are used primarily in the beginning steps of finishing procedures for composites and ceramics.

Tungsten Carbide Finishing Burs

Tungsten carbide is a very hard material (harder than steel) material used to fabricate carbide tools with cutting that do not dull quickly. Tungsten carbide finishing burs come in several shapes, with designs ranging from 7 to 30 cutting flutes (Fig. 13.9).

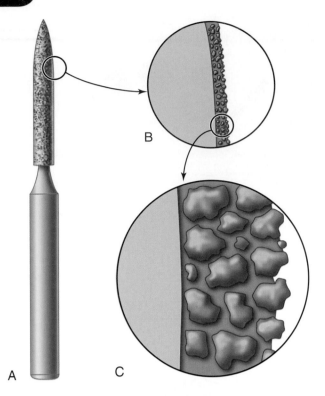

FIG. 13.8 (From Heymann H, Swift E, Ritter A: *Sturdevant's Art & Science of Operative Dentistry* (ed 6). St. Louis, 2013, Elsevier.)

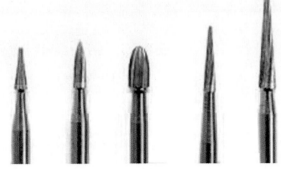

FIG. 13.9 (Courtesy of AXIS Dental Sàrl.)

The higher the number of flutes the bur has, the finer is the ultimate finish. A bur that contains only seven flutes will have a very aggressive cutting action. These burs rank up to 9 on the Mohs scale and are used primarily for finishing. They are used to cut preparations or to finish composite restorations.

Aluminum Oxide (Corundum), Emery
Aluminum oxide (corundum; 9 on the Mohs scale) is a synthetic abrasive that is often manufactured as a white or tan powder. The powder form is used in sandblasting restorations in preparation for cementation and air abrasion. It is used in bonded and coated rotary devices. Aluminum oxide–impregnated rubber wheels are called *Burlew wheels*. This popular abrasive comes in several grit sizes and has largely replaced emery. It is used to smooth enamel or to finish metal alloys and ceramic materials, and to polish highly filled and hybrid composite restorations and porcelain restorations.

Sand
Sand is a natural abrasive composed of quartz and silica. This abrasive rates a 7 on the Mohs scale and is manufactured as coated disks and handheld strips used in the finishing process.

Silicon Dioxide
Silicon dioxide has a Mohs ranking of 6 to 7 and is commonly found in prophylaxis paste for heavy stain

removal and on rubberized cups and points used for finishing and polishing composite restorations.

Pumice
Pumice is volcanic silica manufactured as a loose abrasive. Superfine, flour of pumice (Mohs hardness scale, 6) is extremely fine and a major component of many prophylaxis pastes used to polish tooth structure, dental amalgam, and acrylic bases. Fine, medium, and coarse pumice are primarily used in dental laboratory procedures and should not be used on natural tooth structures.

Tin Oxide
Tin oxide (6 on the Mohs harness scale) is an extremely fine abrasive that is used extensively as a final polishing agent for enamel and restorations. This abrasive is usually found as a powder that is mixed with water or glycerin (Fig. 13.10).

Rouge
Rouge is iron oxide with a Mohs hardness value of 5 to 6. It is frequently found in block form, which then is run onto a rag wheel to polish precious and semiprecious metal alloys in the laboratory. Rouge is not used intra-orally (Fig. 13.11).

Calcium Carbonate
Calcium carbonate, also called *chalk* or *whiting*, is a mild abrasive with a low Mohs ranking of 3. It is found in prophylaxis paste and dentifrice. It is used to polish teeth, metal restorations, and plastic materials.

Sodium Bicarbonate
Sodium bicarbonate has a very low Mohs ranking of 2.5 to 3 and is used as a cleaning agent in toothpaste and in supragingival air polishing (Fig. 13.12).

Glycine
Glycine is an amino acid with a Mohs ranking of 2 and is used as a cleaning agent in supra-gingival and sub-gingival air polishing (Fig. 13.13).

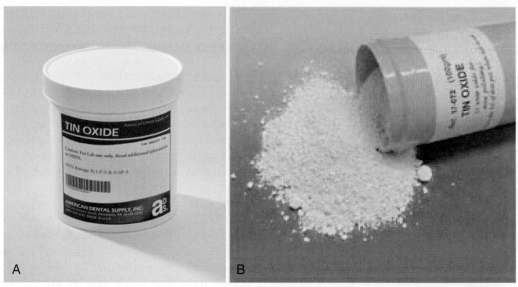

FIG. 13.10 (**A,** Courtesy of American Dental Supply, Inc. **B,** Courtesy of How to Clean Marble.)

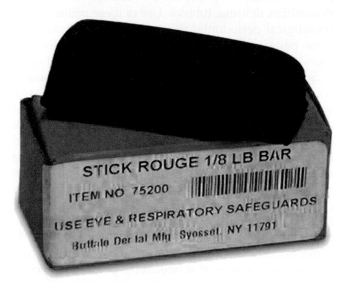

FIG. 13.11 Stick rouge to be utilized on a rag wheel in the dental laboratory to polish precious and semi-precious metal alloys. (Courtesy Buffalo Dental Manufacturing Co. Inc.)

Potassium and Sodium

Potassium and sodium have very low Mohs rankings of 0.4 and 0.5. These agents are nonabrasive and are used in toothpaste and desensitizing agents.

PREPARATIONS USED FOR ABRASION

Prophylaxis (Prophy) Paste

Prophylaxis (prophy) paste is a mixture of 50% to 60% abrasive materials such as pumice and tin oxide and lubricants. Prophy paste may be 20 times more abrasive to dentin and 10 times more abrasive to enamel than commercially prepared dentifrice. Preservatives, flavoring agents, coloring agents, and therapeutic agents are added. The abrasive powder is diluted with a lubricant to reduce the rate of abrasion and the amount of frictional heat produced. The lubricant also helps keep the

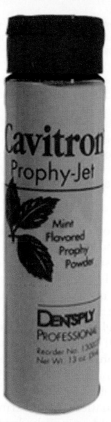

FIG. 13.12 Sodium bicarbonate utilized for supra-gingival air abrasion. (Courtesy Dentsply Sirona.)

preparation in a paste form by preventing hardening on exposure to air. Preservatives are included to prolong shelf life, and coloring and flavoring agents are added to increase patient acceptance. Fluoride is added to many preparations and is claimed to be a therapeutic agent in the prevention of caries, but studies have shown it not to be effective in the amount and concentration used.

Prophylaxis pastes are supplied as coarse grit (5 μm) to superfine grit (2 μm) commercially prepared pastes for polishing and cleaning of tooth structures. Coarse prophylaxis

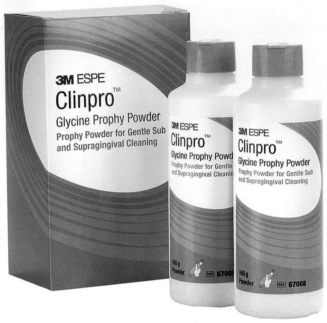

FIG. 13.13 Glycine powder utilized for supra-gingival and subgingival air polishing. (The photograph is reproduced herein with permission. © 3M 2020. All rights reserved.)

paste can produce scratches on polished surfaces of restorations such as gold, amalgam, and composite.

> **Caution**
>
> Remember: Polishing materials should be harder (but by only one to two Mohs hardness rankings) than the surface to which they are applied. Cleaning materials should be equal to or less hard than the surface to which they are applied.

Polishing of tooth surfaces should remove soft deposits (biofilm) and polishable stains without damage to hard or soft tissues. Studies of the amount of tooth structure removed with prophy paste and rubber cup polish have been questioned due to the variables associated with the studies. No scientific proof shows how much enamel is removed during polishing or if it is removed at all due to the polishing process. These results led to the philosophy of "essential selective polishing," which is now regarded as the most appropriate approach in selecting the suitable polishing agent for the clinical situation and determining which teeth and surfaces should be polished with said agent. All teeth stained or unstained may be polished; it is just a matter of selecting the appropriate agent to complete the polishing procedure. It is essential to first evaluate the type of tooth structure (enamel, dentin, cementum), the state of demineralization, and/or the type of restorative material (metal, porcelain, composite) present before a polishing or cleaning agent is selected.

> **Caution**
>
> A significant amount of roughening of composite, porcelain, and gold restorations is produced even by fine prophy pastes.

When considering prophy pastes, select the least abrasive paste possible, or a nonabrasive paste, to remove existing stains and soft deposits. These abrasives should be applied as wet as possible with a light, intermittent touch and at low speed. Whenever coarse or medium paste is selected, it should be followed by the use of fine paste in a new or cleaned prophy cup. Unstained teeth should not be polished with abrasive agents but rather a nonabrasive cleaning paste.

Various prophy pastes have been developed with additives to assist in remineralization and to reduce tooth sensitivity. MI Paste (GC America) contains Recaldent (casein phosphopeptide-amorphous calcium phosphate) (See Fig. 7.14), which allows teeth to remineralize and repair the very early stages of decay. NuCare (Sunstar Butler) with NovaMin (Sultan Healthcare) contains bioactive glass particles that release calcium, sodium, phosphate, and silica ions in the presence of water/saliva. These ions combine to form a hard and strong hydroxycarbonate apatite layer to occlude, and thereby desensitize, dentinal tubules. Use of these pastes before nonsurgical periodontal therapy may be indicated for those patients whose sensitivity to scaling is not profound enough to warrant the use of local anesthetics.

Specialty products are recommended for today's cosmetic restoration when the use of traditional paste will damage the surface, resulting in a less than ideal appearance. NUPRO Shimmer (Dentsply Sirona) is not designed for stain removal due to the particle size in the paste being so fine they are not course enough to remove stain; however, they do produce a high shine on the already polished restoration. Clinpro Prophy Paste (3M ESPE) uses abrasive variability in its formulation; this abrasive begins as a coarse material to remove stain and then quickly breaks down to a fine paste to provide luster. Soft Shine (Waterpik Technologies) is made from micron-fine particles that effectively polish all types of composite and ceramic restorations. Traditional prophy paste is not recommended for use on esthetic restorative materials; use agents that have been specially formulated for esthetic restorative surfaces.

Dentifrice (Toothpaste)

Similar to prophylaxis paste, toothpaste contains a mixture of abrasive materials to clean tooth structures and restorations, and enhance resistance to discoloration and plaque accumulation. These commercial preparations contain 20% to 40% abrasive agents, coloring agents, flavoring agents, and therapeutic agents. The abrasive agents improve the efficiency of the toothbrush in the removal of stains, food debris, and biofilm. They also increase light reflected by the enamel. The lowest possible abrasive rankings are desirable to prevent removal of softer tooth structures and restorations (Fig. 13.14). Sodium bicarbonate and calcium carbonate are the most common abrasives used in commercial preparations of dentifrice. Therapeutic agents that benefit the tooth structures such as fluorides,

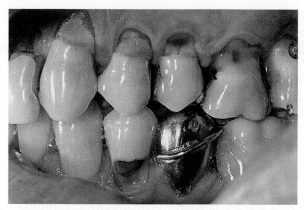

FIG. 13.14 Toothbrush abrasion; notice that the effects of abrasion are also seen on the amalgam restoration. (Courtesy of Dr. Steve Eakle.)

tartar control agents, desensitizing and remineralizing agents, and agents that remoisturize dry mouths are also delivered through dentifrices.

The American Dental Association (ADA) Seal of Acceptance on toothpaste products indicates that the abrasive particles in the dentifrice do not exceed the maximal acceptable abrasiveness, and that scientific data verify claims made by the manufacturer (Table 13.2). The U.S. Food and Drug Administration (FDA) regulates the amount and type of abrasive that is placed in dentifrice.

Benefits of Dentifrices

- Assist in the reduction of biofilm
- Assist in the reduction of stains
- Assist in the reduction of dental caries
- Assist in the reduction of dentin hypersensitivity
- Assist in the remineralization of tooth structures
- Assist in the remoisturizing of dry mouth
- Assist in the reduction of calculus formation

Factors Contributing to Dentifrice Abrasion

- Type of abrasive in the dentifrice
- Amount of abrasive used
- Stiffness of the toothbrush bristle
- Toothbrushing method used by the patient
- Frequency and duration of toothbrushing
- Amount of saliva present
- Type of restorations present
- Amount and location of exposed root surfaces present

Denture Cleansers

The use of a toothbrush with water and a mild cleaning agent (Fig. 13.15) is sufficient to remove most plaque, surface stains, and food debris from removable prosthetic appliances. Immersion of the prosthesis into commercially prepared denture cleansers that loosen stains and deposits then can be rinsed or brushed away is also appropriate. A dental ultrasonic agitating device may be used to improve the efficiency of a commercially prepared immersion agent. Commercially prepared stain and tartar agents are beneficial in the removal of calculus from the prosthesis.

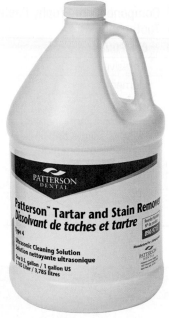

FIG. 13.16 In-office tartar and stain remover. (Courtesy of Patterson Dental.)

⚠ Caution

A well-thought-out infection control protocol must be in place to prevent contamination of a removable prosthesis and ultrasonic cleaner.

Procedure for Cleaning a Removable Prosthesis in the Dental Office with an Ultrasonic Cleaner and Immersion Agent

1. Completely submerge the prosthesis in a sealed bag such as a ziplock bag or use an autoclavable beaker filled with an immersion agent (tarter and stain remover) (Fig. 13.16).
2. Follow the manufacturer's directions for correct dilution of the immersion, amount of time for immersion, and agitation in the ultrasonic, typically 10 to 15 minutes.
3. Remove the prosthesis and rinse thoroughly with water. Be careful to avoid contamination of the prosthesis and the liquid in the ultrasonic basin.
4. Remove loosened debris with a denture brush.

Commercial denture cleansers should be nontoxic, nonabrasive, and harmless to the components of the prosthesis. Full acrylic prostheses can be soaked in dilute alkaline or acid commercial preparations. Prostheses with metal components should not be placed in dilute acid solutions or hypochlorites (bleach) because of the resultant corrosion of these components.

💡 Clinical Tip

Patients should always be reminded to use products specifically developed for home care of these removable prostheses and never to use regular toothpaste, powdered household cleansers, or bleach when cleaning their removable appliances at home, including dentures, partial dentures, orthodontic appliances, mouth guards, and whitening trays.

Table 13.2	Components of Prophy Paste and Toothpaste	
PROPHY PASTE	**COMPONENT**	**TOOTHPASTE**
50%-60%	Abrasive	20%-40%
20%-25%	Humectant	20%-40%
10%-20%	Water	20%-40%
—	Foaming agent—sodium lauryl sulfate (SLS); removed from many dentifrices because of patient sensitivity	1%-2%
2%-3%	Flavoring/coloring agents	2%-3%
1%-2%	Therapeutic (fluoride)	1%-2%

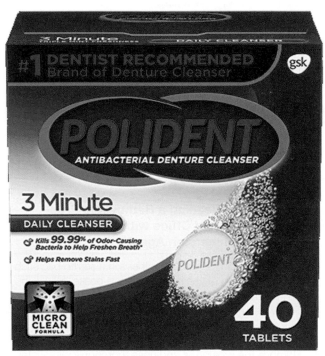

FIG. 13.15 Polident denture cleansing agent. (Courtesy of GlaxoSmithKline.)

FINISHING AND POLISHING PROCEDURES

Finishing and polishing procedures follow a similar sequence. Sufficient amounts of material are removed to reproduce the anatomic contours of the restoration/prosthesis, and finer and finer cuts are then made into the material with diminishing abrasive agents until it takes on a smooth, shiny, mirror-like surface. The benefits of a properly finished and polished restoration/prosthesis include decreased biofilm retention, resistance to tarnish/corrosion, increased longevity of the restoration, decreased attrition of natural tooth surfaces during chewing, improved esthetics, and improved health of surrounding tissues. It is important that the appropriate clinical decision be made as to the choice of abrasive agents, the properties of the surface, and the order in which the abrasives are applied, and that attention be given to thorough removal of each abrasive agent before a finer one is used. If abrasive agents are left on structures or on delivery equipment, they continue to abrade even though a finer abrasive is currently being applied. Some abrasive agents are designed for both finishing and polishing because of the presence of components with abrasive variability. One-step diamond micropolisher cups and points are appropriate for both finishing and polishing. The clinician must be careful of heat generated by the use of rotary instruments, controlling this by applying pressure and speed intermittently, and using water or air for cooling purposes.

In addition, care must be taken to consider the anatomic form of the tooth. The finished and polished restoration should have a smooth, continuous line flush with the tooth surface. When restorative margins end at or near the root, instrumentation near or on this cavosurface margin may result in ditching or gouging of the softer cementum surfaces. Contours of teeth must be re-created and should not be flattened or overly rounded. The contact area need not be polished. Polishing this area may remove material, resulting in an open contact that can lead to impaction of food, causing damage to the periodontium, or may contribute to caries formation.

The provision of finishing and polishing procedures for tooth structures and restorative materials by the oral health care auxiliary is dependent on the scope of practice regulations established by each state.

> **! Caution**
>
> Some intraoral finishing and polishing procedures are not allowed by auxiliary under certain circumstances or with specific types of equipment according to state dental practice acts.

MARGINATION AND REMOVAL OF FLASH

Before finishing or polishing an amalgam or composite restoration, the clinician should check the integrity of the cavosurface margins for prematurities (overhanging margins) and deficiencies (Fig. 13.17). The detrimental effects of overhanging margins on hard and soft tissues are well documented. The overhanging margin acts as a niche for microorganisms that contribute to periodontal disease and caries, prevents the efficient use of dental floss, and increases inflammation. The process of removing restoration prematurities to bring the restoration flush with the cavosurface tooth structure is called **margination**. This process may vary from removal of feathered **flash** to removal of overhang (ledges created by overhanging cervical margins). The decision to remove excessive

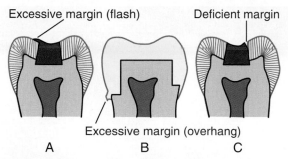

Excessive margin (flash)   Deficient margin

Excessive margin (overhang)

A   B   C

FIG. 13.17 Line drawing of **(A)** excessive occlusal margin (flash); **(B)** excessive proximal margin (overhang); and **(C)** deficient occlusal margin.

Table 13.3	Indications and Contraindications for Air Polishing
INDICATIONS FOR AIR POLISHING	**CONTRAINDICATIONS FOR AIR POLISHING**
Patient with supra-gingival extrinsic stain	Patient with respiratory disease
Patients with biofilm accumulation	Patient with sodium restriction diets when sodium bicarbonate is powder of choice for stain removal
Patients with biofilm induced inflammation	Patient with limited swallowing Patient with difficulty breathing Patient with communicable infections Immunocompromised patients Patient taking potassium, antidiuretics, or steroid therapy.

Hand cutting instruments, such as an amalgam knife, scalers and files, or rotary cutting diamonds burs and carbide burs, are used. When using hand instruments for margination, use very sharp instruments and work apically to the margin of the restoration, using a shaving motion in diagonal overlapping strokes and keeping the instrument in contact with the tooth surface. Avoid trying to remove too much of the overhang, in a single stroke. An ultrasonic scaler, or slow-speed rotary handpiece with abrasive points and cups, may be used to remove overhanging margins. Follow this with hand cutting instruments and finish with abrasive strips, and then check the results with floss and an explorer.

 Caution

If it is determined that the overhanging margin or flash is too large for safe and effective removal by the auxiliary, the patient should be scheduled for an appointment with the dentist, who will perform this procedure or replace the restoration.

material from a restoration is based on clinical and radiographic findings. Careful evaluation of the restoration is necessary to determine whether margination is indicated or the restoration needs to be replaced (see the accompanying box "Indications for Margination"). Margination may be indicated if the **overhang** is small, the contact is intact, and there is no indication of caries. Margination is not generally within the scope of practice for the dental assistant, and although it is within the scope of practice for the dental hygienist in many states it should not be considered a routine procedure. Careful consideration as to the type and amount of restorative material present must be made before undertaking this procedure. Margination by the dental hygienist may be performed with hand cutting instruments, with a slow-speed rotary device, or with ultrasonic instruments although instruments may not effectively or safely remove large overhanging margins. Extreme care must be used to preserve the integrity of the existing restoration and to prevent damage to adjacent tooth and tissue structures.

AMALGAM

It is generally recommended that amalgam restorations be polished no sooner than 24 hours after placement. The slow final setting of traditional amalgams and potential for chipping the margins of even the new high-copper amalgams prevent immediate polishing (see Chapter 10). In addition, as many older types of amalgams age, the results of creep and corrosion produce surfaces that may benefit from periodic polishing procedures. This does not seem to be a problem for the newer high-copper amalgams. The amount of finishing and polishing required depends on the care taken in carving and burnishing the amalgam at the time of placement and the effects of the oral environment on older restorations (Fig. 13.18).

FINISHING AND POLISHING AMALGAM RESTORATIONS

Polishing of amalgam should begin by evaluating cavosurface margins for excess material, and remove as indicated (Procedure 13.1). Finishing is next, using abrasive devices to remove severe scratches and surface defects. Bonded and coated abrasives greater

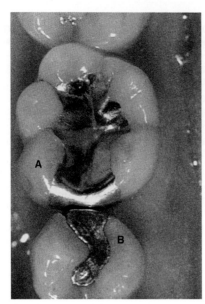

FIG. 13.18 **A,** Polished amalgam restoration. **B,** Unpolished amalgam restoration.

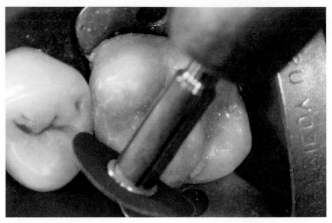

FIG. 13.19 (From Heymann H, Swift E, Ritter A: Sturdevant's Art & Science of Operative Dentistry (ed 6). St. Louis, 2013, Elsevier.)

than 25 µm in particle size or special multifluted finishing burs are used. Polishing that is accomplished with bonded, coated, or loose abrasives ranging in particle diameter from 20 µm to submicron-sized gives the amalgam restoration a mirror-like luster. Care must be taken whenever rotary instruments are used to avoid the generation of excessive heat and aerosols. The use of water through an air-water syringe or from the handpiece and proper evacuation are recommended.

COMPOSITE

Composite restorations are finished and polished in three steps as part of the restorative procedure (Procedure 13.2). Marginal and occlusal excesses are first removed in initial finishing with diamonds or multifluted carbide burs. Intermediate finishing is accomplished with flexible disks (Fig. 13.19), cups, and strips, beginning with coarse and sequentially proceeding to superfine. Final polishing is accomplished with a submicron aluminum oxide–based polishing paste applied with soft cups or felt pads (see the accompanying box, "Finishing and Polishing Composite Restorations").

Finishing and Polishing Composite Restorations

Initial finishing: Bonded and coated rotary abrasives, 100 µm or larger, or multifluted carbide or diamond finishing burs

Intermediate finishing: Bonded and coated rotary abrasives <100 µm but >20 µm

Final polishing: Bonded and coated abrasives or polishing paste from 20 to 0.3 µm to produce a final luster.

Traditional prophy paste, air polishing, and the use of ultrasonic scalers are not recommended for most esthetic restorations. If the composite has developed extrinsic staining, it may need to be polished after placement. Fine abrasives are used in progression from fine to finest, with care taken to change the delivery device and rinse thoroughly between each polishing. The procedure should remove only the outermost stained surface and should produce a lustrous finish.

GOLD ALLOY

Precious and nonprecious crowns, inlays, and onlays are finished and polished in the dental laboratory before they are delivered to the dental office for final fitting and cementation. In the process of final fitting, minor adjustments made with abrasive stones and diamonds may be necessary. It is important that the resultant scratches are removed before final cementation. Burlew wheels on a slow-speed handpiece are used, followed by rouge on a rag wheel (Fig. 13.11).

CERAMICS (PORCELAIN)

Ceramic restorations (including porcelain) achieve a glassy smooth surface from the glazing procedure at high temperatures (see Chapter 9). Occasionally, they need some adjustment and are finished and polished in the dental laboratory. Adjustments made chairside during the fitting of these restorations are done with diamonds. The resultant roughened ceramic surface after clinical adjustment has been shown to increase wear of opposing tooth structure. Clinicians must properly finish and polish ceramic restorations after making adjustments. Rubber polishing points and wheels designed for ceramics are used for finishing, and diamond polishing paste (Fig. 13.20) is used for the final polish of the restoration to an enamel-like luster.

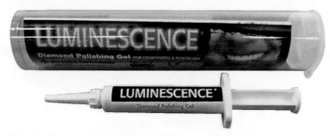

FIG. 13.20 Diamond polishing paste utilized for the final polish of ceramic restorations. (Courtesy Abrasive Technology, Inc.)

! Caution

Heat generated during adjustment may also result in cracking of ceramic—always use low speed and low pressure to minimize heat generation and cracking.

Characteristics of a Properly Finished and Polished Restoration

- Smooth anatomic contours
- Contact areas intact with normal form
- Embrasures spaced correctly
- Refined margins
- Smooth surfaces
- Restored function
- Eliminate biofilm retention irregularities
- Restored gingival health

Chairside Adjusting and Polishing of Acrylic Denture Bases

After the placement of a new denture or partial, a reline of the prosthesis or when weight loss occurs, a patient may need to have a denture or partial adjusted due to sore spots or over-extensions of the acrylic flanges into the vestibule or posterior of the mouth that makes the appliance hard to wear. The dentist will evaluate the denture for any necessary adjustments and make those adjustment at chairside. The first step is to trim any excess material with an acrylic bur (Fig. 13.21, far left). (See Chapter 17 for detection of sore spots with Pressure Indicator Paste or Colored Transfer Applicators.)

Once the appropriate amount of material has been removed the dentist will polish the denture by using a series of abrasives and rubber points to eliminate the roughness caused by the burs and more abrasive points (see Fig. 13.21, points are in order by abrasivity, blue most abrasive to yellow least abrasive). In order to ensure scratches are not left in the surface of the appliance which could harbor bacteria, the dentist will incrementally move from the most abrasive material to the least abrasive material. This will leave a smooth surface on the appliance.

POLISHING DURING ORAL PROPHYLAXIS (CORONAL POLISH)

Before the coronal polishing procedure is begun, a careful tactile evaluation of tooth surfaces must be done to

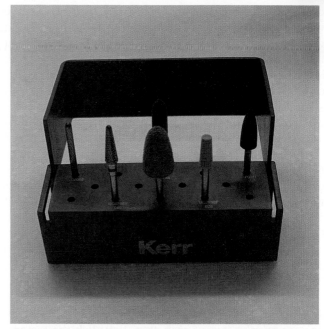

FIG. 13.21 Acrylic finishing and polishing kit utilized for chairside polishing of a partial or complete denture. (Courtesy of Matt Crimaldi.)

correctly identify and remove calculus. If a restoration is incorrectly identified as calculus and is aggressively scaled, the restoration may be removed or altered to the point of needing replacement. In addition, all restorative materials must be identified to prevent undesired removal, damaging of margins, or scratching of the surface by traditional, commercially prepared prophy paste (see Chapter 2 for identification of restorative materials). Adverse effects on the tooth surface with the use of prophy paste and the philosophy of selective polish are discussed earlier in this chapter [see the Caution box in the section "Prophylaxis (Prophy) Paste"]; polishing must be a carefully considered part of the oral prophylaxis. The clinician must consider the tooth structure as well as restorative surface when choosing the most appropriate polishing or cleaning agent.

AMALGAM

Low-copper amalgam restorations will tarnish and corrode over the years (see Chapter 10). Polishing during oral prophylaxis may greatly benefit these restorations. Rubber cups or bristle brushes with commercially prepared prophy paste are used on occlusal and smooth surfaces and dental tape on proximal surfaces. The contact area should not be polished, as contact with the adjacent tooth may be lost.

COMPOSITE

Composite restorations, which become stained after placement, may be polished as part of a regular maintenance appointment. The use of ultrasonic and sonic scalers and air-polishing devices should be avoided on or around these restorations because these instruments may damage the surface of the restoration. The use of traditional prophy pastes may cause excessive wear; typically these restorations should be polished with aluminum oxide polishing paste. It is important that composite restorations be polished only if stain is present, and that appropriate manufacture's recommended materials are selected and used to avoid scratching or altering the surface of the softer composite materials. Begin stain removal with the least abrasive products. If the stain is not easily removed with fine paste, proceed to more aggressive grits or rubber polishing points and finishing disks. Pay close attention to the restoration's contour and marginal integrity, always keeping the rotary instrument moving using a light, sweeping intermittent motion. Complete the polishing procedure using light pressure with a very wet, specialized polishing paste on a soft felt pad. Total polishing time should not exceed 30 seconds on any stained surface.

Remember to proceed sequentially from most abrasive to least abrasive polishing material, using a clean or new prophy cup at each step, to polish the restoration. Staining at the margins may also represent microleakage (see Chapter 6, Fig. 6.3) that penetrates under the restoration. These stains cannot be polished away (Procedure 13.2).

GOLD ALLOYS AND CERAMICS

Ceramics and gold alloys are extremely resistant to staining (see Chapter 9). If scratches or irregularities are present, they are usually due to instrumentation that has scratched the outer glaze of the ceramic or high polish of the gold. Regular prophy paste is not recommended for polishing ceramic restorations because of possible removal of the glaze layer. Specialty pastes (such as Proxyt) are available that contain microfine particles that are not harmful for polishing porcelain veneers and crowns (Fig. 13.22).

RESIN/CEMENT INTERFACE

Margins on resin-bonded ceramic restorations are more susceptible to staining because of the properties of resin cements. Stains accumulating at the ceramic/cement interface must be evaluated carefully for actual staining or microleakage.

IMPLANTS

The clinician must be careful not to abrade the surface integrity of titanium implants (see Chapter 12). Biofilm may be removed with special titanium hand instruments, plastic sheaths for ultrasonic scalers, and nonabrasive cleaning paste (such as Proxyt) or tin oxide. Air polishing with glycine is also appropriate for removal of soft deposits on implants.

AIR POLISHING AND AIR ABRASION

The use of air to propel very small particles (microparticles) as a replacement for rotary cutting instruments (a process called air abrasion) has not proven to

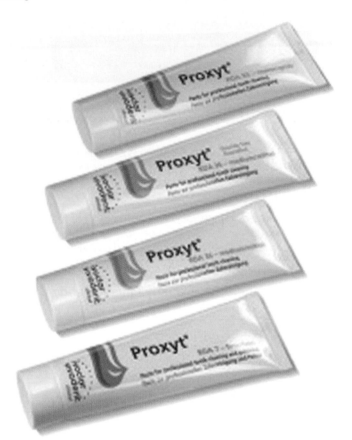

FIG. 13.22 Proxyt polishing paste. (Courtesy of Ivoclar Vivadent.)

be as successful as originally expected and is seldom used in modern practices. Air polishing, however, is very successful and widely used to remove extrinsic stains and biofilm. If used, clinicians should follow manufacturers' recommendations for precautions in safety and contraindications in individual clinical applications.

Supragingival Air Polishing

Supragingival air polishing uses several forms of powder (sodium bicarbonate, aluminum trihydroxide, glycine, erythritol, calcium sodium phosphosilicate, or calcium carbonate) plus flavoring agents, air, and water at a pressure of approximately 40 to 60 pounds per square inch (psi) as a fast, effective, and efficient means of removing stains and soft deposits from enamel surfaces and in pits and fissures. Glycine and erythritol powders have been found to produce less surface damage on restoratives than sodium bicarbonate powders; however glycine does not remove stain and is only effective in biofilm removal. Calcium sodium phosphosilicate powder has been found to have desensitizing results in cases of dentinal hypersensitivity, and aluminum trihydroxide powders contain harder particles that should not be used on most esthetic restorations.

Proper technique is essential to remove stain and biofilm while controlling contaminated aerosols and preventing soft tissue damage. The closer the tip of

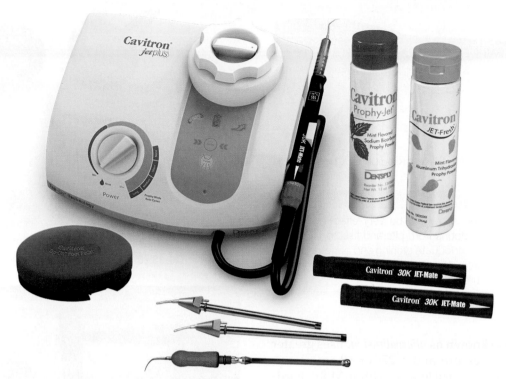

FIG. 13.23 Supra-gingival air polishing unit. (Courtesy of Dentsply International [York, PA].)

the air-polishing unit is to the tooth surface the greater the amount of aerosols produced. The nozzle of the air-polishing unit should be kept in a constant circular motion 3 to 4 mm from the tooth surface, at an angle of 60 to 80 degrees on smooth surfaces and a 90 degree angle on occlusal surfaces. Most research continues to recommend caution near restorations, particularly composite, resin cement, and porcelain surfaces (Fig. 13.23).

Air polishing is less abrasive than traditional prophy paste, as the particles used in air polishing have a Mohs hardness ranking of 3 versus the ranking of 6 found in some traditional prophy pastes. Air polishing is not contraindicated for use on enamel and may be less damaging to cementum or dentin than traditional polishing. In addition, air polishing can be safely used on titanium implants and orthodontically banded/bracketed teeth.

Subgingival Air Polishing

Subgingival air polishing is the process of polishing the anatomical crown and clinical root surface using fine particles under air pressure of approximately 40 pounds per square inch to remove biofilm subgingivally. Subgingival air polishing improves periodontal health by detoxifying root surfaces in shallow to moderate or deep periodontal pockets. The powder approved in the United States for use in the in the subgingival air polishing unit is glycine (Mohs ranking of 2). Other forms of powder (sodium bicarbonate, aluminum trihydroxide, calcium sodium phosphosilicate, or calcium carbonate) should not be used as they are more abrasive than the glycine, which can cause

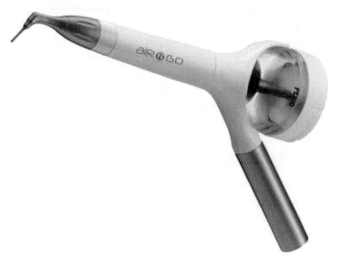

FIG. 13.24 Subgingival air polishing unit. (Courtesy of Acteon Group.)

damage to the tooth structure and the junctional epithelium (Fig. 13.24).

As with supragingival air polishing, proper technique is essential with Subgingival air polishing to prevent the spread of dental aerosols and air-polishing powders. Glycine powder can be used in most air polishing devices; however, a subgingival nozzle is required to reach the depth of the sulcus. The nozzle is inserted into the pocket at a 90-degree angle to the long axis of the root until resistance is met, then moved back from the base of the pocket about a 3 mm distance. At this time the tip is activated, dispensing glycine and water under pressure to remove biofilm. The tip should not be activated for longer than 5 seconds per root surface.

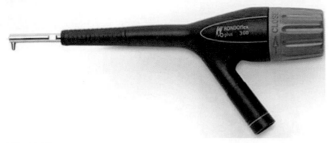

FIG. 13.25 Air abrasion tip. (Courtesy of KaVo Dental [Charlotte, NC].)

 Clinical Tip

Air polishing has been shown to be very effective in the removal of stains and debris from pits and fissures. Debris in the fissures prevents adequate etching and penetration of sealant into the fissures. Air polishing eliminates this cause for many pit and fissure sealant failures.

Air Abrasion

Air abrasion, also known as *microabrasion*, uses greater compressed air pressure and a 27- or 50-µm aluminum oxide powder particle size with a Mohs hardness ranking of 9. This process is used for chairside cleaning of cast appliances before cementation, intraoral repair of ceramic and composite restorations, and preparation of tooth surfaces before bonding. Air pressure of 40 to 160 psi and a controlled adjustable-tip orifice allow aluminum oxide particles to strike a tooth or restoration with enough force to effectively abrade the surface. Cutting can be controlled to remove minimal amounts of tooth and restorative structure (Fig. 13.25).

 Caution

The use of appropriate clinician and patient safety equipment and control of aerosols with high-volume evacuation are critical for both air polishing and air abrasion.

LABORATORY FINISHING AND POLISHING

Some appliances and restorations such as complete and partial dentures and gold crowns must be polished after adjustments have been made to them. The adjustments can be made at chairside and some polishing devices are available for chairside use (see Fig. 13.21). However, many clinicians utilize rag wheels and/or felt tips or wheels in the dental office laboratory to complete the final polishing of these appliances and restorations (prior to cementation) (Fig. 13.26).

RAG WHEEL

The rag wheel is a polishing device made of muslin or cloth clamped or sewn together in the shape of a

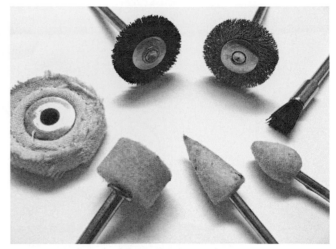

FIG. 13.26 (Courtesy of T. Rand Collins MD.)

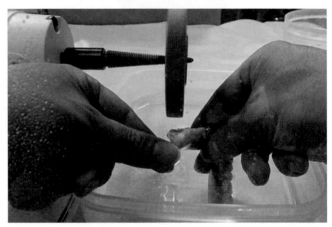

FIG. 13.27 Polishing acrylic on partial denture. (Courtesy of Masanari Oshima.)

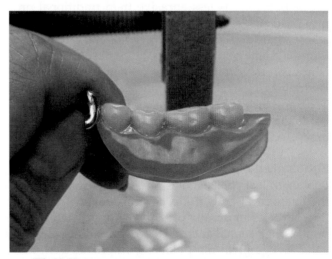

FIG. 13.28 Polished acrylic. (Courtesy of Masanari Oshima.)

wheel. They come in a variety of sizes that can be used with a laboratory handpiece or dental lathe. A polishing agent is added to the rag wheel and used for buffing or polishing acrylic appliances such as denture and partial denture bases (Figs. 13.27 and 13.28).

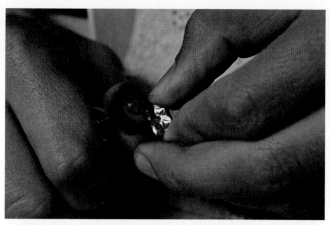

FIG. 13.29 U.S. Air Force Senior Airman Justin Rhodes, 20th Dental Squadron dental lab technician, polishes a gold crown at Shaw Air Force Base, S.C., May 15, 2012. Rhodes is a native of Owensboro, KY. (U.S. Air Force photo by Airman Nicole Sikorski/Released.)

FELT CONES AND WHEELS

Felt cones and wheels are polishing devices made of felt in the shape of cones and wheels that can be used with a laboratory handpiece or dental lathe. The abrasive agent is added to the felt polishing device and used to smooth restorations and appliances (Fig. 13.29).

SAFETY/INFECTION CONTROL

Aerosols are created whenever a rotary device and moisture are used. These aerosols can provide a means for disease transmission. The use of rotary devices may produce particulate matter and vapors from the substrate being abraded. Silica particles from restorations and mercury vapors pose potential health risks. In addition, splatter from abrasives can produce serious eye damage. These particles are released into the air and are hazards to dental personnel and their patients. The use of precautionary personal protective equipment, including a mask and eye protection, is essential for the dental team. Protective eyewear is highly recommended for the patient as well. The use of pre-procedure antimicrobial rinses has been shown to reduce microbial aerosols, and high-speed evacuation is recommended instead of a saliva ejector.

> **! Caution**
>
> - Maintain dental laboratory asepsis by sterilizing or disinfecting all wheels and rotary cutting devices
> - Use fresh, dry powders for each procedure, and remove contaminated portions of stick or block abrasives
> - Maintain adequate ventilation to efficiently remove particulates from the air

PATIENT EDUCATION

Composite restorations and resin-bonded ceramic restorations are particularly susceptible to staining. Effective oral hygiene techniques and awareness of dietary staining and stain-producing habits can prevent a certain amount of surface discoloration. Thorough removal of biofilm from restorative surfaces will prevent staining associated with bacterial accumulation.

Patient education on the effects of staining foods, particularly colored beverages such as coffee, tea, soft drinks, and wine, and on the result of tobacco stain on composite restorations and tooth surfaces, should be part of the original restorative procedure, as should regular recall appointments. Patients with exposed cementum and dentin are particularly susceptible to staining and the effects of abrasives. In an attempt to improve the color of their teeth, patients may use home remedies or excessively abrasive commercial products. The consequences often are toothbrush abrasion and wear of restorations and tooth surfaces. Patient education should include the use of approved abrasive agents. The maintenance of esthetic restorations and tooth structure is a collaborative effort between the patient and the clinician. Good patient education and the evaluation of teeth and restorations for appropriate polishing and finishing will increase oral esthetics and patient satisfaction.

SUMMARY

The decision to abrade a surface to contour, finish, polish, or cleanse a structure requires careful consideration. The clinician must have knowledge of the properties of the material being abraded, the abrasive, and the factors that affect abrasion. The process of abrasion can produce undesirable effects if not carefully controlled. Appropriate use of abrasion can also produce a surface that will contribute to the esthetics and longevity of the restoration and the health of surrounding oral tissues.

INSTRUCTIONAL VIDEOS

See the Evolve Resources site for a variety of educational videos that reinforce the material covered in this chapter.

Procedure 13.1   Finishing and Polishing a Preexisting Amalgam Restoration

See Evolve site for Competency Sheet

Consider the following with this procedure: safety glasses are recommended for the patient, PPE is required for the operator, ensure appropriate safety protocols are followed, and check your local state guidelines before performing this procedure.

EQUIPMENT/SUPPLIES (FIG. 13.30)

1. Mirror and explorer
2. Air-water syringe
3. Articulating paper
4. Isolation materials
5. Slow-speed handpiece and attachment
6. Finishing burs, stones, disks, and cups
7. Dappen dish
8. Pumice or polishing paste
9. Disposable rubber cup and brush
10. Tin oxide

NOTE: Polish amalgam no sooner than 24 hours after insertion to allow the amalgam to develop its maximal strength.

PROCEDURE STEPS

Examine the cavosurface margins of the entire restoration for excess material.

NOTE: Remove excess material to prevent plaque accumulation or gingival irritation.

1. Check occlusion with articulating paper and clinically for premature occlusal contact; look for equal intensity of the articulating paper markings.

NOTE: Premature occlusal contact can cause sensitivity and excessive wear on the restoration or opposing teeth; the dentist will need to adjust the occlusion.

2. Remove proximal cavosurface excesses with an amalgam knife or a similar sharp instrument, using short, overlapping strokes (Fig. 13.31).
3. Isolate the restoration with cotton rolls and saliva ejector.
4. Use pointed stones for the occlusal surface and a disk or cup for smooth surfaces, beginning with the coarsest abrasive (i.e., a brown cup or "brownie") and then with finer abrasives ("greenies" and finally "super greenies") (Fig. 13.32 and 13.33). Adapt the side of the stone to the restoration and tooth.
5. Use slow to low-moderate speed, always moving the stone from tooth to amalgam to prevent ditching the cavosurface margin.
6. Use a light sweeping intermittent motion while keeping the finishing instrument moving to avoid excessive heat and mercury vapor production. Maintain a wet environment to reduce heat.
7. Rinse the area thoroughly when changing abrasives to prevent the more abrasive particles from abrading the surface.

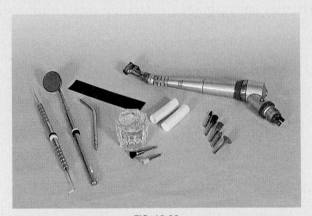

FIG. 13.30

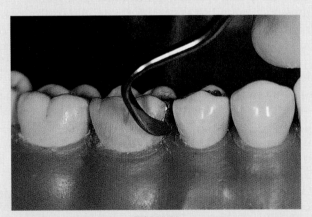

FIG. 13.31

8. Use the rubber cup and brush with a slurry of pumice and then tin oxide (Fig. 13.34).

9. Keep the cup or brush in motion at all times, using light intermittent strokes and moderate speed.

10. Rinse thoroughly between the use of pumice and tin oxide.

11. Polish the proximal surfaces with a handheld finishing strip or pumice and dental tape.

12. Wrap the strip around the tooth contours to avoid flattening of proximal contours (Fig. 13.35).

13. Do not polish through the contact area. Polishing through the contact area can create a weak or open contact.

14. NOTE: The final product is shown in Fig. 13.36.

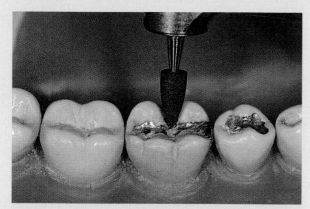

FIG. 13.32

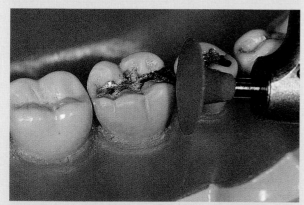

FIG. 13.33

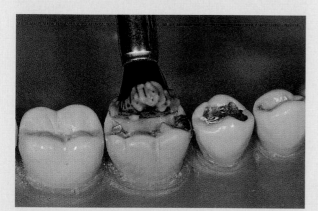

FIG. 13.34

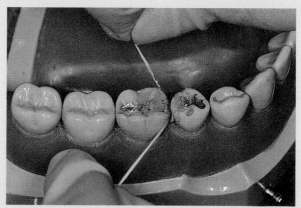

FIG. 13.35

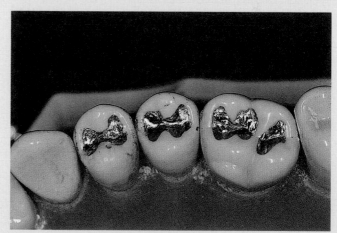

FIG. 13.36

Procedure 13.2 Polishing a Preexisting Composite Restoration

See Evolve site for Competency Sheet.

Consider the following with this procedure: safety glasses are recommended for the patient, PPE is required for the operator, ensure appropriate safety protocols are followed, and check your local state guidelines before performing this procedure.

EQUIPMENT/SUPPLIES (FIG. 13.37)

1. Mirror and explorer
2. Air-water syringe
3. Isolation materials
4. Slow-speed handpiece and attachment
5. Abrasive finishing disks
6. Sterilizable mandrel
7. Abrasive flexible wheels and points
8. Polishing paste
9. Rubber cup

NOTE: Initial contouring, finishing, and polishing are done immediately after insertion.

PROCEDURE STEPS

1. Examine the restoration for staining.
   NOTE: Do not polish if stain is not present.
2. Isolate the area with cotton rolls and saliva ejector.
3. Remove cavosurface flash with a sharp scaler, a #12 scalpel blade, or a gold knife.
4. **NOTE:** A gold knife, also called a finishing knife or amalgam knife, has a small, thin blade designed to carve restorative materials.
   NOTE: Avoid deeply scratching the restorative material. A shaving motion is used rather than bulk removal, as bulk removal may result in voids at the margins if excess composite is removed.
5. Use, in order, coarse to fine abrasive disks on a sterilizable mandrel or flexible wheels and rubber points, rinsing after each application (Fig. 13.38 and 13.39).
   NOTE: Rinse thoroughly to completely eliminate coarser particles before polishing with finer abrasive disks, to prevent overabrasion.
6. Use a light sweeping intermittent motion from enamel to restoration (Fig. 13.40).

NOTE: This pattern of movement prevents ditching of restorations at the margins.

7. Keep the rotary device in motion at all times.
   NOTE: Smooth surfaces can be polished using cups and disks; occlusal surfaces are better reached with points (Fig. 13.41).
8. Complete the polish with sequentially applied abrasive paste on a rubber cup.
   NOTE: This must be an abrasive paste designed for polishing composites; begin with coarse and proceed through superfine.

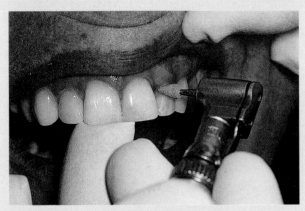

FIG. 13.38

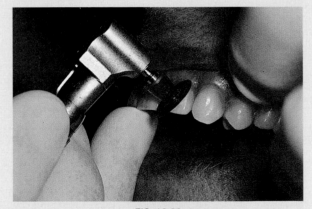

FIG. 13.39

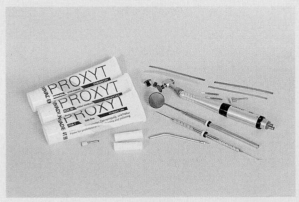

FIG. 13.37

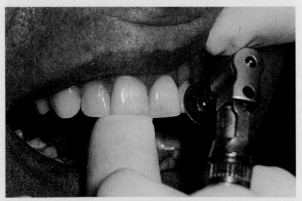

FIG. 13.40

Procedure 13.2   Polishing a Preexisting Composite Restoration

9. Polish proximal surfaces with handheld polishing strips or polishing paste and dental tape (Fig. 13.42).

NOTE: These strips must be very thin to prevent loss of the proximal contact.

10. Avoid flattening of proximal contours.

NOTE: Keep the rotary polishing device or abrasive strip contoured to the shape of the tooth.

11. Rinse thoroughly and evaluate for smoothness and luster.

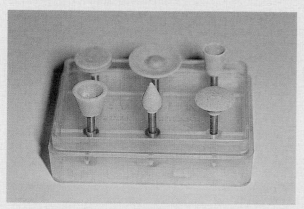

FIG. 13.41

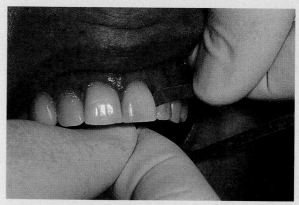

FIG. 13.42

Get Ready for Exams!

Review Questions

Select the one correct response for each of the following multiple-choice questions.

1. The goal of finishing and polishing of restorations includes:
   a. The removal of excess material
   b. The smoothing of roughened surfaces
   c. The production of better esthetics
   d. All of the above

2. Cleaning of teeth is primarily meant to:
   a. Remove excess material
   b. Smooth roughened surfaces
   c. Remove soft deposits
   d. Recontour surfaces

3. The depth and space between cuts made by an abrasive are determined by:
   a. The properties of the abrasive
   b. The properties of the substrate being abraded
   c. The contour of the restoration
   d. Both a and b

4. Which of the following represents the correct hardness ranking, from hardest to softest?
   a. Gold, amalgam, composite, enamel
   b. Enamel, amalgam, gold, composite
   c. Composite, enamel, gold, amalgam
   d. Amalgam, enamel, composite, gold

5. All of the following will increase the rate of abrasion *except*:
   a. Increased pressure
   b. Decreased speed
   c. Use of larger abrasive particles
   d. Use of more abrasive particles than substrate

6. Which powder is best for subgingival air polishing practices?
   a. Sodium bicarbonate
   b. Aluminum trihydroxide
   c. Glycine
   d. Calcium carbonate

7. To control the numbers of abrasive particles that contact the surface:
   a. The operator should increase the speed
   b. The operator should decrease the pressure
   c. The operator should use a lubricant
   d. The operator should not use rotary instruments

8. Loose abrasives:
   a. Are safe-sided
   b. Are used on cups and brushes
   c. Come in various shapes
   d. Use sterilizable mandrels

9. A substance used to prevent a dentifrice from drying is called a(n):
   a. Humectant
   b. Binder
   c. Detergent
   d. Alkaline peroxide

10. After polishing a patient's teeth you notice scratches on a gold crown; the following most likely contributed to these scratches:
    a. Use of an inappropriate polishing agent
    b. Corrosion of the crown
    c. Improper toothbrushing
    d. None of the above would contribute to scratches on the crown

Continued

11. Your patient has older amalgam restorations present, and you have determined that these restorations could benefit from amalgam polish. Give the correct sequence in the use of rubber abrasive points:
    a. Brownies, super greenies, greenies
    b. Brownies, greenies, super greenies
    c. Supper greenies, greenies, brownies
    d. Greenies, super greenies, brownies

For answers to Review Questions, see the Appendix.

Case-Based Discussion Topics

1. *Discuss how the operator uses knowledge of the factors that affect abrasion to control the polishing sequence of* an amalgam restoration, a composite restoration, and a gold restoration.

2. *List two materials used to polish stains from the coronal surfaces of teeth, and discuss the contraindications to using various abrasives on tooth surfaces.*

3. *Case Study Question*
A 30-year-old computer programmer comes to the dental office complaining of catching dental floss on a new class II distal occlusal (DO) composite restoration on tooth #29. Examination reveals excess composite at the gingival margin and an overcontoured distofacial surface of this restoration.
Discuss instruments, materials, and techniques for correcting the problem.

BIBLIOGRAPHY

American Dental Hygienists' Association (ADHA): *Association Position Paper on the Oral Prophylaxis.* Available at https://www.adha.org/resources-docs/7115_Prophylaxis_Postion_Paper.pdf.

Anusavice KJ, Shen C, Rawls HR: *Phillips' Science of Dental Materials* (ed 12). Philadelphia, 2013, Saunders.

Barnes CM: Polishing esthetic restorative materials. *Dimensions of Dental Hygiene,* 8(24):26–28, 2010.

Barmes CM: Shining a new light on selective polishing. *Dimensions of Dental Hygiene,* 10(3):42–44, 2012.

Barnes CM: *Air Polishing: A Mainstay for Dental Hygiene, ADA Continuing Education Recognition Program.* PennWell Publications, St. Louis, July 2013. Available at https://www.yumpu.com/en/document/read/22671110/air-polishing-a-mainstay-for-dental-hygiene-ineedcecom.

Bird D, Robinson D: *Modern Dental Assisting* (ed 12). Missouri, St. Louis, 2018, Elsevier.

Calley K: Maintaining the beauty and longevity of esthetic restorations. *Dimens Dental Hygiene,* 7:38–41, 2009.

Darby M: *An Evidence-Based Approach to Cleansing and Polishing Teeth.* The American Academy for Oral Systemic Health, 2012. Available at https://aaosh.org/evidence-based-approach-cleansing-polishing-teeth/.

Darby M, Walsh M: *Dental Hygiene Theory and Practice* (ed 4). Missouri, 2015, Elsevier Saunders.

Daubert D: Subgingival air polishing. *Dimensions of Dental Hygiene,* 11(12):69–73, 2013.

Davis K: *Biofilm Removal with Air Polishing and Subgingival Air Polishing, ADA Continuing Education Recognition Programpennwell publications,* 2013. Available at https://fliphtml5.com/jarv/ijwq/basic.

Davis K: *Do You Know About Air-Flow Perio? RDH Magazine* 2013. Available at https://www.rdhmag.com/articles/print/volume-33/issue-1/coumns/glycine-powder-aids-in-periodontal-biofilm-removal.html.

Felix L, Mossman S: Dental hygienists play key roles in advising patients on restorative options and helping them maintain them. *Dimensions in Dental Hygiene,* 15(3):30–31, 2017.

Gutkowski S: The trek to positive polishing, mastering the challenge to actually use air polishers. *RDH Magazine,* 6:68–70, 2013.

Mopper K: Contouring, finishing, and polishing anterior composites, *Inside Dentistry,* 7(3):62–70, 2011.

Mossman SL: Material selection and maintenance. *Dimensions of Dental Hygiene,* 12:63–67, 2014.

Pence S: Polishing basics. *Dimensions of Dental Hygiene,* 11(26):28, 2013.

Pence S: Polishing particulars. *Dimensions of Dental Hygiene,* 11(26):28, 2013.

Robinson D, Bird D: *Essentials of Dental Assisting,* (ed 6). Missouri, 2017, St. Louis, Elsevier.

Sorensen JA: Finishing and polishing with modern ceramic systems. *Inside Dentistry,* 2:10–16, 2013.

Wilkins E: *Clinical Practice of the Dental Hygienist* (ed 12). Philadelphia, 2017, Lippincott, Williams & Wilkins.

Chapter Objectives

Upon completion of this chapter, the student should be able to:

1. Compare the various types of cements for:
   - Pulpal protection
   - Luting
   - Restorations
   - Surgical dressing
2. Describe the properties of cement, and explain how these properties affect selection of cement for a dental procedure.
3. Identify the components of the various dental cements.
4. Describe how the components of various dental cements affect the properties of the cement.

5. Compare the advantages and disadvantages of each cement.
6. Describe the manipulation considerations for mixing cements.
7. Describe the procedure for filling a crown with luting cement.
8. Describe the procedure for removing excess cement after cementation.
9. Apply the mixing technique for each type of cement.

Key Terms

Cavity Varnish a thin layer of resinous material placed on the floor and walls of the preparation to seal the tubules and minimize microleakage

Liner a thin layer of material placed to protect the pulp from the chemical components of dental materials, from oral fluids and microorganisms associated with microleakage, to stimulate reparative dentin, or to act as a pulp capping

Base a thick layer of cement used to protect the tooth from chemical and thermal irritation and to support restorations in deep cavity preparations

Secondary Consistency thick, putty-like, condensable physical state of a material which can be rolled into a ball or rope, suitable for use as a base

Buildup a thick layer of cement or restorative material used to replace missing tooth structure in a badly broken-down tooth and to act as support for a restoration such as a crown

Luting cementing two components together such as an indirect restoration cemented on or in a tooth, including inlays, crowns, bridges, veneers, orthodontic brackets and bands, and posts and pins

Permanent lasting indefinitely

Temporary/Provisional referring to materials expected to last from a few days to a few weeks

Intermediate referring to materials expected to last from a few weeks to a year

Sedative soothing; acting to relieve pain

Primary Consistency less viscous, easily flowing state of a material which can be can be drawn out to a 1-inch string with a spatula lifted from the center of the mass, suitable for luting

Adhesion the attractive forces of atoms or molecules that join two surfaces together

---

Few materials in dentistry are used as frequently or with as many applications as dental cements. There are an impressive number of dental cements available, and each may have specific or multiple uses. No single cement is universally acceptable for all applications; rather, various cements are available whose properties and manipulation make them an appropriate choice for a given application. There are cements specifically targeted for use in orthodontics, endodontics, surgery, and implants. Many dental cements have inferior strength and high solubility when compared

with other restorative materials and, with the exception of resin and glass ionomer cements, have little or no adhesive properties. Even with these limitations, cements are used in a wide variety of dental procedures. The clinical demands of different types of prosthetic restorations, ranging from gold crowns, PFM (porcelain-fused-to-metal) crowns, all-ceramic crowns, indirect composite resins, and CAD/CAM (computer-assisted design/computer-assisted machining) products, have made the selection of cements more challenging. With the multitude of cements available, it is easy to become confused as to which cement should be selected for a given situation. In most cases, the dentist will select the cement for a procedure on the basis of mechanical as well as biological factors. It becomes the dental assistant's responsibility to manipulate the cement to the proper consistency within the recommended mixing time. Many expanded function auxiliaries are also placing the cement, seating the crown and removing the excess at the end of a procedure. The dental hygienist may be placing and removing cements and instrumenting against the cement surface during periodontal procedures. It is important that the oral health practitioner have a thorough understanding of cement uses, properties, limitations, and manipulation to effectively use and work around these materials.

DENTAL CEMENTS

Cement can be defined as a substance that binds two surfaces together rigidly. In dentistry cement, when set, is a hard, brittle material with a wide range of applications such as lining a cavity preparation, as a temporary or permanent filling or securing a crown in place. Typically, cement is formed by mixing two components together, often a powder and liquid or two pastes that becomes a viscous liquid or mass that hardens. Luting agents are cements used as adhesives to secure indirect restorations to the tooth.

CLASSIFICATION

Dental cements have been classified by their uses and properties into three categories by the International Standards Organization and the American Dental Association.

Type I Cements. These cements are luting agents that glue crowns, bridges, onlays and inlays to the tooth or cement or bond orthodontic bands or brackets in place. These cements can be permanent (long-term) or provisional (temporary).

Type II Cements. These cements are used for provisional or intermediate restorations or long-term in the case of glass ionomer cements. Cements used as dental sealants are also in this group.

Type III Cements. These cements are used for bases or liners for cavity preparations.

USES OF DENTAL CEMENTS

Dental cements have a variety of uses. These include pulpal protection and sedation, luting of indirect restorations, provisional restorations, intermediate intracoronal restorations, root canal sealers and surgical dressings (Table 14.1).

Pulpal Protection

The bacterial effects of caries, the biological response to chemicals contained in restorative materials, and even the cutting of tooth structure may cause pulpal irritation. Pulpal irritation can also occur as the result of thermal conductivity of metal restorations placed near the pulp, and when the dentin remaining over the pulp is too thin to withstand compressive, tensile, and shearing stresses. Many of the chemicals contained within the materials used to restore teeth have the potential to cause irritation. Older amalgam formulations were prone to more corrosive products leaking into the tubules of the tooth structure, causing discoloration. Cavity varnishes, liners, and bases act as protective layers between the dentin and the restorative material (Fig. 14.1). There has been a dramatic reduction in the use of pulpal protection materials as resin bonding technologies and high-copper amalgams have replaced these older types of restorations.

TABLE 14.1   Uses of Dental Cements

USES OF CEMENTS	CEMENT
Cavity liner/pulpal cap	Calcium hydroxide
Pulpal medicament/low-strength base	Zinc oxide eugenol
High-strength bases	Reinforced zinc oxide eugenol, zinc phosphate, zinc polycarboxylate, GIC, RMGIC, resin-based cements
Crown buildups	RMGIC, composite resins
Permanent cementation	
Cast crowns, inlays/onlays, and bridges	Zinc phosphate, zinc polycarboxylate, GIC, RMGIC, resin-based
Porcelain, ceramic or composite veneers, inlays, onlays, and all-ceramic crowns High-strength ceramics	Resin cements, self-adhesive resin cements RMGIC, adhesive resin, self-adhesive resin
Endodontic posts	Zinc phosphate, GIC, RMGIC, adhesive resin, and self-adhesive resin
Orthodontic bands	Fluoride-added zinc phosphate, polycarboxylate, GIC, RMGIC
Orthodontic brackets	GIC, RMGIC, Resin
Provisional cementation	Zinc oxide eugenol or noneugenol, zinc polycarboxylate, resin provisional cement
Provisional restorations	Reinforced zinc oxide eugenol, polycarboxylate, zinc phosphate, GIC, RMGIC
Surgical dressing	Zinc oxide noneugenol

GIC, glass ionomer cement; *RMGIC*, resin-modified glass ionomer cement.

Cavity varnish. **Cavity varnish** is not cement, but it acts as a protective barrier between the tooth preparation and restoration (see also Cavity Varnish in Chapter 10 Amalgam), varnish formulations are solutions of natural resins (copal) or synthetic resins dissolved in a solvent such as alcohol, ether, or chloroform. The varnish is applied in two or three layers over the surface of the preparation. The solution is placed in a thin film, allowing evaporation of the solvent to occur in 5 to 15 seconds before application of the second layer. An air stream can speed up the evaporation of the solvent. The resin layer protects the pulp by sealing the tubules from the penetration of irritating chemicals found in some restorative materials and/or acidic luting agents such as zinc phosphate cement. This resin varnish is thought to reduce the amount of microleakage and staining at the restoration/tooth interface. Copal varnishes, although popular for many years, are no longer widely used today. They were used extensively under amalgam restorations, but studies showed that they washed out, leaving a microscopic gap between the amalgam and the cavity preparation. Today's resin bonding agents, which also seal enamel and dentinal tubules, have largely replaced the use of varnish.

Liners. A **liner** is a thin layer of protective material that is placed over the dentin to seal the tubules from chemical or bacterial irritants.

Calcium hydroxide is used as a liner in cavity preparations in which the remaining dentin over the pulp is minimal. When close to the pulp or very small exposures are suspected, this material is used as an indirect or direct pulp-capping agent or as a dressing after vital pulpotomy procedures on primary teeth. Components of a popular two-paste system include calcium hydroxide, zinc oxide, and glycol salicylate (e.g., Dycal, Dentsply). A light-cured form of the paste-paste system is also available, and because of its resin content it is a bit stronger than the other liners. With paste-paste systems, equal amounts of catalyst and base are mixed to a creamy consistency. Calcium hydroxide powder in an aqueous suspension is another form of the material used for pulp capping or vital pulpotomies.

> **Mixing Calcium Hydroxide (Dycal) for Cavity Liner**
>
> **Mix:** Equal lengths of base and catalyst pastes on paper pad for 10 seconds to a uniform color
> **Working time:** 2 minutes 30 seconds
> **Setting time:** 3 minutes 30 seconds

Calcium hydroxide has an alkaline pH about 11 and can neutralize some acids. This alkali stimulates secondary dentin when in direct contact with the pulp, providing a barrier between pulp and restoration. It has some antimicrobial activity, meager thermal insulating properties, and provides minimal strength to support the forces of condensation. Under amalgam restorations calcium hydroxide paste slowly leaches out over time as it is water-soluble.

Bases. A **base** is cement that is applied in a layer about 1-2 mm thick over the dentin to provide thermal and chemical insulation to the pulp and provide support to restorations in deep cavity preparations. Some bases may act as a pulpal medication as well. Bases may be classified as low strength or high strength.

Zinc oxide – eugenol (ZOE) is considered to be a low-strength base material. Unless it is reinforced with other materials such as polymethylmethacrylate (PMMA) fibers to make it stronger, it typically will not be used to support a restoration. The eugenol in ZOE does have some soothing effects on the pulp. An unreinforced ZOE base is often used more like a liner and is placed in a thin layer which as a consequence will provide little thermal insulation. It is supplied as a powder (zinc oxide) and liquid (eugenol) or in a paste-paste formulation (e.g., Cavitec, Kerr Corporation). Equal lengths of the two pastes are extruded from tubes, mixed to a uniform consistency, and applied in a thin layer over the desired area. ZOE will be discussed in detail later in the chapter.

High-strength bases have approximately four times the compressive strength of low-strength bases and liners. They have the strength needed to support restorations in deep preparations. Cements used as bases are mixed to **secondary consistency**—a thick putty-like consistency that is condensable and can be rolled into a ball or rope. Bases placed at a thickness of 0.75 mm or greater provide protection from the thermal conduction of metallic restorations and galvanic shock. When the cavity preparation is so deep that there is 2 mm or less of remaining dentin over the pulp, many clinicians will choose to provide mechanical support for the restoration by first placing a cement base. The restorative material is placed after the initial set of the base has occurred.

Some high-strength bases are provided as hand-mixed powder and liquid or premeasured capsules of powder

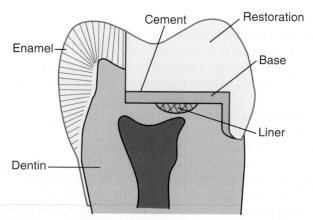

FIG. 14.1 Line drawing of layers of cement, base and liner, under a restoration.

and liquid that are mixed by trituration. Others are provided as paste-paste systems in tubes with automixing tips. Examples of cements used for high-strength bases include reinforced ZOE (IRM, Dentsply), zinc phosphate (Fleck's Cement, Keystone Industries), zinc polycarboxylate (Durelon Maxicap, 3M ESPE), glass ionomer (Fuji II, GC America), resin-modified glass ionomer (Fuji II LC, GC America), and resin (a dentin bonding agent and usually a flowable composite). Zinc phosphate cement is acidic, so a liner or varnish may be needed under it to protect the pulp in deep preparations. Resin-modified glass ionomer cement is one of the most popular materials used as a base material, because it is not irritating to the pulp, bonds to tooth structure, releases fluoride, and is strong. When placed in a thin layer resin-modified glass ionomer cement can also be used as a liner.

 Clinical Tip

Because of their fluoride release and low solubility, light-cured resin-modified glass ionomer cements are a popular choice as general cavity liners or bases. Some of the new bioactive formulations release calcium ions to promote hydroxyapatite and secondary dentin growth.

Mixing Reinforced ZOE (IRM, Dentsply) for a Base

Mix: Dispense a ratio of 1 level scoop to 1 drop of liquid on a paper pad or glass slab. Use a stiff spatula to mix ½ the powder into the liquid, then add the remaining powder in 1 or 2 increments. Spatulate thoroughly to produce a thick mix. Wipe the mix with the spatula vigorously 5 to 10 seconds to produce a smooth, stiff mix. Total mixing time about 1 minute.
Working time: 3.5 to 4 minutes
Setting time: 5 minutes from the start of mix
    Setting time is accelerated by increased temperature, humidity, and powder/liquid ratio.

Buildup

A **buildup,** much like a high-strength base, provides mechanical support for a restorative material when an excessive amount of tooth structure is missing. The remaining tooth structure first needs to be rebuilt to better support the restorative material or to act as a foundation before crown preparation. With placement of a cement buildup, the compromised tooth is reinforced (Fig. 14.2). Resin-modified glass ionomer and resin cements are the strongest of the cements. Typically, resin cement is not used in thick layers as a buildup, but composite resin restorative material serves well for this purpose. Resin-modified glass ionomer cement is frequently used as a buildup material when only a portion of the coronal tooth structure is missing so that there is still remaining sound tooth structure to support the crown. Its desirable features are its strength (compared to the conventional cements), chemical bond to the mineral component of enamel and dentin, good seal to the tooth, and fluoride release.

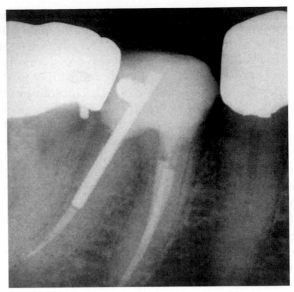

FIG. 14.2 Radiograph of a cement buildup over endodontically treated tooth #30, to reinforce the remains of the tooth in preparation for crown placement. (Courtesy of Steve Eakle, University of California, San Francisco [San Francisco, CA].)

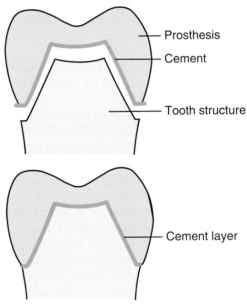

Prosthesis

Cement

Tooth structure

Cement layer

FIG. 14.3 Line drawing of a seated crown and the cement filling the restoration/tooth interface.

Luting of Indirect Restorations

A luting agent is a material with low viscosity, which placed between the prepared tooth and restoration, sets, and firmly attaches the restoration to the tooth (Fig. 14.3).

Orthodontic Bands and Brackets

Orthodontic bands and brackets are retained on teeth for several months or even years. Brackets are usually bonded directly to the enamel with resin cements (see Fig. 14.4 and Chapter 5 Principles of Bonding, Procedure 5.3), whereas bands are cemented without bonding.

    The cement must adhere tenaciously to the enamel and the orthodontic band to provide leverage for tooth movement and when the band is removed have

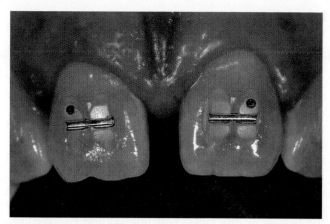

FIG. 14.4 Orthodontic brackets bonded directly to enamel with resin cement. (From Powers JM, Wataha JC: *Dental Materials: Properties and Manipulation*, ed 10, St. Louis, 2013, Mosby, p. 87.)

minimal effect on the tooth surface. Demineralization of the tooth surface due to solubility of cements and resultant leakage of bacteria between the bands and the tooth surface has often led to white spots on the enamel or caries. This concern has been minimized to some extent with fluoride-releasing, anticariogenic glass ionomer (e.g., Ketac Cem, 3M ESPE) and resin-modified glass ionomer cements (e.g., GC Fuji Ortho, GC America).

Metal, plastic, and ceramic brackets can be bonded to the enamel with resin cements. The enamel is treated with phosphoric acid, rinsed, and dried before application of bonding agent. Then, resin cement is applied to the bracket and seated on the primed enamel. Self-etching primers could be used as well, but some of them do not etch the enamel as well as phosphoric acid. Self-, light- and dual-cured cements are available. It is possible to use light-cured cement under metal brackets by positioning the curing light at 45 degrees to the bracket from all angles on the facial, then curing from the lingual as well.

Restorative Material

Permanent, Intermediate, and Provisional (Temporary). Because of their lower strength and wear resistance and higher solubility, cements are not frequently chosen as **permanent** restorations. The exceptions are glass ionomer cement (GIC) and resin-modified glass ionomer cement (RMGIC), which, because of their release of fluoride and chemical bond to tooth structure, are used for class V restorations of root caries in adults and for restoration of primary teeth (see Chapter 6 Composites, Glass Ionomers, and Compomers). The formulations of glass ionomer cement and resin-modified glass ionomer cement as restorative materials are different and much thicker than the GIC or RMGIC luting cements. The luting cements must have a low film thickness to allow the restoration to seat fully.

As **provisional (also called temporary)** and **intermediate** restorations, dental cements are mixed to secondary consistency (Procedure 14.1). The choice

of cement for this type of restoration is largely based on the particular clinical situation. Provisional restorations are used for emergency situations when appointment scheduling does not allow sufficient time to place a permanent restoration. Provisional restorations are placed when a tooth is symptomatic or when deep caries removal is required. By placing a **sedative** provisional restoration, the dentist is able to evaluate the response of the pulp before reappointing for a permanent restoration. Provisional and intermediate restorations are used to restore teeth awaiting treatment such as inlays, between endodontic appointments, or when extensive treatment plans require several weeks or months of coverage before treatment can be completed.

See Chapter 18 Provisional Restorations for a discussion of provisional luting and intracoronal cement provisionals.

Root Canal Sealers

There are many types of cement that can be used along with gutta percha or without it to seal the canal space when doing root canal therapy. The sealers are available as two pastes that can be packaged in syringes or premeasured capsules or powder and liquid which are hand mixed on a pad or glass slab. The sealer materials may encompass a wide range of components such as calcium hydroxide, zinc oxide with eugenol or non-eugenol substitute, resins, glass ionomer, calcium silicate, or mineral trioxide aggregate. Some of the materials are also used for vital pulpal therapy. They all have different properties, handling characteristics, working and setting times. Manufacturers' specifications must be followed carefully.

Surgical Dressings

As surgical dressings, cements are used to provide protection and support for the surgical site, to provide patient comfort, and to help control bleeding. The periodontal surgical dressing was developed in 1923 by Dr. A W Ward. His product was called Ward's Wonder Pac and it consisted of zinc oxide, eugenol with added alcohol, pine oil, and asbestos fibers (today's product no longer contains asbestos). Over time it became apparent that eugenol acted as an irritant to the tissues and was damaging to exposed bone. Current products have shifted away from the use of eugenol.

The most widely used product in the USA is Coe Pak (GC America). It is a two-paste system—base and catalyst. The base contains zinc oxide as the main component with oils as plasticizers (make it flexible), gums to give it body for handling, and lorothidol as a fungicide. The catalyst paste contains coconut fatty acids that are thickened with rosin and chlorothymol as an antibacterial agent. It is available in regular and fast set and hard set formulations. It also comes as manual mix or automix delivery (Fig. 14.5).

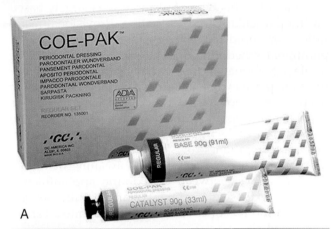

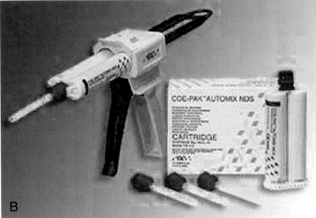

A

B

FIG. 14.5 Surgical dressing in 2-paste systems. **A,** Tubes of hand-mixed material. **B,** Pastes in automix system. (Courtesy Coe Pak, GC America.)

Preparing the Surgical Dressing

For the hand-mixed dressing, equal lengths of base and catalyst pastes are dispensed onto a non-porous paper pad. They are mixed with a tongue blade (disposable) or spatula to a soft putty-like consistency of uniform color. The setting time can be accelerated by immersing the mixed putty-like material in warm water. When the mix is no longer tacky, it can be shaped into two ropes about the width of a little finger. These materials tend to stick to gloves, so a lubricant such as KY Jelly (Reckitt Benckiser), petroleum jelly, or water should be applied to the gloves before handling. Starting at the distal of the surgical site a rope is spread over the tissues on the facial and lingual and pressed into the interproximal areas. The dressing is mechanically retained by gently forcing the material into the embrasure spaces and under the contacts (Fig. 14.6). The material should not extend more than 2 mm beyond the surgical site. If needed, the patient (or the operator if the patient is too numb) should move the cheeks, lips, and tongue in a range of motions to shape the edges of the dressing (a process called muscle trimming or molding). This helps to prevent the hardened material from irritating tissues and dislodging the dressing after it has set. The occlusion should be checked to assure that the dressing is not interfering. Use a plastic instrument or other suitable instrument to keep the dressing from extending above the height of contour of the teeth. Some materials become hard and others remain somewhat flexible depending on their formulation.

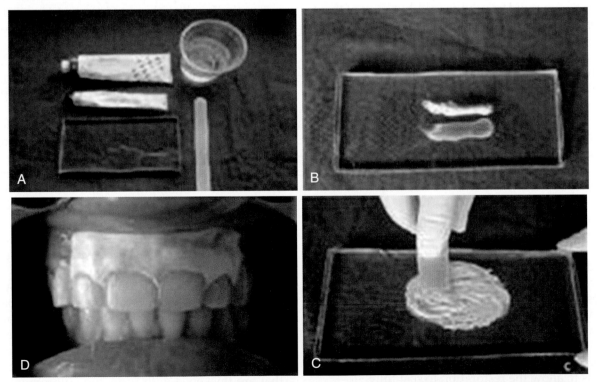

A

B

D

C

FIG. 14.6 Mix and application of surgical dressing (Coe Pak, GC America). Clockwise: **A,** Tubes of material, mixing slab, and disposable spatula. **B,** Base and catalyst pastes dispensed on a slab. **C,** Mixed pastes. **D,** Dressing applied to the surgical site. (From Kathariya R, Jain H, Jadhav T: To pack or not to pack: the current status of periodontal dressing. J Appl Biomater Funct Mater, 13(2):e73–e86, 2015.)

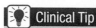
Clinical Tip

When mixing surgical dressing material use a wooden tongue blade. It can be discarded when done. The material is sticky and difficult to remove from a spatula.

Removing the Dressing

After the tissues have healed it is time to remove the dressing. A blunt instrument is used under the edge of the dressing with gentle lateral pressure to loosen the pack. The clinician must be aware of the location of sutures and avoid breaking the sutures away with the dressing. Large pieces of the dressing are lifted with cotton forceps and the surgical site is cleaned with a dilute solution of hydrogen peroxide or sterile water (Fig. 14.7). Occasionally, all or part of a dressing will come off prematurely and need to be reapplied.

Criteria for a Well-Placed Dressing

- Does not dislodge or disturb the placement of any surgical sutures
- Smooth, with as little bulk as possible
- Covers the surgical site with minimal overextension
- Interlocked interdentally to provide stability

TYPE I CEMENTS: LUTING AGENTS

Luting cements can be placed into two broad categories: non-adhesive and adhesive cements.

Non-adhesive cements: Retention of the restoration is enhanced by filling the interface between the restoration and the prepared tooth with a hard setting cement, much like hard-setting household cements.

Adhesive cements: Stronger than non-adhesive cements, adhesive cements fill the interface and provide micromechanical and/or chemical retention between the tooth substrate and restorative materials.

Luting restorations with traditional cements using mechanical retention was the only means of cementation until the mid-1960s when dentin bonding with acid-etch systems was developed, leading to today's *adhesive dentistry*. Zinc polycarboxylate and glass ionomer cements with some degree of chemical adhesion to tooth structure were also introduced about that time.

PROPERTIES OF LUTING CEMENTS

Properties of luting cements differ from one type of cement to another. No cement is ideal for every clinical situation. Although one type of cement may be appropriate for a single crown, it may not be ideal for a multiple-unit bridge; some cements work well on metal surfaces, but others are more appropriate for ceramic or porcelain surfaces. Ideally, the cement should adhere to the tooth structure as well as the restorative material. The clinician must consider both physical and biological properties when selecting cement for a specific dental procedure. The most important properties are as follows: strength, solubility, viscosity (affecting film thickness), biocompatibility, anticariogenic properties, retention, esthetics, radiopacity, and ease of manipulation (Table 14.2).

Ideal Properties of a Luting Agent

- Adhesion to tooth structure
- Adhesion to restorative material
- Adequate strength to resist functional forces
- Not soluble in oral fluids
- Ability to achieve low film thickness
- Biocompatibility with oral tissue
- Anticariogenic properties
- Radiopacity
- Ease of manipulation
- Esthetics and color stability

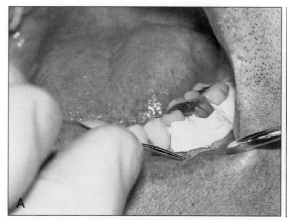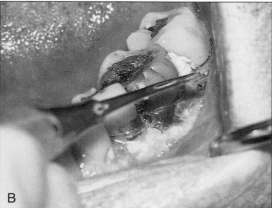

FIG. 14.7 Removal of surgical dressing. **A,** Instrument under the edge of the dressing to loosen it. **B,** Use an instrument to remove pieces of the dressing from the interproximal spaces. (From Robinson DS, Bird DL: *Essentials of Dental Assisting,* ed 6, St. Louis, 2017, Elsevier.)

TABLE 14.2   Properties of Luting Cements

PROPERTY	GIC	RMGIC	RESIN	ZINC PHOSPHATE	ZINC POLYCARBOXYLATE	ZOE
Strength	Moderate	Moderate	High	Low	Low	Low
Solubility	Moderate	Low	Very low	High	High	High
Film thickness	Low	Low	Low	Low	Low, medium	Low, medium
Postoperative sensitivity	Moderate	Low	Low	Moderate	Low	Low
Fluoride release	High	High	None	None	None	None
Adhesion	Moderate	Moderate	High	None	Moderate	None
Esthetics	Good	Good	Good	None	None	None
Manipulation*	Moderately easy	Easy	Moderate	Difficult	Moderately easy	Easy

GIC, Glass ionomer cement; *RMGIC*, resin-modified glass ionomer cement; *ZOE*, zinc oxide eugenol cement.
*Encapsulated and automix forms are easy to manipulate.

Strength

The cement's resistance to deformation or fracture under an applied force is a measure of its mechanical properties. Cements must be strong enough to resist the forces of mastication and the dynamics of the patient's mouth and occlusion. Compressive, tensile, and flexural strengths are important considerations for differing cement applications. Bond strength is important in high-stress areas.

Caution

Cements are brittle materials with good compressive but more limited tensile and flexural strength.

The strongest cements are resin cements, and the weakest is zinc oxide eugenol. Cements used for permanent luting and high-strength bases need good compressive, tensile and flexural strength. As can be seen in Table 14.2, resin-based cement is high in mechanical strength and fracture toughness, and polycarboxylate cement is low in both. Many cements consist of a combination of powder and liquid; their ratio determines many of their properties. The strength of cement is controlled primarily by the amount of powder used in the prepared mix. In general, an increase in the powder-to-liquid ratio increases the strength of the cement. However, excessive powder or liquid can weaken the cement.

Solubility

One of the greatest challenges for dental cements is the tendency to dissolve in oral fluids, leading to marginal ditching, microleakage, recurrent caries, and failure of the restoration. Solubility is important whenever the cement is expected to remain exposed to mouth fluids for prolonged periods. Many cements will disintegrate in the oral environment over time. Increasing the amount of powder incorporated into the liquid can reduce the solubility of the cement. However, there are limits since it may increase the viscosity and film thickness. High resistance to oral solubility helps to maintain the marginal seal. Bonded, resin-containing cements are nearly insoluble.

Viscosity and Film Thickness

The consistency, or viscosity, of mixed cement refers to its thickness and ability to flow. Cements used for permanent or temporary luting of fixed prostheses, other indirect restorations, and endodontic posts must be able to flow to a thin film thickness to allow the restoration to seat properly and completely. On the inside of a crown a small space is created in the laboratory to allow room for the cement. Without this space the crown would not seat fully. Also, if the film thickness is too thick, the restoration will not seat fully, leaving cement exposed at the margins. This will result in the need for excessive occlusal adjustment and the increased likelihood of cement washing away at the margins leading to tooth sensitivity, recurrent decay, and staining.

For primary consistency, also known as *luting consistency*, cements should be able to be mixed thin—to about the consistency of honey with a film thickness of 25 μm or less (see Procedure 14.2).

Clinical Tip

Low film thickness is critical to fully seating and retaining indirect restorations.

The cement must be able to flow easily and completely throughout the interface between the restoration and preparation. To be considered an effective luting cement, American Dental Association (ADA) specifications require the cement to be able to flow to a film thickness of 25 μm or less. As a comparison, a human hair is about 20 to 50 μm. Resin-based cements and resin-modified glass ionomer cements are thixotropic, meaning they will flow under pressure. When cementing with any of these cements the patient should be instructed to bite down on a stick during initial set to force the material into all intracoronal areas.

Mixing cement to secondary consistency requires the addition of powder to increase strength and bring the cement to a thick, putty-like consistency (see Procedure 14.1). Cements mixed to secondary consistency are used as bases and restorations, provisional or permanent.

Several factors influence the consistency of mixed cement. Temperature has a great effect; a lower temperature will slow the setting reaction, giving the clinician more working time and allowing incorporation of more powder into the liquid.

 Caution

Although the amount of powder incorporated into the mix has a direct relationship to strength and solubility, it may substantially increase the viscosity of the mixed cement, making it unsuitable for cementation of a restoration.

Biocompatibility and Anticariogenic Properties

Cements must be safe to use on patients. Where a specific type of cement may be appropriate in one circumstance, it may be inappropriate in another. Cement may be suitable for use in a conservative preparation, but then cause sensitivity and even pulpal necrosis in a deep preparation. Some cements are composed of a combination of zinc oxide powder or powdered glass mixed with an acid. The pH of the acid both at placement and after complete setting is a matter of concern due to postoperative pulpal sensitivity associated with the acid exposure. Other causes of pulpal sensitivity include unsealed dentinal tubules, trauma to the pulp during preparation, and bacterial leakage under the provisional restoration. Careful attention to powder-to-liquid ratios, dispensing technique, and mixing recommendations can minimize sensitivity from cements. Cement with low risk for postoperative sensitivity should be selected when susceptibility to sensitivity is a concern. Eugenol, found in the liquid of zinc oxide eugenol cements, has an obtundent (i.e., soothing, sedative) effect on the pulp due to its good sealing ability, antibacterial properties, and neutral pH.

 Clinical Tip

Many products include fluoride in their formulations; it is important to distinguish between fluoride release and fluoride-containing products. Fluoride released from powdered glass formulations found in glass ionomer cements has an anticariogenic property for reducing secondary caries. Products that do not release fluoride do not have an anticariogenic effect.

Retention and Adhesion

Good adhesion is a critical component of restorative dentistry, as good adhesion helps to increase retention of the restoration and minimize microleakage.

Adhesion is the bonding of dissimilar materials by the attractive forces of atoms or molecules and includes two types of adhesion: mechanical and chemical.

Mechanical adhesion: Mechanical adhesion is based on the interlocking of one material with another; an excellent example is Velcro.

Chemical adhesion: Chemical adhesion occurs at the molecular level, when atoms of the two materials swap electrons (ionic bonding) or share outer electrons (covalent bonding).

In many dental applications, chemical adhesion and mechanical adhesion occur together. We now have a much better understanding of the surface characteristics of enamel and dentin and the requirements needed to obtain good adhesion to them. The most recently developed dental cements, using resin adhesive technologies, strive to achieve a micromechanical and chemical bond between the tooth and the restoration. Several things may weaken the strength of the adhesion between two materials, including differences in the coefficient of thermal expansion of the two materials, dimensional changes that occur during setting of the adhesive agent, and contamination of the substrates by water and saliva and/or by residual enamel and dentin cutting debris from tooth preparation, known as the "smear layer."

 Clinical Tip

Good adhesion will not occur unless there is a good fit between the restoration and the tooth preparation.

There are three possible reasons for failure of an adhesive: structural, adhesive, and cohesive failure. Structural failure occurs as a result of internal failure within the tooth structure; the tooth itself breaks away from the restoration, leaving the restoration intact. Adhesive failure is a failure of the bond, and it occurs when the adhesive layer separates from the tooth structure causing the restoration to dislodge from the tooth. Cohesive failure is a measure of the strength of the bonding material itself, and it occurs when there is failure within the adhesive layer; this may also result in dislodging of the restoration with the cement layer still present in the restoration and on the tooth preparation (Fig. 14.8). Failure of the adhesive can result in failure of the restoration, leakage occurring between the tooth structure and restoration, and the formation of secondary caries.

The acid-etch bonding system is the basis of today's adhesive dentistry. In this process, the main mineral component of enamel and dentin, hydroxyapatite, is removed from the surface of the tooth structure with an acid etchant to create roughness

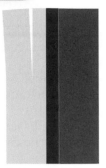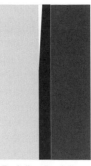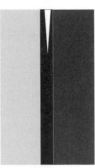

| A. Structural failure | B. Adhesive failure | C. Cohesive failure |

FIG. 14.8 Failure mechanisms of adhesive bonding. The blue line is the adhesive, to the left is tooth structure and to the right is the restoration. **A,** Structural failure occurs within the tooth structure (or the restoration). **B,** Adhesive failure occurs between the adhesive and the tooth structure (or the adhesive and the restoration). **C,** Cohesive failure occurs within the adhesive itself.

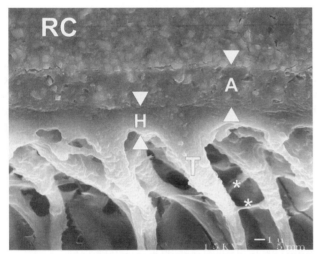

FIG. 14.9 Scanning electron micrograph of tooth-restoration interface bonded with dental adhesive. A, adhesive layer. H, hybrid layer with T, resin tags. RC, resin composite restoration. (From Frankenberger R, Perdigão J, Rosa BT, et al: "No-bottle" vs "multi-bottle" dentin adhesives—a microtensile bond strength and morphological study. *Dent Mater, 17:373–380, 2001.)*

and micropores. When resin bonding agents or self-adhesive cements are applied to the etched surfaces resin monomers of the bonding agent or cement fill the micropores and roughness to create resin tags that micromechanically lock the substrate to the restoration (Fig. 14.9).

 Caution

A bond will not occur if the surfaces being bonded are not completely clean and dry. Enamel should be dry and dentin free of excessive moisture or saliva. Over-drying of the dentin can cause sensitivity and a weaker bond in some techniques.

Esthetics

Cements are available in a variety of shades and opacities. Typically, resin cements are used for bonding porcelain veneers, ceramic or composite inlays and onlays, and ceramic full crowns.

Radiopacity

Radiopacity is an important property in the measure of the success of a cement. High radiopacity will allow the cement to show when examined with x-rays so that it will not be mistaken for caries or a void. Good radiopacity will also make excess cement easier to see; this is particularly important in the case of implants and in restorations with deep subgingival margins.

Selecting a Luting Cement

When choosing a luting cement, the clinician must consider which of the following indirect restorations are being used:
- Metal and metal-based restorations—crowns, bridges, inlays, or onlays
- Glass-ceramic restorations
- High-strength ceramic restorations
- Indirect composite restorations

The restorative material itself may be the primary determinant for the cement selection. For example, some glass-ceramic restorations need to be bonded to the tooth in order to enhance their strength, but a high-strength ceramic such as zirconia can be cemented with non-adhesive cement. Other considerations include the amount of mechanical retention from the form of the preparation and whether the patient has parafunctional habits (i.e., bruxing). In order for the cement to be successful, the tooth preparation must have adequate retention and resistance form. While adhesive cements can enhance retention of the restoration, they cannot overcome the negative influence of an over-tapered, non-retentive preparation and extreme bruxing forces.

CLASSIFICATION OF LUTING CEMENTS

Luting cements not only serve to retain a restoration to the tooth but also help to prevent microleakage by sealing the interface between the tooth and the restoration. Retention of the restoration to the tooth can be by mechanical means, chemical interaction with the tooth, or a combination of the two. Luting cements may be chosen as permanent cements or provisional (temporary) cements depending on the clinical need.

Luting cements can be classified according to their composition. That is, they are water-based, resin-based, or oil-based.

Functions of Luting Cements

The two main functions of luting cements are:
1. to seal the interface between the tooth preparation and the restoration
2. to augment the retention of the restoration

WATER-BASED LUTING CEMENTS

Water-based cements undergo an acid–base setting reaction. The cements are typically a liquid (the acid) and a powder (the base). When they are mixed together they undergo a chemical reaction that neutralizes the acid and base. The cation (H^+) of the acid and the anion (OH^-) of the base combine to form water and the remaining components form a salt. It may take several hours for the setting reaction to reach completion and the acidity to become neutral.

Zinc Phosphate Cement

Zinc phosphate, the oldest of the cements, was introduced in 1879. Zinc phosphate cements because of their acidic nature have produced problems with post-cementation hypersensitivity. These cements are also soluble and among the cements in use today are weaker cements. For these reasons, zinc phosphate cements are not widely used. If used, they are applied as permanent luting agents under metal-based indirect restorations and for cementation of orthodontic bands. The incorporation of additional powder into the mix makes them strong enough for high-strength bases, and they provide thermal insulation for the pulp. A popular brand of zinc phosphate cement is Fleck's Cement (Keystone Industries).

Composition. The powder of zinc phosphate cement is principally zinc oxide (90%) and magnesium oxide (10%); fluoride is added by some manufacturers to aid in the prevention of caries under orthodontically banded teeth. The liquid is made from phosphoric acid and water. When the cement powder is incorporated into the liquid, an exothermic chemical reaction occurs, that is, heat is produced. Attention to proper mixing technique is required to minimize this reaction. The setting and exothermic reactions of zinc phosphate cement are controlled by time and temperature. Incremental incorporation of the powder into the liquid allows for controlled dissipation of heat. Mixing over a large area of a cooled glass slab also dissipates the heat. The glass slab should be cooled to be effective in dissipating heat, but not to below the dew point (approximately 18 °C [65 °F]), at which water condensation would shorten the setting time. Use of a frozen slab can greatly increase the incorporation of powder and can increase the working time, helpful when several orthodontic bands are cemented.

Properties. Initially, the acidity (pH about 2.5) of zinc phosphate cement is low and becomes neutral within 24 to 48 hours. The initially low acidity may irritate the pulp in deep preparations (usually those with less than 1 mm of remaining dentin over the pulp) resulting in post-cementation hypersensitivity or in rare occasions, even pulpal necrosis.. Pulpal protection in deep cavity preparations is recommended with cavity varnish, liners, bases, or dentin bonding systems.

Strength, solubility, and film thickness are important properties. The internal surface of indirect restorations such as PFM or gold crowns, inlays, and onlays are sandblasted to enhance retention. The cement flows into irregularities in the roughened surface of the restoration and onto the prepared tooth surface, locking the two together. The low film thickness of properly mixed cements allows for the intimate contact necessary for good retention. Zinc phosphate cement has adequate strength and rigidity for cementation of single-unit and long-span bridges, but it is weaker than resin or hybrid ionomer cements. Ceramic restorations are not cemented with zinc phosphate cement, because it does not bond the ceramic to the tooth and thus puts the brittle ceramic restoration at risk of fracture. Zinc phosphate cement's solubility is clinically acceptable but greater than that of most other cements. This greater solubility has made it less favorable with clinicians for the cementation of orthodontic bands.

Zinc Phosphate

ADVANTAGES
- Over a century of clinical use
- Low film thickness
- Inexpensive
- High rigidity

DISADVANTAGES
- Initial pulpal irritation and postoperative sensitivity
- Mechanical bond only
- Technique-sensitive proportioning and mixing
- Relatively high solubility
- Weaker than most other cements

Manipulation. Zinc phosphate cements are dispensed in a powder/liquid system and are mixed on a cooled glass slab with a metal cement spatula. The powder is shaken before it is dispensed into four to six portions on one end of the slab, and the liquid is dispensed in drops at the other end of the slab. The powder is added slowly in small increments to the liquid. With smaller initial increments the acidity is reduced and the reaction is retarded. Each increment is mixed for 10 to 15 seconds, for a total of 60 to 90 seconds of mixing. The cement is mixed in a figure-eight motion over a large area of the cooled slab to absorb the heat of the exothermic reaction, neutralize the acid, and allow more powder to be incorporated. Proper luting consistency is achieved when the mixed cement strings 1 inch above the slab from the mixing spatula. (See Procedure 14.2.)

Excess cement should be removed from interproximal areas before the cement sets. A knotted strand of dental floss is a helpful tool when dragged back and forth across the margins several times. The excess at accessible margins should be allowed to set before removing it. Ideally, varnish or another surface sealer should be applied to the margins after the excess is removed to allow maturation of the set and decrease solubility.

 Clinical Tip

Zinc phosphate cements are difficult to remove from mixing surfaces; glass slabs and spatulas should be wiped clean before the cement sets. Set cement may be removed with the use of ultrasonic cleaners or a solution of baking soda and water.

Mixing Zinc Phosphate Cement for Luting

Mix: On cool glass slab mix 4 to 6 small increments of powder into liquid for 10 to15 seconds each increment over a large area to dissipate heat. Mix for a total of 60 to 90 seconds until smooth and creamy. It should string 1 inch from the spatula.
Working Time: 2 minutes
Setting Time: 5.5 minutes

Zinc Polycarboxylate Cement

Zinc polycarboxylate cements (introduced in 1968) were the first cements developed with an adhesive bond to tooth structures. These cements have been used for final cementation of indirect restorations; today they are used primarily as long-term temporary cements.

Composition. Zinc polycarboxylate cements are supplied as a powder/liquid system and set through an acid–base reaction. The powder is similar to that of zinc phosphate cement and is mostly zinc oxide with magnesium oxide, bismuth, and aluminum oxide. The liquid is an aqueous solution of polyacrylic acid. The polyacrylic acid produces minimal irritation to the pulp. Some manufacturers are supplying premeasured capsules for mixing in a triturator.

Properties. The viscosity of zinc polycarboxylate cement is higher than that of most other cements. However, on vibratory action on the restoration during seating the cement flows to an appropriate film thickness. The liquid of this cement should not be dispensed before mixing time, as the loss of water by evaporation can make it more viscous.

These cements have lower compressive strength (55 MPa) and higher solubility when compared with glass ionomer and resin cements. Zinc polycarboxylate cements cause little irritation to the pulp even when the remaining dentin layer is as thin as 0.2 mm. They are useful for cementing indirect restorations, for bases, liners, and temporary fillings. They are radiopaque, so excess interproximal cement can be seen on an x-ray.

Retention of polycarboxylate cements is both chemical and mechanical, making this cement useful for retention of indirect restorations. The chemical adhesion to the tooth is created by free carboxylic acid groups interacting (chelating) with calcium ions in the tooth structure. The bond is achieved only if the cement still exhibits a glossy appearance when the restoration is seated. The bond is not as strong as that obtained with resin cements combined with bonding agents. The working time can be extended with the use of a cooled glass slab.

Zinc Polycarboxylate

ADVANTAGES
- Adheres to tooth structures
- Nonirritating to the pulp
- Inexpensive

DISADVANTAGES
- Higher solubility
- Lower strength
- Shorter working time
- Early increase in film thickness can inhibit seating of the restoration

Manipulation. Polycarboxylate cements are dispensed in a powder/liquid system and are mixed on a glass slab or a nonabsorbent paper pad with a metal cement spatula. The powder is dispensed with the manufacturer-supplied scoop, and the viscous liquid is dispensed with a dropper or a unit-marked syringe. Never increase the amount of liquid, as this will dramatically reduce the strength of the cement. Add the powder to the liquid, and mix for 30 seconds until the mix is creamy. The cement must be used immediately because of the short working time. The cement is no longer usable when it loses its gloss and becomes stringy. (See Procedure 14.3.) Two common brands are Durelon (3M ESPE) and HyBond Polycarboxylate (Shofu Dental Corporation).

Mixing Polycarboxylate Cement for Luting

Mixing: Mix all powder into liquid at once for 30 seconds until creamy
Working Time: 2.5 minutes. Do not use when it loses its gloss and becomes stringy
Setting Time: Regular set—10 minutes; Fast set—5 minutes

 Clinical Tip

As with other cements, cleanup of mixing surfaces and spatula should be done while zinc polycarboxylate cement is still soft.

Glass Ionomer Cements

Glass ionomer cements (introduced in 1972) were derived from silicate cements and polycarboxylate cements. Originally developed as an alternative to silicate cements for esthetic restoration of anterior teeth, glass ionomer cements have become one of the most versatile cements used today. Similar to the polycarboxylate cements, these cements chemically bond with tooth structures through chelation with calcium ions, although retention is primarily through micromechanical retention. Glass ionomer cements also contain aluminum fluorosilicate glass, giving them the ability to release and replenish fluoride. Glass ionomer cements are used as permanent luting agents for indirect restorations, luting of orthodontic bands, restorative materials (see Chapter 6), high-strength bases, and core buildups. Although the cement is able to chemically bond to metals such as noble, non-noble, and stainless steel and tooth substrate, it is not able to bond to glazed porcelain. In many instances, the same product can be mixed to different viscosities for different uses. This simplifies product selection and inventory control. Glass ionomer cements include both traditional GICs and resin-modified glass ionomer cements (RMGICs).

Traditional Glass Ionomer Cements

Composition. The cement is supplied as a powder and liquid system. The powder is aluminum fluorosilicate glass with barium glass added for radiopacity (Fig. 14.10). The liquid is polyacrylic acid copolymer in water. When the powder and liquid are mixed, the polyacrylic acid attacks the glass to release fluoride ions. Fluoride improves the translucency of the otherwise opaque material and improves the material's strength.

Properties. Glass ionomer cements are biologically compatible with the pulp when manipulated properly. Mild to severe postoperative sensitivity has been reported. Overdrying of the preparation, moisture contamination during the first 24 hours of setting, and hydrostatic pressure on fluid in the dentinal tubules when seating a crown have all been indicated as possible sources of this sensitivity. Fluoride release during the life of the cement is bacterio-static, may have an anticariogenic effect, and may act to remineralize tooth structure attacked by bacterial acids. GIC acts as a fluoride reservoir. It can release fluoride but can also absorb fluoride from oral sources such as fluoride-containing toothpaste or mouthrinse and release it at another time. Strength, solubility, and film thickness are comparable with other permanent cements. Its compressive strength is over 100 MPa but its brittle nature causes it to be weak in tension, about 6 MPa.

An increase in solubility has been demonstrated with moisture contamination during the first 24 hours. Teeth restored with glass ionomer restorations, bases, and core buildups must be properly isolated for the 6- to 8-minute setting time. The margins of the cemented crown must be coated with the supplied coating agent or varnish until the initial set is achieved. Faster setting materials are less sensitive to the solubility issue. The best bond to enamel and dentin can be achieved for GIC and RMGIC by first removing the smear layer created by cavity preparation debris. To remove the smear layer, mild acid such as 10% polyacrylic acid is applied to the preparation for 5 to 10 seconds and rinsed off. Leaving the acid on longer will begin to remove mineral from the tooth surface and weaken the bond since the glass ionomer cement bonds to mineral.

Traditional Glass Ionomer Cements

ADVANTAGES
- Chemical adhesion to tooth and metal
- Fluoride release
- Easy to mix
- Moderate strength

DISADVANTAGES
- History of postoperative sensitivity
- Sensitive to moisture or drying during setting
- Does not bond to glazed porcelain
- Marginal solubility

Manipulation. These cements are dispensed in a powder/liquid system or in premeasured capsules. Hand mixing of the powder and liquid is similar to that of polycarboxylate cement. Premeasured capsules are very popular because of their ease of use and consistency of mix (e.g., Ketac Cem Aplicap, 3M ESPE or GC Fuji I Capsule, GC America) (Fig. 14.11). When using the premeasured capsules, follow the manufacturer's directions on activating the capsule and mixing in the triturator. After mixing the capsule is mounted in a gun-type applicator and has a delivery tip for dispensing of the mixed cement. The mix should be used right away and mixes that become thick or lose their glossy appearance should be discarded. For *GC Fuji I Capsule* the mixing time is 20 seconds with a working time of 2.5 minutes and

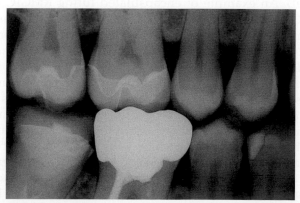

FIG. 14.10 Radiograph of the interface between restorations and teeth filled with radiopaque cement in upper right molars.

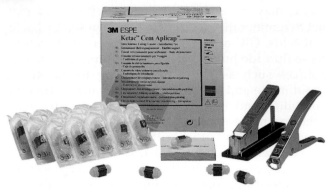

FIG. 14.11 Glass ionomer cement kit with premeasured capsules, activator and delivery gun. (Ketac Cem Aplicaps, Courtesy 3M ESPE.)

a setting time of 2 minutes and 50 seconds. Glass ionomer luting cements are self-curing (see Procedure 14.4).

Mixing Glass Ionomer Cement for Luting

Mix:
1. Premeasured capsules: mix in triturator according to manufacturer's instructions
2. Powder-liquid: mix level scoop to 1 or 2 drops (varies by manufacturer) incorporating all of the powder into the liquid until smooth mix is achieved.

Working Time: About 3 minutes depending on product
Setting Time: 5-7 minutes depending on product
Note: *If the mix loses its glossy appearance, do not use it*

Resin-Modified Glass Ionomer Cements

Resin-modified glass ionomer cements (also called hybrid glass ionomer cements) were introduced in 1995. Resin was added to traditional glass ionomer cement to help improve its properties. For luting they can be used for metal-based restorations, endodontic metal posts, orthodontic bands and brackets, or stronger ceramics such as zirconia or lithium disilicate.

Composition. The composition of resin-modified glass ionomer cement (RMGIC) is similar to that of traditional glass ionomer cement, but it is modified by the addition of resin. The cement is supplied as a paste-paste formulation or powder and liquid. The powder is similar to traditional GIC but has chemicals added to catalyze the light-cure or chemical-cure reaction of the resin component. The liquid contains water-soluble methacrylate monomers, tartaric acid, water, and 2-hydroxyethyl methacrylate (HEMA) as well as initiators for light-curing.

The set of the material occurs by two mechanisms: an acid–base reaction and a resin polymerization reaction that can be light-cured, chemical-cured, or both (dual-cured). The polymerization reaction occurs first and can be initiated by exposure to a curing light, or in darkness occurs by self-cure of the resin. The acid–base reaction is slower and continues for some hours after the material has hardened.

Properties. The added resin helps to improve the compressive and tensile strength and to decrease solubility. These cements do not have the susceptibility to early moisture contamination that traditional glass ionomers have because of the resin component. They have excellent film thickness. Fluoride release is the same as that of traditional glass ionomer cements. RMGIC expands as it absorbs moisture after setting. The expansion is greater in some RMGICs than others, and some non–high-strength all-ceramic restorations fractured after they were cemented with RMGIC because of excessive expansion. (See Chapter 9 Ceramics.) The most problematic of those RMGIC have been removed from the market.

Resin-Modified (Hybrid) Ionomer Cements

ADVANTAGES
- Good strength
- Fluoride release
- Insoluble
- Chemical adhesion to tooth
- Less postoperative sensitivity
- Excellent film thickness

DISADVANTAGES
- Recommended for luting only high-strength all-ceramic restorations or metal-based restorations

---

Manipulation. The powder and liquid can be hand mixed, but the most popular version is the premeasured capsule. The capsule is activated to allow powder and liquid to join and is mixed in a triturator as specified by the manufacturer (see Procedure 14.4). The capsule has a dispensing tip so the mixed cement can be placed directly into a crown (or cavity preparation in the case of the restorative material). An example of encapsulated luting RMGIC is GC Fuji Plus (GC America). When handling the glass ionomer cement a no-touch technique is mandatory since the liquid contains HEMA, a known contact allergen.

Resin-modified glass ionomer luting cements are also available in two-paste systems: one system has a cartridge that delivers each paste separately to be hand mixed (e.g., RelyX Luting Cement, 3M ESPE) and the other system has a cartridge with an automixing tip making mixing and dispensing easy and convenient (RelyX Luting Plus, 3M ESPE; FujiCEM 2, GC America). For FujiCEM 2 the working time is 2 minutes 15 seconds and setting time in the mouth is 4 minutes 30 seconds.

Clinical Tip

To avoid postoperative dentin hypersensitivity when using a RMGIC, it is important **not** to overdry and desiccate the preparation before cementation.

RESIN-BASED LUTING CEMENTS

Resin cements were introduced in the mid-1980s and are basically composite resins modified to have lower viscosity. They are used for bonding of ceramic restorations, conventional crowns and bridges, and for direct or indirect bonding of orthodontic brackets. Low-strength ceramic restorations (especially porcelain-based materials) must be bonded to the tooth with resin cements to reduce their risk of fracturing under functional stresses. However, high-strength (zirconia and some lithium disilicate, e.g., e-Max, Ivoclar Vivadent) crowns are very strong and can be cemented with RMGIC (see Chapter 9). Resin cements help increase retention of crowns placed onto clinically short teeth or teeth with less than ideal preparation taper.

Composition

Resin-based cements are similar in composition to composite restorative materials. Filler particle size is kept very small, similar to microfills, microhybrids, or nanohybrids (see Chapter 6). Initiators of polymerization are added to change the setting mechanism. Pigments are added to aid in tooth color matching.

Properties

Resin cements are virtually insoluble in the oral cavity. They have superior bond strength to enamel and dentin, wear resistance at exposed margins, and high compressive strength.

Methods of Cure

Polymerization (curing) of resin cements occurs by three possible mechanisms: chemical-cure (self-cure), light-cure, or dual-cure. Some materials are cured by only one of these methods, while others may use both light-curing and self-curing methods; that is, they are dual-cured.

Chemical-Cured. With chemical-cured resins the set is initiated when the components are mixed together. No light or heat is needed. They are useful where light-curing is not possible as with thick or opaque ceramic restorations, metal restorations, or endodontic posts. Limited number of shades and translucencies are available with chemical-cured resins. Chemical-cured resin cements are more radiolucent than the other types of resin cements making it difficult to detect excess cement on radiographs. Careful removal of excess cement should be done before the cement reaches its final set.

Light-Cured. Light-cured resin cements require a light of a certain wavelength to activate photo-initiators that start the polymerization process (see Chapter 6, section on Light Curing). Light-cured materials allow the operator to have extended working time and decide when to initiate curing. When removing excess cement some clinicians use a "wave" technique (also called tack cure) whereby they wave the curing light over the resin margins for a few seconds to cause the resin to gel but not reach its final set. This "tacks" the restoration in place and allows for easier clean up of the excess cement. Light-cured cements are popular for thin porcelain veneers or in easily accessible parts of the mouth. Light-curing will not work well when the restoration is too opaque or too thick to allow the light to transmit to all of the cement. Light-cured resin cements are the most color stable compared to chemical- or dual-cured cements.

Dual-Cured. Because of the afore-mentioned limitations with light curing, materials are available that have a combined chemical-cure and light-cure. Usually the chemical-cure is slow to allow for adequate working time and the light initiates the cure. In areas where the light cannot reach, the chemical-cure will take the set to completion. Dual-cured resin cements are very popular but have the drawback of potentially discoloring over time because of chemicals called aromatic amines that help in the setting process. The highest degree of polymerization occurs when light-curing is used to initiate the setting process.

Categories of Resin Cements

Resin cements can be categorized into four main groups:
- Esthetic resin cements
- Adhesive resin cements
- Self-adhesive resin cements
- Provisional resin cements

Esthetic Resin Cements. Esthetic resin cements are low viscosity resins derived from composite resin. They are only lightly filled with very small particle fillers and are mostly low viscosity resin to maintain a low film thickness. They are strong, radiopaque, and have good bond strength to tooth and restoration when proper surface preparation is performed.

Some of these esthetic cements are manufactured as a single paste that is light-cured. They are used extensively for cementation of porcelain veneers and for ceramic and indirect composite resin restorations that are somewhat translucent. Because of their translucency, the final color of the restoration can be impacted by the color of the underlying cement. These light-cured cements provide the operator with almost unlimited working time to seat and position multiple veneers at one time. They are, however, rather light sensitive so the overhead operatory light should be positioned away from the mouth once the veneers have been seated. Head lamps used with loupes should be turned off. Esthetic resin cements can also be used for bonding of orthodontic brackets.

Other esthetic resin cements are manufactured as two-paste systems (base and catalyst) that come in dual-barrel syringes with automixing tips. These cements are dual-cured and that assures a final cure in all aspects of the restoration, especially in those restorations with thicker or opaque parts that the curing light cannot penetrate.

Esthetic resins are not adhesive in nature. Hence, they require the use of enamel and dentin bonding agents on the tooth and silane coupling agents or special primers on the ceramic or composite restoration in order to bond the restoration to the tooth. The enamel and dentin is usually prepared by the etch-and-rinse technique before bonding agents are applied. Internal surfaces of ceramic restorations are etched with hydrofluoric acid or sandblasted before the application of silane or primers.

When esthetic cements are used to cement porcelain veneers, the surface to which they are being bonded is mostly enamel and the etch-and-rinse technique is preferred. Acidic (self-etching) primers are easier to use by eliminating etch and rinse steps, but they do not etch enamel as well as the etch-and-rinse technique. (See Chapter 5 Principles of Bonding.)

Esthetic resins are made in a variety of tooth colors and translucencies to aid in achieving a desirable esthetic outcome. Usually, a shade is chosen to approximate the shade of the restoration, so that the appearance of the restoration is not altered by the underlying cement as light passes through the restoration and reflects off the cement. On occasion, it is necessary to mask the color of the dentin, especially if it is discolored. In this situation, an opaque cement of the appropriate shade is selected.

Many manufacturers provide try-in paste. This water-soluble, non-setting paste is matched to the base shade of the cement and is used to temporarily hold the restoration in place while the operator confirms the shade of the final product. Commercially available esthetic resin cement kits include Nexus (Kerr Dental), RelyX ARC (3M/ESPE), and Calibra (Dentsply) (Fig. 14.12).

Clinical Tip

Try-in paste is used to confirm the final shade of the restoration and to hold the restoration in place while the dentist and the patient inspect its form and esthetics.

Adhesive Resin Cements. Adhesive resin cements have wide applications for luting metal, ceramo-metal, and all-ceramic restorations but are not used for porcelain veneers. They are strong, radiopaque cements

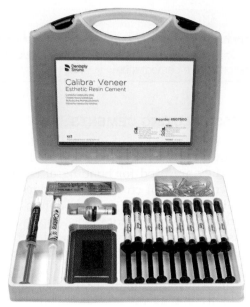

FIG. 14.12 Esthetic resin kit for luting ceramics such as porcelain veneers. Kit contains etchant, bonding agent, and several colors of try-in paste and resin cement. (Calibra Esthetic Resin Cement, Courtesy Dentsply Sirona.)

with low film thickness and strong bonds to properly prepared tooth and restoration surfaces. Adhesive resin cements when used with bonding agents have the capability of bonding to metal as well as ceramic restorations. Ceramic restorations are prepared for bonding by either sandblasting or etching with hydrofluoric acid, and then silane is applied. Internal surfaces of metal restorations are sandblasted. A special primer is used on the metal or ceramic. The adhesive cement is typically a dimethacrylate resin (with glass filler particles) which bonds to the primer. It is formulated in self-cure or dual-cure modes.

Other resin systems may be used. C&B Metabond (Parkell) uses a 4-META (methyl methacrylate) resin and contains adhesive monomers that can bond to metal. Panavia 21 (Kuraray Co.) uses a phosphorylated methacrylate monomer (MDP) that aids bonding. Panavia requires the use of a protective gel on the margins of the restoration to exclude oxygen so the cement can set completely. The resins used in these two products are attracted to metal oxides on the surface of base metal alloys.

Adhesive resin cements are available in universal, translucent, or opaque colors and are formulated in paste-paste automix systems.

While the use of self-etching primers greatly simplify the bonding process by reducing the number of steps and potential operator errors compared to the etch-and-rinse technique, it is still vitally important to carefully follow manufacturer's instructions. Do not mix and match primers and adhesive resins from different manufacturers, because there may be incompatibility that will weaken the bond or inhibit full setting.

> ❗ **Caution**
>
> Carefully follow manufacturer instructions for use of resin cements and bonding agents. Do not use bonding agents from one manufacturer with resin cement from another manufacturer. There may be incompatibility of materials that prevent full setting of materials or weaken the bond.

Self-Adhesive Resin Cements. While adhesive resin cements require separate bonding agents to bonding to tooth or restoration surfaces, self-adhesive resin cements eliminate the need for separate etching and priming for bonding. This is achieved by combining acidic monomers with the adhesive diacrylate resin. The acidic monomers have a low pH and etch the tooth. The negatively charged acidic monomers form ionic bonds with positively charged calcium ions in the tooth. During setting of the self-adhesive resin the acidic monomers undergo a change in pH from very acidic (pH 2) to less acidic (pH 5 to 6) as glass filler particles react with the acidic monomer and fluoride is released. The smear layer is incorporated into the cement rather than being dissolved and rinsed away as with the etch-and-rinse technique. The cement must be completely cured, because uncured resin will be acidic and irritate the pulp. The advantage for the clinician is a reduction in the number of clinical steps required. There is no need for etching, rinsing, or drying the tooth structure. This also reduces the risk of over- or under-drying the dentin and reduces post-cementation sensitivity.

The disadvantage of self-adhesive resin cements is that they do not achieve bond strengths as great as esthetic or adhesive resin cements. The bond to dentin is of moderate strength, but the bond to enamel is not as good. Self-adhesive resin cements should not be used where a strong enamel bond is needed as with cementation of orthodontic brackets or porcelain veneers unless a separate selective acid etching of enamel is also used. With selective enamel etching, phosphoric acid is applied to enamel only for 10-20 seconds before the self-adhesive resin is applied. Phosphoric acid should be kept off the dentin because etching it lowers the bond strength of self-etching resins to dentin.

The application of the mixed cement is very simple. It takes only a single step much like the application of zinc phosphate cement – mix and apply. Examples of self-adhesive resin cements include MaxCem Elite Chroma (Kerr Dental) (Fig. 14.13), Smart-Cem 2 (Dentsply), and Rely-X Unicem (3M/ESPE). These materials are supplied as dual-cured formulas. They are packaged in auto-mix syringes with two pastes or capsules with dispensing tips. A new self-adhesive resin cement has been introduced that is called a universal cement (Panavia SA Cement Universal, Kuraray Noritake), because it has incorporated two monomer technologies that allow it to bond to glass-based ceramics without etching and applying silane and to non-glass ceramics without the need for a separate special primer.

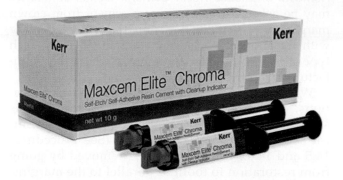

FIG. 14.13 Self-adhesive resin cement with a dual-barrel syringe to which an auto-mixing tip can be attached. (MaxCem Elite Chroma, Courtesy Kerr Dental.)

> ## Types of Restorations and Methods of Curing
>
> **LIGHT-CURED**
> - Porcelain veneers less than 1.5 mm thick
> - Orthodontic retainers not containing metal
> - Periodontal splints not containing metal
>
> **DUAL-CURED (LIGHT ACTIVATED AND CHEMICALLY ACTIVATED)**
> - Ceramic or indirect resin inlays, onlays, crowns, and bridges
>
> **CHEMICAL-CURED (SELF-CURED)**
> - Metal-based inlays, onlays, crowns, and bridges
> - Full metal crowns and bridges
> - Endodontic posts
> - Ceramic or indirect resin inlays, onlays, crowns, and bridges

> ❗ **Caution**
>
> Light-cured and dual-cured resin cements should be protected from ambient light in the operatory as it may initiate the curing process.

Cementation of Ceramic Restorations with Resin Cement

Try-In of Ceramic Restoration. Before cementation the restoration is tried on the crown preparation or in a cavity preparation (inlay/onlay) to confirm esthetics and adjust the fit as needed. The internal surface of the restoration will be contaminated after try-in and must be cleaned. Additionally, the surface of the ceramic must be prepared for bonding. Some clinicians use a solution of acid (typically hydrofluoric acid) for ceramics or sandblasting depending on which ceramic system is used. Some ceramics should not be acid treated but require special primers. (See Chapter 9 for a discussion of the preparation of the internal surfaces of ceramic restorations for cementation.) If the laboratory has pre-etched the ceramic restoration, do not re-etch it after try-in. Use alcohol or a commercial ceramic cleaner such as *Ivoclean* (Ivoclar Vivadent).

Removal of Excess Resin Cement. Dental auxiliaries may be asked to remove excess cement from crown margins after seating. It is important to be familiar with the proper consistency recommended for each type of cement intended for removal. Check the manufacturer's recommendations.

When cementing permanent ceramic restorations, excess resin cement should be removed as soon as seating is completed and before the chemical set or light cure is complete. (See Procedures 14.5 and 14.6.) Excess cement is removed by going from restoration to tooth or parallel to the margins. Avoid moving from tooth to restoration as cement may be pulled away from the margins leaving an opening.

Some clinicians prefer to "tack-cure" the resin cement to aid in removal. The tack-cure is best used for translucent restorations, because the light can penetrate the restoration and the gel set will be the same inside and outside the restoration. That way cement won't be pulled from under the margins when removing the excess. Once the excess cement has been removed, light-curing is completed.

Self-cured resin cements are best used for metal or opaque ceramic restorations. Remove the excess cement when it just begins to stiffen. The resin under the margins will be partly set to the same degree as the excess outside the restoration. Removal of the excess at this stage will avoid pulling cement from under the margins.

The set of some resin cements (Panavia 21, for example) is more strongly inhibited by oxygen, so the manufacturer recommends coating the margins with glycerin or other gel to exclude oxygen during the set. Knotted floss can be used interproximally to remove excess cement before it sets. It is possible that all excess cement will not be removed before it sets. Having a good knowledge of the tooth morphology is helpful in knowing where to look for residual cement, because concavities on the crown/root or root furcations can tend to retain excess cement. Explorers, scalers, curettes, and scalpels are helpful in removing excess cement. A good, solid finger rest and short strokes are a must when using a scalpel for cement removal to avoid slippage and soft tissue trauma. Residual excess cement will act as a plaque trap with risks of recurrent caries, gingival inflammation, or periodontal infection with bone loss. Some clinicians prefer to take a radiograph after cementation if excess cement is suspected. Many resin cements are radiopaque and can be seen on the radiograph. Cement on the proximal surfaces is easier to detect on the radiograph than buccal and lingual surfaces, because the bulk of the tooth structure can hide the cement from view.

 Clinical Tip

It is important to pay attention to the manufacturer's directions regarding bonding of the tooth surface and preparation of the restoration surface to achieve a strong bond and to eliminate postoperative sensitivity.

 Caution

Removal of excess resin cement is difficult if the material is allowed to set completely; follow the manufacturer's directions for removal. Excess cement is easy to remove after a few seconds of exposure to a curing light, but difficult to clean up if cured too long.

Resin-Based Cements

ADVANTAGES
- High strength
- Insoluble
- Low wear
- Excellent adherence to tooth structure
- Can bond all-ceramic restorations
- Esthetic shades available
- Low chance of postoperative sensitivity

DISADVANTAGES
- The introduction of water or oral fluids at any point during the bonding procedure can lead to lowered bond strength
- Self-adhesive resin cements should not be applied on exposed pulp or dentin that is close to the pulp
- Requires additional steps in preparation of internal restoration surfaces
- Removal of excess cement may be difficult

Provisional Resin Cements

Provisional resin cements are used to temporarily retain provisional crowns, bridges, or other indirect provisional restorations. They are formulated to have low compressive and tensile strengths, so the provisionals can readily be removed. Some provisional resin cements are formulated to have higher compressive strength for cases where longer term provisionals are needed (e.g., UltraTemp REZ, Ultradent Products). They are not bonded so clean up of the prepared tooth is simple. Because they shrink on setting, microleakage is slightly greater than with other provisional cements. They eliminate the problem associated with eugenol from ZOE provisional cements. Residual eugenol from provisional crowns cemented with zinc-oxide/eugenol can adversely affect the set of resin cements used for the final restoration.

Provisional resin cements are composed mostly of dimethacrylate resin with glass filler particles. They are compatible with other resin systems such as bonding agents, composites, and resin build-up materials. They are available in paste-paste systems in cartridges or syringes with auto-mixing tips, so mixing and dispensing

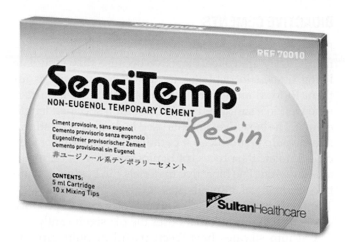

FIG. 14.14 Provisional resin cement kit containing cartridge of resins (base and catalyst), automixing tips, and mixing/dispensing gun. (SensiTemp Resin, Courtesy Sultan Healthcare.)

is easy. They come with self-, light-, or dual-cure capability. Some of the self-cure cements are available in regular or fast set modes. Examples of commercial available products include TempBond Clear (Kerr Dental), Premier Implant Cement (Premier Dental Products), and SensiTemp Resin (Sultan Healthcare) (Fig. 14.14).

Compomer Cements

Compomer cements are considered to be a subset of resin cements. Compomer cement are somewhere between resin cements and glass ionomer cements in their composition since they contain some of the components from each type. Compomer is a composite modified by polyacid, so that it releases fluoride like GIC (but to a lesser extent) and is strong and wear resistant like composite. It has both the slow acid–base reaction similar to GIC and the polymerization reaction of resin. It can be self-cured, light-cured, or dual-cured. The self-cure occurs in about 3 minutes in the mouth. The luting compomer comes in a powder-liquid formulation. Some versions are not adhesive to tooth structure like glass ionomer. So, to gain adhesion a bonding agent is needed. However, Dyract Cem Plus (Dentsply) is a product that is self-adhesive. Compomer luting cements are not widely used.

OIL-BASED LUTING CEMENTS

Zinc Oxide Eugenol

Zinc oxide eugenol cements, commonly referred to as ZOE cements, have been widely used for many years. Generally, ZOE cements do not have the strength needed to serve as permanent cements or high-strength bases. So, they are mainly used for provisional cementation, provisional and intermediate restorations, low-strength bases, and as root canal sealers and periodontal dressings.

Composition. Various ZOE cements are available in powder/liquid and paste/paste systems. In the two-paste system, one is labeled a base and the other a catalyst. The principal ingredient of the powder is zinc oxide and it can contain up to 8% other zinc salts which act as accelerators. The liquid, eugenol, has the distinct smell of cloves, because it is a derivative of oil of cloves. It is a weak acid and up to 2% acetic acid may be added as an accelerator. Zinc oxide and eugenol when mixed together undergo an acid–base reaction. If acetic acid has not been added, then water is needed to initiate the reaction.

In systems using two pastes, as for provisional cements, vegetable or mineral oil is added to the zinc oxide powder to create one paste and fillers are added to eugenol to create the other paste. The paste with zinc oxide will be white and the eugenol paste will be amber in color.

Because eugenol can interfere with the set of resins, ZOE should not be used as a base or provisional cement if composite resin or resin bonding agents will be used. However, if the surface of the enamel or dentin is cleaned thoroughly before bonding, the effect of the eugenol is removed. After the provisional crown is removed and excess cement removed, cleaning the preparation with flour of pumice and a prophy cup or brush is an effective way of removing the small bits of residual ZOE cement.

Formulations are made without eugenol and are called *non-eugenol zinc oxide cements.* They are used as provisional cements (e.g., TempBond NE by Kerr Dental) for provisional crowns when resin cement is planned for the permanent restoration.

Properties. Eugenol has long been known for its sedative effect on the pulp, largely caused by its antibacterial effects and its good marginal seal. It can be irritating when in direct contact with oral mucosa or pulp. The mixed ZOE has a neutral pH of 7, which makes it very biocompatible with tooth structure.

ZOE cements are not as strong as other permanent luting agents and are rarely used for this purpose. Thus, they are ideally suited for provisional cementation. Their weaker tensile strength allows them to be easily removed at a second appointment, when a permanent restoration is to be placed. ZOE cement has a compressive strength of 26 MPa which falls below the ISO 3107 standard of 35 MPa for permanent luting cements. When EBA (2-ethoxybenzoic acid) is added to the eugenol in a 2:1 ratio and 30% alumina is added to the powder to reinforce it, much more powder can be incorporated into the liquid and the resultant mix is much stronger (72 MPa compressive strength). Resin fibers (20% polymethyl methacrylate) are also added to increase strength and wear resistance making them suitable for intermediate restorations (e.g., IRM, Dentsply Sirona) and high-strength bases.

The film thickness of ZOE cements is between 16 and 28 μm and when alumina is present it approaches 57 μm (25 μm and below are more ideal for luting). ZOE cements are susceptible to hydrolysis and a significant amount of its volume can be lost in a 6 month period. So, they do not serve well for long-term provisional restorations. Glass ionomer and resin-modified glass ionomer cements perform much better as long-term provisional restorations.

Powder/liquid and paste/paste systems are easily manipulated. The set, strength, and viscosity are controlled by the incorporation of powder into the liquid or, in the paste/paste system, by a change in the ratio of base to catalyst.

Zinc Oxide Eugenol

ADVANTAGES
- A wide variety of uses
- Sedative to the pulp
- Easily manipulated
- Low cost

DISADVANTAGES
- Low strength
- High solubility
- Unable to be used under composite restorations and indirect restorations cemented with resin or resin-modified glass ionomer cements (RMGICs)

Manipulation. When two-paste ZOE are used, equal lengths of accelerator and base pastes are placed on a paper mixing pad or glass slab and are mixed until a uniform color is achieved. If the powder/liquid system is used, the powder bottle is shaken and the powder is measured with the manufacturer-supplied scoop. The liquid is dispensed in the corresponding number of drops. The powder is incorporated into the liquid until the desired consistency is achieved. Heavy spatulation with a metal spatula allows for the incorporation of more powder; this additional powder will greatly enhance the strength of the cement. (See Procedure 14.1.)

 Clinical Tip

ZOE cements are difficult to remove from mixing surfaces; glass slabs and spatulas should be wiped clean before the cement sets. Set cement may be removed with alcohol or orange solvent.

Timeline of the Introduction of Dental Cements

1850s: Zinc oxide eugenol
1870s: Zinc phosphate
1950s: Methylmethacrylate resin (poor performance)
1960s: Zinc polycarboxylate, Bis GMA resin, and glass ionomer
Early 1990s: Resin-modified glass ionomer, compomer, and adhesive resin
Early 2000s: Self-adhesive resin

BIOACTIVE CEMENTS

Bioactive cements are a relatively new category of cements. They are called bioactive because they stimulate living tissues. In dentistry the test for bioactivity is for them to form an apatite-like substance on their surface when left in a simulated body fluid for a specified length of time. The bioactive cements used in dentistry can stimulate the pulp to produce a reparative dentin bridge or they can stimulate the process of remineralization of demineralized dentin. The bioactive materials can be divided into two groups: calcium silicates and calcium aluminates. They both have acid–base setting reactions and produce an alkaline byproduct that raises the pH significantly.

Calcium silicates have been useful in pulp capping and vital pulpotomies. The first of these materials to be widely used in endodontics is mineral trioxide aggregate (MTA). Introduced in the 1990s as ProRoot MTA (Dentsply), MTA is chemically similar to Portland cement. It has a number of properties that contribute to wound healing: 1. it is alkaline in nature because it forms calcium hydroxide as it sets creating an antibacterial environment, 2. it releases calcium ions that help repair dentin, 3. it bonds and seals the area, and 4. it stimulates formation of secondary dentin and hydroxyapatite. The shortcomings of MTA are that it is difficult to handle, has a very long setting time, and a low compressive strength (about 50 MPa). Newer improved materials have emerged with new applications. TheraCal LC (BISCO Dental Products) is a light-cured resin-modified calcium silicate used as a liner and Biodentine (Septodont) is used as a base under direct restorations to stimulate dentin repair.

Calcium aluminate cements are usually hybrid materials containing calcium aluminate and glass ionomer. The calcium aluminate portion is responsible for the development of a high pH during setting, strength, reduced microleakage, and stability. The glass ionomer portion is responsible for its viscosity, early setting time, and early strength. Due to their strength (compressive and shear bond), retention, low solubility, and low film thickness (about 15 μm), they make excellent permanent luting agents for all metal, ceramo-metal, or high-strength ceramic crowns and bridges (e.g., Ceramir C&B, Doxa Dental). They do not require surface treatment of the tooth such as etching, priming, or conditioning. They are available in premeasured capsules with delivery tips.

HANDLING OF CEMENTS

STORAGE

Cements should not be stored in warm or humid areas of the dental office. If you are refrigerating your cement, it should be taken out of the refrigerator at least 1 hour prior to use so it can reach room temperature.

PRECEMENTATION CHECK

Prior to mixing the cement the crown or other indirect restoration should be tried in/on the prepared tooth. In many states dental assistants and hygienists licensed in expanded functions can prepare the restoration for cementation by performing many of the following procedures:

1. If the crown is not immediately seating all the way, the first thing to check and adjust is the proximal contacts.
2. If it is still not seating completely, the inside of the crown should be checked (using a variety of materials and techniques for marking spots that bind on the preparation) and adjusted.
3. Next, the margins should be checked with a fine-tipped explorer to see that they are flush with the prepared margins of the tooth. If they are not flush, then re-check the contacts and interior of the crown. If no problems are found with the fit, the discrepancies may be caused by a poor impression or a lab error (which would necessitate starting with a new impression).
4. Then, check and adjust the occlusion.
5. Confirm that the patient is happy with the appearance of the crown and the bite feels comfortable.
6. Re-polish as needed and clean the interior of the crown in preparation for cementation.

MIXING

It is important that cements be mixed to their appropriate consistency in accordance with manufacturers' recommendations, with meticulous attention to detail. Cements that are mishandled may lead to difficulties in seating, retaining the restoration, or even pulpal sensitivity. Cements may be hand mixed or may come in premeasured capsules mixed in a triturator or mixed as material is extruded through automixing tips attached to dual-barrel syringes.

Even skilled hand mixing may incorporate air that is thought to lead to the reduction of bond strength between the restoration and the tooth substrate. Also, inaccurate ratios of powder and liquid can be dispensed from scoops and liquid droppers. If hand mixing is chosen, the amount of time taken to mix the cement must be carefully monitored as too much mixing time may make the cement too viscous while too little time may cause the cement not to be mixed thoroughly (Fig. 14.15). Cements mixed in capsules or via automix systems provide the following advantages: consistent mix, reduced clean-up, reduced cross contamination, and avoids incorporating air in the mix.

Clinical Tip

There are many types of cement available and each one has multiple uses and differences in mixing techniques so that it is very important to **ALWAYS** follow the manufacturer's instructions for storage, mixing, and handling.

Caution

Light-cured cements may not be appropriate for deep preparations: the ultraviolet (UV) light may fail to activate some of the material, leaving part of the cement unset. Dual-cured products help to eliminate this problem.

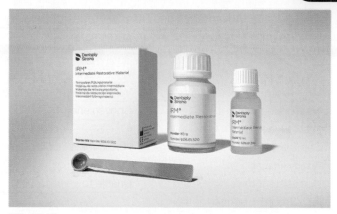

FIG. 14.15 Zinc oxide eugenol hand-mixed powder/liquid *(IRM Intermediate Restorative Material)*. It has resin fibers added to increase strength and wear resistance and is used as an intermediate restoration. (Courtesy Dentsply Sirona.)

Advantages and disadvantages of each delivery system are listed in Table 14.3.

WORKING AND SETTING TIMES

Working time and setting time are considerations in the choice of cement and mixing mechanism. A longer working time is needed for cementation of longer span bridges versus single crowns and a shorter setting time is desirable for difficult-to-isolate areas. Patient considerations and the dental team's mixing and delivery skills play a part in the selection of appropriate cement. The dental auxiliary is responsible for delivering the cement at the proper consistency within very definite time frames. A skilled auxiliary must be able to routinely mix a variety of cements rapidly to their proper consistency.

Cement Manipulation Considerations for Cements in Powder and Liquid Form

1. Keep powder and liquid separated when dispensing.
2. Fluff powder before dispensing by gently rolling the container in your hand to aerate.
3. Use scoop provided by the manufacturer and ensure scoop of powder is level, not heaping.
4. Section the powder into increments according to the manufacturer's directions; when increment size varies, the smallest increments are mixed first.
5. Dispense the liquid by holding the dispenser vertically before squeezing to obtain uniform drops.
6. Close caps of powder and liquid containers immediately after dispensing to avoid evaporation and contamination.
7. Incorporate powder and liquid thoroughly when mixing. If incremental mixing is used, each increment must be completely incorporated before the next is added.
8. Use moderate pressure on the spatula when mixing.
9. Use both sides of the spatula blade.
10. Mix cement in a "stropping" motion.
11. Gather all the material together to test the viscosity.

TABLE 14.3 Advantages and Disadvantages of Delivery Systems

HAND MIXING	AUTOMIXING	PREDOSED CAPSULES
Advantages		
Vary viscosity	Consistent mix	Consistent mix
Vary volume of material mixed	Vary volume of material used	Convenience
No extra equipment	Convenience	Disposable, less asepsis
Less expensive		Less cleanup required
Can mix shades if needed	No air voids incorporated in the mix	No air voids incorporated in the mix
Disadvantages		
Inconsistent mix	Unable to vary viscosity	Unable to vary viscosity
Air voids incorporated in the mix		
Less convenient	Additional equipment needed	Volume of capsule is fixed
More cleanup required	Cannot blend shades, more expensive	Cannot blend shades, requires extra equipment, more expensive

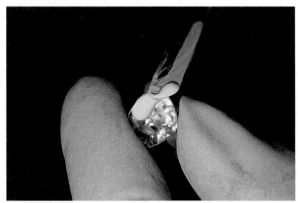

Fig. 14.16 Loading a crown—wipe the blade of the spatula against the margin of the crown.

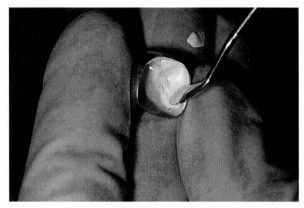

Fig. 14.17 Loading a crown—using a flat-bladed instrument, cover all the walls with a thin, even coating of the cement.

> **⚠ Caution**
>
> Light-cured cements should not be used if there is a potential for incomplete set of the cement under a dental prosthesis because the curing light cannot reach the cement to activate curing.

LOADING THE RESTORATION

The dental assistant may be responsible for filling the crown with a luting cement before transferring it to the dentist. The techniques described in the accompanying box ("Loading a Custom-Made Crown for Cementation") will ensure that the cement is evenly loaded in the crown, and that the margins are coated internally.

> **Loading a Custom-Made Crown for Cementation**
>
> 1. Gather cement from the mixing surface with the blade of the spatula or a plastic instrument.
> 2. Wipe the blade against the margin of the crown (Fig. 14.16).
> 3. Cover all the interior walls of the crown with a thin, even coating of cement, making sure it is free of air bubbles (Fig. 14.17).
> 4. Do not fill the prosthesis to more than one-quarter the inner volume; overfilling the prosthesis may prevent complete seating.
> 5. Transfer the crown cement-side down on the palm of your hand for the dentist to pick up and seat.

> **Reasons Cement May Keep a Crown from Seating Fully**
>
> 1. Too much cement is present in the crown and hydraulic pressure does not allow excess cement to flow out.
> 2. The cement mix is too thick (viscous) and the cement does not flow readily.
> 3. The cement is starting to set and will not flow.
> 4. Cement was selected with a film thickness that is too great for luting.

> **⚠ Caution**
>
> Crowns that have long walls and a narrow diameter, such as crowns for lower incisors or for premolars, should not be filled with too much cement. Just a thin layer of cement should be applied to the walls of the restoration's interior (intaglio) to allow cement to flow out when the crowns are seated. With too much cement, hydraulic pressure may prevent the cement from flowing out and the crown from seating completely.

REMOVAL OF EXCESS CEMENT

Some cements should not be removed until completely set, such as zinc phosphate cement; others may be best removed when the cement reaches a rubbery or gel consistency, such as resin-modified glass ionomer cement;

and others when the cement is tack-cured, that is, light-cured resin cement. (Removal of excess resin cement was previously discussed.) Follow the manufacturer's directions for appropriate consistency at removal. Cement consistencies vary from rock hard to rubbery.

1. Remove cement in bulk when possible.
2. Use a piece of knotted floss to remove cement from interproximal areas before it sets. Draw the floss out under the contacts rather than coming back up through the contact, which might dislodge the crown.
3. Use a scaler or curette followed by an explorer to remove excess cement from subgingival surfaces, taking care to not scratch the surface of the restoration or gouge the margins where the tooth and restoration meet.

Timing of Excess Cement Removal after Luting a Crown

(Follow the manufacturer's directions for appropriate consistency at removal). Remove interproximal cement before set
  In general:
Zinc phosphate—let cement set completely
Zinc polycarboxylate—let cement set completely. Do not try to remove when rubbery
Zinc oxide eugenol—let cement set completely
Glass ionomer cement—some versions can be removed at the gel stage
Resin-modified glass ionomer cement—Expose excess to curing light for 1 second, then remove at gel stage or let it self-cure and remove at gel stage
Resin cements—remove excess *before* they set completely, often after 1 second tack cure.

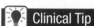 **Clinical Tip**

When removing excess cement before it is fully set, be sure to secure the crown against the tooth so your manipulation does not lift the crown.

CEMENT-ASSOCIATED PERI-IMPLANT DISEASE

Excess cement remaining after placement of an implant is positively associated with peri-implant disease. Biofilm-related infections can result in the removal of the implant in severe cases. The American Academy of Periodontology (2013) has reported a prevalence of peri-implantitis in three studies ranging from 6.61% to 36.6%. There are several factors associated with these infections, including cement residue. Radiographs do not always reveal this residual cement, especially on buccal/lingual surfaces. Margins that are subgingival exhibit a greater amount of undetected cement. Cement-related bone loss may occur quickly or be delayed for several years (Fig. 14.18).

At the time of the cementation of the implant restoration, a titanium scaler or curette should be used for removal of excess cement. Titanium instruments are strong enough to remove the set cement but are soft enough to avoid scratching the implant surface. Plastic or graphite instruments may leave tiny bits of their material embedded in rough surfaces of the implant that may themselves contribute to peri-implantitis. The

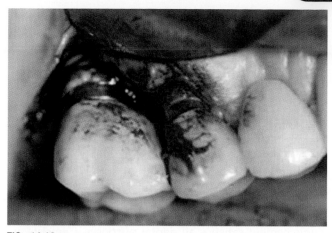

FIG. 14.18 Excess cement remaining subgingivally has become a chronic bacterial plaque trap causing bone loss around the dental implant. See cement on the distal surface wrapping around to the facial surface. (Courtesy Drs. Nick Shumaker and Leslie Paris. From Slim L: Cement-associated peri-implantitis, *RDH Magazine*, 33(12), 2013.)

dental hygienist should evaluate each implant carefully to monitor probe depths, clinical and radiographic signs of inflammation, and/or the presence of cement residue.

 Caution

Complete removal of excess cement is essential to maintain gingival health.

CLEANUP, DISINFECTION, AND STERILIZATION

The removal of cement before it is set provides for easier cleanup of mixing slabs, spatulas and delivery instruments. Instruments and equipment that come in contact with cement should be cleaned as soon as is reasonably possible, using alcohol-saturated gauze squares. If immediate cleanup is not possible, use an ultrasonic cleaner with cement removal solution. If barriers have not been used, equipment such as triturators, cement activators, the outside of cement bottles, and dispensing scoops and syringes must be properly disinfected. Sterilization of mixing and delivery instruments is necessary. Glass and plastic mixing slabs are recommended because they can be sterilized in heat sterilizers. Paper pads, although convenient, are a source of contamination; there is no reliable way to combat this other than using only one sheet at a time (very difficult to mix on this). Porous paper pads absorb some of the cement liquid and alter the powder to liquid ratio.

CARE AROUND MARGINS

Proper instrumentation during prophylactic procedures and appropriate delivery of some therapeutic agents such as fluoride are important considerations for the continuing care of the fine line of cement at margins of indirect restorations. Care must be taken to avoid gouging or ditching the cement during hand instrumentation. Although the cement margin may be very small (25 μm), even minute breaks are a place for biofilm to form and initiate microleakage and secondary caries. Ultrasonic and sonic scalers should be avoided on margins of cemented restorations whenever possible, because they may cause fracturing of the cement. Air polishers may abrade cement at restoration margins. Fluoride application on glass ionomer and resin-based cement margins should be limited to neutral sodium fluoride, because acidulated fluoride products may attack the cement.

SUMMARY

A restoration may be esthetically pleasing and functional at the time of cementation, but if problems occur with retention, postoperative sensitivity, and recurrent caries, patients will most likely ask questions as to why the treatment failed and how good the dentist's skills are. No single cement satisfies all dental purposes. Cements are chosen to match the physical properties of the restorative material being used, and the requirements of each clinical situation. The allied oral health practitioner is responsible for handling, mixing, and delivering the cement to the dentist. Proper cement manipulation is important in determining the quality of a cement's physical properties. In addition, the use of instruments on a cement margin can directly affect a restoration's longevity. Procedures for placement of provisional restorations are important to the success of future permanent restorations. It is essential the auxiliary is knowledgeable in the uses, properties, handling characteristics, and precautions for all cements used in the dentist's office.

INSTRUCTIONAL VIDEOS

See the Evolve Resources site for a variety of educational videos that reinforce the material covered in this chapter.

Procedure 14.1 Zinc Oxide Eugenol Cement (ZOE): Primary and Secondary Consistency

See Evolve site for Competency Sheet.

Consider the following with this procedure: *safety glasses are recommended for the patient, PPE is required for the operator, ensure appropriate safety protocols are followed, and check your local state guidelines before performing this procedure.*

EQUIPMENT/SUPPLIES (FIG. 14.19)

- Cement paste/paste or cement powder/liquid and dispensers
- Paper mixing pad or glass slab
- Flexible cement spatula

PROCEDURE STEPS: PRIMARY CONSISTENCY

1. Dispense the recommended amount of base paste and accelerator paste onto a mixing pad.
   NOTE: One-half inch of each is usually enough for a single crown restoration.
2. Mix the materials, using both sides of the flat blade in a "stropping, pushing" motion.
3. The mix is in primary consistency when it is smooth and creamy and after gathering together lifts 1 inch off the mixing surface (Fig. 14.20).
4. Whenever possible, immediately clean the spatula with gauze.

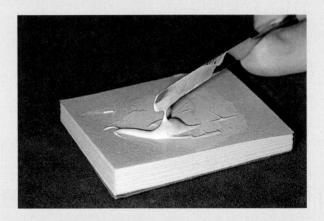

FIG. 14.20

PROCEDURE STEPS: SECONDARY CONSISTENCY (FIG. 14.21)

1. Fluff the powder, and measure onto one end of the mixing surface.
   NOTE: Aerated powder provides for a more accurate measurement.
2. Shake the liquid, and dispense at the opposite end of the mixing surface.

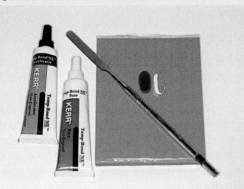

FIG. 14.19

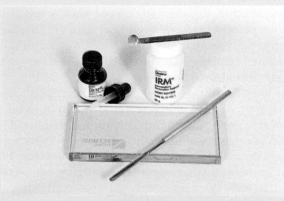

FIG. 14.21

Procedure 14.1 Zinc Oxide Eugenol Cement (ZOE): Primary and Secondary Consistency—cont'd

NOTE: Hold the dispenser vertical while dispensing to obtain uniform drops.

3. Incorporate the powder into the liquid in two increments or all at once according to the manufacturer's directions (Figure 14.22).

NOTE: Incorporate as much powder as possible into the liquid (Figure 14.23).

4. Mix the materials, using both sides of the flat blade in a "stropping, pushing" motion.

5. The cement will be in secondary consistency when it can be rolled into a ball and is no longer tacky (Fig. 14.24).

6. Whenever possible, immediately clean the spatula with moist gauze.

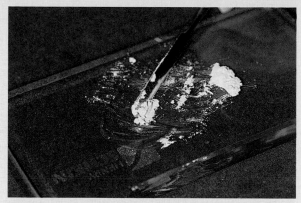

FIG. 14.23

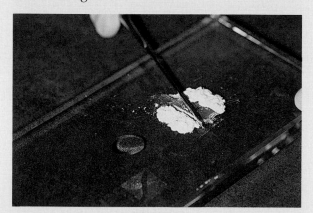

FIG. 14.22

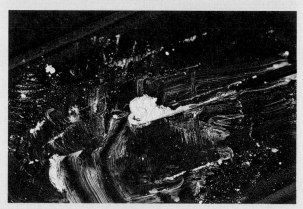

FIG. 14.24

Procedure 14.2 Zinc Phosphate Cement: Primary Consistency

See Evolve site for Competency Sheet.

Consider the following with this procedure: safety glasses are recommended for the patient, PPE is required for the operator, ensure appropriate safety protocols are followed, and check your local state guidelines before performing this procedure.

EQUIPMENT/SUPPLIES (FIG. 14.25)

- Cement powder
- Cement liquid and dispenser
- Cool glass slab
- Flexible cement spatula

PROCEDURE STEPS

1. Obtain a cooled glass slab.

NOTE: The frozen slab method may be used for multiple orthodontic bands or long-span bridges.

2. Fluff the powder, and dispense the recommended amount onto one end of the slab.

3. Divide the powder into four to six increments to include smaller and larger increment sizes.

NOTE: Smaller increments are incorporated first.

4. Shake the liquid, and dispense the recommended amount at the opposite end of the slab.v

NOTE: Hold the dispenser vertical while dispensing to obtain uniform drops (Fig. 14.26).

5. Incorporate the first increment into the liquid.

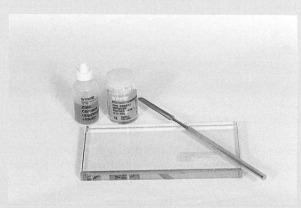

FIG. 14.25

Continued

Procedure 14.2　Zinc Phosphate Cement: Primary Consistency—cont'd

NOTE: Hold the spatula blade flat against the mixing surface. Use both sides of the spatula in a sweeping "figure-eight" motion over a large area of the slab (Fig. 14.27).

6. Each increment is completely incorporated and is mixed for 20 to 30 seconds, beginning with the smallest and progressing through the largest.

NOTE: Adding increments of powder and completely incorporating each into the mix will help to neutralize the acid, control the setting time, and allow for completion of the exothermic reaction before use (Fig. 14.28).

7. Place the spatula blade at a 45-degree angle to the slab, and gather the mass together to test the consistency.

NOTE: For primary consistency, the material should be smooth and creamy. Draw the spatula up from the mix; the cement should follow the spatula, breaking after 1 inch (Fig. 14.29).

8. Clean the spatula and slab with moistened gauze and disinfect or sterilize.

NOTE: If the cement is allowed to harden on the slab or spatula, it may be removed in an ultrasonic cleaner or by soaking in a solution of baking powder.

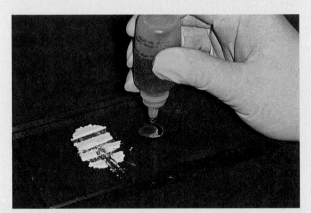

FIG. 14.26

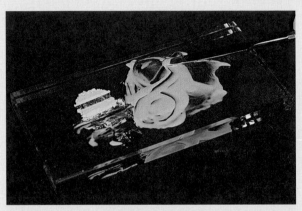

FIG. 14.28

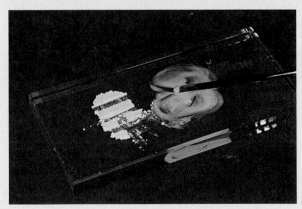

FIG. 14.27

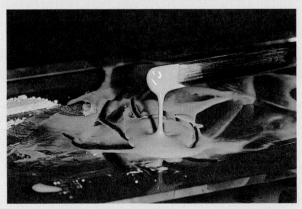

FIG. 14.29

Procedure 14.3　Zinc Polycarboxylate Cement: Primary Consistency

See Evolve site for Competency Sheet.

Consider the following with this procedure: *safety glasses are recommended for the patient, PPE is required for the operator, ensure appropriate safety protocols are followed, and check your local state guidelines before performing this procedure.*

EQUIPMENT/SUPPLIES (FIG. 14.30)

Cement powder and dispenser
Cement liquid and dispenser
Paper mixing pad or glass slab
Flexible cement spatula

Procedure 14.3   Zinc Polycarboxylate Cement: Primary Consistency—cont'd

PROCEDURE STEPS

1. Fluff the powder, and measure onto one end of the mixing surface.
   NOTE: Aerated powder provides for a more accurate measurement.
2. Shake the liquid, and dispense at the opposite end of the mixing surface.
   NOTE: Hold the dispenser vertical while dispensing to obtain uniform drops, or, if using a syringe dispenser, be careful to note the number of lined increments to dispense.
3. Incorporate the powder into the liquid in two increments or all at once according to the manufacturer's directions.
4. Mix the materials, using both sides of the flat blade in a "stropping, pushing" motion.
5. The mix is in primary consistency when it is smooth and creamy and after gathering together lifts 1 inch off the mixing surface.

NOTE: The consistency is somewhat thicker than that of other cements and appears glossy (Fig. 14.31). The cement is too thick and starting to set if it produces thin stringy "cobwebs" when lifted off the mixing surface (Fig. 14.32). Do not use that mix if it loses its glossy appearance.
6. Whenever possible, immediately clean the spatula with moist gauze.

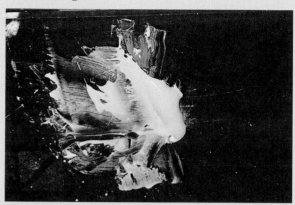

FIG. 14.31

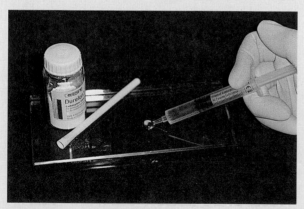

FIG. 14.30

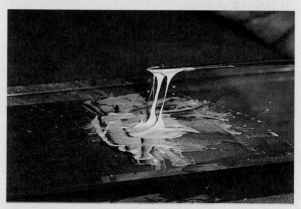

FIG. 14.32

Procedure 14.4   Glass Ionomer Cement: Predosed Capsule

See Evolve site for Competency Sheet.

Consider the following with this procedure: *safety glasses are recommended for the patient, PPE is required for the operator, ensure appropriate safety protocols are followed, and check your local state guidelines before performing this procedure.*

EQUIPMENT/SUPPLIES (FIG. 14.33)

- Premeasured capsule of cement
- Cement activator
- Triturator
- Cement dispenser

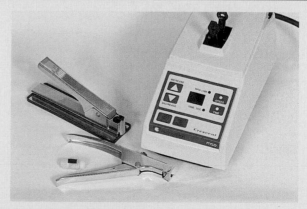

FIG. 14.33

Continued

Procedure 14.4   Glass Ionomer Cement: Predosed Capsule—cont'd

PROCEDURE STEPS

1. Place the premeasured capsule into the cement activator and press down on the handle.

   NOTE: The activator breaks the seal between the powder and the liquid in the capsule, allowing the materials to meet. Make sure you use sufficient pressure to feel the seal break (Fig. 14.34).

2. Place the capsule into the triturator and set for the recommended amount of time, usually 10 to 15 seconds.

   NOTE: The capsule is similar to an amalgam capsule and needs to be secured in the arms of the triturator before mixing (Fig. 14.35).

3. Remove the capsule from the triturator and immediately place into the cement dispenser; advance the mixed cement to the end of the dispensing tip (Fig. 14.36).

4. Load the crown directly from the dispenser (Fig. 14.37).

5. Discard the capsule and disinfect the activator and triturator. The dispenser may be sterilized.

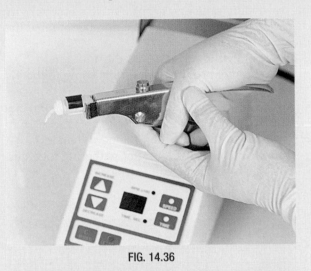

FIG. 14.36

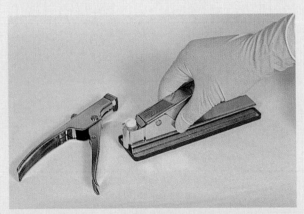

FIG. 14.34

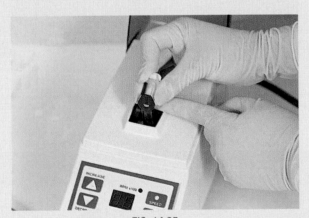

FIG. 14.35

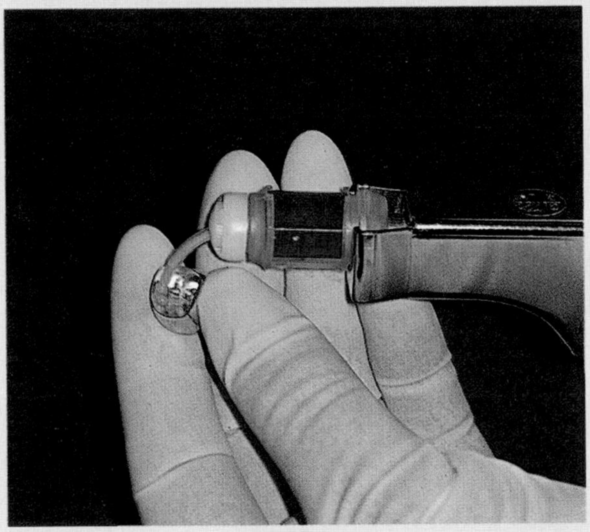

FIG. 14.37

Procedure 14.5   Resin-Based Cement for Indirect Restorations: Ceramic, Porcelain, Composite

See Evolve site for Competency Sheet.

Consider the following with this procedure: safety glasses are recommended for the patient, PPE is required for the operator, ensure appropriate safety protocols are followed, and check your local state guidelines before performing this procedure.

EQUIPMENT/SUPPLIES

- Tooth conditioner (etchant)
- Primer/bond (universal) adhesive
- Disposable applicator
- Dispensing dish
- Cement/adhesive
- Blunt instrument

PROCEDURE STEPS

1. Clean preparation of all provisional material.
   NOTE: Eugenol-containing materials should not be used in provisional coverage.
2. Clean the dentin with a rubber cup and nonfluoride cleaning paste.
   NOTE: Fluoride should not be used before bonding.
3. Rinse thoroughly and lightly air dry.
4. Clean and dry and prepare the internal surface of the restoration.
   NOTE: Organic debris accumulated during try-in must be removed; this can be done by several means, including the use of an ultrasonic cleaner and phosphoric acid etchant. Microetching is recommended for preparation of the internal surface of the restoration.

5. Apply tooth conditioner according to the manufacturer's directions.
   NOTE: The use of a fine needle tip attached to the syringe of the conditioner will allow control of the conditioner to prevent etching of areas prone to postoperative sensitivity.
6. Rinse and blot dry, leaving a moist glistening surface.
   NOTE: Blot drying provides the correct amount of "wetness" on the tooth surface while avoiding desiccating the tooth surface.
7. Isolate the area to prevent saliva contamination.
   NOTE: If saliva contamination occurs, repeat steps 5 and 6.
8. Apply primer/bond adhesive agent to the tooth and internal surface of the restoration according to the manufacturer's directions (Fig. 14.38). shows the etch-and-rinse procedure to maximize bond strength with a significant amount of enamel remaining in the preparations for these veneers.
9. The universal adhesive is applied to the teeth and scrubbed for 20 seconds with a microtip (Fig. 14.39).
10. Dispense the desired shade of cement base paste into the restoration and seat the restoration.
11. Initiate the set with a curing light until the cement reaches the gel phase and then remove the excess cement (Fig. 14.40).
12. Review the final results, showing the veneers in place (Fig. 14.41).

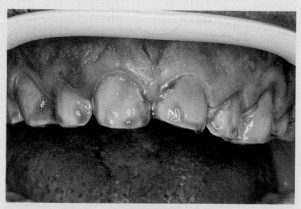

FIG. 14.38

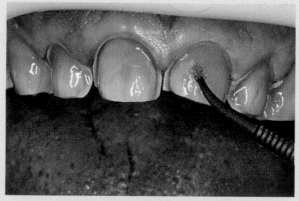

FIG. 14.39

Continued

Procedure 14.5   Resin-Based Cement for Indirect Restorations: Ceramic, Porcelain, Composite—cont'd

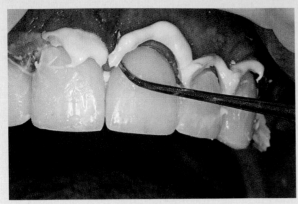

FIG. 14.40

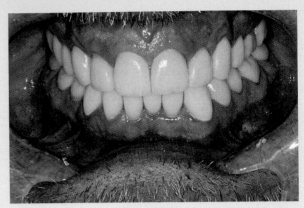

FIG. 14.41

Figures 14.38 - 14.41 from Blank JT: 3M ESPE's RelyX Ultimate Adhesive Resin Cement: A cement for nearly any indirect indication, www.dental-productsreport.com.

Procedure 14.6   Self-Adhesive Technique for Indirect Restorations: Ceramic, Porcelain, Composite

See Evolve site for Competency Sheet.

Consider the following with this procedure: *safety glasses are recommended for the patient, PPE is required for the operator, ensure appropriate safety protocols are followed, and check your local state guidelines before performing this procedure.*

Shown is the cementation of a ceramic crown with a self-adhesive resin cement.

EQUIPMENT/SUPPLIES

- Matrix
- Self-adhesive resin cement (Fig. 14.42).
- Light-cure delivery system
- Floss; explorer or scaler

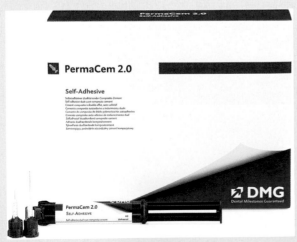

FIG. 14.42

PROCEDURE STEPS

1. Follow steps 1-3 in Procedure 14.5.
   NOTE: When using self-adhesive cements the etching and bonding steps are not done (Fig. 14.43).
2. Try in the crown and confirm fit at margins, contact areas and bite. (Fig. 14.44).
3. Prepare the internal surface (intaglio) of the crown by sandblasting (Fig. 14.44).
4. Rinse thoroughly and dry the crown (Fig. 14.45).
5. Place the mixing and delivery tips on the cement cartridge. Express cement and coat the walls of the crown with a thin layer of cement and fully seat the crown with finger pressure or have patient bite on a cotton roll (Fig. 14.46).
   NOTE: Do not overfill the crown with cement. Hydraulic pressure may prevent the crown from seating fully.
6. The cement is dual-cured, so wave the curing light over the margins of the crown for 2 seconds to gel the cement. Remove the excess cement with a scaler

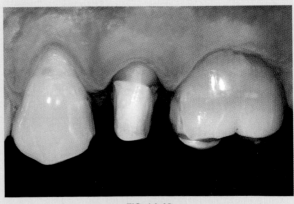

FIG. 14.43

Procedure 14.6   Self-Adhesive Technique for Indirect Restorations: Ceramic, Porcelain, Composite—cont'd

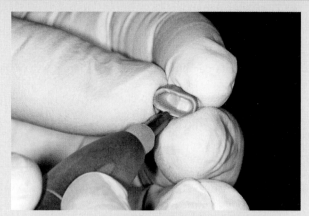

FIG. 14.44

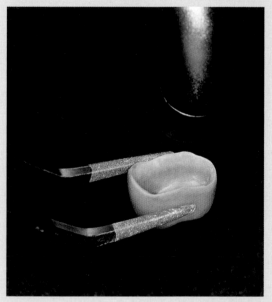

FIG. 14.45

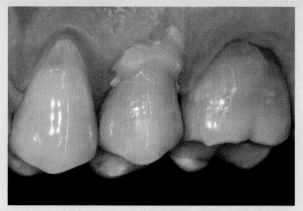

FIG. 14.46

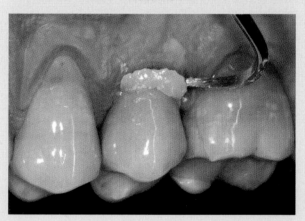

FIG. 14.47

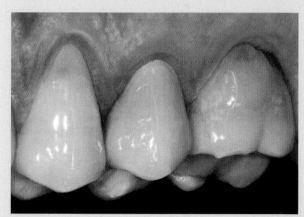

FIG. 14.48

or explorer. Used knotted floss to remove excess cement from the interproximal area (Fig. 14.47).

NOTE: The removal of excess cement before curing is necessary; a short light-cure to cause the cement to gel allows for easier removal. Pay special attention to interproximal areas, using knotted floss to remove excess cement. Once the cement has fully set it is very difficult to remove, especially from interproximal areas.

7. Check the cure marginal fit, contact areas and adjust occlusion as necessary (Fig. 14.48).
8. Check the radiograph to confirm seating and cement removal
9. Finish and polish any areas that have been adjusted.

TRY-IN OPTION: BEFORE PREPARATION OF THE TOOTH FOR BONDING

1. Dispense the appropriate shade of try-in paste onto a mixing pad. Load the restoration and seat onto the preparation.

NOTE: Try-in paste is matched to the cement base material and is used to obtain the correct shade of cement. Restoration "try-in" particularly for anterior crowns is recommended before final cementation to ensure acceptance of restoration esthetics.

2. Once the restoration fit and esthetics are verified, the try-in paste is removed from the preparation and the restoration is cemented, using one of the techniques already described.

Figures 14.42 - 14.48 courtesy of DMG America, Englewood, NJ.

Get Ready for Exams!

Review Questions

Select the one correct response for each of the following multiple-choice questions.

1. Cements mixed to primary consistency are used for
   a. High-strength bases
   b. Luting
   c. Core buildups
   d. Surgical dressings

2. It may be necessary to place an insulating base under restorations to
   a. Encourage sclerotic dentin formation
   b. Protect the pulp from sudden temperature changes
   c. Reduce acidity
   d. Calcify the dentinal tubules

3. The test for a properly mixed zinc phosphate luting cement is
   a. Putty consistency
   b. Granular consistency
   c. Checking whether cement will break and form a drop at the end of the spatula
   d. Checking whether cement will hold a thin string, breaking when the spatula is raised an inch

4. Which cement should *not* be used for temporary cementation of crowns to be permanently cemented with resin cements?
   a. Zinc polycarboxylate
   b. Zinc phosphate
   c. Zinc oxide eugenol
   d. Any cement is appropriate

5. Which cement exhibits an exothermic reaction during mixing?
   a. Glass ionomer
   b. Zinc phosphate
   c. Resin cement
   d. Calcium hydroxide

6. Which dental cements use the bonding procedure before placement of the dental cement?
   a. Zinc phosphate and polycarboxylate
   b. Zinc oxide eugenol and glass ionomer
   c. Resin
   d. Calcium hydroxide and zinc oxide eugenol

7. When luting a crown, it is important to
   a. Have a film thickness that allows for complete seating
   b. Have a film thickness that provides proper insulation
   c. Have a film thickness for complete filling of the crown
   d. None of the above

8. Many cements should *not* be dispensed until ready to mix because of
   a. Dehydration from exposure to air
   b. Contamination from moisture in the air
   c. Materials coming in contact with each other
   d. All of the above

9. Which dental cement bonds to dentin, is "kind" to the pulp, and resists recurrent decay?
   a. Zinc oxide eugenol
   b. Polycarboxylate
   c. Calcium hydroxide
   d. Glass ionomer

10. Zinc phosphate cement is mixed over a large area of the glass slab to
    a. Help lengthen the working time
    b. Help neutralize the chemicals
    c. Help dissipate the exothermic reaction
    d. All of the above

11. Proper instrumentation at cement margins includes
    a. Avoiding gouging or ditching cement margins
    b. Using ultrasonic scalers to remove deposits on resin-based cement margins
    c. Use of air polishing on resin-based cement margins
    d. All are correct

12. Light-cured cements may be used for luting
    a. Non-metal orthodontic retainers
    b. Porcelain veneers less than 1.5 mm thick
    c. Porcelain or gold inlays
    d. A and B

13. Which cement should *not* be used under a composite restoration because of the oil content of the liquid?
    a. Zinc phosphate
    b. Glass ionomer
    c. Calcium hydroxide
    d. Zinc oxide eugenol

14. Adhesion is molecular attraction between materials with
    a. Similar molecules
    b. Dissimilar molecules
    c. Irregular surfaces
    d. None of the above

15. The latest generation of adhesive systems incorporates a
    a. 1-step system
    b. 2-step system
    c. 3-step system
    d. 4-step system

16. Newly mixed polycarboxylate cement should no longer be used for luting when
    a. the mix is shiny
    b. the mix flows readily
    c. the mix is creamy
    d. the mix is stringy or web-like

17. Adding resin to glass ionomer cement does all of the following except one. Which one?
    a. increases the fluoride release
    b. increased compressive strength
    c. decreases solubility
    d. increases tensile strength

18. Failure to remove all excess cement from subgingival margins may cause all of the following except one. Which one?
    a. aphthous ulcers
    b. periodontal infection

Get Ready for Exams!—cont'd

   c. bone loss
   d. recurrent caries
For answers to Review Questions, see the Appendix.

Case-Based Discussion Topics

1. A 22-year-old administrative assistant is scheduled for a gold crown preparation. She has been seen in your office previously for a crown and experienced some difficulty with sensitivity while the provisional crown was in place.
Which cement would be the best choice for luting the temporary crown, and why?

2. A 40-year-old accountant is scheduled for cementation of an all-ceramic crown on tooth #5. The provisional crown has been cemented with a noneugenol zinc oxide cement.

Why was this cement chosen for the provisional coverage, and which cement would be the best choice for the permanent crown?

3. A 9-year-old is scheduled for cementation of orthodontic bands.
Which cement would be the best choice, and why?

4. You are asked to mix a final luting cement and fill a crown with it in preparation for seating. Although the crown seated completely on try-in, when the dentist attempts to seat the cement-filled crown, the margins remain open and the crown is high.
What might be the explanation for this situation?

5. Your office is considering going to a premeasured cement system.
What situations can you foresee in which this system may be problematic?

BIBLIOGRAPHY

American Academy of Periodontology: Academy report: peri-implant mucositis and peri-implantitis: a current understanding of their diagnoses and clinical implication. *J Periodontol*, 84:436–443, 2013.

Anusavice KJ, Shen C, Rawls HR, editors: *Phillips' Science of Dental Materials (ed 12).*, Philadelphia, 2013, Saunders.

Baghani Z, Kadkhodazedeh M: Periodontal dressing: a review article. *J Dent Res Clin Dent Prospects Autum*, 7(4):183–191, 2013.

(No authors listed) Periodontal dressing. *J Integrated Dent August*, 1(1):1–12, 2012.

Cao Y, Bogen GB, Lim J, et al.: Bioceramic materials and the changing concepts in vital pulp therapy. *J Cal Dent Assoc*, 44(5):279–289, 2016.

Christensen G: Success with cements, self-etching primers. *Dental Products Report*, 64–68, 2001.

Fruits T, Coury T, Miranda F, et al.: Uses and properties of current glass ionomer cements: a review. *Gen Dent*, 44:410–415, 1996.

Gutkowski S: Minimal intervention: making it stick: cements in dental hygiene. *RDH Magazine*, 28:36–37, 2008.

Helpin M, Rosenberg H: Resin-modified glass ionomers in pediatric dentistry. *Practical Dental Hygiene*, 33–35, 1996.

Jeffries SR: Bioactive dental materials. *Inside Dentistry*, 12(2), 2016. https://www.aegisdentalnetwork.com/id/2016/02/bioactive-dental-materials.

Jivraj SA, Reshad M, Donovan T: Selecting luting agents. *Inside Dentistry*, 9(2), 2013.

Kathariya R, Jain H, Jadhav T: To pack or not to pack: the current status of periodontal dressing. *J Appl Biomater Funct Mater*, 13(2):e73–e86, 2015.

Kaufman L: Proper clean-up: removing excess/residual resin-based dental cement. *Dental Learning*, August 3, 2017. Available at http://www.dentallearning.net/proper-clean-removing-excessresidual-resin-based-dental-cement

Leinfelder KF: Should I change the type of cement I use? *J Am Dent Assoc* 130:1492, 1999.

Miller M: *Resin Cements and Resin Ionomers, (vol. 13).* Houston, 1999, REALITY Publishing. 505 to 544.

Notarantonio A: How to bond all-ceramic crowns [video]. *Dental Products Report*, May 2013. Available at http://www.dental-productsreport.com/dental/article/how-bond-all-ceramic-crowns-video.

Pameijer CH: A review of luting agents. *Int J Dent*, 2012:752861, 2012.

Powers JM, Sakaguchi RL, editors: *Craig's Restorative Dental Materials*, (ed 13)., St. Louis, 2012, Mosby.

Schmidt SJ: Temporary cements revisited. *Inside Dental Assisting*, 11(2), 2014. https://www.aegisdentalnetwork.com/ida/2014/04/Temporary-Cements-Revisited.

Slim L: Cement-associated peri-implantitis. *RDH Magazine*, 33(12), 2013. http://www.rdhmag.com/articles/print/volume-33/issue-12/columns/cement-associated-peri-implantitis.html.

Strassler HE, Morgan RJ: Cements for PFM and all-metal restorations, *Inside Dentistry* 9(11), 2013. https://www.aegisdentalnetwork.com/id/2013/11/cements-for-pfm-and-all-metal-restorations?page_id=297.

Strassler HE, Morgan RJ: Cements for today's all-ceramic materials, *Inside Dentistry* 9(12), 2013. https://www.aegisdentalnetwork.com/id/2013/12/cements-for-all-ceramic-materials.

Strassler HE, Morgan RJ: Provisional–temporary cements: techniques to facilitate placement of provisional restorations. *Inside Dental Assisting*, 8(4), 2012. https://www.aegisdentalnetwork.com/ida/2012/08/provisional-temporary-cements.

Chapter Objectives

Upon completion of this chapter, the student should be able to:

1. Describe the purpose of an impression.
2. Describe the three basic types of impressions.
3. Explain the importance of the key properties of impression materials.
4. Explain why alginate is an irreversible hydrocolloid.
5. List the supplies needed to make an alginate impression and explain how they are used.
6. Select trays for alginate impressions for a patient.
7. Mix alginate, load and seat the tray, and remove the set impression.
8. Evaluate upper and lower alginate impressions, in accordance with the criteria for acceptability.
9. Disinfect alginate impressions and prepare them for transport to the office laboratory.
10. Troubleshoot problems experienced with alginate impressions.
11. Compare similarities and differences among the physical and mechanical properties of polyvinyl siloxane (PVS) and polyether impression materials.
12. Discuss the advantages and disadvantages of using polyether impression material for a crown impression.
13. Explain the difference between a hydrophobic and a hydrophilic impression material.
14. Evaluate cord placement and gingival retraction for acceptability.
15. Use ferric sulfate astringent to control gingival bleeding before making an impression.
16. Make a registration of a patient's bite in centric occlusion.
17. Assemble the cartridge of impression material with mixing tip and load into the dispenser.
18. Explain what a digital impression is and how it is used.
19. Describe the advantages and disadvantages of digital impressions.
20. Disinfect PVS and polyether impressions and prepare them for transport to the dental laboratory.

Key Terms

Diagnostic Casts positive replicas of the teeth and surrounding oral tissues and structures produced from impressions that create a negative representation of the teeth; commonly called *study models* and used for diagnostic purposes and numerous chairside and laboratory procedures

Preliminary Impression an impression of the dentition or edentulous arch and surrounding tissues taken as a precursor to other treatment; often used to make casts (models) of oral structures for planning, and to construct custom trays or provisional restorations

Final Impression a detailed impression of oral structures used to make an accurate cast from which restorations or prostheses are made

Bite Registration an impression of the upper and lower teeth in the patient's normal bite relation

Dimensional Stability ability of a material to maintain its size and shape over a period of time

Accuracy ability of a material to adapt to and flow over the surfaces of the oral structures to record fine detail

Tear Resistance ability to avoid tearing when the material is in thin sections

Colloid glue-like material composed of two or more substances in which one substance does not go into solution but is suspended within another substance; it has at least two phases: a liquid phase called a *sol* and a semisolid phase called a *gel*

Hydrocolloid a water-based colloid used as an elastic impression material

Reversible Hydrocolloid an agar impression material that can be heated to change a gel into a fluid sol state that can flow around the teeth, and then cooled to gel again to make an impression of the shapes of the oral structures

Irreversible Hydrocolloid an alginate impression material that is mixed to a sol state and as it sets converts to a gel by a chemical reaction that irreversibly changes its nature

Agar a powder derived from seaweed that is a major component of reversible hydrocolloid

Sol liquid state in which colloidal particles are suspended; by cooling or a chemical reaction, it can change into a gel

Gel a semisolid state in which colloidal particles form a framework that traps liquid (e.g., Jell-O)

Alginate a versatile irreversible hydrocolloid that is the most used impression material in the dental office; it lacks the accuracy and fine surface detail needed for impressions for crown and bridge procedures

Elastomers highly accurate elastic impression materials that have qualities similar to rubber; they are used extensively in indirect restorative techniques, such as crown and bridge procedures

Imbibition the act of absorbing moisture

Surfactant a chemical that lowers the surface tension of a substance so that it is more readily wetted; for example, oil beads on the surface of water, but soap acts as a surfactant to allow the oil to spread over the surface

Polysulfide an elastic impression material that has sulfur-containing (mercaptan) functional groups; it has also been referred to as *rubber base impression material*

Condensation Silicone a silicone rubber impression material that sets by linking molecules in long chains but produces a liquid by-product by condensation

Addition Silicone a silicone rubber impression that also sets by linking molecules in long chains but produces no by-product; the most commonly used addition silicones are the polyvinyl siloxanes

Polyvinyl Siloxane (PVS) (Also Referred to as Vinyl Polysiloxane) very accurate addition silicone elastomer impression material; it is used extensively for crown and bridge procedures because of its accuracy, dimensional stability, and ease of use

Polyether a rubber impression material with ether functional groups; it has high accuracy and is popular for crown and bridge procedures

Astringent a chemical used in tissue management during gingival retraction to control bleeding and constrict tissues

Flash a common term for the cuff of impression material that extends apical to the margin of a crown preparation and represents an impression of the root or unprepared tooth

Digital Impression detailed digital images of the preparation, surrounding and opposing teeth, and tissues taken by a digital scanner for the purpose of making a restoration

Intraoral Scanner a type of camera that takes digital images (typically in continuous video form) of oral structures for CAD/CAM procedures, such as crown preparations.

In dentistry, an impression material is used primarily to reproduce the form of teeth, including existing restorations and preparations made for restorative treatments, as well as the form of the arches and other oral hard and soft tissues for removable prostheses. Impression materials are also used by maxillofacial prosthodontists to make molds of facial defects resulting from cancer and trauma, so that they can construct facial prostheses to restore facial form. Many different types of impression materials have been developed over the years, allowing the dentist to select materials according to the demands of the treatment and the oral environment. Participation in the making of impressions is one of the most frequently performed patient contact functions of the dental assistant and is performed increasingly by the dental hygienist. It is important that both have an understanding of the clinical applications, handling characteristics, physical properties, and limitations of these materials. They must also know proper techniques and materials for disinfecting the impressions. In some states, dental auxiliaries can be licensed in expanded functions that include making final impressions for crowns and bridges, implants, and partial denture procedures.

OVERVIEW OF IMPRESSIONS

Making impressions of oral structures is almost an everyday occurrence in a busy dental practice. Selection of the impression material will be influenced by what the impression will be used for. To replicate oral structures, the impression materials must be in a moldable or plastic state that can adapt to the teeth and tissues. Usually, the impression material in its plastic state is loaded into a tray for carrying it to the mouth and supporting it so that it does not slump and distort. Within a specified period of time, the impression material must set to a semisolid, elastic, or rigid state. Elastic

impression materials are used more extensively than rigid materials, because elastic materials flex from tissue undercuts when removed from the mouth, whereas rigid materials cannot. The completed impression forms a negative reproduction of the teeth and tissues. When plaster or stone is poured into the impression and hardened, the replica that is formed is a positive reproduction of the teeth and tissues (see Chapter 16 Gypsum and Wax Products). The replica is called a *cast* or *model*. In the initial diagnosis and treatment planning phase, the dentist may request that the dental assistant or hygienist make impressions of the teeth and surrounding structures, so that **diagnostic casts**, commonly called *study models*, can be made for further study when the patient is no longer present. When an impression is made of a tooth that has been prepared for a restoration, the replica of the prepared tooth is called a *die* and is used for fabrication of the restoration in the dental laboratory. Fig. 15.1 shows an impression

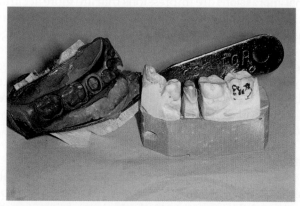

FIG. 15.1 A double-bite impression and the cast from the impression with a die of the crown preparation that can be removed by the technician to facilitate the creation of a wax pattern.

and the mold and die made from that impression. Use of the die allows the dentist or laboratory technician to perform the procedure by the indirect technique. With the indirect technique, the restoration is not made directly on the tooth, as with the direct placement of amalgam, but is constructed in the laboratory (indirectly) and later is cemented on the tooth.

TYPES OF IMPRESSIONS

Dental impressions can be categorized into three basic types based on how they will be used. These types include the following:
1. Preliminary impressions
2. Final impressions
3. Bite registration (occlusal) impressions

While the dentist has a wide variety of materials to choose from to make these impressions, in the modern practice the choice will likely be alginate, silicone rubber (polyvinyl siloxane), or polyether. It is possible that no impression material will be used; instead, a digital image of the oral structures may be used. Digital impressions are discussed separately (see "Digital Impressions," below).

Preliminary Impressions

Preliminary impressions, as the name implies, are made as a precursor to another treatment. Casts made from them are often used for planning purposes such as for diagnostic casts (study models). Preliminary impressions may be used to make working casts from which custom trays or provisional (temporary) restorations can be made or to create casts for pre- and post-treatment records. On occasion, what starts out to be a preliminary impression can also be used as the final impression. For example, a cast made from an alginate impression to design a removable orthodontic appliance may be accurate enough to send to the laboratory for fabrication of the appliance. Alginate is a useful, inexpensive material that is excellent for preliminary impressions but lacks the detail and accuracy to be used for a crown impression.

Final impressions

Final impressions are impressions that are more accurate in their replication of the oral structures. To provide a good fit and marginal integrity for a crown, bridge, or implant a very detailed and accurate impression of the preparation and surrounding structures is needed. A detailed replication of the oral tissues is needed to fabricate well-fitting partial and complete dentures as well. Polyvinyl siloxane and polyether are the two most commonly used materials for final impressions.

Bite registration

A replication of the patient's bite is needed to establish the proper relation between a restoration or prosthesis and the opposing teeth. An impression is made that captures this relationship (see Procedure 15.4), so that it can be used in the office or sent to the dental laboratory where the restoration will be fabricated. **Bite registrations** are also used to help mount diagnostic casts in their proper relationship on an articulator. Although wax has been used for bite registration for decades (see Procedure 15.5), polyvinyl siloxane is currently more popular for this purpose. A wax bite registration is easily distorted.

TYPES OF IMPRESSION MATERIALS

Impression materials can be categorized into two major groups:
1. Elastic materials
2. Inelastic materials

Elastic impression materials include the hydrocolloids (agar and alginate), polysulfides, silicone rubber materials (condensation and addition; e.g., polyvinyl siloxane), polyethers, and a hybrid of polyether and polyvinyl siloxane. Of the elastic materials agar hydrocolloids, polysulfides, and condensation silicone rubbers are not used much anymore. Alginate, polyvinyl siloxane (PVS), and polyether are the most commonly used elastic impression materials. Alginate is used extensively for preliminary impression whereas PVS and polyether are used primarily for final impressions.

Inelastic materials are the older impression materials and include dental compound, impression plaster, zinc oxide eugenol, and impression wax. Because of the superior properties of the elastic materials, inelastic materials are seldom used in dentistry today (although some dentists still use stick compound for border molding custom trays for denture impressions).

Key Properties

Although impression materials must have a degree of strength, their key properties are as follows:

Accuracy: When the impression is made the impression material must closely adapt to and flow over the surface of the tooth preparation and tissues to record the minute details in order to be accurate. The material will tend to flow if it has low viscosity and there is pressure on the material as the tray is seated.

Tear resistance: After the impression material sets, it must have good tear resistance to prevent tearing during removal from the mouth. With a crown impression the material in the gingival sulcus is very thin and would tear if the tear resistance was poor.

Dimensional stability: After the impression is removed, the set material must remain dimensionally stable; otherwise, casts and dies poured from it would be inaccurate.

IMPRESSION TRAYS

Impression trays are used to carry the impression material to the mouth and to support it until it sets, is removed from the mouth, and is poured into dental plaster or stone. Trays should be rigid to prevent distortion of the impression. They can be made for arches with teeth or for edentulous ridges.

STOCK TRAYS

Impression trays can be pre-manufactured trays, called *stock trays,* which are purchased in a variety of sizes (small, medium, large, and extra large) for both adults and children (Fig. 15.2). Stock trays can be metal or plastic, and each of these can be solid or perforated. Perforated trays have holes in their sides and bottom to help retain impression material as it extrudes through the holes and locks into place. Solid trays often have raised borders on the internal surfaces that help lock in the impression material. These are called "rim-lock" trays.

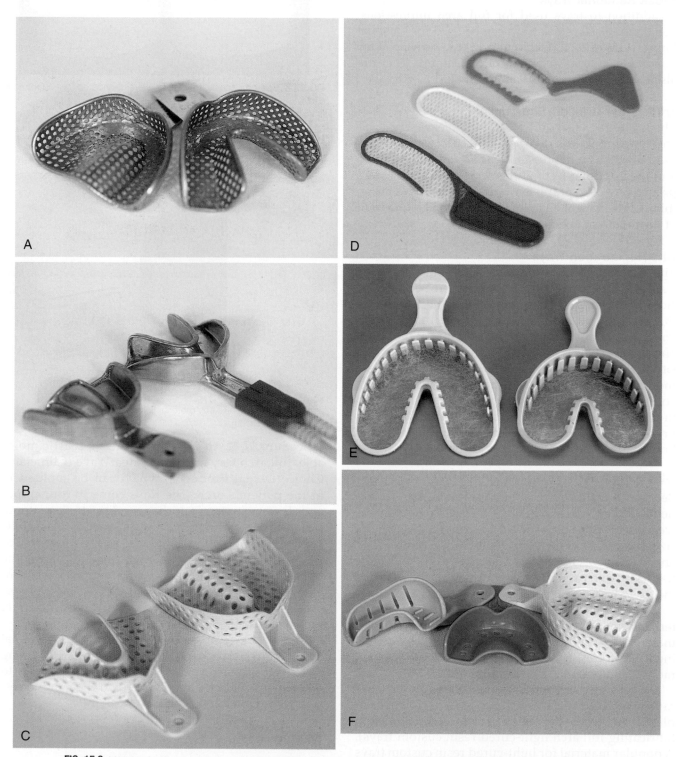

FIG. 15.2 Variety of metal and plastic stock impression trays. **A,** Full arch metal perforated trays. **B,** Rim-lock metal tray with option for water cooling (tray on the right has water hose attached). **C,** Disposable plastic perforated trays. **D,** Bite registration trays. **E,** Triple trays take impression of prepared teeth, opposing teeth, and bite. **F,** Quadrant (*left*), anterior section (*middle*), and full arch (*right*) trays. (From Bird DL, Robinson DS: *Modern Dental Assisting* (ed 11). Philadelphia, 2015, Elsevier.)

Impression materials used in solid trays require the application of an adhesive to further retain them and prevent distortion of the impression if they should partially pull out of the tray. Plastic trays are inexpensive and disposable, whereas metal trays are more expensive and must be cleaned and sterilized between uses.

Stock Sectional Trays

In addition to trays used for full arch impressions, metal and plastic stock trays can be used for sectional impressions as well. Sectional trays can be shaped for quadrants, anterior segments or half-mouth. They are also used for bite registration impressions.

Triple Trays (Closed-Bite Trays)

The triple tray (also called *closed-bite, double-bite, dual-arch,* or *check-bite tray*) is a stock sectional tray that is used to make an impression of the teeth being treated and the opposing teeth at the same time and, if used properly, will capture the correct centric occlusion (bite) of the patient. Quadrant trays will fit a quadrant of the mouth or one-half of an arch.

Bite Registration Trays

Bite registration trays are typically U-shaped plastic frames with a thin fiber mesh stretched between the sides of the frame. The mesh retains the impression material (called *bite registration material*) and is thin enough so as not to interfere with closure of the upper and lower teeth in proper bite relationship. Bite registration material is placed on both sides of the mesh, the frame is positioned over the teeth to be recorded, and the patient closes into the normal bite relationship until the material sets (see Figs. 15.67 through 15.70 in Procedure 15.4). They can encompass a full arch or be limited to a quadrant or anterior section.

CUSTOM TRAYS

Because of the wide variation in size and shape of patients' arches, stock trays may not fit some patients well. Ideally, the tray should conform to the length, size, and height of the arch, depth of the palatal vault, and position of the teeth. To get the best fit it may be necessary to custom make the tray to fit the patient's mouth (Fig. 15.3).

Custom trays used with elastomeric impression materials provide a uniform thickness of the impression material producing dimensional stability and reducing inaccuracies. The result is highly accurate working models and ultimately, well-fitting restorations.

Custom trays are usually constructed in the laboratory with chemical-cured, light-cured, or thermoplastic resins (see Procedure 15.1 for information on fabricating full arch light-cured resin custom trays). A popular material for light-cured resin custom trays is Triad VLC Tray Material, Dentsply Sirona (Fig. 15.4). The technique for fabricating custom chemical-cured acrylic trays is presented in Chapter 17,

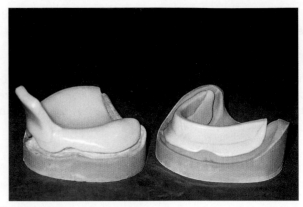

FIG 15.3 Custom acrylic trays that were fabricated on edentulous casts.

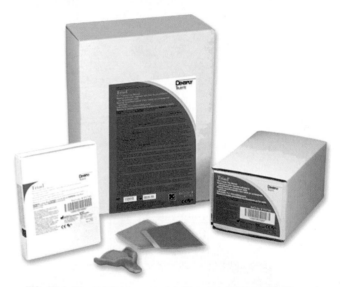

FIG. 15.4 Triad VLC tray material. (Courtesy of Dentsply Sirona.)

Procedure 17-1. An example of thermoplastic moldable, full arch tray material is HeatWave (Clinician's Choice Dental Products), which can be molded to fit the patient's arch. The trays come in four upper and lower anatomical shapes. The tray material softens after 1 minute in a water bath that is 71 °C (160 °F) and can be adapted to an existing cast or shaped by hand to fit the patient's arch. Molding the tray will adapt better, providing many of the benefits of a chemical- and light-cured custom tray; use less impression material; and provide more accurate impressions.

Custom trays can be made for full arch or sectional impressions. A stock tray can be customized by lining it with a putty impression material that is adapted to the dental arch of the individual, and then an impression is made in this customized stock tray.

HYDROCOLLOIDS

A **colloid** is a glue-like material composed of two or more substances in which one substance does not go into solution but is suspended within another substance. **Hydrocolloids** are water-based colloids that function as elastic impression materials. The two hydrocolloids used in dentistry are agar hydrocolloid (or **reversible hydrocolloid**) and alginate hydrocolloid (or **irreversible hydrocolloid**). Much like gelatin, when **agar** powder is mixed with water, it forms a glue-like suspension that entraps the water, making a colloidal suspension called a **sol**. Heating it will disperse the agar in the water faster. When the agar sol is chilled, it will **gel**, becoming semisolid or jelly-like (like Jell-O). When the agar gel is heated, it will reverse its state back into a liquid suspension (sol). Therefore it is a reversible hydrocolloid. Alginate powder will also form a sol that gels. However, with alginate, a chemical reaction occurs that prevents it from reversing back to a gel when heated. Therefore it is an irreversible hydrocolloid.

REVERSIBLE HYDROCOLLOID (AGAR)

Reversible hydrocolloid was introduced into dentistry in 1925 and was the first elastic material to gain popularity. It overcame many of the problems with inelastic materials (see the section "Inelastic Impression Materials,") in that it could take accurate impressions of teeth and arches with tissue undercuts and could be removed from the mouth without injuring the patient or breaking. Its main clinical use is for impressions of operative and crown and bridge procedures. It also has uses in the laboratory for the duplication of casts (models). Its use has declined over the years as elastic (rubber) impression materials have been introduced. Detailed information about reversible (agar) hydrocolloid can be found on the Evolve website at www.evolve.elsevier.com/Hatrick/materials.

IRREVERSIBLE HYDROCOLLOID (ALGINATE)

Alginate, also called *alginate hydrocolloid* or *irreversible hydrocolloid,* is by far the most widely used impression material. It is inexpensive, easy to manipulate, requires no special equipment, and is reasonably accurate for many dental procedures. Alginate is used for making impressions for diagnostic casts, partial denture frameworks, and repairs of broken partial or complete dentures, as well as for fabrication of provisional restorations, fluoride and bleaching trays, sports protectors, preliminary impressions for edentulous arches, removable orthodontic appliances, and a multitude of other uses. However, it is not accurate enough for the final impressions for inlay, onlay, crown, and bridge preparations. It does not capture the fine detail of the preparation needed for a precise fit of such restorations. Also, it is thick and does not flow well into embrasures or occlusal surfaces. Final impressions are made with more accurate materials such as one of the elastomers (polyvinyl siloxane or polyether). Final impressions are used to make detailed replicas of the prepared teeth from which precisely fitting restorations will be made.

Common Uses of Alginate Impressions

- Diagnostic casts (study models)
- Preliminary impressions for complete dentures
- Partial denture frameworks
- Opposing casts for crown and bridge treatments
- Repairs of partial and complete dentures
- Provisional (temporary) restorations
- Custom trays for home-use fluoride or bleaching
- Sports protectors and night guards
- Removable orthodontic appliances

Composition and setting reaction. The main active ingredient in alginate is potassium or sodium alginate, which makes up 15% to 20% of the powder. Proportions of ingredients vary from manufacturer to manufacturer and with fast-, regular-, and slow-set materials. It is produced from derivatives of seaweed. See Table 15.1 for the components of alginate and their functions. The "dustless" alginate powders have organic glycols or glycerin added to keep powder from becoming airborne when it is dispensed. The dust contains silica particles, and they are a potential health hazard if inhaled.

When alginate powder is mixed with water, calcium sulfate dihydrate reacts with sodium alginate to form calcium alginate. Calcium alginate is insoluble and causes the sol of mixed powder and water to gel. Because this occurs by a chemical reaction, it cannot be reversed back to the sol state as can agar hydrocolloid. It is a fairly rapid chemical reaction, so trisodium phosphate is added as a retarder to delay the reaction. The amount of retarder that is added will control the time of the set and will differentiate between fast- and regular-set alginates. Diatomaceous earth is added as a filler to increase stiffness and strength and to prevent the surface from being sticky. Potassium sulfate is added to keep the alginate from interfering with the set of the gypsum products used to pour the impression. Some manufacturers have added chemicals to the alginate that change color as the chemical reaction progresses to indicate when it is time to insert the impression, and the color changes again when it is time to remove the impression.

Working time. Regular-set alginates have a working time (from start of mix to seating in the mouth) of 2 to 3 minutes, and fast-set alginate has a working time of 1.25 to 2 minutes (American Dental Association [ADA] specification no. 18 sets the minimum at 1.25 minutes). The longer the time used to mix the alginate, the faster it must be loaded into the tray and seated in the mouth.

Setting time. Regular-set alginates set in 2 to 5 minutes, and fast-set alginates set in 1 to 2 minutes. Setting time

TABLE 15.1	Composition of Alginate Impression Material	
MATERIAL	**PERCENTAGE (APPROXIMATE)**	**PURPOSE**
Sodium or potassium alginate	15%-20%	Colloidal particles as basis of the gel
Calcium sulfate dihydrate	14%-20%	Creates irreversible gel with alginate
Potassium sulfate	10%	Ensures set of gypsum materials
Trisodium phosphate	2%	Retarder to control setting time
Diatomaceous earth	55%-60%	Filler to increase thickness and strength
Other additives:	Very small quantities	
• Organic glycols • Flavoring agents • Coloring agents • Disinfectants		To reduce dust when powder is handled To improve taste of material To provide pleasant colors To cause antibacterial action

can be lengthened by using cold water or shortened by using warm water. Adjusting the powder-to-water ratio can affect the set but also adversely affects the physical and mechanical properties and therefore is not recommended. It is advisable to leave the impression in the mouth for an additional minute after it appears set, because the tear strength and the ability to rebound from undercuts without permanent deformation increase during this time.

Clinical Tip

For patients with sensitive teeth, alginate mixed with cool water can be painful. Use regular-set alginate with warm water. The working and setting times will be shortened, but the patient will be more comfortable.

Important Properties of Alginate

Permanent deformation. Alginate will be compressed when it is removed from undercuts in the mouth. The greater the compression, the more likely it is that the alginate will be permanently deformed to some degree. A certain thickness of alginate (2 to 4 mm) is needed between the impression tray and the teeth or tissue undercut; alginate that is too thin will deform more and will tear more easily. As with reversible hydrocolloid, when an alginate impression is removed it should be done with a rapid "snap" to prevent the deformation of critical surfaces. If 8 to 10 minutes are allowed to elapse from the time an alginate impression is removed from the mouth until pouring the model, some recovery or rebound will occur from the deformation. That deformation which does not recover is the *permanent deformation,* and it will be recorded in the poured gypsum cast as a distortion. As long as the distortion is small, it may not be clinically significant. Usually, the time needed for disinfecting the impression is at least 10 minutes, and most of the rebound will have occurred by then.

Dimensional stability. Alginate is very sensitive to moisture loss and will shrink as a result. Once the impression is removed from the mouth, it should be rinsed and

disinfected (Procedure 15.6), wrapped in a damp (not dripping wet) paper towel, and sealed in a zippered plastic bag. (An alternative to wrapping in a damp paper towel would be to put a few drops of water in the plastic bag. Alginate could imbibe water from a towel that is very wet and swell.) Enclosing the impression this way will create an environment with 100% humidity to minimize water loss from the alginate. Some moisture will be lost from the impression even in 100% humidity from syneresis. Syneresis occurs with many gels that are left standing, whereby they contract and some of the liquid is squeezed out of the gel, forming a wet film on the surface. This loss of water changes the properties of the material. Ideally, the impression is poured after it is disinfected. If the impression must be stored until it can be poured a few hours later, then it must be kept at 100% humidity (as with the zippered plastic bag and a few drops of water). The longer that pouring is delayed, the more likely that some distortion will occur in the alginate.

Tear strength. The tear strength of alginate is more important than its compressive strength because most commercial alginates far exceed the minimal allowable value for compressive strength. Alginate mixed with too much water will be weaker and more likely to tear on removal from the mouth. Thin sections of alginate are also prone to tearing. In addition, slow removal of the alginate from the mouth will contribute to tearing. If the impression can be left in the mouth for an additional minute beyond the point when it is set, it will increase in tear strength. When properly handled, alginate has adequate tear strength for most purposes for which it is used. Some alginates have silicone polymers added to increase the strength.

MAKING ALGINATE IMPRESSIONS

Objective

The objective of impression making is to reproduce the oral structures with acceptable accuracy while practicing good infection control and maintaining patient comfort. The dental assistant and the dental hygienist can make alginate impressions. They will need to prepare the patient for the impressions and to dispense, mix, and load alginate into trays. After removal of the impression, the assistant or the hygienist disinfects and properly handles the impression until it is poured with the appropriate gypsum material. She also may be responsible for clearing residual alginate from the mouth and face of the patient.

Tray Selection

Stock trays work well with alginate because they provide plenty of room for an adequate thickness of alginate. Alginate must be tightly adapted to the tray to be accurate. If the alginate pulls loose from the tray, a distortion will occur. If a tray is set on the bench top, unsupported alginate extending from the back of the tray may lift a portion of the impression and dislodge it from the tray. A perforated tray can be used because the alginate oozes through the perforations and locks into place. A solid tray can also be used if an adhesive made for alginate (e.g., TAC, Bosworth) is applied to the inside of the tray before the alginate is loaded. Solid rim-lock trays should also have adhesive applied because alginate will occasionally pull free from the rim-lock on removal of the impression. If disposable plastic trays are used, they should be rigid. Flexible plastic trays have the potential to distort under the weight of the wet gypsum during pouring or when used in areas of undercuts in the mouth.

A properly selected full arch tray will cover all of the teeth and will extend into the facial and lingual vestibules without impinging on the tissues. It will extend posteriorly to include the retromolar area for a mandibular tray and the hamular notch area for a maxillary tray. It will be deep enough to provide at least 2 mm of space for alginate beyond the incisal and occlusal surfaces of the teeth and wide enough to allow approximately 5 mm of alginate between the sides of the tray and the tissues. On occasion, standard stock trays will not cover all of the desired areas for the impression and must be modified with utility wax to create appropriate extensions of the tray and support the alginate. A common area for this to occur is the third molar area of an individual with large jaws. Wax may also be added to the mid-palatal area of the tray to support the alginate when the patient has a very deep palatal vault (see Fig. 15.52, Procedure 15.2). Usually, the patient is asked to rinse the mouth to remove loose debris and thick saliva before the impression is made. An antimicrobial rinse may be used to reduce the number of oral pathogens.

Dispensing

Manufacturers supply measures for powder and water for their alginates. Use the appropriate ones and adhere to the recommended proportions of powder and water to maintain the desired physical properties

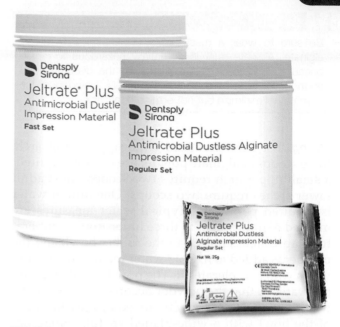

FIG. 15.5 Alginate packaged in bulk in a plastic drum or premeasured packets equivalent to two scoops with many manufacturers. (Courtesy of Dentsply Sirona.)

of the alginate. Powder measures (also called *scoops*) will vary among manufacturers, so do not interchange them with other manufacturers' scoops. The same principle applies to water measures.

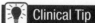 **Clinical Tip**

Water and powder measures can vary in size among manufacturers. If your office uses more than one brand of alginate, color-code the measures so they are not intermixed.

During shipping or prolonged periods of sitting, the powder may pack tightly and some of the ingredients may settle out, so that they are not evenly distributed throughout the powder. Because of the compacting of powder particles, the amount of powder scooped will be greater than the manufacturer intended when developing the measuring scoop. When the compacted powder is incorporated into the recommended volume of water, the resulting mix will be too thick and will often set too rapidly. To prevent this from happening, containers of alginate such as cans or plastic containers should be turned end-over-end a few times to decompress (fluff) the powder and mix the ingredients. Some alginates are supplied in premeasured, watertight packages with a quantity suitable for a medium-sized arch (equivalent to two scoops with most manufacturers) (Fig. 15.5). This packaging is more expensive, but some practitioners find it to be convenient, to provide a more consistent mix, and to minimize cross-contamination.

> ⚠️ **Caution**
>
> Be sure to wear a mask while dispensing and mixing alginate. Alginate dust is potentially hazardous to inhale because it contains silicon dioxide in the diatomaceous earth fillers, as well as other chemicals. Using dustless alginate will minimize but not eliminate this risk.

Mixing. For a moderate to large upper adult arch, three scoops of alginate powder are usually required; a small upper arch requires two scoops. Most adult lower arches require two scoops. One unit of water is required per scoop. Typical water measures are marked to indicate up to three units. Room temperature tap water is placed in the rubber bowl, and the powder is added to it. Cold water retards the set, and warm water accelerates it. The powder is stirred into the water so that the powder becomes wet. Next, the wet powder is aggressively mixed against the sides of the bowl with a wide-bladed spatula. Some operators prefer to rotate the bowl in one hand while mixing with the other. Some offices use mechanical mixing machines for rapid mixing, ease of use, and a consistent mix (Fig. 15.6). The rubber bowl is attached to the mechanical mixer that spins the bowl. With both mechanical and hand-mixing, the water-powder mixture is forced against the sides of the bowl to further incorporate the powder into the water and to force out entrapped air. Mixing should be completed within 45 seconds for regular-set alginate and within 30 seconds for fast-set alginate. The completed mix should have a creamy consistency (see Fig. 15.6, C). If it appears grainy, it has not been mixed thoroughly.

Loading the tray. Mixed alginate is picked up on the spatula and pushed into the depth of the tray. This action forces out air, thus preventing large voids in the impression. The alginate should be loaded in large increments as quickly as possible. Using a small number of large increments reduces the chance for entrapped air. The tray should be loaded

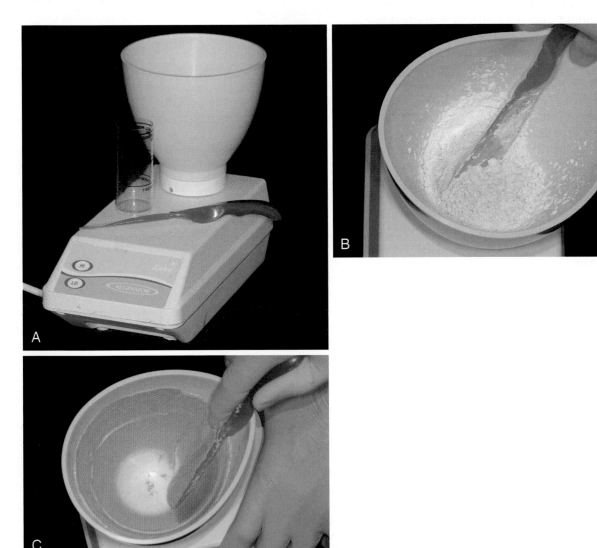

FIG. 15.6 Mechanical mixer used to mix alginate for an impression A. Mechanical mixer with water measure and spatula B. After water is added to the powder in the bowl, a spatula is used to wet all of the powder C. Spatula presses the wet powder against the rotating bowl until a smooth, creamy mixture is achieved (From Powers JM, Wataha JC: *Dental Materials: Properties and Manipulation* (ed 11). St. Louis, 2017, Elsevier.)

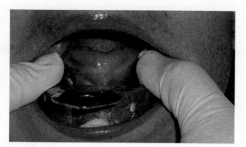

FIG. 15.7 Mandibular tray seated and patient has lifted the tongue to allow alginate to flow into the lingual vestibule and to shape the lingual frenum attachment. (Courtesy of Gwen Essex.)

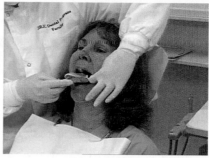

FIG. 15.8 To place the maxillary impression the right-handed operator stands in the 11 o'clock position (1 o'clock position for left-hander) and retracts the right corner of the mouth with the side of the tray while retracting the left corner of the mouth with the mirror or index finger of the other hand. (From Robinson DS, Bird DL: *Essentials of Dental Assisting* (ed 6). St. Louis, 2017, Elsevier.)

until the alginate is even with the top of the sides of the tray. A wet, gloved finger is used to smooth the surface of the alginate and to create a shallow trough over the ridge area of the alginate (see Fig. 15.54 in Procedure 15.2) that reduces the chance for entrapped air and helps to orient the tray over the teeth when it is seated.

Seating the tray. Once the tray is loaded, the operator should take some alginate from the bowl on the gloved index finger and wipe it on the occlusal surfaces and embrasures of the teeth to force air out from the occlusal grooves and embrasure spaces. If regular-set alginate has a 2-minute working time and the alginate was mixed for 45 seconds, the operator has 75 seconds to load the tray, wipe the alginate on the teeth, and seat the tray. For fast-set alginate, the operator has about 45 seconds for the same process after mixing for 30 seconds. On warm days, the tap water may be warmer than usual and may accelerate the set. Conversely, on cold days, cooler tap water may retard the set.

For the lower impression, the operator is usually standing in front of the patient to one side at approximately the 7 o'clock position for right-handers and 5 o'clock for left-handers. The right side of the tray is used to retract the left corner of the mouth, and a finger or mouth mirror retracts the right corner (opposite sides for left-handers) (see Fig. 15.55 in Procedure 15.2). The tray is rotated into the mouth, aligned over the teeth with the tray handle in the midline, and seated in the posterior first. The tray is then seated in the anterior, and as it is being seated over the incisors, the lower lip is pulled out of the way to allow alginate to flow into the anterior vestibule. The patient is asked to lift the tongue to the roof of the mouth momentarily and then to relax it (Fig. 15.7). This tongue motion allows alginate to flow into the lingual vestibule and defines the lingual frenum attachment. The tray is stabilized by the index and middle fingers of the right (or left) hand over the right and left sides of the arch.

The procedure is similar for the upper arch with the following modifications. A right-handed operator stands just behind the patient at the 11 o'clock position and retracts the right corner of the mouth with the side of the tray while retracting the left corner of the mouth with the mirror or index finger of the other hand (Fig. 15.8). Left-handed operators should reverse

the positions and stand at the 1 o'clock position, retract the left corner of the mouth with the side of the tray and retract the right corner of the mouth with a mirror or index finger of the other hand. The tray is rotated into position, aligned over the teeth, centered with the midline, seated in the posterior first, and gently seated toward the anterior to allow alginate to flow forward and not back into the palate. Trays can also be placed while the patient is in the supine position. A right-handed operator can seat the lower tray from the 8 o'clock position and the upper tray from the 11 or 12 o'clock position, and left-handed operators from comparable positions on the opposite side (4 o'clock for lower and 12 or 1 o'clock for upper). The patient should be seated upright after the tray is placed to minimize the collection of saliva and alginate at the back of the throat. For both upper and lower impressions, the posterior aspect of the tray should be inspected for proper seating and for excess alginate. Excess alginate should be swept away quickly with the mouth mirror or a cotton swab to prevent a gagging or breathing problem for the patient.

Clinical Tip

Controlling the gag reflex:
1. Place topical anesthetic on a cotton swab, and put it on the back of the tongue for 1 to 2 minutes, or spray the back of the mouth with topical anesthetic spray.
2. Place utility wax on the posterior extent of the upper tray to help contain the material.
3. Use fast-set alginate. Accelerate the set with warm water, if you can work fast enough to load and seat the tray.
4. Properly proportion the water and powder so that the mix is not too runny.
5. Do not overfill the tray.
6. Seat the tray in the posterior first, then anterior. Look at the palatal area and clear excess material with a quick sweep of the mouth mirror.
7. Position the patient's head forward slightly so that saliva will not pool in the back of the throat, and use a saliva ejector to keep the mouth clear.
8. Use distraction (e.g., have the patient lift one leg during the impression and hold it up, and breathe slowly and deeply through the nose).

Removing the tray. Alginate left in the mixing bowl can be checked for completeness of set. The impression should be left in the mouth for approximately 1 minute after the set, because it gains in tear strength during this time. This may not be possible with patients who gag easily. When you are ready to remove the tray, use a finger at the top of the side of the tray to apply pressure to break the seal while pulling the tray quickly away from the teeth with a snap. Protect the teeth in the opposing arch with fingers placed on top of the tray.

Handling the impression. The impression should be rinsed thoroughly under running water to remove adherent saliva. Next, it should be evaluated to determine whether the impression is acceptable for its anticipated use. If determined to be acceptable, the impression is held inside a plastic bag (to prevent the inhalation of disinfectant spray) and sprayed with a suitable disinfecting solution. An alternative to spraying the impression is to immerse it for 10 minutes in a suitable disinfectant. Immersion for up to 30 minutes in 1% sodium hypochlorite or 2% glutaraldehyde has been shown not to significantly affect the dimensions (by swelling) or surface detail of alginate.

A laboratory knife is used to remove excess, unsupported alginate from the back of the tray. Any pooled fluid is drained or shaken off because the alginate can imbibe moisture and swell. It is placed into a zippered plastic bag labeled with the patient's name with a few drops of water or a damp paper towel until ready to pour (Fig. 15.59, Procedure 15.2). Ideally, the impression should be poured within an hour, because it is not dimensionally stable.

CRITERIA FOR CLINICALLY ACCEPTABLE ALGINATE IMPRESSIONS

Alginate impressions should be evaluated immediately after they are removed from the mouth and rinsed. The determination should be made at this point as to whether or not the impression should be repeated, so it can be done while the patient is still seated and the operatory is set up for it. An acceptable impression will cover all areas of interest (teeth, ridge form, muscle attachments, palate, etc.). The structures should be recorded with sufficient detail to be clearly identified and should not have a grainy surface, which is usually the result of inadequate mixing. There should be minimal voids caused by entrapped air, especially in areas critical to the use of the impression (e.g., occlusal surfaces if a night guard will be made). The alginate should be fully seated in the tray and should not have pulled free or distorted (Fig. 15.9). The impression should be free of debris. Table 15.2 lists criteria used to assess an alginate impression for clinical acceptability. When problems are found with an impression, refer to Table 15.3 for a troubleshooting guide that suggests possible causes and solutions for a variety of problems.

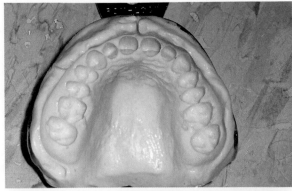
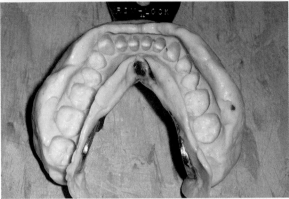

FIG. 15.9 Acceptable upper and lower alginate impressions that have met the established criteria. (Courtesy Dr. Steve Eakle.)

TWO-CONSISTENCY ALGINATE SYSTEM

A relatively new development with alginate is a two-consistency system (AccuDent XD, Ivoclar Vivadent). Compatible alginates with two different viscosities are used together to make impressions with improved accuracy and surface detail. This combination is particularly useful for complete and partial denture impressions. The light-bodied gel flows well from the large diameter tip of the delivery syringe but does not slump. It is placed into the peripheral vestibule of the upper or lower arch and acts as a border molding material. The thick tray gel completes the impression of the remainder of the arch while supporting the syringe gel (Fig. 15.10). The two materials meld together without seams. The tray material resists flowing and is more likely to stay in the tray and out of the patient's throat avoiding the gag reflex in many patients.

The two materials come in premeasured packaging and they are fast setting. However, the syringe material has a slightly longer setting time to allow it to be mixed first, loaded into the syringe and put aside while the tray materials is mixed and loaded into the tray. The tray material undergoes a color change to indicate when setting has started.

ELASTOMERS

Elastomers are highly accurate elastic impression materials that have qualities similar to rubber and hence are often called *rubber materials*. They are used extensively in restorative dentistry for fabrication of metal

TABLE 15.2	Criteria for an Acceptable Alginate Impression

Both Maxillary and Mandibular Impressions

All teeth and alveolar processes recorded
Peripheral roll and frenums included
No large voids and few small bubbles present
Good reproduction of detail
Free of debris
No distortion
Alginate firmly attached to tray

Maxillary Impression

Palatal vault recorded
Hamular notch area included

Mandibular Impression

Retromolar areas included
Lingual extensions recorded

castings, ceramic restorations, bridges, implant restorations, partial denture frameworks, and complete dentures. The four types of elastomers are as follows:

- Polysulfides
- Condensation silicones
- Addition silicones (polyvinyl siloxane)
- Polyethers

The two most widely used elastomers are polyvinyl siloxane (PVS) and polyether. More recently a hybrid material, vinyl polyether, has been introduced that combines the best properties of polyethers and polyvinyl siloxane. The elastomers share a general formulation that includes a flexible matrix which contains filler to reduce the effects during setting that polymerization shrinkage has on dimensional stability and accuracy. They also have in common a polymerization reaction that involves formation of long-chain polymers and

TABLE 15.3 Troubleshooting Alginate Impressions

PROBLEM	CAUSE	SOLUTION
Premature set	Too much powder in mix Prolonged mixing/loading time Water or room too warm	Fluff powder in container; use correct measures for powder and water Use timer to gauge working time Use cool water to slow the set
Slow set	Water too cold Too much water	Use warmer water Use correct water/powder measures
Grainy, lack of surface detail	Incomplete mix of powder and water	Wet all of powder, and mix to creamy consistency
Incomplete coverage of teeth or tissues	Tray too small or too short for arch Tray incompletely seated	Select larger tray or extend borders with rope wax Use a mouth mirror to check for complete seating of the tray
Voids on occlusal surfaces	Trapped air when tray is seated	Wipe alginate on occlusal surfaces before seating tray
Large voids at vestibule or midpalate	Trapped air Not enough alginate in tray Improper seating of tray Lip in the way	Place alginate in vestibule or palate before seating tray Use adequate amount of alginate Seat tray in posterior first, allow alginate to flow forward into vestibule, seat tray in anterior Pull lip out to create room for alginate
Small voids throughout	Air trapped in mix during spatulation	Press alginate against sides of bowl when mixing with wide-blade spatula to force out air
Distortion or double imprint	Impression removed too soon Tray moved while alginate was setting	Check residual alginate in bowl for set; let stand an additional 1 minute Hold the tray steady until set; do not have patient hold the tray
Torn alginate	Impression removed too slowly Thin mix	Remove impression quickly with a snap Use proper proportions of water and powder
Excess alginate at back of tray	Tray seated in anterior first, then posterior, forcing alginate out the back Tray overfilled with alginate	Seat tray in posterior first, forcing alginate anteriorly Load tray level with sides Create shallow trough for teeth Remove excess alginate from the back of the tray

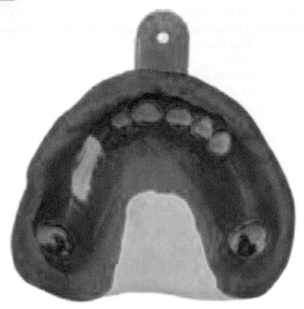

FIG. 15.10 Maxillary impression with the two consistency alginate system for a partial denture framework. The syringe material (orange) has been used to establish the peripheral borders and to capture an imprint of the rest seats for the framework. (AccuDent XD, Courtesy of Ivoclar Vivadent.)

cross-linking of chains. Because they are not water based, they are not as sensitive as the hydrocolloids to water loss or **imbibition** (water uptake). The shelf life is typically 12 to 18 months. Storage of these materials in a refrigerator will lengthen the shelf life. Stored materials should be allowed to return to room temperature before use unless an extended working time is needed.

USE OF ADHESIVE

The rubbery nature of elastomers means that they do not adhere well to solid metal or custom acrylic impression trays. An adhesive is placed in the tray to prevent the set material from separating from the tray and causing distortion (Fig. 15.11). Each type of elastomer has its own adhesive with which it is compatible; therefore adhesives should not be interchanged among different types of materials. The tray adhesive should be applied in a thin layer and allowed to dry. If the adhesive is not applied well in advance of use of the tray, then a stream of air can be used to accelerate the drying process.

ELASTIC RECOVERY

Because of their rubbery nature, elastomers have a certain amount of elastic recovery, or "rebound," from deformation. Rebound reduces distortion in the cast that is poured from the impression. PVS impression material has the best elastic recovery of the elastomers.

WETTABILITY

Elastomers generally are not wet well by water (and are therefore called *hydrophobic*), because water forms a high contact angle with them (see Fig. 5.2 in Chapter 5 Principles of Bonding). In other words, water beads on their surface much like raindrops on a newly waxed car. Of the elastomers, the polyethers are the most hydrophilic, or wettable. Wettability can be seen clinically

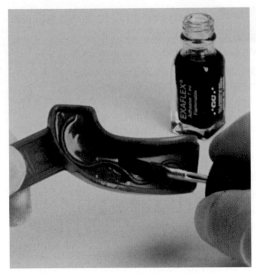

FIG. 15.11 Adhesive is applied to the interior of the tray to aid in retaining the elastomeric impression material. (From Rosenstiel SF, Land MF, Fujimoto J: *Contemporary Fixed Prosthodontics* (ed 4). St Louis, 2006, Elsevier.)

when impression materials are able to capture the detail of a tooth preparation when the surface is moist (but not submerged in water or saliva). It also means that wet gypsum materials will flow better into the fine details of the preparation when the impression is poured.

> **Clinical Tip**
>
> Each type of impression material has its own specific tray adhesive. Do not use an alginate tray adhesive for an elastomer. Likewise, do not interchange polysulfide adhesive with an adhesive for polyvinyl siloxane or polyether material.

POLYSULFIDES

Polysulfides are the oldest of the elastomers and are commonly referred to as "rubber base." They are more dimensionally stable and have greater tear strength than alginate or agar hydrocolloids. They are more accurate than alginate but not as accurate as the other elastomers. Polysulfides have been used successfully for crown and bridge impressions and for partial and complete denture impressions. They cannot be used in automixing cartridges and must be hand mixed. They are messy and have an unpleasant sulfur odor. When polyethers and polyvinyl siloxanes came on the market, most practitioners abandoned the polysulfides for these more accurate, dimensionally stable, and pleasant materials. Polysulfides are still used by some for impressions for complete dentures. Detailed information for the polysulfides can be found at the Evolve website at www.evolve.elsevier.com/Hatrick/materials.

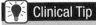

> **Clinical Tip**
>
> Alginate can be used in a moist field, because it is hydrophilic. For the most part, elastomers are hydrophobic. Polyethers are the most hydrophilic of the elastomers and are more forgiving of a little moisture, but not to the degree of the hydrocolloids. A well-isolated field for elastomers is essential.

SILICONE RUBBER IMPRESSION MATERIALS

Two types of silicone impression materials have been developed and are named according to the type of polymerization reaction they undergo during setting: condensation reaction or addition reaction.

Condensation Silicone

Condensation silicone was developed in the 1960s as an alternative to the messy, smelly polysulfide and was first used in the 1960s is useful for crown and bridge procedures. It has more desirable characteristics than polysulfide, such as ease of mixing, pleasant taste, no odor, and shorter working and setting times. The material sets through a condensation reaction that produces ethyl alcohol as a by-product. The ethyl alcohol is rapidly lost by evaporation, leading to a relatively high dimensional instability from shrinkage. Condensation silicones have been replaced by the more accurate and stable addition silicones.

Addition Silicone

The **addition silicone** impression materials were introduced in the 1970s and are an improvement over the condensation silicone materials. Their properties provide greater dimensional stability and accuracy. They are clean and easy to use, with no foul odor or taste. As a result of these improvements, they have become the most popular materials for crown and bridge procedures. They are also among the most expensive of the impression materials.

POLYVINYL SILOXANE (VINYL POLYSILOXANE)

Polyvinyl siloxane (PVS) or vinyl polysiloxane (VPS) is an additional silicone impression material that undergoes a polymerization reaction of chain lengthening (called an *addition reaction*) and cross-linking with reactive vinyl groups that produces a stable silicone rubber. The addition reaction does not produce a liquid by-product that can evaporate and cause shrinkage as with the condensation silicones. PVS has the smallest dimensional change (0.05%) on setting of the elastomers and hydrocolloids. PVS materials have high elastic recovery after removal from undercuts, and they resist tearing (high tear strength).

Some PVS materials produce hydrogen gas through a secondary reaction. If the impression is poured during the first 2 hours when the hydrogen is being released, the cast that results will have a very porous surface and will be unsuitable for most procedures. To counter the release of hydrogen, manufacturers have incorporated scavengers such as palladium powder, to absorb the hydrogen before it gets to the surface.

PVS impressions can be poured in stone several times and are dimensionally stable for a least a week without distortion. For this reason, many practitioners will send the impression with a prescription to the dental laboratory, where the impression may be poured several days later. The PVS materials exhibit little flow (deformation when subjected to a load after setting). This accounts for their accuracy even after repouring.

Hydrophobic Nature

PVS impression materials are hydrophobic by nature and must be used in a dry field. A little moisture on the prepared tooth will result in loss of surface detail in the impression, because the impression material cannot displace the moisture and establish close contact with the surface (it has a high contact angle and low wetting of the surface). Some PVS materials are called *hydrophilic* by their manufacturers, but in actuality they are hydrophobic materials to which a wetting agent (a soaplike **surfactant**) has been added, so that they can tolerate the presence of a small amount of moisture. In a newly placed impression it takes several seconds for the surfactant to move to the surface. Initially, the material is not hydrophilic when it first contacts the teeth and tissues but becomes more moisture tolerant as the surfactant rises to the surface. This delay in the emergence of the surfactant means that the preparation needs to be dry when the wash material is placed. However, the set impression will be more receptive to pouring with die stone.

Viscosities of the Material

PVS is manufactured in light, extra light, regular (or monophase), and heavy viscosities. A monophase viscosity is available from most manufacturers that is used as both a tray material and a syringe material. It is not as viscous as the tray material but is thicker than the light body material, yet it flows well enough to be used in a syringe to be injected around a tooth preparation. Some PVS materials are also available in a two-part putty form, consisting of base and catalyst putty. Powdered silica is added as a filler to give thickness to the base or catalyst pastes or putties.

Surface Detail

The accuracy of an impression material is measured by how well it captures the surface detail of a structure. To capture the surface detail the material must wet (have a low contact angle) and flow over the surface well. Low-viscosity materials (wash/syringe materials) wet and flow better than high-viscosity (tray/heavy body) materials and, therefore capture more detail.

Dispensing System

The most popular dispensing system for the light, extra light, regular, monophase, and heavy materials involves a cartridge with two chambers—one with base and one with catalyst. A mixing tip fits on the end of the cartridge (Fig. 15.12). A hand-operated gun-type dispenser or a motor-driven dispenser (see Fig. 15.16) pushes both the base and the catalyst through the mixing tip at the same time. They pass through an intertwined spiral that mixes appropriate amounts of each material together thoroughly by the time they exit the end of the tip. These mixing devices ensure the proper ratio of the two materials without the creation of bubbles or voids, which are common with hand-mixing. It is important for the operator to make certain that the orifices of the cartridges are cleaned of any residual set material that might block the flow of base or catalyst before applying the mixing tip. Otherwise, proper proportions of base and catalyst may not be mixed.

One manufacturer (Dentsply Sirona) packages the wash material in a small unit dose called a *digit* (see Fig. 15.12). The digit has enough material for a single unit restoration and has a shorter, smaller mixing tip to minimize waste. The digit is mounted in a palm-sized syringe and the material is delivered directly to the preparation. There is also a larger digit available with enough material for about three preparations.

> **Clinical Tip**
>
> Before placing the automixing tip on the impression cartridge, express a small amount of the material to make sure the openings for the two chambers are not blocked by set material.

Working and Setting Time

Because of the popularity of the PVS materials, manufacturers have put much effort into improving their properties to make their products more appealing than those of their competitors. The working time of PVS (from start of mix until it can no longer flow) is approximately 2 minutes. The setting time is the time measured from the start of mix to the time the material is hard and can be removed from the mouth. Setting times have been adjusted so that the practitioner has an assortment of materials with fast or regular set. Setting times vary among manufacturers and range from approximately 2 minutes (fast set) to 6 minutes (regular set). The working and setting times are affected by temperature. On a warm day the materials may set faster. Working and setting times can be increased by refrigerating the material before use.

Some newer materials (e.g., Imprint 4 VPS Super Quick; 3M ESPE) have been introduced with a setting time of 75 seconds. To achieve this fast set a chemical reaction occurs after the working time has passed that warms the material quickly to body temperature, which accelerates the set.

Putty/Wash Techniques

Some clinicians like to use putty for the tray material and a light body wash material to syringe around the prepared teeth. They feel that with subgingival margins on the preparations, the stiff putty causes hydraulic pressure that forces the wash material into the gingival sulcus to better capture the margins in the impression. These materials can be used with two different techniques.

One-step technique. With the one-step technique, the putty is mixed and loaded into a tray by the assistant while the operator injects the syringe material around the prepared teeth. An indentation (about the size of the prepared tooth) should be made in the putty in the area of the preparation to allow wash material to cover the preparation without being displaced by the putty. The tray is seated while the putty and syringe material are still unset, allowing them to bond together.

> **Clinical Tip**
>
> With the one-step putty/wash impression technique, be sure to make an indentation into the putty in the area of the preparation. Otherwise, the stiff putty will displace much of the wash material from the prepared tooth.

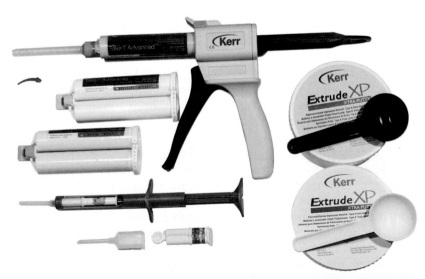

FIG. 15.12 Polyvinyl siloxane impression material in a variety of viscosities (light, regular, heavy body) in cartridges with mixing tip and mixing gun (*top left*) with unit-dose impression material (digit; Dentsply Caulk/Dentsply International) in a delivery syringe (*bottom left*) and putty (base and catalyst) in plastic jars (*right*).

Two-step technique. With the two-step technique, the putty in essence is used to create a custom tray within a stock tray. In the first step, the putty is mixed and placed in a stock tray. It is seated over the teeth with a plastic sheet placed between the putty and the teeth to create room for light body material. Some practitioners prefer to cut away some of the putty after it has set to create space for the light body material rather than using the plastic sheet. In the second step, light body material is syringed around the prepared teeth, and some is injected into the space in the putty created by the teeth. The tray with the putty is seated over the teeth.

> **⚠ Caution**
>
> With the two-step putty/wash technique, putty should *not* show through the wash material in the impression of the preparation. Show-through areas are pressure spots where the preparation hit the putty. The putty will compress while the tray is in the mouth, and then rebound after the tray is removed. This will cause distortion in the impression.

Potential putty/wash distortions. Both one-step and two-step putty techniques can result in distortions in the impression if care is not taken. Because putty does not flow well, the one-step technique may result in voids or a pulled appearance of the wash material when wash and putty do not flow and join together completely. With the two-step technique, because the putty is set before the wash is added, any areas where the putty shows through the wash material potentially have distortion. The flexible set putty may have been compressed by contact with tooth structure and then rebounded to its original shape when the impression was removed from the mouth. This is particularly critical if it occurs in the area of the prepared tooth. To avoid these problems with putty, some clinicians use a one-step technique in which putty has been replaced with a heavy body tray material that flows better.

> **💡 Clinical Tip**
>
> PVS putty should *not* be mixed while latex gloves are worn. Sulfur products from the gloves can interfere with the set of the material. Washed hands covered with vinyl gloves should be used.

Putty used for a matrix. Putty also has many uses at chairside and in the laboratory. Putty is used in many offices to capture an imprint of a tooth before it is prepared for a crown. After preparation, the imprint is used as a matrix to form a provisional (temporary) crown with tooth-colored acrylic resin. Many practitioners use the heavy body material in the tray instead of putty; others select a monophase material to place in the tray and to syringe around the teeth. The monophase material is formulated to have enough body to stay in the tray, yet is fluid enough to inject around the teeth. It does not flow as well as the light or extra light materials, however.

Removing the set impression. First, determine that the impression materials are fully set. Removing the impression prematurely can cause distortion Read the manufacturer's instructions on setting time. Immediately after seating the impression, place a small portion of the tray and wash materials on the bracket table. When they have set, the materials in the mouth should also be set because the heat of the patient's mouth should accelerate the set.

Remove the impression quickly to minimize the potential for plastic deformation (permanent deformation) of the impression. Removing the impression causes it to be stretched and compressed. The gingival sulcus, interproximal areas, and areas of undercuts will produce the most stretching and compression. Elastomers handle this stress best if applied quickly and released. So, quick removal of the tray applies stress quickly and allows it to release without deforming. However, it takes a few minutes for complete recovery to occur. For PVS materials it is best to wait 20 to 30 minutes before pouring the impression. Prolonged stretching or compression will produce permanent distortion and result in an inaccurate cast or die.

Bite registration. A registration of the patient's bite is typically made using elastomers (PVS or polyether) or wax.

PVS bite registration. PVS is used for bite registration because of its accuracy, dimensional stability, and ease of use. It offers no resistance to biting down; therefore it does not risk shifting the direction of the patient's bite as a hard material might. It can be used for this purpose in two ways:

1. Most practitioners prefer to use automatic mixing cartridge systems and to inject material from the mixing tip directly onto the occlusal surfaces of the mandibular teeth. They then have the patient close into centric occlusion (Fig. 15.13). Bite registration materials are viscous materials that stay in place when applied to the occlusal surfaces of teeth. This property makes it easier to register the bite and remove the material from the mouth, because it has not slumped and flowed all over the teeth.

2. Some practitioners use a bite tray (Fig. 15.2, D) that is usually a disposable plastic frame with a gauze-like material stretched between the arms of the frame. Material is dispensed on both sides of the gauze, the frame is seated over the teeth, and the patient closes into centric occlusion until the material sets (see Procedure 15.4). The tray supports the bite registration better than without it. These materials are formulated with a rapid setting time of 1 to 2 minutes. When set they are relatively stiff materials that exhibit very little flow under loading forces and remain dimensionally stable for at least a week, unlike wax bite registrations, which can warp after removal from the mouth with temperature changes or applied loads.

Polyether can be used in the same manner.

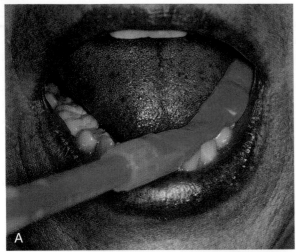

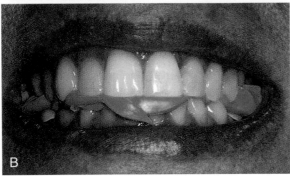

FIG. 15.13 Bite registration. **A,** Applying bite registration material to the teeth. **B,** Patient closed into centric occlusion.

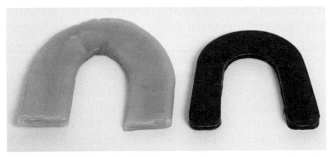

FIG. 15.14 Wax bite wafers. On the left is a wafer made by the heating and folding baseplate wax and on the right is a preformed commercially available wax wafer.

Wax bite. Wax is a less expensive material used by some clinicians to register the bite (see Procedure 15.5). Baseplate wax or utility wax can be softened by heating and then folded several times into a wipe rope about 4 or 5 mm thick that is bent into the shape of an arch (horseshoe-shaped). Premade horseshoe-shaped bite wafers are commercially available (e.g., Coprwax, Kulzer and Bite Wafers, Hygienic) and come with or without a thin aluminum foil between two layers of wax (Fig. 15.14). The foil prevents biting all the way through the wax.

Mismatch between PVS Bite and Cast from Alginate Impression. Because PVS material captures so much more detail and flows better than alginate, there will be a mismatch between the PVS bite registration and a cast made from an alginate impression. The differences are particularly acute in the occlusal, buccal, and lingual embrasure areas of the teeth. With PVS the embrasures will be sharply detailed and the PVS material will flow deeper into the embrasures in the bite registration, whereas with alginate the impression of the embrasures will be more rounded and shallower because alginate does not flow as well, and the cast will be lacking in detail in those areas. When the PVS bite registration is placed on the cast, it will not seat fully (Fig. 15.15). If the opposing cast is mounted against the preparation cast with that registration, then the bite will be propped open and the crown will be high in the mouth.

To prevent this mismatch problem, trim the bite registration with a scalpel to leave just an imprint of the occlusal surfaces and about 1 mm beyond and remove any sharp extensions of PVS into the occlusal embrasures. Also be sure to remove from the casts any blebs (beads of stone) created by trapped air in the impression. Making these adjustments should allow the bite registration to seat fully on the cast.

PVS alginate substitutes. Relatively inexpensive PVS materials (e.g., AlgiNot [Kerr Dental], Algin-X [Dentsply Sirona], and Counter-Fit [Clinician's Choice Dental Products]) have been developed as substitutes for alginates. They are much more dimensionally stable for long periods and do not need to be poured right away. Therefore, an impression of the opposing arch could be sent to the laboratory with the final crown impression without worrying about it drying and distorting, as with alginate. The PVS materials do not have to be wrapped in wet paper towels to avoid moisture loss and can be repoured several times. They have applications for diagnostic casts (study models) and as a matrix for a provisional crown or bridge. Because they are dimensionally stable, the matrix can be disinfected and stored, in case the patient breaks the provisional crown or bridge and a new one needs to be made.

Silicone die technique. Some practitioners use a specially formulated addition silicone material in an automatic mixing cartridge system to make dies for indirect composite inlays. A tooth is prepared for a composite inlay, and an alginate impression is made of the preparation. The silicone die material is injected into the alginate impression, and it sets within 2 minutes. That die can be used to prepare the composite inlay at chairside. The completed inlay is cemented into the preparation with resin cement (see Fig. 6.20 in Chapter 6 Composites, Glass Ionomers, and Compomers). This procedure is relatively quick. It saves the dentist a laboratory bill, the need to clean, disinfect and prepare an operatory for a second visit, the need to place and remove a temporary filling, and it saves an additional trip and local anesthetic injection for the patient.

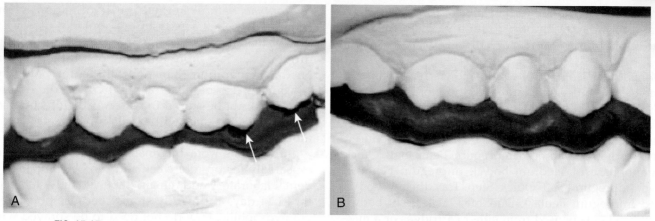

FIG. 15.15 Mismatch between cast made from an alginate impression and bite registration made with PVS. **A,** Casts not fully seated in the bite registration in the molar area. **B,** Casts seated after trimming cast and bite registration.

Polyethers

Polyethers are elastic impression materials that came to the European market in 1965 and gradually became popular in the United States. They are very accurate materials with good flow and tear strength and are excellent for use in crown and bridge procedures. They are more hydrophilic than PVS. The hydrophilicity gives polyethers good wetting properties for making detailed impressions in the presence of a small amount of moisture, making them particularly useful for impressions of preparations with subgingival margins. They do not release hydrogen gas and can be poured immediately with gypsum products without the formation of bubbles on the surface of the cast. They have excellent mechanical properties with good elastic recovery, and they do not shrink.

Consistency and setting reaction. Polyethers are supplied as light, medium, and heavy body viscosities. Equal lengths of material are dispensed from two unequal-sized tubes of base and catalyst onto a mixing pad, or the materials are provided in cartridges with auto-mixing tips, similar to the PVS materials. The base is a moderately low molecular weight polyether with a cation reactive group. The catalyst contains aromatic sulfonic acid that reacts with ethylene terminal groups, which polymerize by a reaction that causes rings of polyether copolymer to open and link together in long chains. When they go through their final reaction, they set very quickly. The catalyst can cause skin and tissue irritation. Therefore thorough mixing of the base and catalyst is necessary to avoid any irritation of the oral tissues.

Mechanical mixing. In addition to tubes or cartridges, both polyethers and PVS impression materials come in large pouches of base and catalyst that are placed into a mechanical mixer (Pentamix; 3M ESPE) and delivered directly into the impression tray (Fig. 15.16). The mixer handles a much larger volume of material than

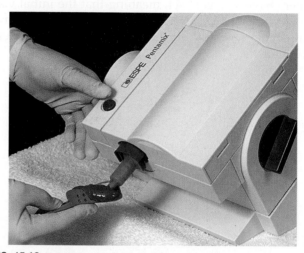

FIG. 15.16 Polyether impression material mixed and dispensed from the mixing machine (Pentamix; 3M ESPE) directly into a tray.

cartridges used in the automatic mixing guns and is more economical.

Properties. The original polyethers were the stiffest of all of the rubber impression materials; as a consequence, they were difficult to remove from the mouth in the presence of undercuts. In 2000 newer formulations of polyether (e.g., Impregum Penta Soft; 3M ESPE) were introduced that are much more flexible and have a more pleasant taste (Fig. 15.17). They are easier to remove from the mouth, and it is easier to separate the cast from the impression without breaking teeth.

Block out undercuts. With all of the elastomers, undercuts around bridge pontics, open embrasures around periodontally involved teeth, large bony tori and fixed implant fixtures should be blocked out with utility wax. This will prevent the impression material from flowing under them and locking the impression tray in the mouth (Fig. 15.18). It is a very unpleasant experience for both the patient and the practitioner to have locked-in impression trays cut apart with burs to remove them from the mouth.

Working and setting times. Polyethers have working and setting times comparable to those of PVS materials. Regular set materials have a working time of 2 to 3 minutes and a setting time (total time from start of mix) of 5 to 6 minutes. In 2005, 3M ESPE introduced fast setting polyethers (Impregum Penta Soft Quick [monophase or medium body], Impregum Penta H and Impregum Soft Quick Step Tray [heavy body], and Impregum Penta L DuoSoft Quick [light body]) that can be dispensed from either cartridges or a mixing machine. For these fast set materials the working time is 1 minute and the setting time is 4 minutes. Polyethers have a "snap" set, meaning that the initial viscosity remains the same throughout the working time but changes rapidly during the remainder of the setting process.

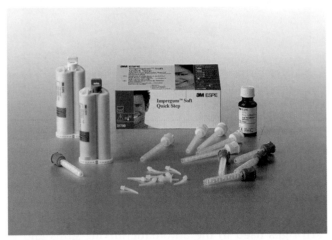

FIG. 15.17 Softer formulation of polyether impression material. Kit contains 3 cartridges of tray (heavy-body) material and a cartridge of syringe (light-body) material, bottle of tray adhesive, mixing tips and delivery tips that snap on to the end of the mixing tips. (Impregum Soft Quick Step, Courtesy of 3M ESPE.)

Hydrophilic nature. Permanent deformation is low compared with the polysulfides but not as low as that of the silicones. This material is somewhat hydrophilic, so it is more forgiving of a little moisture on the preparation than polysulfides or polyvinyl siloxanes. Also because of this hydrophilic nature, they must not be stored in water or disinfecting solution, because they will swell from the uptake of moisture.

Impressions from this material can be poured up repeatedly for up to a week and can be shipped to a dental laboratory and remain dimensionally stable for up to 14 days if properly stored. Because polyethers are hydrophilic, they do not need to be sprayed with surfactant before they are poured with stone. The fact that their polymerization does not produce volatile by-products contributes to their dimensional stability. Table 15.4 compares features of elastic impression materials.

VINYL POLYETHER SILICONE HYBRID

In the early part of the 2000s, a new class of elastomers was introduced. The new material is a hybrid of PVS and polyether. The purpose of the hybrid is to obtain the best features of each type of material. The material is composed of polyether and siloxane groups combined in a polymer. The polyether component makes the material hydrophilic, so it can tolerate a little moisture around the preparation and can be poured easily without the need to spray the impression with a surfactant. The siloxane component provides dimensional stability and recovery from deformation (caused by removal of the impression from the mouth). The material flows well and has high tear strength. It is available in regular and fast sets and in five viscosities, including light and extra light, monophase, heavy, and rigid heavy body. An example of this hybrid is EXA'lence (GC America).

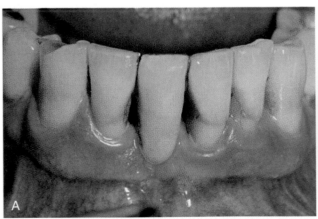
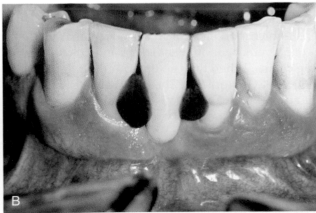

FIG. 15.18 Wax to block out undercuts. **A,** Teeth with gingival recession that has created large embrasure spaces where impression material may lock in place. **B,** Soft, red utility wax placed in spaces to prevent impression material from entering.

TABLE 15.4	Features of Elastic Impression Materials						
IMPRESSION MATERIAL	**COST**	**SURFACE DETAIL**	**DIMENSIONAL STABILITY**	**TEAR STRENGTH**	**EASE OF USE**	**POUR WITHIN**	**ABILITY TO RE-POUR**
Alginate	Low	Lowest	Low	Low	High	1 hr	No
Addition silicone (polyvinyl siloxanes)	High	High	Highest	Medium	High	1 wk	Yes
Polyether	High	High	High	Low to medium	High	1 wk	Yes

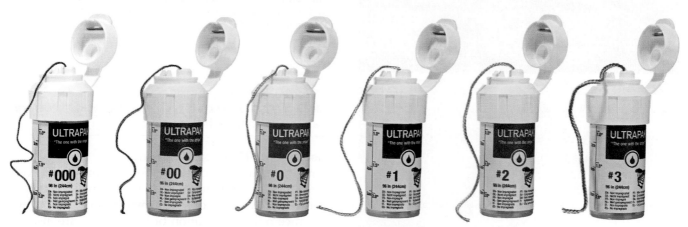

FIG. 15.19 A series of sizes of knitted gingival retraction cord (Ultrapak, Courtesy of Ultradent Products.)

COMPONENTS OF IMPRESSION MAKING FOR CROWN AND BRIDGE PROCEDURES

Both dental assistants and hygienists frequently are involved in the impression-making process. Those that are licensed in extended functions may actually pack retraction cord, use astringents, and make the impressions for crowns and bridges. All of those involved in assisting with the impression or with making it need to be knowledgeable about the materials and the process.

GINGIVAL RETRACTION

Retraction of the marginal gingiva is often needed for impressions of teeth prepared for restorations such as crowns and bridges, especially when the preparation extends subgingivally. The objective of gingival retraction is to provide a space in the gingival sulcus of adequate dimensions to receive the wash (syringe) material so that the entire margin can be captured in detail and at least 0.5 mm of the tooth (usually the root) beyond the margin.

Methods of Retraction

There are several ways to achieve the desired space in the sulcus for the impression material. Methods include use of cord, retraction paste, or a minor surgical procedure with a laser or electrosurgery to produce a small trough in the sulcus.

Retraction Cord

Placement of gingival retraction cords is among the most common methods of displacing the gingival tissue away from the tooth preparation to create space for the impression material. Cord placement should not cause damage to the gingival tissue or tear the epithelial attachment of the gingiva to the root. It should produce mild lateral displacement of the free gingival tissue.

Retraction cords come in a variety of forms and thicknesses. The cords can consist of twisted strands of cord material, braided strands, or woven or knitted strands. The various thicknesses of the cord are numbered to aid selection. Typically, the smaller the number, the smaller the diameter of the cord. For example, 000 cord is very small and number 3 is very large (Fig. 15.19). Cords can also be plain or impregnated with an astringent.

Bleeding should be controlled before attempting to place retraction cords. Bleeding control can be accomplished in several ways: (1) a local anesthetic containing epinephrine can be injected into each gingival papilla to constrict the blood vessels; (2) an astringent can be applied to the sulcus to stop the bleeding; or (3) coagulation can be obtained with a laser or by electrocautery.

Prepacking the Sulcus

Bleeding caused by trauma to the gingiva from the bur during preparation of the tooth can be minimized by packing a cord of medium diameter before finalizing

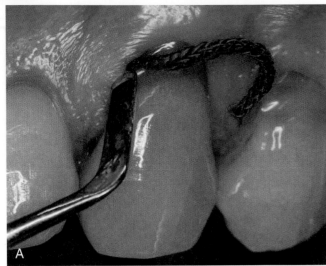

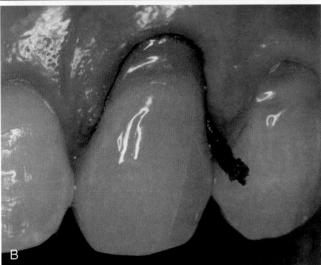

FIG. **15.20** Prepacking the gingival sulcus. A. Cord is being packed into the gingival sulcus B. Cord is placed prior to an operative procedure to place a restoration in the sensitive root abrasion lesion. It keeps the gingival tissue away from the rotating bur and helps prevent bleeding. (From Heymann H, Swift E, Ritter A: *Sturdevant's Art & Science of Operative Dentistry* (ed 6). St. Louis, 2013, Elsevier.)

the margins. The cord displaces the gingiva away from the tooth and provides some protection for it (Fig. 15.20). It also begins the retraction process, making it easier to pack the cords for the impression.

Cord Packing Instruments

There are many instruments designed for packing retraction cord. Cord packers are two-ended with each end at a different angle to the other to allow placement of the cord all the way around the tooth. The degree of offset of the angle of the blade to the handle can vary among manufacturers (Fig. 15.21). Cord packers can be smooth on the end or serrated. The packing blade should be thin enough to fit into the sulcus without damaging the tissue but not so thin that it cuts the tissue. The type of cord packer selected is based mostly on operator preference. The tooth preparation should have adequate separation from the adjacent tooth to allow the packer to access the sulcus.

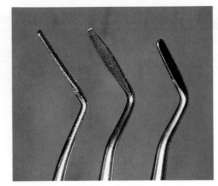

FIG. **15.21** Cord packers with different degrees of offset of the blade to the handle. (From Rosenstiel SF, Land MF: *Contemporary Fixed Prosthodontics* (ed 5). St Louis, 2016, Elsevier.)

> 💡 **Clinical Tip**
>
> Bleeding of the gingival tissue is the number one reason for an inadequate impression. It must be controlled *before* attempting to make the impression.

Astringents/Hemostatic Agents

Astringents are topically applied chemicals that constrict tissues and are useful in gingival retraction. Because they also constrict small blood vessels and produce mild coagulation of blood, they are also hemostatic agents. They are commonly applied to the tissues on a cotton pledget or on retraction cord, or are scrubbed into the tissues with a cotton-tipped cannula attached to a syringe (Fig. 15.22).

The two most common astringents/hemostatic agents are aluminum chloride (Hemodent [Premier Dental Products], Gingi-Aid [Belport], and ViscoStat Clear [Ultradent]) and ferric sulfate (Astringedent or ViscoStat; Ultradent). Racemic epinephrine (Orostat; Belport) is an effective astringent and vasoconstrictor but is used less frequently, because it can spike blood pressure and increase the heart rate. This can be potentially dangerous for patients with hypertension or cardiac problems.

Astringents and hemostatic agents used to control bleeding in the gingival sulcus will adversely impact the surface detail of a PVS impression. Ferric sulfate may also interfere with the set of the material. Astringents should be washed off the tooth before applying wash material.

> ❗ **Caution**
>
> Racemic epinephrine should be used with caution for patients with hypertension or cardiac problems. Cord soaked in racemic epinephrine and applied to the gingival sulcus can spike the blood pressure and increase the heart rate!

Two-Cord Retraction Technique

A gingival retraction technique using two cords has become popular. A small cord is placed first in the sulcus. The function of this cord is to help control bleeding and

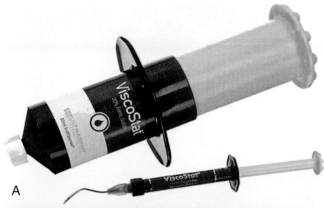

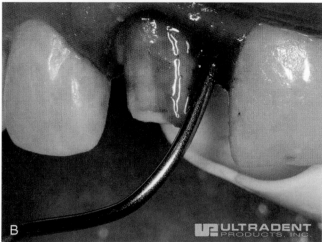

FIG. 15.22 Astringent is used to control bleeding gingival tissues prior to making the impression (ViscoStat, Ultradent Products). A. Large syringe of astringent is used to fill individual smaller syringes. B. Ferric sulfate astringent is scrubbed into the bleeding tissue with a cotton-tipped cannula to form blood clots over the capillaries.

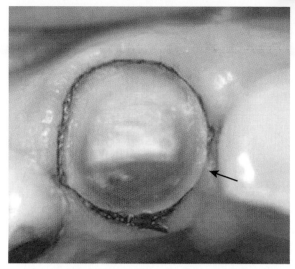

FIG. 15.23 Retraction cord improperly placed: Gingiva rests against the tooth in one portion *(lower right)*.

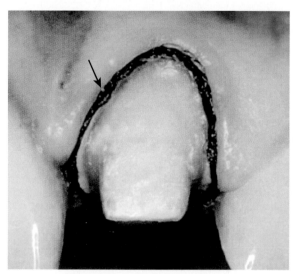

FIG. 15.24 Retraction cord has come partly out of the sulcus and rests on the margin *(upper left)*. The cord should be tucked back in the sulcus to ensure adequate retraction.

minimize the flow of gingival fluid from the sulcus. Often the first cord is dampened with an astringent before it is placed. Once it is in the sulcus any overlapping edges are cut so it fits end-to-end. The second (top) cord is larger in diameter and does the bulk of the retraction. The largest cord that fits into the sulcus should be used. It should be placed so that it is at the level of the margin or slightly apical to it. The top cord should have some overlap so that a "tail" of cord sticks out of the sulcus. This provides something easily grasped when the cord is to be removed. If the sulcus is very shallow, it may not be possible to use two cords. In this case, an appropriately sized single cord should be used to achieve retraction.

Evaluation of Cord Placement

Once the top cord is in place, cord placement should be evaluated. First, the working field should be well isolated, and isolation should be maintained throughout the impression-making process. If the prepared tooth is wet and the cords become wet, they will be slippery and very difficult to place in the sulcus. In addition, if isolation is not maintained after the cords are placed,

they tend to float out of the sulcus and retraction will be lost. Next, an inspection is made of the top cord. It should be at the level of the margin (unless the margin is supragingival) and should be visible 360 degrees around the tooth. If gingival tissue is leaning over the cord, it should be retracted by placement of an additional piece of cord or a cotton pledget in that area. The cord should remain in place for approximately 5 to 8 minutes to achieve good retraction. Time is needed for the cord to stretch the gingival fibers to relax the gingiva away from the preparation, and any astringent/hemostatic agent used needs time to produce hemostasis.

Cord Retraction Checklist: Before proceeding to making the impression your checklist should include (1) good isolation, (2) no bleeding, and (3) cord at the level of the margin and visible entirely around the tooth (Figs. 15.23 and 15.24).

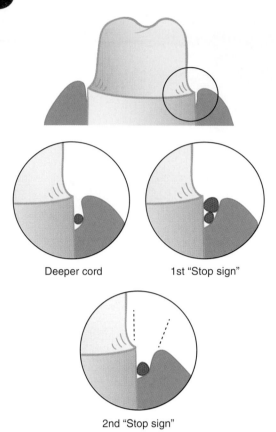

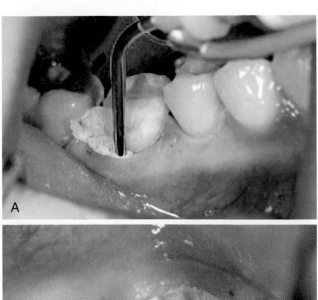

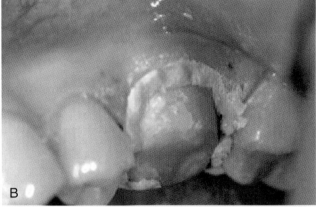

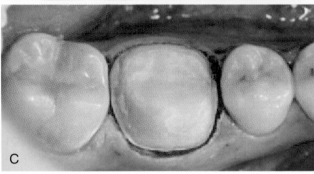

FIG. 15.25 Evaluation points (stop signs) for cord placement and gingival retraction. Top: Prepared tooth before cord placement. Left: Small cord placed to help control gingival fluids and bleeding. Right: Top cord is placed to displace gingival crest away from the margins of the prepared tooth. At this point cord placement is evaluated (1st "stop sign"). Bottom: Top cord has been removed. At this point the retraction is evaluated (2nd "stop sign"). If evaluation at either "stop sign" indicates a problem, it should be corrected before proceeding to the next step. (Courtesy of Dr. John Ino, University of California, San Francisco, CA.)

Evaluation of Retraction

While waiting for the cord to retract the gingiva, use this time to reorganize the working surface for making the impression. Move aside any instruments and materials that are not needed for removing the cord and making the impression. Think about which part of the preparation may be most difficult to access with the wash material. Usually, this is the site to start syringing the wash material first. However, when working on maxillary posterior teeth with the patient supine, start syringing on the distal surface. If you start on the mesial surface, the wash material may flow by gravity over the rest of the preparation and obscure your view of the distal surface and may also entrap air.

When you are ready to remove the top cord, dampen the cord slightly so it does not stick to tissues and cause bleeding when it is removed. Grasp the "tail" of the cord with cotton forceps and gently peel the cord out of the sulcus to minimize the risk of bleeding.

Now, evaluate whether or not the gingiva is adequately retracted. You should be able to see a space between the gingiva and the margin. There should be no bleeding. The bottom cord should have remained apical to the

FIG. 15.26 Clay retraction material (Expasyl; Courtesy of Kerr Corporation, Orange, CA) contains aluminum chloride astringent. **A,** Isolate, dry thoroughly, and inject material slowly into sulcus. **B,** Leave material in sulcus for 2 minutes. **C,** Wash material away and dry. Retraction has been obtained.

margin. If any of these criteria are not met, do not proceed! The odds are small that your impression will be successful. Do not waste time and materials by trying to force an impression in a site that is not ready. If there is inadequate space, repack the cords and determine whether a larger cord is needed. If there is bleeding, pick up a syringe of astringent (ferric sulfate is a good one for this) and scrub the tissues with the cotton-tipped applicator. Rinse and dry the tooth, and look to see whether bleeding has stopped. If not, you may need to inject (where allowed by State Law) a local anesthetic with epinephrine into the papillae. If the bottom cord has lifted, pack it back down. Once these criteria have been met you are ready to start the impression process.

The width of the space created in the gingival sulcus after the cord is removed should be at least 0.3 to 0.4 mm.

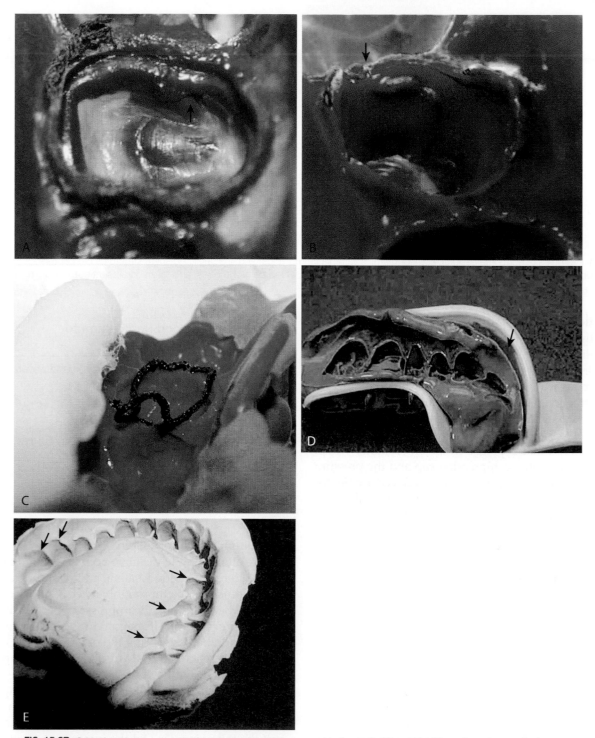

FIG. 15.27 Critical errors in an impression. **A,** A large void is present in the wall of the molar. The adjacent premolar impression has shiny rounded margins lacking detail from contamination with blood. **B,** A portion of the margin is missing. **C,** The bottom cord from a two-cord technique was not packed apical to the margin and is caught in the impression of the margins. **D,** The set impression material has separated from the tray likely from inadequate tray adhesive. **E,** Facial (left molars) and lingual (right molar and premolar) pulls of material. Syringe material was starting to set before the tray was seated.

A sulcus width less than 0.2 mm can cause distortion or tearing of wash material at the margin. Other reasons for tearing of the wash material include the following: a very deep sulcus, bleeding that causes flaws in the impression material, sharp edges of the preparation, and roughness of the preparation that increases the force needed to release the impression material from the surface.

See Fig. 15.25 for an illustration of "stop signs" or evaluation points for cord placement and gingival retraction. The first "stop sign" is after placement of the cord. Evaluate its placement. The second "stop sign" is after removal of the top cord. Evaluate whether retraction is adequate. Do not proceed with the impression until each step is adequately performed!

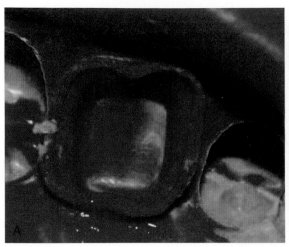 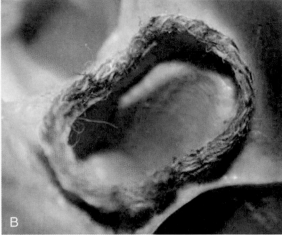

FIG. 15.28 Examples of good impressions. **A,** Clear margins with "flash," no voids, and fine detail. Adjacent structures are captured well. **B,** Bottom cord has been retained in the impression but is not sitting on the margins. Good detail, no voids, and "flash" is present at the margins. (Courtesy of Steve Eakle, University of California School of Dentistry [San Francisco, CA].)

Retraction Paste, Silicone, or Gel

Alternatives to cord for gingival retraction are retraction paste, silicone (PVS), or gel. The first of these materials to be introduced was Expasyl (Kerr Dental); it is a clay-like material with aluminum chloride as an astringent. Other retraction pastes include Traxodent (Premier Dental Products), Retraction Capsule (3M ESPE), Access Edge (Centrix), and Dryz (Parkell). GingiTrac (Centrix) is a PVS material that is placed in the sulcus, after which the patient bites on a compression cap and the pressure causes retraction. Racegel is a gel produced by Septodont. The materials are delivered to the gingival sulcus by way of a blunt needle cannula or a fine delivery tip on a capsule, much like a composite resin delivery capsule. The material displaces the gingiva laterally, and the astringent produces some tissue shrinkage and helps to control bleeding. The material remains in place a minimum of 2 minutes, and then is rinsed out thoroughly and dried before placing the wash material (Fig. 15.26).

MAKING THE IMPRESSION

(See Procedure 15.3 for detailed instructions.)

Criteria for a Successful Impression

A final impression made for a restoration such as a full crown must meet certain criteria in order to be considered useable. First, the impression must capture the fine detail of the prepared tooth, especially at the margins. This is important so that the restoration is sealed at its interface with the tooth. A lack of detail at the margins may result in an ill-fitting restoration with recurrent caries or continued tooth sensitivity. The impression should be free of voids, folds, pulls, and tears. The impression should capture an accurate representation of the other teeth and tissues in the impression site. If the impression is a double-bite impression (using a triple tray), it should capture the opposing teeth and a representation of the patient's acquired bite (where their teeth ordinarily fit together).

> ### Criteria for a Good Impression for a Restoration
>
> - Rigid tray selected and tried in for fit and coverage
> - Adhesive applied to tray
> - Material mixed well
> - Tray adequately filled with material
> - Impression free of voids, tears, pulls—no critical errors
> - Fine detail of preparation, margins with "flash" (impression beyond the margin)
> - Accurate representation of other teeth and tissues in the impression site
> - Teeth do not contact tray

Evaluating the Impression

Before attempting to evaluate an impression, it must be rinsed to remove blood, saliva, and debris. The impression should then be thoroughly dried. Continue to wear gloves when handling the impression, because it has not been disinfected yet. If magnifying loops are available, they should be used. Bring the operatory light over the impression at about a 70-degree angle to the plane of the teeth to cast a slight shadow on portions of the impression. These shadows will help you read the impression better than a bright light brought directly overhead. Rotate the impression to read all aspects of it. Ask yourself the following: (1) Did the impression capture all of the teeth and tissues needed for the restoration? (2) Can I see the preparation clearly? (3) Is the margin visible clearly all the way around the tooth? and (4) Has the impression captured at least 0.5 mm of the unprepared tooth just apical to the margins (producing a cuff of syringe material that is often referred to as the "**flash**").

Some flaws may be present in the impression. Most impressions are not perfect. It is important to know which of the flaws represent critical errors (must remake the impression) and which ones are minor errors that will still allow the impression to be used for the fabrication of the restoration.

Critical errors include the following:

- A portion of the margins is missing or torn.
- The margins look shiny and rounded rather than clearly demarcated. This is usually caused by moisture (blood, saliva, or fluid from the sulcus) on the margin.
- A fold or crease is present in the margin or wall of the preparation. A fold occurs at the junction of two portions of materials that do not flow together, for example, when syringing around the preparation with wash material, the material at the start and that at the end of the circling process do not flow together. Surface tension along the two walls of material may not allow them to join. When syringing around the tooth, push through the material first laid down with new material rather than stopping when the two ends meet.
- A pull (or drag) is present in the area of the preparation. A pull occurs when the wash material starts to set before the tray is placed. When the tray is seated, the partially set wash material is pulled or dragged by the heavy-bodied tray material. This represents a distortion.
- A large void is present in the preparation or the teeth needed to articulate with the opposing cast to establish the proper bite relationship. Any void, large or small, on the margin is a critical error. Voids on the margins are often caused when the syringe tip loses contact with the tooth surface. As the syringe tip bounces away and comes back to the tooth, some air is trapped in the wash material. A good resting point for the hand is needed to stabilize it while placing the syringe material (such as a finger rest).
- Set impression material has separated from the tray. This will cause a distortion.
- Lack of a good union between the heavy-body or putty material used in the tray and the light-body/syringe material placed around the teeth (often caused by one material starting to set before the other material is placed)

See Fig. 15.27 for clinical images of critical errors in impression making

Minor errors include the following:

- Small voids (<1 mm) not on the margin
- Small folds not on the walls or margins of the preparation
- A pull on buccal or lingual surfaces of teeth that are away from the preparation
- A slight separation of the material from the tray at a site not involving the preparation or teeth critical to establishing the occlusal relationship with the opposing teeth.

Fig. 15.28 shows examples of acceptable impressions.

Clinical Tip

When using the two-cord technique, the bottom cord often will come out and be embedded in the impression (Fig. 15.30, B). *Do not* try to remove it! That may tear the impression into the margins. Simply cut off any loose ends. The remaining cord will end up in the cast and can be easily removed when a removable die is made.

Factors That Limit Obtaining an Accurate Impression

- Selecting a poorly fitting tray
- Not using enough tray adhesive or not letting it dry adequately before loading the tray
- Inadequate control of bleeding
- Incomplete retraction of the gingiva
- Selecting impression material for syringing that is too thick to flow around the preparation or into the gingival sulcus
- Using mixed impression material that is starting to set
- Tearing of impression material on removal because the material is too weak or the sulcus was not opened adequately and the material flowing into it was too thin

DIGITAL IMPRESSIONS

You have learned in this chapter that traditional impression materials for crown and bridge procedures are required to be dimensionally stable, accurate in reproducing fine detail, strong in tear resistance, sufficiently flowable, easy to remove, able to rebound rapidly from distortion, pleasing in taste and smell, and easy to disinfect and store. The impression process is technique sensitive and often unpleasant for the patient. Computer-assisted design/computer-assisted machining (CAD/CAM) dentistry (see Chapter 9 Dental Ceramics) introduced the capture of digital images of the preparation, adjacent structures, and opposing dentition and structures, and this process became known as the **digital impression**. The digital impression removes many of the requirements and pitfalls of traditional impressions.

LEARNING CURVE

As with any new technology introduced into the dental practice, the use of digital impressions requires some thought as to how it will be incorporated into the practice, who will use the **intraoral scanner** (the image capture device), who will maintain it and how training and practice will occur. Team members will need time away from daily activities to receive training, and there is a learning curve, so some accommodation must be made to allow team members to practice the new techniques before they can become proficient. Some manufacturers of the intraoral scanners provide training in the dental office and others provide it at their headquarters. With proper training, the dental auxiliary can perform image capture and transmission of the images to the laboratory. Most state dental boards have not yet regulated the use of intraoral scanners by dental auxiliaries. Check to see if any regulations have been implemented in your state.

Intraoral Scanning: Originally, intraoral scanning cameras were part of a complete in-office CAD/CAM system. The digital images captured by the scanner were used with computer software to design the restoration and the design file was sent to an in-office milling unit to cut out the ceramic restoration. Later, stand-alone scanners were developed that could capture the desired images and send the file to a laboratory for processing. Stand-alone scanners do not have the capability to design the restoration, but some scanning systems let the clinician mark the location of the margins. Captured images can be transmitted through a secure Internet portal to a commercial laboratory and copies of the file stored on the computer as a part of the dental record. Not all dental laboratories are equipped for CAD/CAM processing, so there may be designated laboratories to which the images are transmitted. Another variation is to send the images to a central processing center that makes the models from those images and sends the models to a standard laboratory where the restoration is made.

SCANNING DEVICES

Complete in-office CAD/CAM systems with digital scanners, computer with design software, milling device and firing/glazing oven are available (e.g., CEREC AC [Sirona Dental Systems] and E4D Dentist [E4D Technologies]). Stand-alone intraoral scanners are also available for those offices that are not interested in or not ready to embrace in-office fabrication of restorations. These scanning systems include CEREC AC Bluecam and Omnicam (Dentsply Sirona), Planmeca Emerald (E4D Technologies), Lava Chairside Oral Scanner (3M ESPE), iTero Element (Align Technology), CS 3500 and 3600 Intraoral Scanner (Carestream Dental) and TRIOS 3 (3Shape).Most of the scanners are connected to the computing unit by a cord, but some new scanners are cordless (e.g., Trios 3 Wireless Scanner, 3Shape).

Image Capture: Intraoral scanners all are handheld but their methods of capturing images differ. Older scanners captured images by taking multiple still images and stitching them together by software. Newer scanners use streaming video to capture images of the teeth and surrounding structures.

For most single restorations images are needed of the prepared tooth, adjacent teeth and opposing teeth. A buccal bite registration image is used by many scanners to establish the proper occlusal relationship, but the type of bite registration may vary from scanner to scanner. All scanning systems are capable of scanning full arches, not just quadrants.

Use of Powder: Some systems require that the teeth be coated lightly with an opaque powder (usually titanium oxide) to provide contrast for the best image reproduction. The powder provides uniform reflective surfaces so the camera can accurately record the many contours present in the preparations or teeth. Other systems do not need to use the powder because their imaging mechanisms are different.

Scanner Positioning: Some systems require that the intraoral portion of the scanner with the camera portal be held just off the teeth when capturing the images whereas others allow the scanner to rest on the teeth to increase

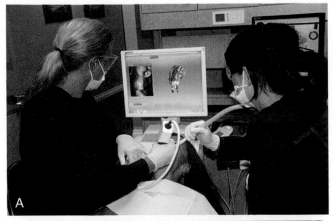
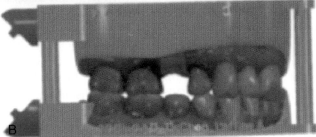

FIG. 15.29 Intraoral digital scanner used by the auxiliaries A. Obtained a digital impression and opposing arch. B. Virtual bite registration (A, from Rosenstiel SF, Land MF: *Contemporary Fixed Prosthodontics*, ed 5, St Louis, 2016, Elsevier. B, from Powers JM, Wataha JC: *Dental Materials: Properties and Manipulation* (ed 11). St. Louis, 2017, Elsevier.)

steadiness for a clear image (Fig. 15.29). Scanning times vary a little from system to system and range from about 3 to 8 minutes, depending on operator skills, the number of teeth being scanned, whether powder is needed, and the demands of the scanning unit.

Correcting the Scan: Some units have an erase software tool that allows the operator to erase a portion of a scan and rescan only that portion. Some clinicians have their assistant scan the arch before the preparation and scan the opposing arch. (It could be done while the patient is getting numb.) The assistant erases the portion of the scan that has the unprepared tooth and then just scans the prepared tooth. The software fills in the prepared tooth in the correct location. There is no need to redo the entire scan.

Open or Closed Software Platform: Some manufacturers have a closed software platform meaning that the scanned images can only be used with that manufacturer's CAD/CAM products (design software and milling). The trend is for manufacturers to use open software platforms that allow images to be transferred and milled on platforms produced by different manufacturers.

From Table 15.5 with scanners from major manufacturers, the trend with the newest versions of intraoral scanners is that they use continuous video to capture images in full color without the use of powder and the captured images can be used with other manufacturers CAD/CAM chairside or laboratory equipment.

TABLE 15.5   Digital Impression Systems

SYSTEM	IMAGING CAPTURE	COLOR IMAGE	DIRECT IMAGE TRANSMISSION TO LABORATORY	POWDER NEEDED	USE WITH ANY MANUFACTURERS' PRODUCTS (OPEN PLATFORM)
CS 3600 (CareStream Dental)	Continuous video	Yes	Yes	No	Yes
CEREC Omnicam (Sirona Dental Systems)	Continuous video	Yes	Yes	No	Yes
Planmeca Emerald (E4D Technologies)	Continuous video	Yes	Yes	No	Yes
Lava Chairside Oral Scanner (3M ESPE)	Continuous video	Yes	Yes	No	Yes
iTero Element (Align Technology)	Continuous video	Yes	Yes	No	Yes
TRIOS 3 (3Shape)	Continuous video	Yes	Yes	No	Yes

Shade Taking: At least one scanning system incorporates shade taking with its ability to take digital intra-oral photographs. The scanner takes the shades of the adjacent teeth during the scan of the prepared teeth eliminating the potential human error in interpreting shades. The shades are mapped out on the images at several locations and can be seen on the computer monitor. This is a time saving feature since it eliminates separate steps for shade taking and writing a shade description for the laboratory.

ADVANTAGES AND DISADVANTAGES OF DIGITAL IMPRESSIONS

Advantages

In addition to not needing impression materials, there is no need for trays, adhesive, disinfectants, pouring impressions, and packaging impressions for transport to the laboratory. A significant advantage is the ability of the clinician to view the preparation magnified on a computer monitor and see it from multiple angles by rotating the image. Undercuts, uneven or rough margins, and areas of under-reduction can be detected and corrected before the image is transferred to the laboratory. The evaluation of the preparation before sending the images to the laboratory eliminates many potential errors that would result in remakes of the restorations. The images themselves can be reviewed and retaken if judged inadequate. In many states this important function can be delegated to a properly trained hygienist or assistant, allowing the dentist to perform other functions. When digital impressions are used in conjunction with an in-office milling device, the restoration can be completed in one visit instead of two (see Fig. 9.3, Chapter 9, Dental Ceramics).

For the patient the impression process is easier, particularly for those patients with a strong gag reflex or severe tissue undercuts or tori. In addition, the time needed for the completed restoration to return from the laboratory is shortened. The images can be transmitted instantly, so the time needed for the laboratory to pick up the impression, pour it, cut out dies, and mount the casts in the proper occlusion is eliminated. A few studies have been done comparing the accuracy of digital impressions to traditional impressions. The studies concluded that digital impressions were as accurate as or better than traditional impressions.

Disadvantages

There are significant costs (between $15,000 and $35,000 for stand-alone systems) involved in purchasing a digital scanner and some training and practice that are needed to efficiently operate it. Laboratories charge a fee for processing digital images. The size of the scanner may present a problem for patients with limited opening, but they would have problems with traditional impressions as well.

Digital Impressions: Advantages and Disadvantages

Advantages
- Creates permanent 3-D color pre- and post-operative models which can be stored and reused indefinitely and do not take up space in the office
- Digital images can be used to point out problems to the patient and better communicate treatment needs
- At least as accurate as traditional impressions, possible better
- Does not need impression materials, adhesive, trays, pouring impressions and packaging them for the lab
- The prepared tooth/teeth can be viewed on the computer monitor and corrections can be made before sending images to the lab or in-office milling
- Images can be sent to the lab instantly
- Scanning can be stopped and restarted at will (e.g., to control moisture)
- Images can easily be re-made if necessary
- Images can be made by properly train dental auxiliaries in most states
- Eliminates messy clean-up
- More comfortable for the patient
- Fewer adjustments needed on the restoration and fewer remakes

Disadvantages
- Cost of the scanner is significant
- Training and practice is needed
- There may be a fee for processing digital images
- Some scanners may be too large to fit in the most posterior regions of small mouths or patients with limited opening
- A very few manufacturers have closed-system software so that the scanner only works with their CAD/CAM systems

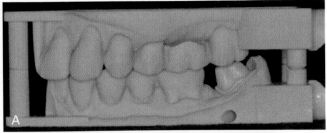

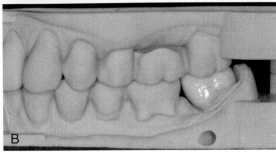

FIG. 15.30 Model and die created from a digital scan that was sent to a 3-D printer A. Digital scan of the quadrant with the crown preparation and opposing quadrant articulated by a digital bite registration B. CAD/CAM ceramic crown is seated on the die (From Powers JM, Wataha JC: *Dental Materials: Properties and Manipulation* (ed 11). St. Louis, 2017, Elsevier.)

SOFT TISSUE MANAGEMENT

Although many of the components of traditional impressions are not needed, there is still a need for management of the gingival tissues. If the margins of the preparation are all supragingival, there may be no need for gingival retraction and likely there will be no bleeding. However, most crown preparations involve the replacement of old restorations where at least some of the margins are at or below the gingival crest. The digital image of the preparation needs to capture the margins and approximately 0.5 mm of tooth apical to the margin (comparable to the desired "flash" in a traditional impression). So, some form of gingival retraction and use of astringents/hemostatic agents (as previously discussed) may be needed. As with any restorative impression good isolation is also required. The preparation must be kept free of blood clots, saliva and debris, as the scanner cannot distinguish between extraneous material and the prepared tooth. This could result in a restoration with faulty margins.

EXPANDED USE OF DIGITAL IMPRESSIONS

As the technology has improved and more clinicians and manufacturers have discovered the capabilities of digital impressions, their applications have expanded beyond uses for traditional crown and bridge procedures. Many clinicians are applying the technology to implant impressions for surgical guides, custom abutments and crowns and for complete denture impressions to produce digital models of the ridges and design software to fabricate dentures. Applications for orthodontic impressions have also being developed such as for orthodontic aligners and appliances. The models needed for these applications can be milled from large blocks of acrylic or generated from digital impression using software-directed 3-D printers that spray fine acrylic particles in layers to build up the models to the desired form (Fig. 15.30).

Offices without Scanners

For clinicians that do not have scanners in their offices, there are still options to have CAD/CAM restorations fabricated. They can make a traditional impression and the laboratory can scan it to create a digital impression or they can pour up the traditional impression to produce a gypsum model that the laboratory can scan and use to design and mill a restoration.

INELASTIC IMPRESSION MATERIALS

Inelastic impression materials in the form of dental impression compound, impression plaster, zinc oxide eugenol, and impression wax are among the oldest impression materials used in dentistry. For the most part, the elastic impression materials have replaced them in modern dentistry.

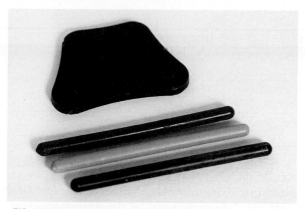

FIG. 15.31 Types of impression compound: cake and sticks.

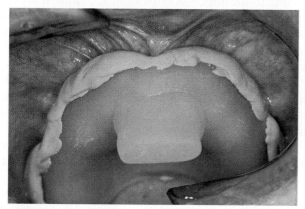

FIG. 15.32 Stick compound used for border molding of a custom impression tray. (Courtesy of Mark Dellinges, University of California School of Dentistry [San Francisco, CA].)

DENTAL IMPRESSION COMPOUND

Uses

Impression compound is a rigid thermoplastic material that softens when heated and becomes firm again at mouth temperatures. Impression compound is most commonly used as thick sheets (sometimes called *cakes*) or sticks (Fig. 15.31). At one time, compound cakes were used in denture impression making, but they are no longer popular for this use.

Some dentists use and some dental schools still teach the use of compound sticks to mold the peripheral borders of a custom tray and to form the palatal seal in impressions for complete dentures (Fig. 15.32). After the peripheral borders have been established, an impression is taken in the tray with one of the elastomers.

IMPRESSION PLASTER

Impression plaster is seldom used today but was used mainly for complete denture impressions. When used as the primary impression material, a wet mix (high water-to-powder ratio) was used to make it more fluid. After it set in the mouth, it was scored with a knife or bur, fractured along the score lines, and removed. The pieces were reassembled in the laboratory, and poured into dental stone to form the cast. Because of the complexity of its technique, impression plaster has been replaced by elastic materials that are easier to use and more accurate.

ZINC OXIDE EUGENOL IMPRESSION MATERIAL

Zinc oxide eugenol (ZOE) impression material, like impression plaster, is seldom used today. In its day, ZOE was favored as an impression material for mucostatic (does not displace the tissues) impressions. When a patient had loose tissue over an edentulous ridge and the operator did not want to displace these tissues with a stiff or heavy viscosity impression material, ZOE was often chosen.

IMPRESSION WAX

Wax is another inelastic material that was used early in dentistry for impressions. Waxes are often stiff at room temperature and become moldable when heated. They lack accuracy for final impressions for restorative treatments and distort easily on removal from tissue undercuts or when affected by temperature fluctuations after removal from the mouth.

Some waxes with low melting temperatures remain moldable at mouth temperatures and are used to correct minor voids in impressions for complete dentures or to build a posterior seal (post dam) for the maxillary denture by adding wax to the impression in the area of the juncture of hard and soft palates, and then reseating the impression in the mouth (see more on waxes in Chapter 16).

INFECTION CONTROL PROCEDURES

DISINFECTING IMPRESSIONS

Dental impressions should always be considered contaminated. They are usually contaminated with saliva or blood, which may contain viral and bacterial pathogens. Although most infectious agents, such as human immunodeficiency virus (HIV), do not survive for long periods of time outside of the body, many pathogens, such as the hepatitis viruses, can survive for several days. When impressions are not disinfected before they are poured, microorganisms can get into the gypsum and survive for a week or longer. Spores can survive much longer.

 Caution

Impressions are potentially infectious. They must be disinfected before being handled in the office laboratory or sent to a commercial laboratory.

Ideally, disinfection of impressions should begin in the operatory through chairside measures once the impression is removed from the mouth. Dental personnel should wear personal protective equipment while handling and disinfecting the impressions. The dental office has the primary responsibility for disinfection. Although the Occupational Safety and Health Administration (OSHA) allows transportation of contaminated items, regulations require proper packaging and labeling of these contaminated items. Dental offices should discuss with the dental laboratory the protocol they will use to disinfect items sent to the laboratory and how restorations returning from the laboratory should be handled.

TABLE 15.6 Disinfection of Impressions

IMPRESSION MATERIAL	COMPATIBLE DISINFECTANTS	IMMERSION TIME
Alginate	Iodophors or chlorine compounds (1:10 dilution of household bleach)	10 (up to 30) minutes or spray
Polyvinyl siloxane	Iodophors, glutaraldehydes, complex phenolics, chlorine compounds	10-30 minutes or spray
Polyether	Iodophors, glutaraldehydes, chlorine compounds	<10 minutes or spray

The material that is to be disinfected must be compatible with the disinfectant used and the procedure employed. Incompatible disinfection materials and procedures can cause significant distortion of the impression and failure of the restoration to fit correctly.

After removal from the mouth, impressions should be rinsed thoroughly with water to remove saliva, blood, debris, and other loosely attached contaminants. Excess water should be shaken off before the disinfectant is used, so as not to dilute it. Disinfectants can be applied by immersion of the impression or by spraying its surfaces. Spraying may be preferred for impression materials that tend to distort with immersion, such as the polyethers and alginate. However, spraying has two main disadvantages. First, it creates airborne particles of the disinfecting chemicals that could be inhaled by the staff or patients. Second, it may not adequately reach all surfaces if severe tissue undercuts are present. Immersion can cause distortion of some impression materials, because they are prone to imbibe water and they swell. Alginate can be immersed in appropriate disinfectants for up to 30 minutes. The length of time these sensitive materials are immersed must be monitored carefully, sometimes a difficult task in a busy office. Impressions should be rinsed after the recommended contact time with the disinfectant to remove residual chemicals that can affect the surface of the poured cast. If impressions are to be transported to the dental laboratory, they should be placed in a closed container or a sealed plastic bag.

 Clinical Tip

Spraying an impression should be done inside a plastic bag or headrest cover to contain the spray and protect the handler from inhaling droplets.

Selecting Disinfecting Solution

Impression materials differ from each other in their composition. Thus each type of impression material may require its own disinfecting solution and procedure. Manufacturer recommendations for disinfection should be followed. Alginate impressions can be disinfected safely with an iodophor or 1% sodium hypochlorite solution for 10 minutes. Elastomeric impressions can be disinfected with a wide range of solutions. However, each

particular material may be adversely affected by some disinfectants. For example, phenols with high alcohol content can dehydrate some of the impression materials. Some solutions may also dissolve the tray adhesive that retains the impression material and cause it to come loose from the tray. The silicone (PVS), polysulfide, and polyether elastomers can be disinfected with 1:213 iodophor (i.e., 1 part iodophor to 213 parts distilled water), 1:10 sodium hypochlorite, or complex phenolics. Silicones and polyethers can also be disinfected with glutaraldehydes. It is important to follow the manufacturer's recommendations as to the use and length of time to apply the disinfectant.

Wax bite registrations, PVS bite registrations, and casts all present different problems for disinfection. Wax may distort when it is immersed. The recommended disinfecting procedure is to rinse, spray, rinse, spray, and rinse again, and then to place it in a container for transport. Most elastomeric bite registration materials can be safely disinfected with the same solutions as their impression material counterparts. See Table 15.6 for disinfecting times and materials for impressions. Procedure 15.6 describes processing methods for impression materials.

DISINFECTING CASTS

On rare occasions, it may be necessary to disinfect the cast produced from an impression that could not be properly disinfected because of the nature of the contaminants or an impression material that could not be immersed in the proper disinfectant. Casts should be completely set and stored for at least 24 hours before disinfection to prevent attack by the chemicals on the surface of the cast. Casts seem to be minimally affected by the use of 1:10 sodium hypochlorite, iodophors, or chlorine dioxide. Casts should be sprayed rather than immersed in disinfecting solutions, because some studies have shown damage to the surface in only a few minutes in water-based solutions. Manufacturers have added antimicrobial agents to some gypsum materials, but studies are not conclusive as to their effectiveness.

STERILIZING IMPRESSION TRAYS

Impression trays must be sterilized properly after their use and after a tray is tried in the patient's mouth for fit. Disposable plastic trays are recommended when they can meet the demands of the impression material being used. Flexible materials require a rigid tray to prevent flexing of the tray and distortion of the material. Because of their thickness and rigidity, some putties can better tolerate flexible plastic trays. Inelastic impression materials also may require rigid trays to prevent them from cracking. Plastic trays that are more rigid have been developed and are commercially available. Custom acrylic trays should be discarded when the procedure has been completed or should be immersed in an acceptable disinfectant if they will be reused at the patient's next appointment. Aluminum, chrome-plated, and stainless steel trays can be sterilized by heated steam or chemical vapors, dry heat, or ethylene oxide after they have been thoroughly cleaned.

SUMMARY

In almost all phases of dentistry, impressions are an integral part of the procedures needed for delivering comprehensive care to patients. In many offices, impressions are made daily, and the various impression materials must be understood by the clinician for correct selection, manipulation, and disinfection of the materials and for pouring of casts. Alginate is still the material of choice for preliminary impressions. With the improvements made in the impression materials over the past several decades, many of the older materials such as agar hydrocolloid, polysulfide, condensation silicone, and the inelastic materials have been replaced by more accurate, dimensionally stable elastic materials. Polyvinyl siloxanes and polyethers are the most popular impression materials for final impressions for restorations and removable prostheses.

Each category of the impression materials has its own handling characteristics, which must be considered. Changes in temperature and humidity will influence the materials in different ways, so operators must take these factors into consideration when making impressions. Dimensional changes over time, water loss and gain, deformation, and rebound are among the many physical and mechanical properties that must also be considered when impression materials are handled and disinfected, if the clinician is to meet the objective of producing as accurate a replica of the oral structures as possible.

Dental auxiliaries who have been properly trained and licensed in their states can pack cord and make final impressions using elastic materials or digital images for crowns, bridges, implants, and removable prosthetics. It is imperative that clinicians have a reliable approach to making impressions, including soft tissue management. They must use definitive criteria to evaluate the cord retraction process and the final impression. They must apply their knowledge about the characteristics and manipulation of the impression materials to troubleshoot problems with an impression so they do not repeat their mistakes.

With the growing use of CAD/CAM technology, digital impressions are being used more and more as an alternative to impression materials. Digital impressions are much easier for the patients, and they eliminate many of the requirements needed in the impression materials, such as dimensionally stability, strength in tear resistance, flowability, ease of removal, rapid rebound from distortion, disinfection, and storage. Digital impressions can be transmitted to the dental laboratory within minutes of capturing the images or may be used to design and mill restorations in the dental office.

INSTRUCTIONAL VIDEOS

See the Evolve Resources site for a variety of educational videos that reinforce the material covered in this chapter.

Procedure 15.1 Fabrication of Custom Impression Tray Using Light-Cured Resin

See Evolve site for Competency Sheet.

EQUIPMENT AND SUPPLIES

- Maxillary or mandibular cast
- Sheet of baseplate wax, Bunsen burner, scalpel or lab knife, sheet of aluminum foil
- Triad TruTray kit with resin sheets, Model Release Agent, Air Barrier Coating, disposable brush
- Lab handpiece and acrylic bur or lab lathe with arbor band, acrylic polishing point
- Triad curing unit (Fig. 15.33).

PROCEDURE STEPS

1. Use a trimmed cast (study model) made from a preliminary impression. Use a pencil to scribe a line around the cast that is approximately 3 mm short of the depth of the vestibule (Fig. 15.34). This will be the border of the tray.

   NOTE: The cast has marks for location of tray stops on the 2nd molars and central incisor.

2. Assemble baseplate wax, cast and aluminum foil to use for wax spacer in the tray (Fig. 15.35).

3. Soften baseplate wax and adapt it over the teeth to act as a spacer (Fig. 15.36).

   NOTE: for an edentulous cast one layer of baseplate wax is usually adequate. (See Procedure 17-1 in Chapter 17 for placement of wax spacers and tray stops on edentulous casts.) When taking an impression for a crown or bridge, some clinicians prefer two layers of wax. The spacer provides for a uniform thickness of impression material within the tray.

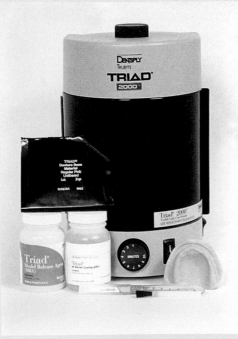

FIG. 15.33

4. Use a scalpel or lab knife to cut the wax back to the marked tray borders.

   Place holes in the wax at the location of the marked tray stops at the 2nd molars and central incisor (Figs. 15.37 and 15.38).

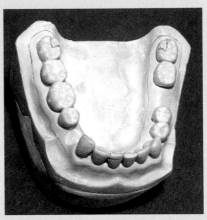

FIG. 15.34 (From Rosenstiel SF, Land MF: *Contemporary Fixed Prosthodontics* (ed 5). St Louis, 2016, Elsevier.)

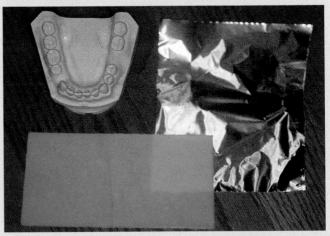

FIG. 15.35 (From Rosenstiel SF, Land MF: *Contemporary Fixed Prosthodontics* (ed 5). St Louis, 2016, Elsevier.)

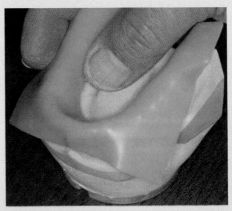

FIG. 15.36 (From Rosenstiel SF, Land MF: *Contemporary Fixed Prosthodontics* (ed 5). St Louis, 2016, Elsevier.)

Procedure 15.1 Fabrication of Custom Impression Tray Using Light-Cured Resin—cont'd

NOTE: Tray stops ensure an even thickness of impression material within the tray.

5. Cover the wax with a sheet of aluminum foil (Fig. 15.39). Remove the excess and smooth the foil (Fig. 15.40).

NOTE: Polymerizing the tray material often produces heat that melts the wax causing it to stick to the tray. The foil makes it easier to remove the wax from the tray after the tray has been light-cured.

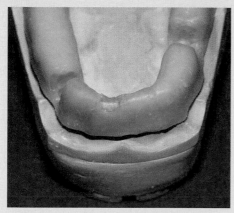

FIG. 15.37 (From Rosenstiel SF, Land MF: *Contemporary Fixed Prosthodontics* (ed 5). St Louis, 2016, Elsevier.)

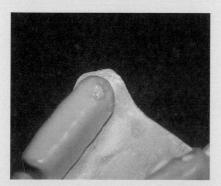

FIG. 15.38 (From Rosenstiel SF, Land MF: *Contemporary Fixed Prosthodontics* (ed 5). St Louis, 2016, Elsevier.)

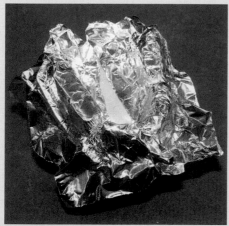

FIG. 15.39 (From Rosenstiel SF, Land MF: *Contemporary Fixed Prosthodontics* (ed 5). St Louis, 2016, Elsevier.)

NOTE: If the foil was not used, the cast and wax should be coated with a thin layer of Model Release Agent. This makes it easier to separate the tray from the cast and remove the wax.

6. Remove the tray material from its light-proof packaging (Fig. 15.41). Insert a small bit of the resin material into the holes created for tray stops and fill the edentulous spaces with resin (Fig. 15.42).

7. Adapt the tray material to the cast using gloved hands spreading it evenly; do not create thin areas (Fig. 15.43).

7. Use a sharp knife or scalpel to remove the excess tray material extending beyond the marked borders. Use a finger to gently rub the tray border to remove wrinkles or sharp edges (Fig. 15.44).

NOTE: Creating smooth borders at this stage save a lot of time later grinding and polishing.

8. From the remaining excess material, shape a handle and place it on the anterior area at the midline. Blend the base of the handle into the tray to get a smooth union of the two (Fig. 15.45).

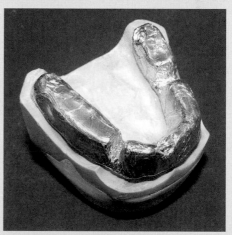

FIG. 15.40 (From Rosenstiel SF, Land MF: *Contemporary Fixed Prosthodontics* (ed 5). St Louis, 2016, Elsevier.)

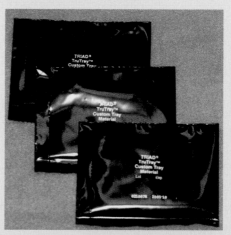

FIG. 15.41 (From Rosenstiel SF, Land MF: *Contemporary Fixed Prosthodontics* (ed 5). St Louis, 2016, Elsevier.)

Continued

Procedure 15.1 Fabrication of Custom Impression Tray Using Light-Cured Resin—cont'd

8. Insert the cast with the tray material into the Triad curing unit and set the timer for manufacturer's recommended curing time (Fig. 15.46).

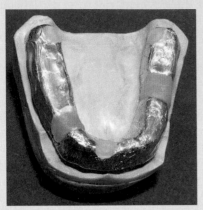

FIG. 15.42 (From Rosenstiel SF, Land MF: *Contemporary Fixed Prosthodontics* (ed 5). St Louis, 2016, Elsevier.)

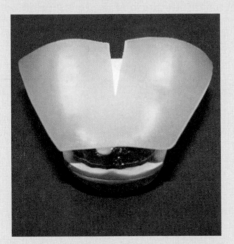

FIG. 15.43 (From Rosenstiel SF, Land MF: *Contemporary Fixed Prosthodontics* (ed 5). St Louis, 2016, Elsevier.)

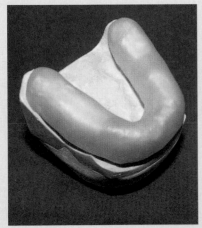

FIG. 15.44 (From Rosenstiel SF, Land MF: *Contemporary Fixed Prosthodontics* (ed 5). St Louis, 2016, Elsevier.)

NOTE: Curing time depends on the type of tray material being used.

9. After initial curing, remove the tray from the cast and remove the softened wax spacer (Fig. 15.47).

NOTE: Heat from the curing lights will soften the wax.

10. Coat the tray with Air Barrier Coating and return it to the curing unit with the tissue side of the tray positioned up. Follow manufacturer's recommended curing times (Fig. 15.48).

NOTE: Resins when cured will have a thin layer of uncured resin on the surface caused by exposure to oxygen in the air. This is the same thing seen with sealants or composites. The air barrier eliminates the oxygen and allows the resin on the surface to cure.

As an alternative to using the air barrier coating, the tray can be scrubbed with a gauze soaked in isopropyl alcohol (rubbing alcohol), and then cleaned with soap and warm water to remove the film of unset resin.

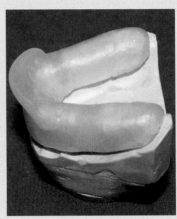

FIG. 15.45 (From Rosenstiel SF, Land MF: *Contemporary Fixed Prosthodontics* (ed 5). St Louis, 2016, Elsevier.)

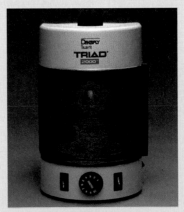

FIG. 15.46 (From Rosenstiel SF, Land MF: *Contemporary Fixed Prosthodontics* (ed 5). St Louis, 2016, Elsevier.)

Procedure 15.1 Fabrication of Custom Impression Tray Using Light-Cured Resin—cont'd

11. Clean the cured tray with a brush and warm (not hot) water and soap to remove residual air barrier.

12. Use an arbor band on a lathe or an acrylic bur in a lab handpiece to adjust the tray borders and remove any sharp edges (Fig. 15.49). Use an acrylic polishing point to smooth the tray borders. Check with your fingers to make sure there are no sharp edges that might be uncomfortable to the patient. Clean trimming debris from the tray.

   NOTE: If additional retention of the impression material is desired beyond that provided by tray adhesive, holes can be cut in the tray.

13. Disinfect the tray in a suitable disinfectant for the recommended time. Rinse and dry the tray and store it in a zippered plastic bag with the patient's name and/or chart number.

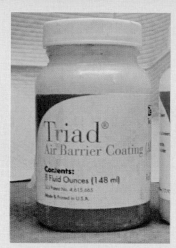

FIG. 15.48 (From Rosenstiel SF, Land MF: *Contemporary Fixed Prosthodontics* (ed 5). St Louis, 2016, Elsevier.)

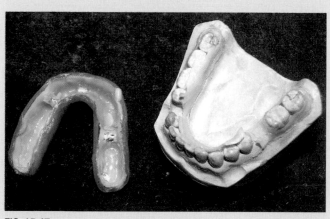

FIG. 15.47 (From Rosenstiel SF, Land MF: *Contemporary Fixed Prosthodontics* (ed 5). St Louis, 2016, Elsevier.)

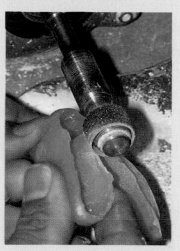

FIG. 15.49 (From Rosenstiel SF, Land MF: *Contemporary Fixed Prosthodontics* (ed 5). St Louis, 2016, Elsevier.)

Procedure 15.2 Making an Alginate Impression

See Evolve site for Competency Sheet.

Consider the following with this procedure: safety glasses are recommended for the patient, PPE is required for the operator, ensure appropriate safety protocols are followed, and check your local state guidelines before performing this procedure.

EQUIPMENT/SUPPLIES (FIG. 15.50)

- Basic setup
- Alginate, powder scoop, and water-measuring cylinder
- Rubber bowl, wide-bladed spatula
- Impression trays (perforated) or solid trays

including rim-locks require alginate adhesive
- Utility wax ropes
- Saliva ejector, disinfecting solution, zippered plastic bag, paper towels

PROCEDURE STEPS

1. *Patient preparation:* Seat the patient. Cover the patient's clothes with a plastic-backed bib. Explain the procedure. Inquire about the gag response and ability to breathe through the nose. Remove dental prostheses unless needed in the impression. Have the patient rinse his or her mouth.

Continued

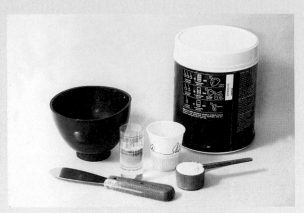

FIG. 15.50

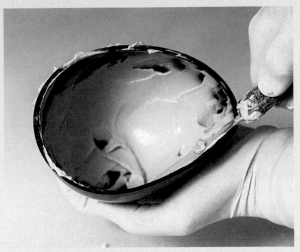

FIG. 15.52

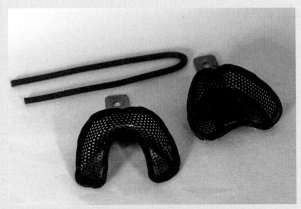

FIG. 15.51

NOTE: If the patient has bridges or fixed implant prostheses, block out with utility wax around pontic spaces likely to lock alginate in place and make removal of the impression difficult. Orthodontic bands, brackets, and arch wires may also need to be blocked out. If the patient has very loose teeth, block out embrasures around these teeth to prevent removing them with the impression. Take precautions for gagging (as highlighted in the clinical tip on controlling the gag reflex). Patients who cannot breathe through the nose may feel threatened if alginate runs out the back of the tray and blocks the airway; therefore seat the tray in the posterior first to force material forward. On occasion, the dentist may want the prosthesis left in during the impression to examine the occlusion later on. Check with the dentist. Rinsing before making the impression removes debris and ropy saliva. An antibacterial rinse will reduce the number of pathogens.

2. *Tray selection:* Quickly examine the patient's mouth, arch size and shape, and palatal depth. Select a tray of the appropriate size. Try it in for fit. Add utility wax as needed for comfort and extension of the tray.

NOTE: If the tray border is short or the palate deep, add wax to extend the tray and support the alginate (Fig. 15.51).

3. *Mixing alginate:* Tumble the container of alginate to fluff powder. Measure three level scoops of powder

for a large upper arch or two scoops for a smaller arch. Two scoops are adequate for the average lower arch. Place in a rubber bowl one measure of room temperature water for each scoop of powder. Add powder to water and stir to wet the powder. Vigorously mix and press the wet powder against the sides of the bowl with a spatula while rotating the bowl with the other hand. The final mix should appear smooth and not grainy (Fig. 15.52).

NOTE: Prepackaged alginate does not require fluffing, because it is already present in the correct proportions. Mix by wiping vigorously against the sides of the bowl to remove entrapped air, and thoroughly mix the powder and water. Water that is cooler than room temperature lengthens working and setting times, whereas warm water shortens these times. Complete the mix within 45 seconds for regular-set or within 30 seconds for fast-set alginate, to allow enough time to load the tray, paint occlusal surfaces, and seat the impression before initial set.

4. *Loading the tray:* Load the tray in large increments, pressing each into the tray until level with the sides. Use a wet, gloved finger to smooth the surface and create a shallow indentation where the teeth will go (Fig. 15.53). Remove excess alginate.

NOTE: Fewer increments will trap less air. Force out entrapped air by pressing alginate into the depth of the tray. Indentation for the teeth helps to orient the tray when seating. Extra material added to the anterior part of the tray helps to fill the vestibule and get a good peripheral roll.

5. *Seating the tray:* Take alginate from the bowl on a finger, and wipe it over the occlusal surfaces and into the embrasures. For upper impression: From behind and to the side of the patient (right-handed—11 o'clock position; left-handed—1 o'clock), retract the right cheek with the posterior corner of the tray and the left cheek with the index finger (reverse for left-handed).

Procedure 15.2 **Making an Alginate Impression—cont'd**

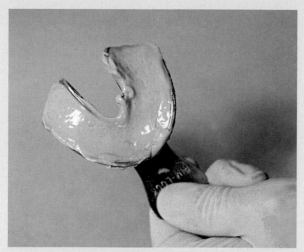

FIG. 15.53

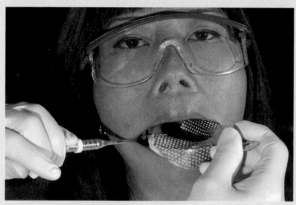

FIG. 15.54

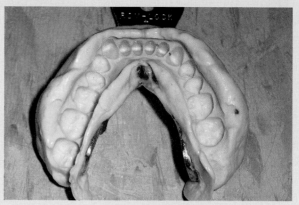

FIG. 15.55

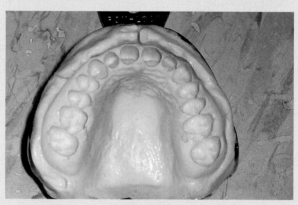

FIG. 15.56

For lower impression: From in front and to the side of the patient (right-handed—8 o'clock position; left-handed—4 o'clock), retract the left cheek with the side of the tray and the right cheek with the left index finger (reverse for left-handed) (Fig. 15.54). Both impressions can be made with the operator seated and the patient reclined, or with the operator standing with the patient upright. If the patient is reclined, seat the patient upright after the tray is placed. For both upper and lower impressions: Rotate the tray into the mouth, and align the tray over the teeth with the handle in the midline. Seat the back of the tray first and complete seating to the anterior as the lip is gently pulled out of the way. Inspect the back of the tray for excess alginate and remove with a quick sweep of the mouth mirror. For lower impression: Have the patient lift the tongue once the tray is seated, and relax it again once alginate has flowed into the lingual areas.

NOTE: Seating the posterior of the tray first allows alginate to flow forward rather than back into the patient's throat. Lifting the lip allows alginate to flow into the vestibule. Quickly removing excess alginate minimizes the gag response. Employ distraction techniques for gaggers. Have them position the head forward, breathe through the nose deeply and slowly, and use the saliva ejector to prevent pooling of saliva.

6. Stabilize the tray until the alginate is fully set. Allow an additional minute before removing the tray.

    NOTE: Check alginate remaining in the bowl to confirm set. Tray movement during setting will cause distortion in the impression. Allowing 1 minute after set helps to increase tear strength.

7. *Removing the tray:* Break the seal by pressing down (or up for a lower impression) on the side of the tray with a finger, or have the patient close his or her lips around the tray handle and blow to puff out the cheeks. Hold the handle in the hand, grasping with the index finger and thumb, and remove the tray with a snap.

    NOTE: Protect the patient's teeth in the opposing arch with fingers of the other hand. Rapid removal minimizes distortion and tearing of alginate.

8. *Handling the impression:* Rinse under running water to remove saliva and debris. Shake out pooled water. Inspect the impression, using criteria for acceptability (see Table 15.3) (Figs. 15.55 and 15.56).

9. *Disinfecting the impression:* Spray thoroughly with disinfectant. Drain off the pooled liquid.

Continued

Procedure 15.2 Making an Alginate Impression—cont'd

NOTE: When the impression is sprayed inside a bag or headrest cover, the aerosol is better contained (Fig. 15.57). Alginate will imbibe liquid and swell, so pooled liquid should be removed.

10. Cut off unsupported alginate at the back of the tray. Wrap the impression in a damp paper towel or place a few drops of water in a zippered plastic bag marked with the patient's name (Fig. 15.58) and seal it.

   NOTE: If the tray is laid on the bench top, unsupported alginate at the back of the tray may lift a portion of the impression and dislodge it from the tray. This will cause a distortion in the impression. If alginate is left in the air, water will evaporate, causing distortion. Ideally, the impression should be poured within 30 minutes, because it is not dimensionally stable for long periods. It will lose water (by syneresis) even in 100% humidity. Allow 10 minutes before pouring to allow the disinfectant to be effective and to allow rebound to occur.

11. Help the patient remove alginate from the face with a damp towel. Have the patient rinse his or her mouth. Inspect the patient's mouth and remove trapped alginate from the embrasures with an explorer and floss.

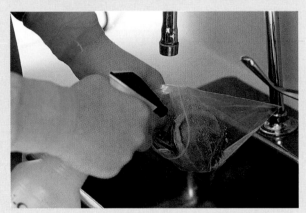

FIG. 15.57

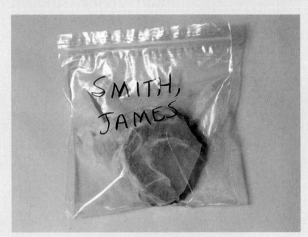

FIG. 15.58

Procedure 15.3 Making a Double-Bite Impression for a Crown

See Evolve site for Competency Sheet.

Consider the following with this procedure: safety glasses are recommended for the patient, PPE is required for the operator, ensure appropriate safety protocols are followed, and check your local state guidelines before performing this procedure.

NOTE: In some states, the dental assistant or hygienist may be licensed to place a retraction cord and make the impression. In states where these functions are not permitted, it is assumed that the dental assistant or the hygienist will assist the dentist.

EQUIPMENT/SUPPLIES (Fig. 15.59)

- Basic crown and bridge setup\
- Double-bite tray (paper insert for metal trays), tray adhesive
- Elastomeric impression material in cartridges: Heavy body tray material and light body syringe material
- Dispenser gun and mixing tips

- Impression syringe

PROCEDURE STEPS

1. Assemble the cartridge in the gun and extrude a small amount of impression material onto a paper towel to ensure that the orifices are not clogged.

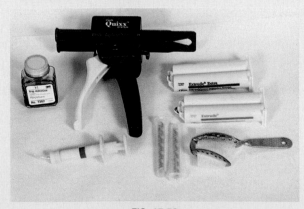

FIG. 15.59

Procedure 15.3   Making a Double-Bite Impression for a Crown—cont'd

Place the mixing tip.

NOTE: Clogged or partially clogged orifices will result in an improper mix of the material, with alteration of setting time and physical properties.

2. Inform the patient of the procedure and have the patient practice closing into centric occlusion (patient's "normal" bite) with the tray in place (Fig. 15.60).

NOTE: Choose opposing teeth that are easily seen, such as the canines on the opposite sides of the mouth, and note their position when they occlude. This relationship will be checked when the impression is made to ensure proper closure.

3. Maintain isolation in the quadrant in which the impression will be made.

NOTE: Saliva can saturate the retraction cord and may cause it to displace from the gingival sulcus.

4. Confirm that cord retraction around the crown preparation is adequate (Fig. 15.61).

NOTE: This is the first "stop sign." The clinician should be able to see the preparation, the cord, and the gingiva displaced from the preparation. In other words, the cord should not be placed so deeply into the gingival sulcus that the gingival crest has collapsed over it and is resting on or near the preparation or the cord should not be placed so shallowly that it is resting on top of the margin.

5. Carefully remove the retraction cord after it has been in place for about 5 minutes (8 minutes if the tissue had been bleeding prior to cord placement). Rinse and dry the tooth.

NOTE: If the retraction cord is dry, lightly wet it before removing it. A dry cord may stick to tissues and cause bleeding when removed. To prevent bleeding, the cord should be gently lifted from the sulcus rather than ripped out quickly.

6. Inspect the gingiva, sulcus, and preparation before proceeding with the impression. Check to see that the tissue is adequately retracted in *all* areas around the preparation, that it is not bleeding, and that the margins of the preparation are free of debris, blood, and astringent. (This is the second "stop sign.")

NOTE: The tissues will stay retracted long enough to control the field. The impression syringe should not be loaded until the field is dry, bleeding is controlled, and retraction is adequate. If a two-cord retraction technique is used in which a smaller cord is left in the sulcus during the impression, check to see that the smaller cord has stayed in place and has not lifted over the margins. If it has lifted, pack it back into place. If blood is oozing from the sulcus, control bleeding by scrubbing the sulcus with ferric sulfate astringent (such as Astringedent; Ultradent) on a small cotton pellet or applicator. Then, rinse residual astringent away, because compounds that contain sulfur can interfere with the set of polyvinyl siloxane impression materials.

7. With the preassembled dispenser gun and mixing tip, load the impression syringe with the light body material. Change cartridges and mixing tips. Load both the preparation and opposing arch sides of the double-bite tray with the heavy body material.

NOTE: The gun-type mixing system ensures a thorough mix with minimal waste of material. For efficiency of time and motion, two guns could be used and preassembled rather than having to unload the light body and load the heavy body with a single gun. Impression putty could be used in place of the heavy starting with the tip just apical to the margin. With the

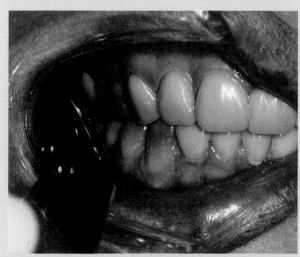

FIG. 15.60

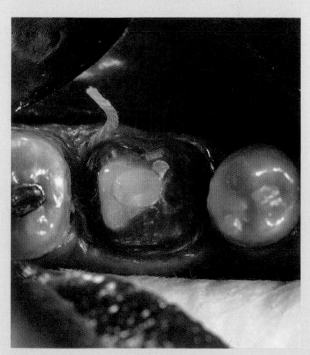

FIG. 15.61

Continued

Procedure 15.3   Making a Double-Bite Impression for a Crown—cont'd

material continually flowing, keep the tip in contact with the tooth while slowly tracing the margin and filling the gingival sulcus. Circle the entire tooth to completely cover the margins, and then continue circling while covering the axial walls and finally the occlusal surface (Fig. 15.62).

NOTE: Establishing a good finger rest will help stabilize the impression syringe. Some manufacturers provide a delivery tip that can be attached to the mixing tip to deliver the light body material directly to the preparation from the cartridge. This method can be awkward in the posterior part of the mouth because the end of the long mixing tip is far away from the operator's hand, making fine control of the tip difficult. Without good hand control, the tip frequently bounces out of contact with the preparation during injection of light body material around the tooth, creating air voids in critical parts of the impression. For retention grooves, the syringe tip should be placed at the bottom of the groove and the groove filled from the bottom to the top.

9. Place the impression tray over the teeth and instruct the patient to close into the rehearsed bite. Check the reference teeth to ensure that the patient has closed into the proper position (Fig. 15.63). Instruct the patient not to shift the bite or open until instructed to do so.

NOTE: A missed bite relation will result in a crown that is grossly high.

10. When the two viscosities of impression material have set, remove the impression. Rinse and dry the impression to remove saliva, blood, and debris.

Inspect it for completeness of the preparation detail. There should be a slight excess of impression material extending beyond the margins and no folds or voids (Fig. 15.64). Minor air bubbles in noncritical areas such as the occlusal surface might be acceptable. Check with the dentist.

NOTE: Folds on axial walls are often the result of material that did not join together at the start and end of the circling process around the tooth, because the material had started to set or because the circle was not completed with new material flowing into first-placed material. Air entrapment resulting in small or large voids is often the result of loss of contact of the syringe tip with the tooth during syringing of the material. If a two-cord retraction technique was used and the cord left in place during the impression comes out attached to the impression, do not attempt to remove it. The impression could tear. Cut off with scissors any loose ends of cord hanging from the impression and leave the cord that is embedded in the impression material.

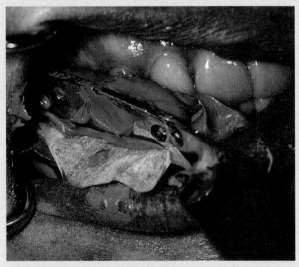

FIG. 15.63

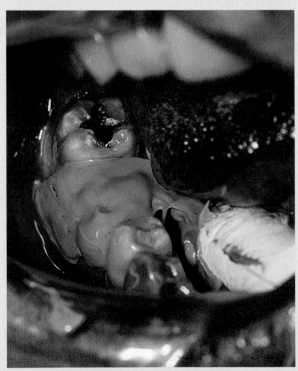

FIG. 15.62

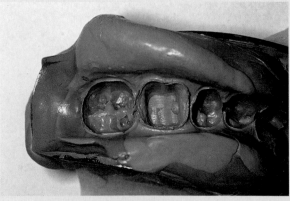

FIG. 15.64

Procedure 15.3 Making a Double-Bite Impression for a Crown—cont'd

11. Hold the impression up to the operatory light and inspect for proper occlusal contacts. The impression material will be very thin where there is contact between opposing teeth, and light can be seen through the material. If contacts are not in the proper locations, a separate bite registration may need to be made.

12. Spray the impression with a suitable disinfectant while it is contained within a plastic bag, seal it in a zippered plastic bag that has been labeled with the patient's name, and transport it to the laboratory (see Figs. 15.59 and 15.60 in Procedure 15.2).

Procedure 15.4 Bite Registration with Elastomeric Material

See Evolve site for Competency Sheet.

Consider the following with this procedure: safety glasses are recommended for the patient, PPE is required for the operator, ensure appropriate safety protocols are followed, and check your local state guidelines before performing this procedure.

EQUIPMENT/SUPPLIES
- Basic setup
- Plastic bite tray
- Elastomeric bite registration material in dual cartridge
- Automatic mixing extruder (gun-type) and mixing tips (Fig. 15.65)

PROCEDURE STEPS

1. Assemble the cartridge in the gun and extrude a small amount of bite registration material onto a paper towel to ensure that the orifices are not clogged.

NOTE: Clogged or partially clogged orifices will result in an improper mix of the materials, with alteration of setting time and physical properties.

2. Place the mixing tip on the cartridge.

3. Inform the patient of the procedure and have the patient practice closing into centric occlusion (the patient's "normal" bite) with the tray in place.

NOTE: Choose opposing teeth that are easily seen, such as the canines, and note their position when they occlude. This relationship will be checked when the bite registration is taken.

1. Dry the teeth to be included in the bite registration.

2. Extrude mixed material onto each side of the bite registration tray until the gauze is evenly covered with material about 2 mm thick (Fig. 15.66).

3. Center the tray over the mandibular teeth to be included and have the patient close into the practiced bite (Figs. 15.67 and 15.68).

NOTE: Now is the time to check the relationship of the opposing teeth (i.e., canines) to see if they are properly occluded.

4. Instruct the patient to hold the teeth together until the material is set (in 3 minutes or less).

NOTE: If the patient moves the teeth during the setting stage, a distortion will likely occur and will often be seen as imprints wider than the teeth.

5. Remove the bite tray when the material is set. Inspect it to see that all of the teeth needed for the registration are included and that there are no major voids (Fig. 15.69).

NOTE: When set, the material should not indent and should feel firm.

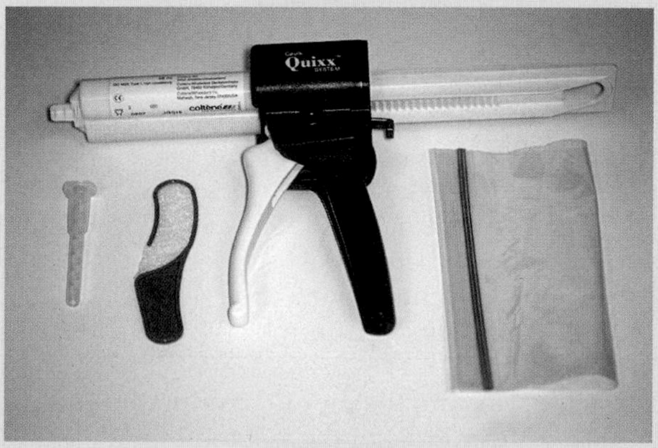

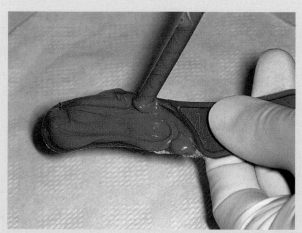

FIG. 15.65

FIG. 15.66

Continued

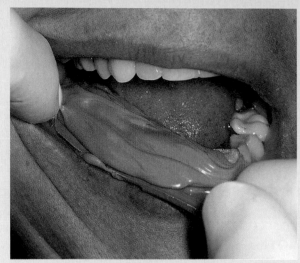

FIG. 15.67

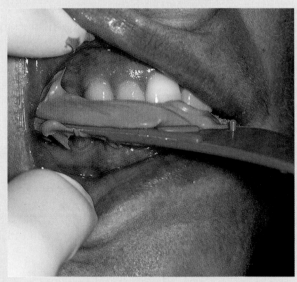

FIG. 15.68

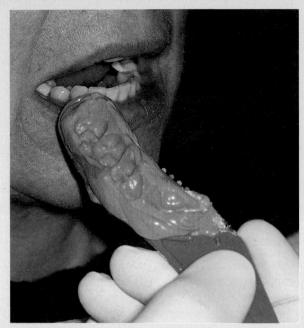

FIG. 15.69

teeth. The gauze with a thin layer of material should be present in these areas.

NOTE: If the material is thick in areas where there should be contact of opposing teeth, the patient may not have closed properly. Inspect the patient's occlusion and compare it with the bite registration. If there is an error, rehearse bite closure and repeat the procedure. If the tray is not inserted far enough posteriorly, the patient may bite on the back edge of tray rather than biting together completely.

7. Rinse the material under running water to remove saliva and debris.
8. Spray the bite registration material with a suitable disinfectant while it is contained within a plastic bag. Seal it in a zippered plastic bag labeled with the patient's name, and transport it to the laboratory.

6. Check for correct occlusion. Hold the bite registration material to the operatory light and see that light shines through in areas of contacting

---

See Evolve site for Competency Sheet.

Consider the following with this procedure: safety glasses are recommended for the patient, PPE is required for the operator, ensure appropriate safety protocols are followed, and check your local state guidelines before performing this procedure.

EQUIPMENT/SUPPLIES (Fig. 15.70)

- Bite registration wax or utility wax
- Heat source
- Laboratory knife

PROCEDURE STEPS

1. Heat utility wax sheets until pliable, and fold several times to get 3 to 4 layers of wax.

NOTE: You will need a thickness of 3 to 4 mm to avoid distortion when removing.

2. Form the wax into a horseshoe shape.

NOTE: You may need to reheat the wax to keep it pliable (Fig. 15.71).

3. Try the wax into the mouth, cutting the ends to fit only to the middle of the last tooth in the arch.

NOTE: If you are using preformed wax bite registration blocks, then you will need to trim them only for length (Fig. 15.72).

4. Seat the patient in the upright position and give him or her instructions on closing.

NOTE: Concerning patients in the supine position: if the patient's mouth has been open for a long time or is numb, the patient may close in an abnormal position.

5. Heat the wax again until softened.

NOTE: If using a flame source, assure the patient that the wax will not burn their tissues (Fig. 15.73).

6. Place the wax horseshoe onto the occlusal surfaces of the maxillary teeth (Fig. 15.74).

7. Instruct the patient to bite gently, yet firmly, into the wax.

NOTE: If the patient bites too firmly, the wax may be distorted and torn. If not firmly enough, the teeth may not make adequate indentations in the wax (Fig. 15.75).

8. Allow the wax to cool in the patient's mouth for 1 to 2 minutes.

NOTE: Use an air syringe to hasten cooling by gently spraying the area around the wax.

9. Have the patient open with a straight snap to avoid distortion of the wax.

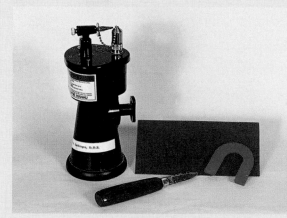

FIG. 15.70

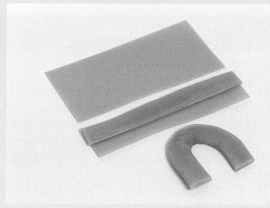

FIG. 15.71

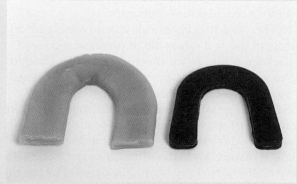

FIG. 15.72

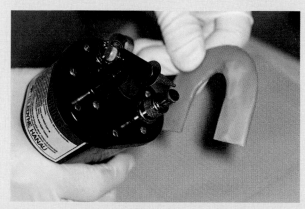

FIG. 15.73

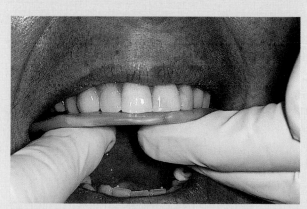

FIG. 15.74

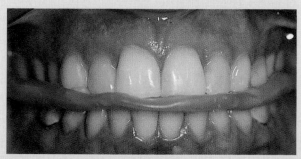

FIG. 15.75

Continued

Procedure 15.5   Wax Bite Registration—cont'd

10. Remove the wax bite registration carefully, being sure not to break or distort the wax (Fig. 15.76).
11. Disinfect the wax bite and store it in a bag labeled with the patient's name.
    NOTE: Follow the manufacturer's recommendations for use of this material. Some disinfecting agents may break down the wax.

12. Store the wax in a cool area (ideally at slightly less than room temperature).
    NOTE: You should try to use the wax as soon as possible to articulate models and to avoid distortion due to relaxation of residual stress (Fig. 15.77).

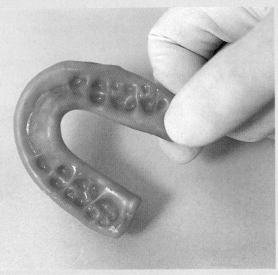

FIG. 15.76

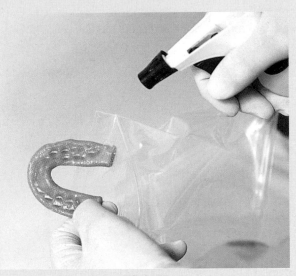

FIG. 15.77

Procedure 15.6   Disinfection of Impression Material or Bite Registration

See Evolve site for Competency Sheet.

Consider the following with this procedure: safety glasses are recommended for the patient, PPE is required for the operator, ensure appropriate safety protocols are followed, and check your local state guidelines before performing this procedure.

EQUIPMENT/SUPPLIES

- Impressions/bite registration
- Various disinfecting solutions in appropriate containers
- Zippered plastic bags

PROCEDURE STEPS

1. Rinse the impression under running tap water and shake off the excess.
   NOTE: Rinsing removes much of the saliva, blood, and other biological debris that can interfere with disinfection.
2. Immerse or spray the impression with an acceptable disinfectant prepared according to the manufacturer's instructions. If spraying, hold the impression within a plastic bag to contain the spray

(see Fig. 15.59 in Procedure 15.2).
   NOTE: Polyethers can be sensitive to immersion. ZOE should not be disinfected with chlorine-containing solutions, because it breaks down the material.
3. Leave the solution on the sprayed impression or leave the immersed impression in solution for the recommended time period.
   NOTE: Polyethers should not be immersed for longer than 10 minutes because they imbibe water and swell. Spraying is preferred.
4. Rinse with water and gently shake off the excess to remove any residual chemicals.
   NOTE: Residual chemicals can adversely affect the surface of the cast when the impression is poured.
5. Package properly for transport (see Fig. 15.60 in Procedure 15.2). A zippered plastic bag is usually satisfactory. Label with the patient's name.
   NOTE: Alginate and agar hydrocolloid should be wrapped in a damp paper towel (or place a few drops of water in the plastic zipper bag) to keep them from losing moisture and distorting. It is not necessary to wrap elastomers. They should be dried after the disinfectant is rinsed off.

Get Ready for Exams!

Review Questions

Select the one correct response for each of the following multiple-choice questions.

1. A dental impression material
   a. Forms a positive imprint of the oral structures involved
   b. Allows the creation of a replica of the structures involved
   c. Is always flexible for easy removal from the mouth
   d. Is used only for crown and bridge procedures and for diagnostic casts (study models)

2. Which one of the following impression materials is transformed from a sol to a gel state when set?
   a. Alginate
   b. Polysulfide
   c. Polyether
   d. Polyvinyl siloxane

3. All of the following are elastic impression materials *except* one. Which one?
   a. Alginate
   b. Polyether impression material
   c. Dental compound
   d. Polyvinyl siloxane (PVS) impression material

4. The types of impression materials that are considered hydrophilic are those that
   a. Have a lot of water in them
   b. Can be immersed in water without absorbing it
   c. Cause water to bead on their surface
   d. Have good surface-wetting characteristics

5. Hydrophobic impression materials
   a. Absorb moisture only after their final set
   b. Are the best type of material to use in the mouth because they repel saliva and blood
   c. Need a dry field to get the best results
   d. Provide the best surfaces on gypsum casts, because they resist the uptake of water during curing of the gypsum

6. Alginate impression material
   a. Is accurate enough to be used for crown and bridge procedures
   b. Has very few uses in the modern dental practice
   c. Is dimensionally stable during the first 24 hours
   d. Can be immersed in an appropriate disinfectant for up to 30 minutes without distorting

7. An irreversible hydrocolloid
   a. Is one that goes from a gel to a sol when it is heated
   b. Is no longer in common use
   c. Is hydrophobic
   d. Cannot reverse from a gel to a sol because a chemical reaction prevents it

8. The elastic recovery (or rebound) of alginate impression material can be increased by which *one* of the following?
   a. Leaving the impression in the mouth for 1 minute beyond its set.
   b. Using a thicker mix of material
   c. Using cold water in the mix
   d. Removing the impression slowly from the mouth

9. Preliminary impressions are useful for all of the following *except* one. Which one?
   a. Diagnostic casts (study models)
   b. All-ceramic inlays
   c. Custom trays
   d. Provisional restorations

10. Three of the following impression materials are the most commonly used. Which *one* is not commonly used?
    a. Polysulfide
    b. Polyether
    c. Polyvinyl siloxane
    d. Alginate

11. The three key properties that materials used for final impressions must possess include all of the following *except* one. Which one?
    a. Accuracy
    b. Dimensional stability
    c. Wettability
    d. Tear resistance

12. Which one of the following impression materials has the lowest tear strength?
    a. Polyvinyl siloxane
    b. Polyether
    c. Vinyl polyether hybrid
    d. Alginate

13. It is important for an accurate impression that the tray not be
    a. Too smooth
    b. Too flexible
    c. Too rigid
    d. Perforated

14. Which *one* of the elastomers has the highest natural (no chemicals added) wettability?
    a. Polyvinyl siloxane
    b. Polysulfide
    c. Polyether

15. As the viscosity of the impression material increases, which *one* of the following properties decreases?
    a. Accuracy
    b. Tear strength
    c. Dimensional stability
    d. Setting time

16. Which of the following elastomers will imbibe water when stored in it and change dimensions?
    a. Polysulfides
    b. Polyethers
    c. Addition silicones

17. Which *one* of the following statements is *true* about the addition silicones?
    a. They are good materials for complete denture impressions but are not accurate for crown and bridge procedures.
    b. They are very dimensionally stable.
    c. They cost about the same as alginate.
    d. They require the use of custom acrylic trays.

18. The least accurate of the elastic impression materials is
    a. Polyvinyl siloxane
    b. Polyether

Continued

　　c. Vinyl polyether silicone hybrid
　　d. Alginate

19. After removing a PVS impression form the mouth it is found that the surface has unset material on it. What can cause this to happen?
　　a. Incomplete mixing of the material
　　b. Residual ferric sulfate astringent on the teeth
　　c. Contamination from latex gloves
　　d. All of the above

20. PVS substitutes for alginate have all of the following advantages *except* one. Which one?
　　a. Dimensionally stable for long periods
　　b. Less expensive than alginate
　　c. Can be re-poured several times
　　d. Do not have to be poured right away

21. At present, the most common conservative method of creating space in the gingival sulcus of a prepared tooth for wash (syringe) material is which *one* of the following?
　　a. Retraction paste
　　b. Retraction cord
　　c. Laser troughing
　　d. Electrosurgical troughing

22. Which *one* of the following astringents has the potential to be dangerous to patients with cardiovascular disease?
　　a. Racemic epinephrine
　　b. Ferric sulfate
　　c. Aluminum chloride
　　d. ViscoStat

23. Reasons the wash material may tear when removing the set impression from the mouth include all of the following *except one*. Which one?
　　a. Narrow sulcus width (<0.2 mm)
　　b. Very deep sulcus
　　c. Sharp edges on the preparation
　　d. Removing the impression with a snap

24. A successful double-bite impression for a crown on tooth #30 includes all of the following *except* one. Which one?
　　a. The margins of the preparation are shiny and rounded.
　　b. The margins and a little of the tooth beyond are captured in the impression.
　　c. No large voids are present in the walls of the preparation.
　　d. Opposing teeth are captured in the proper bite relation.

25. Digital impressions have several advantages over traditional impressions. Which *one* of the following is *not* an advantage?
　　a. Impression material and associated supplies are not needed.
　　b. Digital impressions can be electronically transferred to the laboratory.
　　c. Images of the preparation can be viewed from multiple angles before being sent to the laboratory.
　　d. Gingival retraction is not needed for preparations with subgingival margins.

26. Which *one* of the following impression materials is *least* affected by soaking it in a disinfectant solution for 2 hours?
　　a. Alginate
　　b. Polyether
　　c. Polyvinyl siloxane

27. Disinfecting of impressions
　　a. Is done to protect the patient from surface bacteria
　　b. Must be done for all impressions
　　c. Is done only with impressions for patients with known infectious diseases
　　d. Does not need to be done for the new alginates that have bactericidal chemicals incorporated into them

For answers to Review Questions, see the Appendix.

Case-Based Discussion Topics

1. A 30-year-old retail store manager comes to the dental office to have impressions made for home whitening trays. She indicates that she has a moderate gag reflex.
What impression material is well suited for making whitening trays? What steps can be taken to minimize gagging and to shorten the length of time the impression material remains in the mouth? How should the impression material be handled from the time it is removed from the mouth until it is poured with dental plaster or stone?

2. A dentist practicing in California decides to use the services of a dental laboratory located in New York City. He plans to mail all of his impressions to the laboratory rather than pour them in his office.
What types of impression materials can be used under these circumstances that will still produce accurate casts and dies? Which materials definitely cannot be used? What properties of the materials are most important? How should the impressions be handled before they are shipped to the laboratory?

3. A 53-year-old mail carrier comes to the dental office with a broken facial cusp on tooth #31. Adjacent to #31, the patient has a fixed bridge from #28 to #30 that has a hygienic pontic replacing tooth #29. The dentist will prepare #31 for a porcelain-bonded-to-metal crown, and the dental hygienist or assistant with extended functions will make an impression. Isolation is difficult because the patient salivates profusely, and the gingiva is bleeding because the patient is taking blood thinners. The clinician will be able to control most of the saliva. The bleeding will be greatly reduced when a local anesthetic with a vasoconstrictor is injected into the gingival papillae around the tooth. However, the preparation will not be completely dry.
Which elastomer, by its nature, is somewhat hydrophilic and could be used? Which materials are not naturally hydrophilic but may have surfactants added to make them more hydrophilic? What precautions should be taken before the impression is made to ensure that it can be easily removed from the mouth?

4. The dentist in your office will replace an existing crown on tooth #5 for a young female college student because of recurrent caries under the distal margin. The dentist likes to use a two-step polyvinyl siloxane (PVS) putty/wash technique. You will be asked to prepare an acrylic custom provisional crown for the patient.

How should you prepare for this before the dentist removes the crown, using the materials at hand? What types of impression trays can the dentist use with this technique? Can a polysulfide tray adhesive be used with the PVS putty? How soon does the PVS impression have to be poured? What disinfectants are safe to use with PVS materials?

5. The dentist uses polyether in the office for crown and bridge impressions. This afternoon, a call came in from the dental laboratory indicating that the laboratory's delivery person had been in an automobile accident yesterday; the dies picked up from the dentist's office were broken.

Can the dentist repour the impression and send new dies? Why or why not? Which of the impression materials are good for this purpose? Which elastomer has the greatest accuracy for the longest time?

6. A variety of impression materials may be used in the dental office on a daily basis. It is important to protect all dental personnel who might handle the impressions by proper disinfection. In addition, the accuracy of the impressions might be adversely affected by improper disinfection techniques.

Describe the procedures for disinfecting alginate, polyvinyl siloxane, and polyether impression materials.

7. A dental hygienist licensed with extended functions is preparing to make a PVS impression of tooth #19 for a gold crown. The hygienist has packed cord according to the two-cord technique. The hygienist needed to scrub the gingival sulcus with ferric sulfate astringent to control bleeding.

Before making the impression, what criteria should the hygienist use to determine whether the top cord is properly placed? Once the top cord is removed, what criteria should be used to determine whether the next steps for making the impression can be taken? What should be done to the prepared tooth surfaces once the bleeding has been controlled with ferric sulfate? When the impression has been completed, what criteria will the hygienist use to determine whether the impression can be used for the crown?

BIBLIOGRAPHY

Bayne SC: Impression Materials [PowerPoint presentation]. Available at Open. Michigan website Ann Arbor, MI: University of Michigan. http://open.umich.edu/education/dent/dental-materials/2008/materials or http://www-personal.umich.edu/~sbayne/dental-materials/117-Impression-Materials/Handouts/117-IM-PPT-Handout-CL.pdf.

Bird DL, Robinson DS: Impression materials. In *Torres and Ehrlich's Modern Dental Assisting* (ed. 12). Philadelphia, 2018, Elsevier/Saunders.

Boksman L, Cowie RR: Making polyvinyl impressions: success lies in the details. *Contemporary Dental Assisting*, 28–32, 2007.

Burgess JO: Impression material basics. *Inside Dentistry*, 1(1), 2005.

Burgess JO, Lawson NC, Robles A: Comparing digital and conventional impressions. *Inside Dentistry*, 68–74, 2013.

Burgess JO, Lawson NC, Robles A: Digital impression system considerations. *Inside Dentistry*, 72–76, 2015.

Farah JW, Powers JM, editors: Bite registration materials. *Dental Advisor*, 15:2, 1998.

Merchant VA: Infection control in the dental laboratory environment. In Cottone JA, Terezhalmy GT, editors: *Molinari GT) Practical Infection Control in Dentistry* (ed 2). Philadelphia, 1996, Williams & Wilkins.

Organization for Safety and Asepsis Procedures: Impression disinfection. *OSAP Monthly Focus*, 7:1, 1998.

Powers JM, Wataha JC: Impression materials. In *Dental Materials: Foundations and Applications* (ed 11). St. Louis, 2017, Elsevier.

Sakaguchi RL, Powers JM: Replicating materials—impression and casting. In *Craig's Restorative Dental Materials* (ed 13). St. Louis, 2012, Elsevier/Mosby.

Shull GF: An update on CAD/CAM dentistry. *Dental Learning February*, 4(2):2–8, 2015.

Skramstad M: The clinical application of CAD/CAM technology and materials. *Dental Learning*, 1(6), 2012.

Chapter Objectives

Upon completion of this chapter, the student should be able to:

1. Differentiate between negative and positive reproduction.
2. Differentiate among diagnostic cast, working cast, and dies.
3. Describe the chemical and physical nature of gypsum products.
4. Explain the manufacturing process for gypsum products and how this affects their physical characteristics.
5. Compare the following properties and behaviors of gypsum products: strength, dimensional accuracy, solubility, and reproduction of detail.
6. List the American Dental Association–recognized gypsum products and their most appropriate uses.
7. Explain initial and final set of gypsum and the factors that affect the setting time, setting expansion, and strength.
8. Explain the procedure for mixing and handling gypsum products to create diagnostic casts.
9. Identify the common components of dental waxes.
10. Compare the properties of waxes.
11. Describe the clinical/laboratory significance of each of the properties of waxes.
12. Discuss the three classifications of waxes.
13. Differentiate between direct and indirect waxings and identify which property of dental waxes is most important in their difference.
14. Describe the usual color, form, and use of inlay, casting, baseplate, boxing, utility, and sticky waxes.
15. Prepare model plaster or stone for pouring.
16. Pour the anatomic and base portions of maxillary and mandibular diagnostic casts.
17. Trim maxillary and mandibular diagnostic casts.
18. Obtain a bite registration, using bite registration or utility wax.

Key Terms

Casts hard replicas of hard and soft tissue of the patient's oral cavity, made from gypsum products; also referred to as *models*

Diagnostic Casts casts generally made from dental plaster or stone and used for patient education, treatment planning, and tracking the progress of treatment, as with orthodontic models; these casts are also known as *study models*

Working Casts casts generally made from one of the dental stones that are strong enough to resist the stresses of fabricating an indirect restoration or prosthesis; these casts are also known as *master casts* or *working models*

Dies replicas of the prepared teeth that are generally removable from the working cast

Model Plaster the weakest, most porous form of gypsum product used in dentistry

Dental Stone a stronger, less porous form of gypsum product used in dentistry

Die Stone the densest form of gypsum product used in dentistry

Pouring *pouring the cast* refers to the process of vibrating the flowable gypsum product into an impression; this process must produce a cast that is an exact replica of the structures captured in the impression

Trimming the process of removing excess hardened gypsum from the cast for ease in working with the cast and appearance in presentation

Melting Range a range of melting points of the individual components of wax

Flow the movement of wax as it approaches the melting range

Excess Residue a wax film that remains on an object after the wax is removed

Wax Pattern a duplicate of a restoration carved in wax

Lost Wax Technique a technique for fabricating a metal restoration by encasing the wax pattern in stone and then vaporizing the wax under high temperatures to leave an empty impression space once occupied by the wax; molten metal is then cast into the space and takes the shape of the pattern

Gypsum is a mineral widely found in nature that has been used for making dental casts since 1756. Dental casts and dies are used as replicas of the hard and soft tissues of the patient's oral cavity. First, an impression, the negative reproduction of the patient's mouth, is taken using a soft, elastic material. This

impression is filled with a gypsum material made from a fine powder that is mixed with water to form a flowable mass. Once hardened, this material will be a hard, stable positive reproduction, or cast, of the hard and soft tissues (Fig. 16.1). These hard replicas are used to plan and track the progress of treatment.

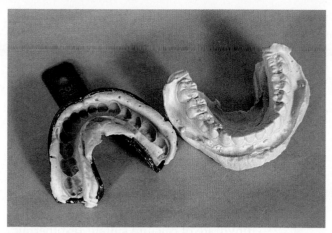

FIG. 16.1 Impressions (negative reproductions) are poured into gypsum to form casts (positive reproductions).

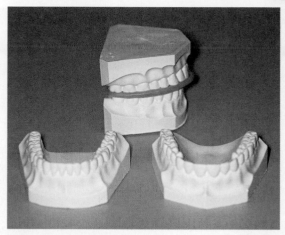

FIG. 16.2 Diagnostic casts made from plaster. (From Bird DL, Robinson DS: *Modern Dental Assisting* (ed 12). St. Louis, 2018, Elsevier.)

They are also used in laboratory procedures, where they serve as the replicas on which dental procedures, either unsafe or too difficult to do directly in the mouth, are performed. The dental auxiliary is frequently called upon to produce these replicas. In some states, the assistant or the hygienist may fabricate intraoral prostheses on these replicas. Both auxiliaries may also find the resultant model useful in presenting information for patient education. The production of gypsum casts requires meticulous attention to detail, a well-thought-out process in their production, and knowledge of the advantages and limitations of each gypsum material for appropriate selection. Inaccurate, incomplete, or weak casts are of little use and are likely to produce costly mistakes in patient treatment procedures.

Dental waxes are used in a wide variety of clinical and laboratory dental procedures. Clinically, they may be used to fabricate direct waxing patterns for cast restorations; alterations and adaptations for impression trays; and wax bite registrations. In the laboratory, they may be used to box an impression before pouring a gypsum product, as baseplates for full and partial dentures, to hold components together before articulation, and to provide indirect patterns for casting.

The dental assistant and hygienist typically will not fabricate the actual direct or indirect wax pattern for a dental casting, but they do need an appreciation for the many steps in the procedure known as the lost wax technique (described later in this chapter). The assistant and the hygienist will frequently manipulate waxes in making alginate impressions, pouring impressions, and making a wax bite registration for articulation of models.

USES AND DESIRABLE QUALITIES OF GYPSUM

Gypsum products are most frequently used to make replicas of the patient's mouth. These replicas are called *diagnostic casts, working casts,* and *dies*. Each of these has a specific purpose in the treatment planning or fabrication of intraoral appliances, prostheses, or restorations.

Diagnostic casts: Also called *study models*, diagnostic casts are used to plan treatment and observe the oral structures of the mouth. Orthodontists use study models extensively as they plan and treat the alignment of the teeth. (Fig. 16.2)

Working casts: Also called *working models*, working casts are used to fabricate appliances such as an orthodontic retainer or bleaching tray or a removable prosthesis such as a partial or full denture. (Fig. 16.3)

Dies: Dies are replicas of individual teeth or groups of teeth and are used to fabricate crowns and bridges. (Fig. 16.4)

Diagnostic casts, working casts, and dies are not required to meet the same use stresses; therefore they do not have the same physical property requirements. The accuracy of each of these replicas is dependent on the accuracy of the impression from which they are poured. The accuracy and use of the replica also depend on the gypsum material used and the properties of this material.

DESIRABLE QUALITIES OF GYPSUM PRODUCTS

There are several desirable qualities for gypsum products used in the making of diagnostic and working casts or dies. These qualities have differing significance depending on the use stresses applied to the product. The importance of qualities such as accuracy, reproduction of fine detail, dimensional stability, hardness, strength, and resistance to abrasion, solubility, ease of use, cost, color, and safety depend on the application of the product. All casts and dies must be accurate, hard, and dimensionally stable under normal conditions of use and storage. Because working casts and dies are used to fabricate intraoral prostheses and restorations they must also have excellent reproduction of fine detail, strength and resistance to abrasion, and minimal solubility. Color is important in the identification of the material and to provide contrast between the die material and the waxed inlay pattern. The amount of expansion of the gypsum material during its set is important to the overall accuracy of the cast. The cost, ease of use, and safety are practical considerations in the manipulation of the product and frequency of its use.

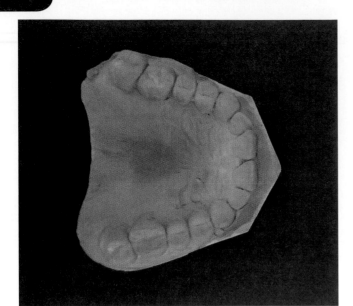

FIG. 16.3 Working cast made of dental stone used to fabricate appliances. (Courtesy of Steve Eakle.)

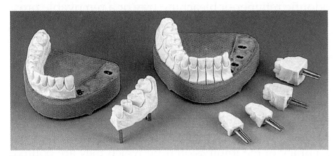

FIG. 16.4 Dies which are replicas of individual teeth used to fabricate crowns and bridges. (Courtesy of Pocket Dentistry.)

PROPERTIES AND BEHAVIORS OF GYPSUM PRODUCTS

CHEMICAL PROPERTIES

Chemically, the mineral gypsum is a dihydrate of calcium sulfate ($CaSO_4 \cdot 2H_2O$), which is mined as solid mass. To form it into a powder, the manufacturer heats this dihydrate, which causes it to lose water. It is then ground to produce a powdered hemihydrate, $CaSO_4 \cdot \frac{1}{2}H_2O$. This process is referred to as *calcination*. When the hemihydrate is again mixed with water, a viscous product capable of flowing is produced. Once this chemical reaction is complete, the hemihydrate is converted back to a dihydrate and becomes again a solid mass. The byproduct of the chemical reaction is heat, so it is called an *exothermic reaction*. The amount of water required to mix with the calcium sulfate hemihydrate is greater than the amount required for the chemical reaction. This excess water produces a mix that can flow into the details of dental impressions. The excess water evaporates on setting, and a mass of interlocking gypsum crystals is produced. Between the gypsum crystals are small voids of air that were once occupied by the water that has evaporated. The amount and size of the air voids remaining are directly related to the final hardness, strength, and

resistance to abrasion of the final product. The components of all gypsum products are chemically the same; the physical differences in the materials are due to the differences in calcination and the resulting amount of water that is drawn off the dihydrate.

Calcination:

Mineralsgypsum (dihydrate of calcicum sulfate)

$$\xrightarrow{\text{heat and/or pressure}} \text{calcium sulfate hemihydrate} + \text{water}$$

Reverse reaction:

Calcium sulfate hemihydrate + water
$$\rightarrow \text{dihydrate of calcium sulfate (exothermic)}$$

> **Clinical Tip**
>
> Plaster contains the most excess water of the various gypsum mixes and therefore produces bigger and more numerous air voids; die stone contains the least excess water and therefore produces fewer, smaller air voids.

PRODUCTION OF GYPSUM PRODUCTS

Production of the various forms of gypsum is basically the same. With some modifications, they are used for several different purposes. Ground gypsum (i.e., calcium sulfate dihydrate) is heated during the manufacturing process until it loses water and becomes calcium sulfate hemihydrate. If the heating process occurs in open vats at a temperature of approximately 115 °C (239 °F), the resulting hemihydrate is porous and irregular in shape. This process will form **model plaster** or β-hemihydrate commonly used for diagnostic casts (study models). If the heating process is done under pressure, in the presence of steam, and at a higher temperature (125 °C [257 °F]), a more uniformly shaped and less porous form of hemihydrate, referred to as **dental stone**, is produced. Dental stone is used for working casts (master casts). By first boiling the gypsum rock in a 30% calcium chloride solution a high-density raw material called *densite* is produced. This densite material is then washed and heated with a greater increase in pressure, and then even more refining of the powder by grinding results in the densest stone known as high-strength or **die stone**. This additional refining makes even more regular particles with better packing ability, thus reducing the amount of water required for mixing and increasing the final density of the product. When high-strength stone is mixed with silica, it forms *dental investment*, a material able to withstand the high heat and stress produced when molten metal is forced into molds to form indirect restorations by the lost wax technique (described later in this chapter).

> **Clinical Tip**
>
> The increase in water necessary to mix a gypsum product also increases the setting time and reduces the strength and hardness of the set gypsum.

PHYSICAL PROPERTIES

Physically, gypsum products are manufactured as plaster, stone, high-strength stone, and gypsum-bonded investment. The main differences in the physical forms are dependent on the variations in size, shape, and porosity of the powders produced by the different manufacturing processes. The larger, more irregular and porous the particles of powder, the weaker and less resistant to abrasion the final product becomes (Fig. 16.5).

Its properties and behavior determine the specific use of the gypsum product. Properties of strength, abrasion resistance, and solubility and behaviors of setting time and expansion vary in importance, depending on the application. Diagnostic casts, for example, are placed under little stress and are usually produced from less expensive materials such as plaster or stone, both of which have lower properties of strength and abrasion resistance. Working casts and dies require materials resistant to greater stresses and thus require higher properties of strength and abrasion resistance and precise accuracy; therefore setting expansion must be carefully controlled.

Strength, Hardness, and Resistance to Abrasion

The morphology of the gypsum particles determines the properties and behavior of the gypsum product. Factors that affect the strength of gypsum products also affect their hardness. Two factors contribute to the strength and abrasion resistance of the final product: the shape of the particles and their porosity; how much water is needed to mix the product. The strength of gypsum products is related to the amount of water, and more critically, excess water, used in producing the study or working cast. Factors that affect the strength of gypsum products also affect their hardness. Because gypsum products require varying amounts of water to wet and incorporate the powder into a workable mixture, it follows that the more water that is used, the weaker the cast will be. Increased porosity of the particles makes it necessary to use more water to convert the hemihydrate particles back to dihydrate particles. A product with less water has a higher density of crystals and is therefore a denser and stronger product. The larger, more irregularly shaped particles are prevented from fitting together densely. For instance, plaster particles are both porous and irregular, requiring more water to mix. The resulting product has more air space because of the less densely packed particles, making plaster considerably weaker than the less porous and more densely packed stone products.

The strength of the gypsum product is an indicator of its ability to resist fracture. Compressive strength of plaster is four times less than that of densite and three times less than that of stone. The tensile strength of plaster is half that of stone. American Dental Association (ADA) specifications require that the material reach minimal compression strength (i.e., wet strength) 1 hour after setting.

 Clinical Tip

To reach maximal strength (i.e., dry strength), the cast may need to set in a dry environment for several hours or overnight.

Dimensional Accuracy

Setting expansion occurs with all gypsum products. Plaster expands the most, at 0.30%, and high-strength stone products the least, at 0.10%. Setting expansion is a result of the growth of crystals as the particles join. Controlling setting expansion is critical for the production of accurate models and dies. It is important that expansion be held to a minimum, particularly when the material is being used to fabricate restorations and dental prostheses. If expansion were excessive, any die fabricated from the gypsum material would eventually result in an oversized restoration. Although some expansion is acceptable for models fabricated from plaster, expansion of die materials would be a source of costly errors. Strict proportioning of water and powder, and of the chemical additives provided by the manufacturer, is required to produce dies with the required level of accuracy. Power-driven, vacuum-mixed, high-strength stone, as produced by dental laboratory technicians, will expand less than if the stone is hand mixed. Setting expansion occurs only during hardening of the gypsum product. No changes occur under normal conditions of use and storage once the product has reached its final set.

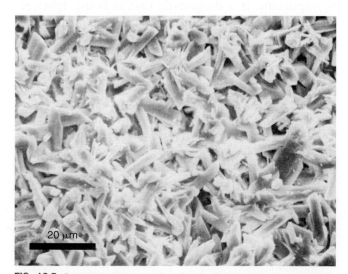

FIG. 16.5 Scanning electron micrograph of the surface of set high-strength dental stone (die stone). The surface is porous with many interlocking crystals of calcium sulfate dihydrate. To the naked eye this surface would appear smooth. (From Powers JM, Wataha JC: *Dental Materials: Properties and Manipulation* (ed 10). St. Louis, 2013, Elsevier, p. 115.)

Reproduction of Detail

The greater the porosity of the final gypsum product, the less surface detail is produced. Even products that have the least amount of porosity have surface irregularities visible at the microscopic level.

Contamination of an impression with blood, food debris, or saliva will affect the surface detail. The impression should be rinsed with water and closely inspected for extraneous materials, and all water used in this rinsing should be thoroughly removed before pouring the impression. Compressed air via the air/water syringe is the best method of removing all the water from the impression prior to pouring.

Compatibility of impression material and gypsum material can influence the quality of surface reproduction. Gypsum materials flow best when there is compatible wetting with the surface of the impression. *Wetting* describes the ability of a material to flow and not bead up, like water on a waxed surface. A decrease in wetting may prevent the gypsum material from flowing into all the details of the impression, leaving air voids from bubbles. Impression materials that are water based work better with water-based gypsum materials: for example, agar and alginate impression materials are water based and generally form the best surface detail with gypsum products. It is always important to follow the manufacturer's directions in selecting gypsum products that are compatible with impression materials.

Silicone, polyvinylsiloxane and polyether impression materials, which are not water based, may benefit from the addition of a surfactant sprayed into the impression before pouring to aid the gypsum in wetting the impression material. The surfactant helps in the wetting of the impression, thus allowing the gypsum material to flow more easily on the impression surface. Spray surfactants should be used sparingly as pooling of the surfactant in the impression will result in chalky areas on the model. A new material on the market distributes surfactant throughout the gypsum product to ensure an equal distribution of surfactant to the entire impression. The product (Wonderadmix; Dental Creations) (Fig. 16.6) helps to eliminate pouring bubbles by breaking the surface tension and allowing the gypsum to glide over the surface of the impression. Wonderadmix is added to the water before the gypsum powder is introduced.

Solubility

Set gypsum products are not highly soluble in water. Solubility is directly related to the porosity of the material; therefore plaster is much more soluble than stone. Exposing models to water for prolonged periods should be avoided (Table 16.1) as they will lose much surface detail as they begin to dissolve.

 Clinical Tip

If gypsum needs to be soaked in water, the soaking should be done in *slurry water*, that is, water saturated with plaster particles to prevent the loss of surface detail.

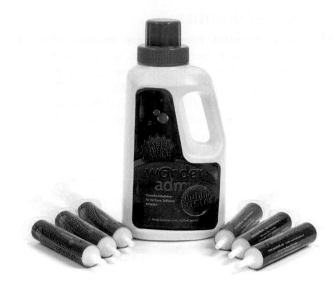

FIG. 16.6 Surfactant which can be added to gypsum to prevent bubbles from occurring. (Courtesy WonderAdmix.)

 Clinical Tip

CAD/CAM technology (see Chapter 9) uses a digital image of the preparation and can avoid the use of stone dies when the restoration is made in one visit without the use of models. Therefore many of the problems mentioned above regarding strength, abrasion, dimensional accuracy, and solubility can be avoided.

CLASSIFICATION OF GYPSUM PRODUCTS

The desired physical properties and behavior necessary for a particular use determine the criteria for selection of a gypsum product. If strength is desired, the choice of a stone or high-strength stone material is important. If a diagnostic cast is being fabricated, plaster or stone is adequate. ADA specification number 25 identifies the following five gypsum products.

IMPRESSION PLASTER (TYPE I)

Impression plaster is rarely used by today's dentists, having been replaced with the less rigid, elastic impression materials. If selected, it would be used as a final impression wash for edentulous arches. Impression plaster may also be used to mount casts on an articulator. A dental articulator is a mechanical device used to place maxillary and mandibular casts in occlusion and in a fixed position (Fig. 16.7). This device is used in the fabrication of removable and fixed prosthodontic appliances.

MODEL PLASTER (TYPE II)

Model plaster is frequently used for diagnostic casts and articulation of stone casts. It has a water-to-powder

Table 16.1   Properties of Gypsum Products

TYPE*	POROSITY	COMPRESSIVE STRENGTH (MPa)	ABRASION RESISTANCE	SETTING EXPANSION
Type II: Model plaster	High	8.8	Low	High
Type III: Dental stone	Moderate	20.6	Moderate	Moderate
Type IV: High-strength/ low-expansion stone	Low	34.3	High	Low
Type V: High-strength/ high-expansion stone	Low	48.0	High	High

MPa, megapascal (1 MPa equals approximately 145 lb/in²); *W/P ratio*, water-to-powder ratio (milliliters of water per gram of powder).
*Type I (impression plaster) is rarely used by today's dentists.

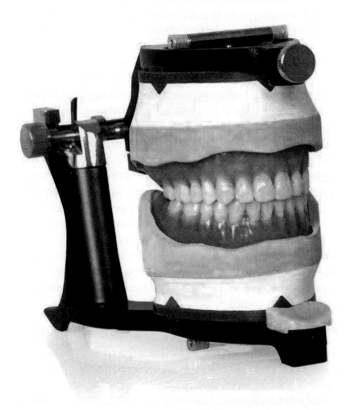

FIG. 16.7 Articulated working casts with full upper and lower removable prosthodontics. (Courtesy of Keystone Industries.)

(W/P) ratio of approximately 0.45 (i.e., 0.45 ml of water per 100 grams of powder), which produces a durable but relatively weak cast when compared with the stone categories. The irregular shapes of the particles prevent them from fitting together tightly. These study casts do not require a significant amount of strength or abrasion resistance. Model plaster is available in fast and regular sets and is easy to manipulate. This product is traditionally produced in a white color to distinguish it from dental stones. Because of its simple manufacturing processes, plaster is the least costly of all the gypsum products.

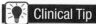 **Clinical Tip**

Model plaster is different from orthodontic plaster, which is a mixture of plaster and stone.

Uses of Diagnostic Casts

- Provide a three-dimensional record of the patient's hard and soft tissues
- Facilitate study of the occlusal relationship of the dental arches
- Facilitate study of tooth size, position, and shape and arch relations
- Facilitate study of hard and soft tissues from the lingual view while teeth are in occlusion
- Provide a record of present conditions for comparison as treatment progresses
- Provide a visual aid for patient education
- Provide a legal record of the patient's arches for insurance, legal suits, and forensics

DENTAL STONE (TYPE III)

Dental stone (e.g., *Hydrocal, USG Corporation*), is ideal for making full or partial denture models, orthodontic models, and casts requiring higher strength and abrasive resistance. Dental stone has uniformly shaped, relatively nonporous crystals. Because of the particle characteristics, dental stone requires less water (W/P ratio = 0.30); its particles therefore pack together more tightly (i.e., the material is denser) and approximately 2.5 times stronger than plaster. Stone is easy to use, moderately expensive, and traditionally colored yellow or white.

DENTAL STONE, HIGH-STRENGTH/ LOW-EXPANSION (TYPE IV)

Type IV materials are often referred to as *die stones* or *densite* because they are especially suited for fabricating wax patterns for cast restorations. A hard, abrasive-resistant surface is necessary to resist the abrasion of sharp instruments used to carve wax on these stone dies. Their crystals are slightly larger and more dense than stone. These products require very strict and detailed handling, are often colored pink or green, have a W/P ratio of 0.23, and are almost two times stronger than type III stones.

DENTAL STONE HIGH-STRENGTH/ HIGH-EXPANSION (TYPE V)

Type 5, a recent addition to the list of ADA gypsum products, has been developed in response to the need for even higher strength, high-expansion dental stones and materials that can withstand the high temperatures (1500 °C [2732 °F]) required by the casting process. The addition of silica, a refractory material, improves the material's resistance to heat and is the reason the material has increased thermal expansion. Higher expansion may seem to be an undesirable property, but it is needed to compensate for the greater casting shrinkage of the newer base metals used for dental castings. These materials are also referred to as *gypsum-based investment*. The increased strength is obtained from a W/P ratio of 0.20. This material, colored blue or green, is the most costly of all the gypsum products.

METAL-PLATED AND EPOXY DIES AND RESIN-REINFORCED DIE STONE

Type IV and V gypsum products are commonly used die materials. These materials are very hard, but they are susceptible to abrasion during carving of wax patterns. Dies are occasionally electroplated with metal to produce better surface detail and make them less susceptible to abrasion. Silver or copper plating can create metal-plated dies that are highly resistant to abrasion. The electroplating process forms a thin shell of metal on the outside of the die.

Epoxy dies use a resin and hardener to produce a die that is harder and has greater abrasion resistance than high-strength stone. These epoxy materials set slowly and may require 16 to 24 hours for setting. Newer fast-set epoxy materials are supplied in an automix system similar to automix impression materials (see Chapter 15 Impression Materials). The epoxy resin and catalyst are forced through the mixing tip directly into the final impression. These fast-set products harden within 30 minutes.

Some gypsum product die stones have resin particles added to reinforce the high-strength stone and make them more abrasion resistant.

INVESTMENT MATERIALS

Investment materials are used to form metal castings through the lost wax technique. These materials, which combine gypsum and silica, can be used to produce models sufficiently strong to allow molten metal to be poured into them. Investment materials have increased expansion on setting; this expansion is necessary to compensate for the shrinkage of metal castings. New controlled expansion liquid is available to replace the use of water for mixing of investment materials. This liquid formulation is used to achieve greater expansion, allowing the dental laboratory technician to achieve optimal fit for a variety of materials.

MANIPULATION OF GYPSUM PRODUCTS

MATERIAL SELECTION

As previously mentioned, the selection of a gypsum product should be based on the desired properties of the material. If a diagnostic cast is being fabricated, dental

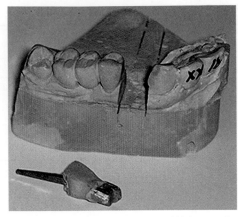

FIG. 16.8 A working cast with a stone base and high-strength stone anatomic portion, and a die made from high-strength stone with metal plating.

plaster is the appropriate choice because of the low physical property requirements and because of its low cost and ease of manipulation. A working cast would require higher strength, accuracy, hardness, and abrasion resistance and therefore would probably be made from dental stone. The dimensional accuracy, strength, and abrasion resistance required for a die would make high-strength stone the best choice. In some instances, a combination of one or more gypsum products is appropriate to curtail cost and increase ease of manipulation. When working models for cast restorations are being made, the die (the replica of the tooth on which, e.g., a crown is being fabricated) is poured of high-strength stone and the remaining teeth and base are poured with type III stone (Fig. 16.8). The entire working model is attached to a dental articulator with plaster.

PROPORTIONING (WATER-TO-POWDER RATIO)

The properties of gypsum products are directly related to their W/P ratio. It is important that the mixed material have sufficient flow to reproduce accurate and minute surface detail; it should be remembered that an increase in the recommended water will result in a thinner mix that takes longer to set but because more water was used, the final product will be considerably weaker, and less accurate. If water is decreased, the mixture will be thicker and may become difficult to manipulate, because it does not produce a flowable mix. Strict adherence to the manufacturer's suggested W/P ratio is recommended (Table 16.2).

 Caution

The W/P ratio has a direct effect on the properties of the resultant product and must be carefully controlled.

Water should be measured with a graduated cylinder and powder weighed on a scale. The use of scoops to measure powder is not recommended because the powder tends to pack down over time as it sits in a container. The use of inappropriate measuring devices and measuring technique will likely lead to one of two results:

- Stone cast with a too-low W/P ratio: The stone will be too thick and detail will be lost.

Table 16.2	Recommended Water/Powder (W/P) Ratios	
Manufacturer Recommended W/P Ratios		
Gypsum Product	Water (in Milliliters)	Powder (in Grams)
Plaster (type II)	45-50 ml (0.45-0.50)	100 g
Stone (type III)	30-32 ml (0.30-0.32)	100 g
High-strength stone (type IV)	19-24 ml (0.19-0.24)	100 g

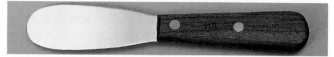

FIG. 16.9 Broad metal gypsum spatula. (From Powers JM, Wataha JC: *Dental Materials: Properties and Manipulation* (ed 11). St. Louis, 2017, Elsevier.)

- Stone cast with a too-high W/P ratio: The stone will be too thin, and its strength may be no greater than that of model plaster.

To avoid either of these scenarios, manufacturers produce pre-weighed envelopes of powder for critical measurements. This method enhances accuracy and saves time but also increases the cost of the material.

MIXING: SPATULATION

Most commonly, plaster and stone are mixed in a flexible rubber bowl with a broad metal plaster spatula (Fig. 16.9); this mixing process is called *spatulation*. Mechanical vacuum mix devices are used when the control of spatulation is critical. The measured amount of water is placed into the mixing bowl and the measured powder slowly sifted into the water within 30 seconds. By sifting powder into water, an even wetting of the powder particles takes place and clumps are avoided. This is the reason for placing the powder in water rather than water into powder. This technique will also minimize the amount of air incorporated into the mix during hand spatulation. The materials are spatulated by first incorporating the powder and water slightly and then vigorously wiping the mix against the sides of the bowl to force out air and ensure wetting of all the powder particles. Spatulation should continue for 1 minute at two revolutions per second until a smooth, homogeneous mix with a glossy surface is produced. An increase in the time and rate of spatulation has a definite effect on setting time and expansion: it will shorten the setting time and increase the rate of setting expansion. Many dental laboratories use mechanical spatulation with a vacuum device to reduce air bubbles and enhance the consistency and accuracy of mixing (Fig. 16.10). Hand spatulation is the most common means of mixing gypsum materials in private dental offices (Procedure 16.1).

INITIAL SETTING TIME AND WORKING TIME

After mixing for 1 minute, the working time begins. During this time, the semifluid mixture is **poured** into the

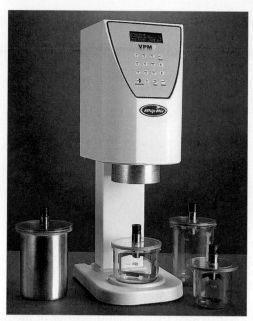

FIG. 16.10 Programmable, power-driven, vacuum-mixing unit, programmed for various types of gypsum products. The powerful vacuum quickly removes air and reduces the risk of bubbles. (Courtesy of Whip Mix Corporation [Louisville, KY].)

impression with the help of a mechanical vibrator (Fig. 16.11) . As the viscosity of the mixture increases, the flow characteristics are decreased and the product loses its glossy appearance. This loss of gloss indicates that the gypsum has reached its initial set. At the time of initial set, the material has no measurable compressive or tensile strength and should not be removed from the mold. For regular-set products, the initial set occurs within 8 to 16 minutes from the beginning of the mix. With a mixing time of 1 minute, this leaves ample working time to pour the impression.

FINAL SETTING TIME

The final set is reached when the material can be handled safely, but it has minimal hardness and resistance to abrasion. At this time, the chemical reaction is complete and the model is cool to the touch, having completed the exothermic reaction. Most manufacturers recommend 45 minutes to 1 hour before the material may be safely separated from the impression. Gypsum products continue to harden and are two to three times harder after 24 hours.

💡 Clinical Tip

Before separating the impression from the cast, ensure that no part of the impression tray is connected to the gypsum. Do not pry or rock in one direction too far, or the cast will likely break because of its lack of tensile strength.

Allowing the impression and cast to remain together for more than 1 hour before separation may have a detrimental effect on the surface characteristics of the cast. Alginate will absorb water from the surface of the cast producing a weaker, more porous surface. The

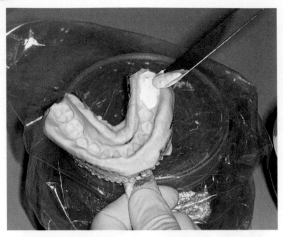

FIG. 16.11 Small increments of plaster flowing slowly from the posterior of an alginate impression on the dental vibrator to ensure air does not get trapped. (From Robinson DS, Bird DL: *Essentials of Dental Assisting* (ed 6). St. Louis, 2017, Elsevier.)

directions provided by the manufacturer of the impression material will indicate how long a gypsum product may remain in contact with the impression material.

 Clinical Tip

If an alginate impression has dried out before the cast has been separated, soak the impression and cast in water for 15 minutes. The alginate will soften, allowing removal of the cast without breaking of the teeth or other anatomic structures. Do not leave gypsum products soaking in water longer than absolutely necessary as they will begin to dissolve.

CONTROL OF SETTING TIMES

It is important to keep in mind that it is impossible to accelerate the final set of a mixture without also accelerating the initial set, thereby reducing the working time. If it is necessary to alter the setting time, this can be accomplished by altering the W/P ratio, spatulation, temperature or amount of accelerators or retarders.

Altering the W/P Ratio

As previously mentioned, an increase in the proportion of water will retard the setting times. However, because an increase by even 1 part water can reduce the strength by as much as 50%, this is not a recommended control. Decreasing the proportion of water will accelerate the setting time, but it also makes the mixture more difficult to manipulate, causing air bubbles and leading to an inaccurate model. Decreasing the amount of water (i.e., decreasing the W/P ratio) is recommended only when the mixture is not being poured into an impression, such as when it is being used as a base to secure models on an articulator.

Spatulation

A longer and more rapid spatulation of gypsum results in an accelerated setting time. This rapid spatulation will also result in increased setting expansion.

Temperature

Within limits, an increase in the temperature of the mixing water will accelerate the setting time. Gypsum is ideally mixed with room temperature water. Increasing the temperature of the water, not to exceed 38 °C (100 °F), will accelerate the set. Any increase in temperature to above 38 °C (100 °F) will have a retarding effect, and at 100 °C (212 °F) no reaction takes place and the gypsum will not set.

Accelerators and Retarders

The most practical way to control setting time is through the manufacturer's addition of chemical accelerators or retarders. Manufacturers add accelerators and retarders to change the solubility of the hemihydrate in water. By increasing the solubility of the hemihydrates, the added accelerator decreases the setting time, and by decreasing the solubility, the added retarder increases the setting time. When accelerators are placed into the gypsum, the manufacturer can cut the time between the initial and final set by 50%. These materials are labeled "fast set." If no accelerators or retarders are placed in the product, the product is labeled "regular set."

The clinician may also add accelerators. Potassium sulfate (K_2SO_4) and set gypsum ($CaSO_4$) particles are examples. The water and crystals from ground set gypsum, commonly retrieved from the runoff water of model trimmers, is called *slurry water*. The dihydrate crystals in the slurry water accelerate the chemical reaction by acting as established sites for crystallization.

Using Clean Equipment and Impressions

When set materials are left in mixing bowls, on spatulas, or on other mixing equipment these materials may inadvertently become part of the fresh mix. The result may be the same as the addition of an accelerator; however, this uncontrolled error will likely also result in an uneven setting of the material. All equipment should be meticulously cleaned after pouring an impression to avoid this mistake.

Blood, saliva, and alginate are organic substances that can retard the set of gypsum. If these organic components are left in an impression, the surface detail of the resulting model may be easily abraded. All impressions must be rinsed free of any organic matter before the impression is poured. Alginate remains in contact with the gypsum product, so it must be noted that even though the outside surface of a cast poured from an alginate impression may seem set, the area adjacent to the teeth needs more time to fully harden.

Remember that when a change is made in the final setting time, a sacrifice is usually made in the working time, strength, or setting expansion of the final product (Table 16.3).

FABRICATING AND TRIMMING DIAGNOSTIC/WORKING CASTS

Diagnostic and working casts have two parts:
(see Fig. 16.12)

Table 16.3	Manipulation Factors		
FACTOR	**WORKING TIME**	**VISCOSITY**	**STRENGTH**
Increase W/P ratio	Increase	Decrease	Decrease
Decrease W/P ratio	Decrease	Increase	Increase
Increase rate of spatulation	Decrease	Increase	No effect
Increase temperature of H_2O	Decrease	Increase	No effect
Decrease temperature of H_2O	Increase	Decrease	No effect

W/P ratio, water-to-powder ratio (milliliters of water per gram of powder).

- *Anatomic portion:* The anatomic portion replicates the hard and soft structures.
- *Art portion* or *base:* The art portion aids in handling and articulating the casts.

The anatomic portion is poured by vibrating small increments of flowable gypsum into the impression. The mixture should be poured slowly in small increments under vibration and allowed to flow from the one tooth imprint to the next, pushing out air ahead of itself as it fills the entire impression, thus eliminating air voids. To conserve costs and make the cast easier to trim, the anatomic portion may be poured with a higher-strength gypsum product and the base poured with a lower-strength product. The art or base portion can be poured by any of three methods (Fig. 16.13) (see Procedures 16.2 and 16.3).

Double-Pour Method

The double-pour technique involves two separate mixes and two separate setting times. The anatomic portion of one or both arches is poured and left in the upright position. Make sure you have slightly over-filled the entire impression, including the palate and borders of the impression. Add a couple of additional small mounds of gypsum to the surface to make a better lock with the base. Approximately 10 minutes after the loss of gloss, a second mix is produced for the art portion(s). This mixture is approximately 1 inch thick and placed on a glass tile in the shape of the impression tray or into a base former. The filled impression is inverted onto the base, with the handle of the tray parallel to the base, and the peripheries of the two portions are joined. Care must be taken to ensure that the base material is thick enough to support the weight of the filled impression so that it does not sink into the base. Avoid manipulating the filled impression once you place it on the base; over manipulation will sink the filled impression into the base. After inverting the impression, excess material may be carefully removed from the base to form a model requiring less time to trim on the model trimmer. Be careful not to allow the base material to contact the impression tray as this will produce a mechanical lock between the tray and set gypsum, making it difficult to separate the tray from the model.

If the cast is being used as a working cast, the anatomic portion is frequently poured with dental

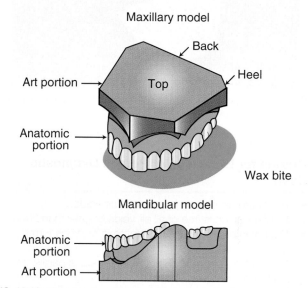

FIG. 16.12 Line drawing of parts and proportions of diagnostic casts. (From Bird DL, Robinson DS: *Modern Dental Assisting* (ed 11). Philadelphia, 2014, Elsevier.)

stone and the base portion is poured with plaster. This gives the anatomic portion sufficient density while allowing for easier trimming of the base portion.

Single-Step Method (Inverted Pour Method)

In the single-step method, one mix of gypsum is produced to pour both the anatomic and art portions of the cast. After the impression is poured, the remaining material is used for the base. This material is placed on a glass tile or into a base former (Fig. 16.13, lower image), the impression is inverted onto it, and the peripheries of the two portions are joined. This method requires better skill and timing. If the mixture is too wet when you finish pouring the impression, the base may flow excessively when the impression is inverted, causing the tray to become locked into the set gypsum. Also, the material in the inverted impression may slump away from the impression, causing distortion of the cast or trapping of air voids. If the mixture in the anatomic portion has reached its initial set when it is inverted onto the art portion, the union between art and anatomic portions will be incomplete.

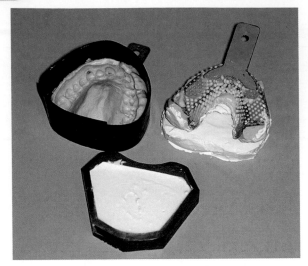

FIG. 16.13 Pouring the art portion of a cast by boxing; model former and inversion on patty base.

Criteria for Evaluation of Poured Diagnostic Casts

- The anatomic portion is free of all air voids.
- The art portion is free of all air voids greater than 2 mm.
- The union between art and anatomic portions forms a continuous surface.
- The occlusal plane, at the premolar area, is parallel to the bottom of the base.
- The base is of adequate thickness but not so thick as to require excessive trimming.
- There is sufficient material extending past the muco-buccal fold and posterior to the casts to replicate all anatomic structures.
- Excess material in the tongue area has been smoothed.,

Boxing Method

In the boxing method, a strip of boxing wax is used to surround the impression, forming a wall into which the gypsum is poured (Fig. 16.13, upper left image). The wax should not distort the impression. It should extend at least 0.5 inch higher than the highest point of the impression and create a base that is parallel to the occlusal plane.

STORAGE

Gypsum products can absorb water from the environment. Humidity and close proximity to water sources will adversely affect the powder. Initially this exposure will accelerate the setting reaction by producing established sites of crystallization. After prolonged exposure, the setting reaction is retarded because of decreased solubility of the crystals by the formation of a dihydrate layer on the hemihydrate particles.

Gypsum should be stored in airtight, moisture-proof containers. To avoid prolonged exposure to moisture, open plaster bins are recommended only if there is rapid turnover of the products.

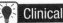 **Clinical Tip**

Avoid reaching into the plaster bin with wet hands or spatula. It will affect the set of the material that has been contaminated.

Products offered in pre-weighed envelopes are commonly used in offices where the turnover of gypsum is low.

CLEANUP

Gypsum mixing and handling equipment must be kept meticulously clean. As previously mentioned, set gypsum particles inadvertently included with freshly mixed gypsum will accelerate the setting time. Bowls, spatulas, mechanical vibrators, and mixing devices should be cleaned of all traces of gypsum as soon as possible after manipulation.

 Caution

Remember that all excess material should be placed in the trash and not rinsed down drains, where it will likely clog pipes. Equipment should then be thoroughly rinsed under running water. Sinks in gypsum-handling areas should be fitted with plaster traps.

INFECTION CONTROL AND SAFETY ISSUES

The need for infection control measures to extend into the dental laboratory has been clearly documented. Routine disinfection of impressions should be done in the dental office. (A discussion of disinfecting agents and procedures for disinfecting impressions are presented in Chapter 15 Impression Materials.) Disinfection of impressions is the best way to prevent the introduction of contaminants into the laboratory area. If this has not been done, the impression and all equipment, such as plaster spatulas and dental vibrators, must be handled with proper personal protective equipment or barriers.

Casts should be completely set and stored for at least 24 hours before disinfecting to prevent attack by the chemicals on the surface of the cast. Casts should be sprayed rather than immersed in disinfecting solutions, because some studies have shown damage to the surface in only a few minutes in water-based solutions. Solutions such as 1:10 sodium hypochlorite, iodophors, or chlorine dioxide have been shown to have minimal effect on cast surfaces when used in this manner. Whenever working with powdered gypsum products a mask should be worn to prevent inhaling the fine powders. A mask should also be worn during trimming of casts as aerosols are produced by the model trimmer that can be inhaled. Protective glasses must always be worn for both the pouring and trimming of casts.

SEPARATING THE IMPRESSION FROM THE CAST

On setting of the gypsum, the impression, tray, and cast must be separated (Procedure 16.4). When the impression is poured, care should be taken to make sure the gypsum does not flow onto the tray, locking it into the set gypsum. To separate the cast, begin by cutting the excess gypsum away from the periphery of the tray. Gently ease a laboratory knife under the tray and lift the tray slightly in several areas. Use the impression material as a cushion to avoid gouging the anatomic portion of the cast. Remember, gypsum products have very low tensile strength. Do not rock the tray back and forth too much; this may result in breaking the teeth of the cast.

Criteria for Evaluation of Trimmed Diagnostic Casts

- Anatomic portion accounts for one-half of the total depth, and the base portion for one-half of the total depth.
- Bases of the maxillary and mandibular casts should be parallel with the occlusal planes and with each other.
- Posterior borders of both casts are at right angles to the base and will stand together when articulated on end.
- Posterior portions include retromolar pads and tuberosities.
- Side borders are perpendicular to the base, symmetric, and trimmed to the depth of the vestibule.
- Anterior borders are perpendicular to the base and are trimmed to the depth of the vestibule.
- Anterior borders of the maxillary cast form a point at the midline and are rounded from cuspid to cuspid for the mandibular cast.
- Mandibular casts have a smoothed tongue space.
- Maxillary and mandibular casts are labeled with the patient's name and date.

TRIMMING

Trimming of models with a model trimmer is done to produce an attractive, symmetric model with easy access to all anatomic portions of the model and a base of sufficient bulk for stability. Bases made from dental stone should be soaked in water for 5 to 10 minutes before trimming to saturate the stone, making it easier to trim. Anatomic portions should never be soaked. Saturation of the teeth may lead to a change in surface texture and, in the case of plaster, may make the teeth more susceptible to chipping.

The cast should be trimmed so that, proportionally, the base makes up one third and the anatomic portion two thirds of the total depth. The occlusal plane should be parallel with the base. The periphery of the largest arch is trimmed first, and then the smaller arch is articulated with a wax bite and trimmed to match (see Procedure 15.5 for a description of wax bite registration). The outer borders should be cut to the depth of the vestibule and should include all muscle attachments, retromolar pads, and tuberosities. If there are facially inclined or rotated teeth, the outside borders should be extended symmetrically to include these anatomic structures. The anterior portion of the maxillary arch is cut to a point at the midline, and the anterior portion of the mandibular arch is rounded from canine to canine (Fig. 16.14) (see Procedure 16.5 for detailed instruction on trimming models).

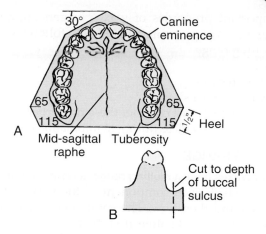
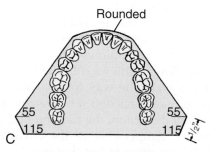

FIG. 16.14 Line drawing of landmarks, angles, and cuts of art portion of diagnostic casts. **A,** Maxillary cast. **B,** Cut to depth of the vestibule. **C,** Mandibular cast. (From Bird DL, Robinson DS: *Torres and Ehrlich Modern Dental Assisting* (ed 9). Philadelphia, 2009, Elsevier.)

⚠ Caution

Exercise care when using the model trimmer. Always wear protective eyewear and mask, establish a flat surface from which to trim, and pay attention to your hand positions. The abrasive wheel can rapidly abrade skin and fingernails! Use even, steady pressure with both hands while trimming. To maintain the abrasive surface of the trimming wheel, maintain an adequate flow of water on the trimming wheel when in use, so that it does not clog with gypsum. Clean the wheel and work surface of all gypsum products immediately after finishing.

COMPOSITION AND PROPERTIES OF DENTAL WAXES

Dental waxes are composed of a mixture of components from natural and synthetic sources. Natural waxes are produced from plants, used in carnauba wax; insects, used in beeswax; and minerals, used in paraffin and ceresin wax. These natural waxes contribute properties to the wax but are rarely used in their pure form. They are combined or mixed with synthetic waxes, gums, fats, oils, resins, and coloring agents. Each component is added to attain the physical properties desirable for the wax application. The components of waxes allow them to be sticky, solid, or liquid depending on the temperature of the wax. Use of the wax will determine properties that are desirable for its application.

Important properties of waxes in general, and of dental waxes in particular, include the following:
- Melting range
- Flow
- Excess residue
- Thermal expansion

The operator must consider these properties when selecting a wax, as well as during manipulation of the wax.

MELTING RANGE

Dental waxes have a **melting range**, a range of temperatures at which each component of the wax will start to soften and then flow. The components with lower melting points will soften first; then, as the temperature is increased, more components will soften and the wax will eventually flow and eventually become a liquid or vaporize. Because wax is unstable, the operator must be careful to prevent its distortion. Controlling the temperature of the wax allows operator control of the viscosity and flow of the wax. In many cases, the operator does not want the wax to flow but only to soften. A flame source is needed if a flowable state is desired. To prevent distortion, the melting range must be higher than the temperature of the environment. This is especially important in hot climates.

FLOW

Flow is the movement of wax as molecules slip over each other. As the temperature of the wax increases, the viscosity of the wax decreases until the wax becomes a liquid. Control of the flow and the melting range is important in manipulating wax. If a wax were capable of flowing at room temperature, it would be very difficult to control. However, even at mouth temperature, there is a point at which flow is undesirable. If you were using a wax for a wax bite registration, you would not want it to flow at mouth temperature, causing distortion of the wax. It is important that the wax not require temperatures much greater than mouth temperature to soften, or it would be uncomfortable when placed in the mouth of the patient. A melting range that is only slightly higher than mouth temperature is desirable for this wax application. For laboratory purposes, waxes may have a much higher melting range. However, even for laboratory purposes, high melting ranges may be undesirable. If you want to use a wax in the boxing of an impression, for example, it is much more desirable to mold the wax, using the heat of your hands or warm water, rather than having to use a flame.

EXCESS RESIDUE

It is important that all wax be removed from the object onto which it is melted. If **excess residue** remains after the wax is removed, this may result in inaccuracies in the object being produced. This is especially important in the lost wax technique, which requires that the wax pattern be completely melted out of the investment mold.

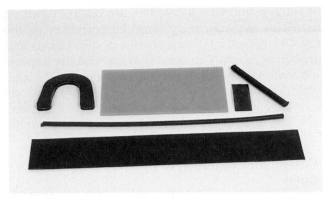

FIG. 16.15 Various forms of wax: Sheets, ropes, and sticks. Impression wax *(top row left)*, baseplate wax *(top row middle left)*, casting wax *(top row middle center)*, inlay wax *(top row middle right)*, utility wax *(middle)*, and boxing wax *(bottom)*.

THERMAL EXPANSION

Waxes expand when heated and contract when cooled; the thermal expansion and contraction of waxes is greater than that of any other dental material. This property is especially important for pattern waxes. If a wax is heated too far above the melting range or is heated unevenly, expansion above acceptable standards will result. Manufacturers provide temperature and handling guidelines for pattern waxes to prevent inaccuracies in the final casting. In addition, if waxes are allowed to stand, dimensional changes occur from the release of residual stress. Wax patterns should be invested within minutes of carving.

CLASSIFICATION OF WAXES

Waxes are grouped as follows:
- *Pattern waxes:* Pattern waxes include inlay wax, casting wax, and baseplate wax
- *Processing waxes:* Processing waxes include boxing wax, utility wax, and sticky wax
- *Impression waxes:* Impression waxes include corrective impression wax and bite registration wax

Manufacturers produce these waxes in several forms. Sticks, sheets, blocks, and tins are used. Waxes have unique coloring to distinguish them in use (Fig. 16.15).

PATTERN WAXES

Pattern waxes are used in the construction of metal castings and bases for dentures. The three types of pattern waxes are inlay wax, casting wax, and baseplate wax.

Inlay Wax

Inlay waxes are used to produce patterns for metal casting through the lost wax technique. There are three ADA specifications for Inlay wax: Type A that can be used directly in the mouth, Type B (type I) and Type C (type II), which are both melted onto a die outside the mouth in the indirect technique. (Table 16.4) (Fig. 16.16). Type A wax, when used directly in the

Table 16.4	Classification of Pattern Waxes, ADA Specification, and General Application.	
CLASSIFICATION OF DENTAL PATTERN WAXES		
NAME OF WAX	**ADA SPECIFICATION**	**USES**
Inlay wax	Type A Type B (type I) Type C (type II)	Direct patterns in mouth Indirect patterns on dies
Casting wax		Construct metal framework of partial and complete denture
Baseplate wax	Type I Type II Type III	Impression in cool climates Impression in warm climates

This Table Identifies the Different Types of Pattern Waxes, the American Dental Association Specification, and Uses of the Wax in Dentistry

mouth, has a much lower melting range to prevent damage to the pulp of the tooth, for the comfort of the patient and the accuracy of the wax on removal. Because direct waxing is performed in the patient's mouth, all the limitations of working in the mouth and patient safety measures must be considered. Because of these limitations, most dentists prefer to use the indirect waxing technique and call on the expertise of a dental laboratory technician to produce the wax pattern and casting. Inlay waxes are supplied in sticks, pellets, and tins, generally in dark colors of red, blue, or green. They are labeled hard, medium, and soft, which refers to their melting ranges. ADA specification number 4 sets standards for pattern waxes: low thermal expansion, complete removal of excess residue, and appropriate melting ranges are important properties.

Casting Wax

Casting waxes are used to construct the metal framework of partial and complete dentures. These waxes come in sheets and preformed pieces for components of partial dentures. The physical properties of casting waxes are similar to those of inlay waxes, with the exception of melting range. Because these waxes are not softened in the mouth, the melting range is important only for laboratory procedures.

Baseplate Wax

Baseplate waxes are sheets (7.5 cm wide by 15 cm long) of wax that generally are pink in color. These sheets are usually layered to produce the contours of the denture and hold the position on which denture teeth are set (Fig. 16.17). There are three ADA specifications for baseplate wax. Type I is softer and utilized in cool climates; Type II has a medium hardness and utilized in warm climates; and Type III is harder and is also utilized in warm climates (Table 16.4). When the sheets of baseplate wax have been layered on resin denture bases to produce the contours of the denture and the denture teeth are

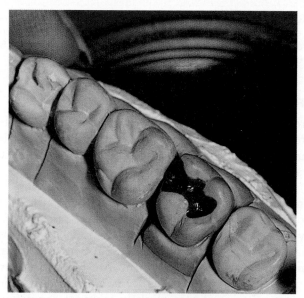

FIG. 16.16 An inlay waxing on a die.

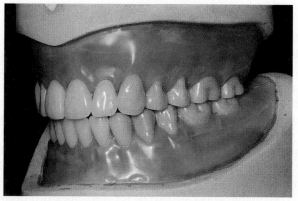

FIG. 16.17 A denture setup on baseplates.

set, the form is then tried into the mouth to establish denture dimensions. The wax must not distort at mouth temperatures. Baseplate wax may also be used for occlusal rims (see Chapter 17 Polymers in Prosthetic Dentistry) and bite registration (see Chapter 15 Impression Materials).

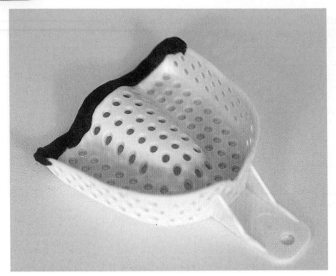

FIG. 16.18 Utility wax used on the posterior of the impression tray to extend the tray and make the fit more comfortable for the patient. (From Bird DL, Robinson DS: *Modern Dental Assisting* (ed 12). St. Louis, 2018, Elsevier.)

PROCESSING WAXES

Processing waxes are used primarily to aid in dental procedures both clinically and in the laboratory. The three types of processing waxes are boxing wax, utility wax, and sticky wax.

Boxing Wax

Boxing wax is used to form the base portion of a gypsum model. A 1.5-inch-wide red , green, or black strip of boxing wax is wrapped around an impression to produce a form into which gypsum is poured. This wax is easily manipulated at room temperature; it is also slightly tacky at room temperature, allowing it to adhere to itself to secure the boxed form.

Utility Wax

Also called *periphery wax*, this wax comes in sticks, long square ropes, and round strips that are easily manipulated at room temperature. They may be used with boxing wax to aid in the pouring of an impression. Utility wax rope is used to adapt the periphery of the impression tray to customize the tray and aid in patient comfort (Fig. 16.18). The wax provides a better fit into the vestibule and control of movement of the impression material.

The pliable wax can also be used to block out undercuts around teeth or tissues prior to impression making to prevent the impression from locking in place (see Chapter 15, Fig. 15.20). However, there is a block out wax on the market that is soft and pliable allowing for easy placement into undercuts on an impression before pouring a model, making baseplates, splints, or injection molding.

Utility wax ropes clear or ivory in colors may be given to orthodontic patients to cover sharp brackets and wires that irritate lips, cheeks and tongue. Utility wax sheets may also be layered to form a horseshoe shape and used for wax bite registrations; however, because they are pliable they can distort easily. These waxes come in various colors of pink, white, and red.

Sticky Wax

Sticky wax comes in orange and red sticks that at room temperature are hard and brittle, but when heated under flame become soft and sticky. Sticky wax is used to adhere components of metal, gypsum, or resin together temporarily during fabrication and repair. Because of its brittle nature at room temperature, even the slightest torque will fracture the wax. This is an important characteristic because it alerts the operator that distortion has occurred during manipulation.

IMPRESSION WAXES

Impression wax and impression wax compounds are thermoplastic materials used to obtain impressions of the oral structures. When heated, they become soft and able to take on a new form in the mouth; and when cooled, they harden and can be removed. These waxes and techniques for using them to take impressions are described further in Chapter 15 Impression Materials. The two types of impression waxes are corrective impression wax and bite registration wax.

Corrective Impression Wax

Corrective impression wax is used in conjunction with other impression materials in the process of taking edentulous impressions. This wax flows at mouth temperature and is used within another impression material to correct undercut areas, to fill in small voids or to help develop a functional posterior palatal seal for maxillary complete denture impressions.

Bite Registration Wax

Bite registration wax is used to produce wax bite registrations for articulation of models. The preformed U-shaped horseshoe shaped wax is often reinforced with metal particles to provide stability. However, similar to corrective impression wax, this wax is susceptible to distortion at temperatures only slightly higher than mouth temperature and must be carefully monitored. Because of this limitation, silicone and other more stable impression materials have largely replaced wax for bite registrations. For fabrication of a wax bite registration, see Procedure 15.5.

OTHER WAXES UTILIZED IN THE DENTAL OFFICE

There are other waxes available on the market for special uses in the dental practice or laboratory setting. They are not included in the categories listed above as they have specialized uses.

Orthodontic Wax

This wax is utilized for patients experiencing pain and irritation while wearing braces. As the teeth are being moved, the orthodontic appliances in the mouth may irritate the soft tissues of the gums and buccal mucosa. The orthodontic wax is applied to the brackets, bands, or wires to prevent poking and scratching of the tissues. The product is clear which will not be readily visible in the mouth. The wax may be provided in a portable container so the patient has access to the material regularly. A small chunk is taken out of the container and flattened out, and then the piece of wax is stuck to the area causing the patient discomfort. The product is safe to ingest as there is a chance a small piece can become dislodged and swallowed.

This wax is a composite material containing powdered aluminum to increase the heat retention, integrity of the compound and provide the properties necessary for efficient modeling. This material is utilized when a dentist is making a new removable denture for a patient. During the jaw-registration stage, the wax is softened over an open flame and place between the record blocks. It will keep the two record blocks together. (See Chapter 17 Polymers for Prosthetic Dentistry, Procedure 17.2). Some clinicians use it in the laboratory as a block put wax.

MANIPULATION OF WAXES

Wax should be softened evenly in dry heat, with warm hands, a warm water bath or by flame. If a wax is softened by flame, it should be rotated above the flame so that it evenly softens or flows. Melted wax should be added in layers onto an object. As previously mentioned, because of changes caused by relaxation of residual stress, wax patterns should be invested within 30 minutes of carving. Waxes such as boxing and utility wax are slightly tacky at room temperature to help them adhere to themselves. They must remain dry if one is to take advantage of this characteristic.

To avoid distortion of waxes, they should be stored at or slightly below room temperature.

LOST WAX TECHNIQUE

Artisans have used the **lost wax technique** for several hundred years. In the 1500s, artisans, in conjunction

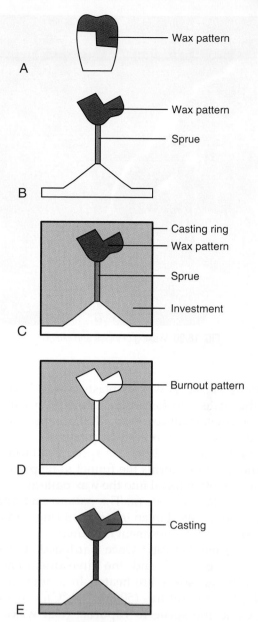

FIG. 16.19 Line drawing series on the lost wax technique. **A,** Wax pattern on a die. **B,** Wax pattern with sprue on a die. **C,** Wax and sprue on sprue base and in investment ring. **D,** Wax pattern vaporized from investment. **E,** Metal casting of wax pattern.

with medical practitioners, invented a method for casting gold for dental restorations in molds; today's techniques are much the same (Fig. 16.19). The process of creating a detailed wax pattern and converting it into a final restoration is known as *casting*. The primary steps in the lost wax and casting procedure are as follows:

1. *Pouring the die:* An exact impression of the preparation is first obtained and poured into a high-strength die stone forming the die.
2. *Waxing the die:* A detailed wax pattern of the restoration is carved on the die including all anatomy, contours, occlusion, and proximal contacts.

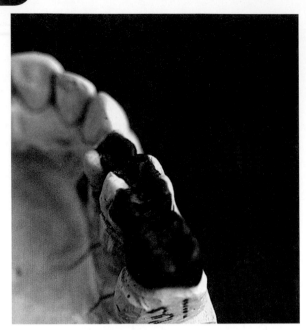

FIG. 16.20 Waxing of inlays and crown.

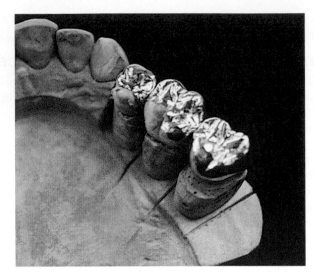

FIG. 16.21 Cleaned and polished metal castings of inlays and crowns.

3. *Spruing the die:* A wax or plastic sprue is attached to the pattern to form the channel into which the molten metal will be forced. Multiple sprues may be used for a more complex wax pattern.
4. *Attaching the sprue base:* The sprue is attached to a sprue base; this forms the funnel to help guide the flow of molten metal into the wax pattern.
5. *Investing the wax pattern:* The pattern and attached sprue are encased in an investment ring into which gypsum-based investment is poured.
6. *Burning out the wax:* Once hardened, the sprue base is removed and the investment-enclosed pattern and sprue are heated in a burnout oven at high temperatures (500 to 700 °C), causing the wax and the sprue to vaporize (lost wax), leaving an impression of the wax pattern in the now-empty space.
7. *Casting the restoration:* The molten metal is moved by centrifugal force through the empty channel formed by the sprue and into the empty wax pattern space.
8. *Final steps:* The metal cools, the sprue is removed, and the casting is cleaned and polished using a series of polishing steps to form a smooth and glossy surface. The polishing procedure must be accomplished without altering the margins, contacts, or occlusion of the restoration. It is now ready to be cemented onto the tooth (Figs. 16.20 and 16.21).

The accuracy of the entire casting process must be carefully executed to produce a clinically acceptable final restoration The lost wax procedure takes several steps, each of which can cause inaccuracies in the final product. Properties of expansion and contraction in the impression material, die stone, wax, investment material, and casting must be controlled to achieve a final restoration that will have intimate contact with the tooth preparation. This accuracy will produce a cement interface of as little as 20 μm, ensuring a precise fit with space for a very fine film of luting cement.

SUMMARY

Gypsum products are used to produce diagnostic and working models of the patient's hard and soft tissues. The properties of strength and hardness, setting expansion, and solubility are directly related to the amounts of water used in their construction. The density of the final product is related to these water amounts and to the size and shape of the particles that are manufactured. Manipulation factors such as the W/P ratio, rate of spatulation, and water temperature used in the mix have a great effect as well. The clinician must have a clear understanding of how these variables can be manipulated appropriately. Pouring of models requires meticulous attention to detail to produce a replica that accurately reflects the hard and soft tissues of the patient's oral cavity.

The dental assistant and dental hygienist may have occasion to use dental waxes in a variety of clinical and laboratory procedures. Although waxes have inherent disadvantages in dimensional stability and control of flow, they are used successfully. The operator must keep in mind the limitations of each wax in order to use it to its best advantage.

INSTRUCTIONAL VIDEOS

See the Evolve Resources site for a variety of educational videos that reinforce the material covered in this chapter.

Procedure 16.1 Mixing Gypsum Products

See Evolve site for Competency Sheet.

Consider the following with this procedure: safety glasses are recommended for the patient, PPE is required for the operator, and ensure appropriate safety protocols are followed.

EQUIPMENT/SUPPLIES (FIG. 16.22)

- Gypsum product
- Scale
- Water (room temperature)
- Water-measuring device
- Flexible mixing bowl
- Broad-blade metal spatula
- Mechanical vibrator

PROCEDURE STEPS

1. Measure the recommended amount of room temperature water into a clean, flexible, rubber mixing bowl.
   NOTE: Increasing or decreasing the water temperature is the preferred way to control the working time.
2. Weigh the recommended amount of gypsum powder onto the scale; use another bowl or weigh onto a paper towel. Make sure to account for the weight of the bowl if you are using this method to transfer powder.

3. Sift the powder gradually into the water, allowing the particles to become wet—about 30 seconds.
   NOTE: This minimizes the amount of air trapped in the mix.
4. Vigorously mix for about 60 seconds by wiping the spatula against the sides of the bowl to incorporate all the powder, removing excess air, until a smooth homogeneous mixture is obtained (Fig. 16.23).
   NOTE: The viscosity of the mix should be sufficient to allow the material to flow only under mechanical vibration.
5. Turn the vibrator on low/medium and place the bowl onto the work surface.
6. Press the sides of the bowl inward with the palms of your hands, at the same time pressing the bowl downward on the work surface of the vibrator to remove all air incorporated during the mixing procedure. The air bubbles will rise to the surface of the mix
   NOTE: This helps to remove air trapped during mixing.
7. Complete the preparation of the gypsum material within 2 minutes.
   NOTE: This includes mixing and initial vibrating and allows for sufficient working time in pouring.

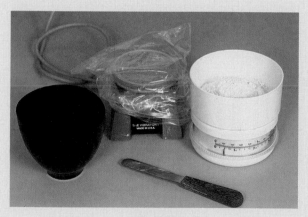

FIG. 16.22

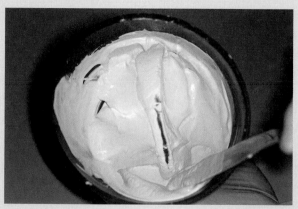

FIG. 16.23

Procedure 16.2 Pouring the Cast: Anatomic Portion

See Evolve site for Competency Sheet.

Consider the following with this procedure: safety glasses are recommended for the patient, PPE is required for the operator, and ensure appropriate safety protocols are followed.

EQUIPMENT/SUPPLIES (FIG. 16.24)

- Mask and safety glasses
- Mechanical vibrator

- Gypsum mixture
- Broad-blade metal spatula
- Small wax spatula
- Disinfected impression

PROCEDURE STEPS

1. Rinse the impression of all traces of disinfecting solution and tap it over the sink until no more water can be shaken out.

Continued

Procedure 16.2   Pouring the Cast: Anatomic Portion—cont'd

2. Holding the handle of the impression tray, place the impression tray onto the working surface of the mechanical vibrator. Rest the tray handle at an angle to the surface of the vibrator.

   NOTE: To facilitate cleanup, cover the working surface of the mechanical vibrator with a disposable cover, such as a plastic bag. Hold the tray at a slight angle to the working table of the vibrator to aid in the flow of the material. The speed of the vibrator should be adjusted only high enough to make the stone flow easily. Too much speed can incorporate bubbles into the mix.

3. Pick up a small increment of gypsum mixture, no bigger than a large pea, on the end of the small wax spatula.

   NOTE: This allows for control of the amount of material flowing into the tooth indentations.

4. Place the increment of mixture at one of the most posterior corners of the impression (Fig. 16.25).

5. Allow the mixture to flow into the tooth indentations from one side to the next of each indentation while controlling the flow of the mixture under vibration to force air out of each indentation.

   NOTE: Air bubbles are formed when the mixture moves too fast over the tooth indentations, trapping air in the impression, or when the mixture will not flow sufficiently to fill the indentations. Use small enough increments to control the flow and tilt the impression as needed to aid the speed of the flow.

6. Continue adding small increments of mixture in the same area while watching the material flow toward the anterior portion of the impression (Fig. 16.26).

7. Tilt the impression forward and continue adding increments across the anterior portion of the impression, making sure to control the flow so that air is not trapped.

8. Tilt the impression toward the opposite posterior portion and continue the addition of increments until the flow reaches the other end of the impression (Fig. 16.27).

9. When all of the tooth indentations are filled with the gypsum mixture, begin adding larger increments until the impression is slightly overfilled (Fig. 16.28).

   NOTE: Lift the impression from the vibrator to prevent the material from flowing over the impression tray.

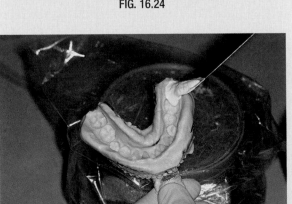

FIG. 16.24

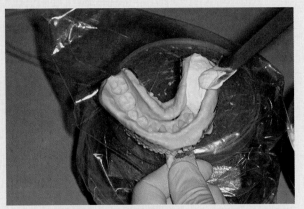

FIG. 16.26

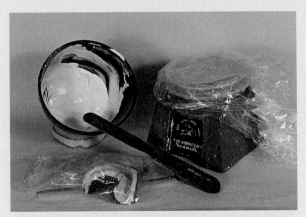

FIG. 16.25

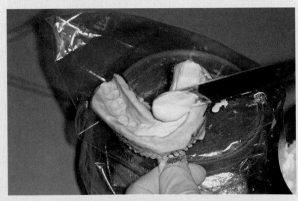

FIG. 16.27

Procedure 16.2 Pouring the Cast: Anatomic Portion—cont'd

10. Vibrate the entire tray for 2 to 3 seconds to settle all increments. Do not smooth the surface of the material.

    NOTE: A roughened surface will allow for better attachment with the base; you may add an additional two or three small mounds of material to the top of the gypsum to help facilitate attachment to the base.

11. Cleanup: Wipe all excess gypsum from the bowl and place it in the trash. Rinse and thoroughly clean the bowl and spatula under running water in a sink fitted with a plaster trap. Remove the plastic bag from the mechanical vibrator and clean the vibrator with a wet paper towel.

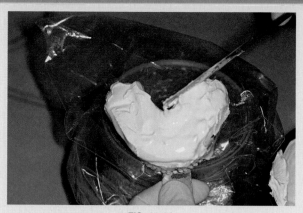

FIG. 16.28

Procedure 16.3 Pouring the Cast: Art (or Base) Portion

See Evolve site for Competency Sheet.

Consider the following with this procedure: safety glasses are recommended for the patient, PPE is required for the operator, and ensure appropriate safety protocols are followed.

EQUIPMENT/SUPPLIES

- Mask and safety glasses
- Glass tile or base former
- Broad-blade spatula
- Gypsum mixture
- Poured impression

PROCEDURE STEPS: DOUBLE-POUR METHOD

1. Allow the poured impression to set for at least 10 minutes.

   NOTE: This prevents the gypsum material from "slumping" away from the impression when it is inverted, causing distortion in the cast.

2. Prepare a mixture of gypsum, using less water for the W/P ratio.

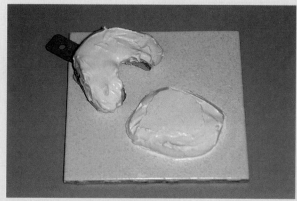

FIG. 16.29

NOTE: This will produce a thicker mix, which is necessary to accommodate the weight of the poured impression when it is inverted. You may use plaster to pour the art portion of a model even if the anatomic portion is poured with a different product. By using plaster, you will save on the cost of the more expensive stone products and if model trimming is necessary, you will save time as plaster trims much more easily than stone.

3. Place the mixture onto the glass tile or into a base former. You should have a mass at least 0.5 inch thick and slightly larger than the dimension of the filled impression and tray (Fig. 16.29).

   NOTE: If using a base former, make sure you choose one large enough for the impression and select the correct arch shape for your impression: pointed for maxillary and rounded for mandibular.

4. Invert the poured impression onto the base, making sure the occlusal plane remains parallel with the base. Use the tray handle and the top of the impression tray as your guide.

   NOTE: If using a base former, you will also need to make sure you keep the midline centered.

5. Very gently move the impression back and forth to bring the anatomic and art portions together. Be careful to prevent the filled tray from sinking into the base.

6. Bring the base material up with a spatula to fill the heels and sides of the impression and along the tray periphery, taking care not to lock the tray in with excess material (Figs. 16.30 and 16.31).

   NOTE: Make sure there are no large air pockets trapped between the art and base portions.

7. Smooth the tongue area of the mandibular impression level with the tray periphery.

Continued

Procedure 16.3   Pouring the Cast: Art (or Base) Portion—cont'd

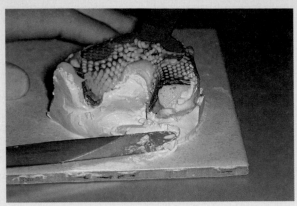

FIG. 16.30

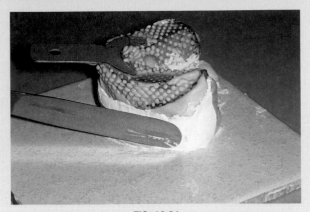

FIG. 16.31

8. You may choose to carefully remove some of the base material to begin to replicate the angle of the trimmed model. This will cut down the amount of time spent trimming the model on the model trimmer. Make sure the model has reached its initial set (loss of gloss) before attempting this.

9. Allow the gypsum to set completely before separating the model for the impression—45 to 60 minutes.

10. When the final set has been reached, the gypsum, impression, and cast are separated.

Procedure 16.4   Separating the Impression from the Cast

See Evolve site for Competency Sheet.

Consider the following with this procedure: safety glasses are recommended for the patient, PPE is required for the operator, and ensure appropriate safety protocols are followed.

EQUIPMENT/SUPPLIES

- Safety glasses
- Laboratory knife
- Plaster nippers

PROCEDURE STEPS

1. Remove the model from the glass tile or base former.
   NOTE: Do not allow agar-type impressions to remain longer than 1 hour without separating, as surface detail will be diminished.

2. Trim all excess gypsum from the tray at the tray edge with a laboratory knife (Fig. 16.32).
   NOTE: Ensure that no part of the tray is connected to the gypsum.

3. Loosen the tray from the impression material by placing the laboratory knife between the tray and the impression material in several areas and gently prying the two apart.

4. Attempt to lift the tray in a upward motion; if the tray does not lift, determine the location of the locked area and remove it with the laboratory knife or plaster nippers (Fig. 16.33).
   NOTE: Remember that gypsum products have very poor tensile strength; too much rocking of the tray will likely result in broken teeth.

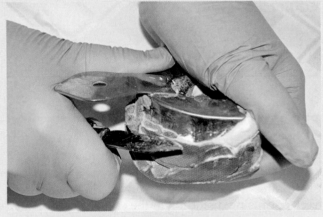

FIG. 16.32

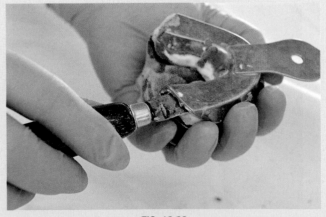

FIG. 16.33

Procedure 16.5 Trimming Diagnostic Casts

See Evolve site for Competency Sheet.

Consider the following with this procedure: safety glasses are recommended for the patient, PPE is required for the operator, and ensure appropriate safety protocols are followed.

EQUIPMENT/SUPPLIES (Fig. 16.34)

- Safety glasses and mask
- Maxillary and mandibular diagnostic casts
- Wax bite registration
- Measuring devices; millimeter ruler and compass
- Pencil
- Laboratory knife
- Plaster nippers
- Model trimmer

PROCEDURE STEPS

1. Soak the art portion of casts for 5 to 10 minutes in water.

   NOTE: Do not allow teeth to soak in water, as this may cause chipping of plaster or surface roughness of plaster or stone. The art portion of the cast should soak for a minimum of 5 minutes.

2. Cut excess gypsum distal to the retromolar pads and tuberosities with plaster nippers (Fig. 16.35).

   NOTE: Excess gypsum in this area may prevent models from being articulated.

3. Remove small bubbles (blebs) of gypsum on the occlusal surfaces with a laboratory knife.

   NOTE: This allows for complete articulation with the wax bite.

4. Check the working table of the model trimmer to make sure it is secure and at a 90-degree angle to the trimming wheel.

5. Adjust water flow over the trimming wheel to allow for sufficient water to clean the wheel.

Base Cut

6. Place the maxillary cast teeth side down on a cushion of layers of paper towels on the laboratory

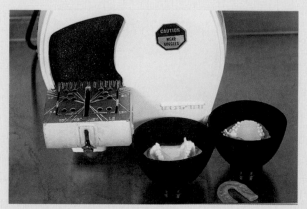

FIG. 16.34

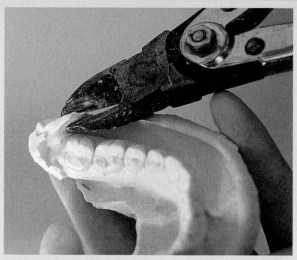

FIG. 16.35

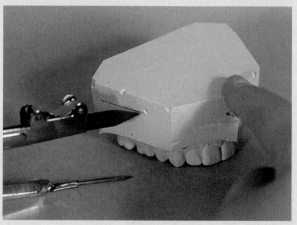

FIG. 16.36

bench and rock forward so that the anterior teeth touch the laboratory bench. The cast should be parallel to the bench top. Measure from the teeth to the base of the cast; the anatomic portion of the cast should be two thirds of the total height, with the art portion accounting for one half of the total height. Mark the models with a compass to this line (Fig. 16.36).

NOTE: The occlusal surfaces are parallel to the laboratory bench, with the anterior teeth touching the surface.

7. Trim the base to the marked line, periodically stopping to evaluate your progress. Remember: You can always continue to cut; if you cut away too much you may need to retake and repour the impression.

   NOTE: You may first need to make a flat back cut to secure casts on the working table of the trimmer.

8. Repeat steps 6 and 7 with the mandibular cast. When occluded the casts should be between 2 and 2.5 inches.

Continued

Side and Back Cuts

9. Measure the back by making a straight line 3 mm behind the retromolar pads of the mandibular cast or tuberosities of the maxillary cast.

10. Trim back to this line (Fig. 16.37). The maxillary and mandibular cast's back cuts should be parallel with one another.

    NOTE: Trim the longest cast first, and then articulate casts with the wax bite, and match the opposite cast's back cut with the models articulated (Fig. 16.38). Do not trim away any anatomy on either cast.

11. Measure the sides 3 mm from the buccal bone at the widest portion of the arch (usually the molar area) and 3 mm at the canine eminence. Mark the cast with a straight edge to connect these points.

12. With the models articulated trim the side cuts symmetrical to these lines (Fig. 16.39). Again the maxillary and mandibular cast's side cuts should be parallel with one another.

    NOTE: Do not trim past the depth of the vestibule.

Anterior Cut: Maxillary Cast

13. Measure 3 mm labial to the midline between central incisors. Measure from the depth of the vestibule or the most facially inclined tooth. Mark the casts with a straight edge to connect this point and the point 3 mm from the canine eminence.

14. Trim the anterior cuts symmetrically to form a midline point.

    NOTE: The maxillary cast forms a point between the central incisors.

Anterior Cut: Mandibular Cast

15. Measure as previously described, 3 mm from several places in the anterior region of the mandibular arch; connect these points with the point of the canine eminence to form a curved line. Trim the anterior cut of the mandible to this curved line.

Heel Cuts

16. Trim the heel cuts at a 90-degree angle to a line formed by connecting the canine eminence point to the side/back cut of the opposite side. The maxillary and mandibular cast's heel cuts should be parallel to one another.

    NOTE: This line is approximately 0.5 inch and symmetric on each side.

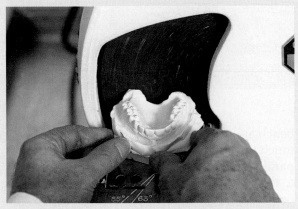

FIG. 16.37

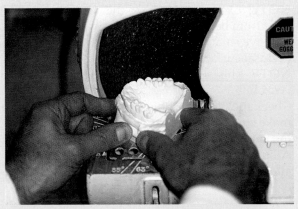

FIG. 16.39

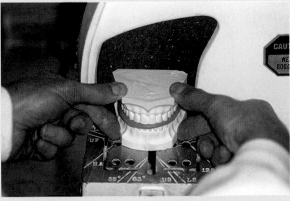

FIG. 16.38

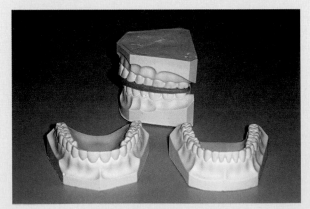

FIG. 16.40

Procedure 16.5 Trimming Diagnostic Casts—cont'd

Optional Steps
Finishing/Polishing

17. Inspect the models for small air voids; small voids may be filled in with a paint brush and a fresh mix of gypsum.
    NOTE: Unless requested by the dentist, do not fill in air voids in areas critical to the case.
18. Trim the contours of the peripheral borders of the model above the mucobuccal fold to form soft scalloped shapes.

19. Using model polish and a soft buffing cloth, polish the cast to a shine (Fig. 16.40).

Labeling/Storage

20. Using an indelible ink marker, label the base or the back cut of the cast with the patient's name and date.
21. Place the cast in a model box labeled with the patient's name, the date of the impression, and the case number.

Get Ready for Exams!

Review Questions

Select the one correct response for each of the following multiple-choice questions.

1. Carefully controlled calcination under steam pressure in a closed container produces:
   a. Plaster
   b. Dental stone
   c. High strength stone
   d. High strength, high expansion stone

2. To decrease the working time of a gypsum product, without changing any physical properties, it is best to:
   a. Decrease the water-to-powder ratio
   b. Increase the rate of spatulation
   c. Increase the water temperature
   d. Decrease the water temperature

3. The main difference between model plaster and dental stone is:
   a. Chemical formula
   b. Solubility in water
   c. Particle size and shape
   d. Accelerators and retarders

4. The most appropriate type of gypsum product to use for orthodontic casts is:
   a. Type I
   b. Type II
   c. Type III
   d. Type IV

5. Initial setting can be detected clinically by:
   a. Loss of gloss
   b. The end of the exothermic reaction
   c. A change in color
   d. Testing to see whether the material is hard enough to separate from the impression

6. The area of the diagnostic cast that records the hard and soft tissues is called the:
   a. Art portion
   b. Base
   c. Anatomic portion
   d. Impression

7. A study model is a positive reproduction. An impression is a negative reproduction:
   a. both statements are true
   b. both statements are false
   c. the first statement is true and the second statement is false
   d. the first statement is false and the second statement is true

8. Material that will act as retarders for the set of gypsum products include:
   a. saliva
   b. set gypsum products
   c. slurry water from the model trimmer
   d. none of the above are considered retarders

9. It is important to consider the following statements when pouring an impression:
   a. Alginate impressions should remain unseparated from the model for only 1 hour.
   b. When the single-step method is used, the material poured into the impression must reach the initial set before the base is poured.
   c. Gypsum should be mixed as wet as possible to allow for sufficient working time
   d. A and B
   e. A and C

10. Diagnostic casts are used for:
    a. patient education
    b. fabricating dentures
    c. fabricating crowns
    d. fabricating orthodontic appliances

11. CAD/CAM fabrication of indirect restorations eliminates the need for:
    a. investing
    b. cutting the preparation
    c. impression taking
    d. A and B
    e. A and C

12. The melting range can best be described as:
    a. The point at which the wax flows
    b. The point at which the wax softens
    c. The required temperature of the heat source
    d. A combination of melting points

Continued

Get Ready for Exams!—cont'd

13. A direct wax pattern is fabricated in the mouth. Which property of the inlay wax is the most important?
    a. Flow
    b. Residual stress
    c. Melting range
    d. Excess residue

14. A wax pattern is invested and burned out by the lost wax procedure. Which property of the inlay wax is the most important?
    a. Melting range
    b. Flow
    c. Residual stress
    d. Removal of excess residue

15. The wax used to form a base into which to pour a gypsum model is:
    a. Boxing wax
    b. Sticky wax
    c. Pattern wax
    d. Baseplate wax

16. Utility wax ropes are used to:
    a. Hold components together for repair
    b. Make forms for wax bite registrations
    c. Make corrections in undercut areas of impressions
    d. Adapt the periphery of impression trays

17. The sprue is used in the lost wax procedure to:
    a. Make the channel into which molten metal is forced
    b. Account for delayed expansion and contraction in the final casting
    c. Hold the wax pattern in the investment
    d. Aid in lowering the melting range of the wax

For answers to Review Questions, see the Appendix.

Case-Based Discussion Topics

1. For each of the following situations, which gypsum material would be the best choice?
   • *The assistant has taken an impression for an orthodontic case study.*
   • *The dentist has taken an impression for a space maintainer.*
   • *The hygienist has taken an impression for a custom bleaching tray.*
   • *The expanded-function assistant has taken an impression for a full gold crown.*

2. How would each of the following situations be best handled?
   • *You need to make a custom tray for an appointment in progress and have just taken the alginate impression. How would you accelerate the setting time of the gypsum product you select?*
   • *You have fast-set plaster in your office and wish to mix enough material to pour two arches. How would you increase the working time?*
   • *Several air voids are present on the surfaces of the teeth. What factors may have caused this?*
   • *When you are working on a cast, the teeth chip and crumble easily. What factors may have caused this?*

3. A gypsum model is articulated with a wax bite registration and is left in the dental laboratory over a hot weekend. The assistant, on coming in on Monday, discovers that the model is no longer in the correct occlusion.
   • *What property of the dental wax most likely caused the problem?*
   • *What could have been done to avoid this problem?*

4. A gypsum model is being poured, using boxing wax. The wax is formed around the impression but will not hold in place.
   What can the assistant do to the wax to help it adhere to itself and the tray?

5. After the preceding problem is corrected, the impression is poured. The hygienist, on separating the boxed model, finds that there is a thin layer of wax on the base portion.
   What property of the wax most likely caused this and what property of the gypsum product contributed to this problem?

6. A final impression for an edentulous case is corrected with corrective impression wax; the impression is then sent to the dental laboratory.
   What precautions must be considered when sending the impression?

BIBLIOGRAPHY

American Dental Association (ADA): Council on dental materials: instruments, and equipment: American Dental Association Specification No. 25. *J Am Dent Assoc*, 102:351, 1981.

American Dental Association (ADA): Council on scientific affairs and ada council on dental practice: infection control recommendations for the dental office and dental laboratory. *J Am Dent Assoc*, 1996.

Bird DL, Robinson DS: *Modern Dental Assisting* (ed 12). Missouri, 2018, Elsevier.

Brukl CE, McConnell RM, Norling BK, et al.: Influence of gauging water composition on dental stone expansion and setting time. *J Prosthet Dent*, 1984.

Darby ML, Walsh MW: *Dental Hygiene Theory and Practice* (ed 4). Missouri, 2015, Elsevier.

King BB, Norling BK, Seals R: Gypsum compatibility of antimicrobial alginates after spray disinfection. *J Prosthodont*, 1994.

Kotsiomite E, McCabe JF: Experimental wax mixtures for dental use. *J Oral Rehabil*, 24:517–521, 1997.

Kotsiomite E, McCabe JF: Waxes for functional impressions. *J Oral Rehabil*, 23:114, 1996.

McCrorie JW: Some physical properties of dental modeling waxes and of their main constituents. *J Oral Rehabil*, 1:29, 1974.

Robinson DS, Bird DL: *Essentials of Dental Assisting*, (ed 6). Missouri, 2016, Elsevier.

Sakaguchi RL, Powers JM: *Craig's Restorative Dental Materials* (ed 13). St. Louis, 2012, Mosby.

von Fraunhofer JA, Spiers RR: Accelerated setting of dental stone. *J Prosthet Dent*, 49:859–869, 1983.

van Noort R: *Introduction to Dental Materials* (ed 4). 2013, Elsevier.

Chapter Objectives

Upon completion of this chapter, the student should be able to:

1. Describe the formation of long-chain polymers from monomers.
2. Explain the effect that cross-linking has on the physical and mechanical properties of polymers.
3. Describe the stages of addition polymerization.
4. Explain the function of a free radical.
5. List the important properties of acrylic resins.
6. Describe the procedure for heat processing a denture.
7. Compare the properties of hard and soft lining materials.
8. List the indications for long- and short-term soft liners.
9. Compare the advantages and disadvantages of chairside and laboratory-processed hard liners.
10. List the indications for the use of acrylic denture teeth versus porcelain teeth.
11. Adjust a denture to relieve a sore spot as permitted by state law.
12. Repair a broken acrylic denture.
13. Use an ultrasonic cleaner for cleaning complete and partial dentures in the office.
14. Educate patients regarding the home care regimen they should follow for complete and partial dentures.
15. Inform patients of the precautions they should take when cleaning their dentures.
16. Fabricate custom impression trays for upper and lower arches.
17. Fabricate record bases for complete dentures, using light-cured material.

Key Terms

Polymers long-chain, high molecular weight molecules produced by chemically linking many low molecular weight monomer molecules

Monomers low molecular weight molecules that are joined to form polymers; as used in dentistry, monomers are usually liquids

Polymerization the act of forming polymers by chemically linking monomers into long chains; the process can be activated by chemicals, heat, or light

Cross-Linked Polymers adjacent long-chain polymers joined by the bonding of short chains along their sides to enhance the properties of the polymer

Addition Polymerization common form of polymerization for dental materials; monomer molecules are added one to another sequentially as the reactive group on one molecule initiates bonding with an adjacent monomer molecule and frees another reactive group (free radical) to repeat the process

Free Radical a reactive group on one end of a monomer that initiates the joining of adjacent monomer molecules to form a polymer

Poly(Methyl Methacrylate) (PMMA) a polymer composed of numerous methyl methacrylate monomers linked together into a long chain. Methyl methacrylate is commonly used in denture fabrication

Plasticizer liquid added to acrylic resin to soften it and make it more pliable

Porosity numerous microscopic holes or voids within a material; often caused during polymerization of resins when monomer vaporizes and is lost; can also be caused by entrapping of air during mixing of powder and liquid

Prosthesis a device used for the replacement of missing teeth and/or soft tissues. It can serve both cosmetic and functional roles

Long-Term Soft Liner a soft liner that is used in patients who have problems with hard acrylic denture bases; it is expected to last for 1 to 3 years

Short-Term Soft Liner a soft provisional (temporary) liner used to improve tissue health; also called a *tissue conditioner;* typically, it lasts from a few days to a few weeks

Hard Liner a rigid reline material used inside a denture to improve the fit and stability

The steady increase in the numbers of older Americans will assure a demand for removable complete and partial dentures. Acrylic resins are polymers that play an important role in removable prosthetics. Acrylic resins are used in the fabrication of complete and partial dentures, as well as maxillofacial prostheses (used to replace missing oral or facial structures). They can be used to simulate the oral mucosa, gingiva, and teeth. They are also used to reline these prostheses to improve their fit and to repair them when they break. CAD/CAM technology has also been applied to *fabrication of complete and partial dentures. Once appropriate records have been attained, prostheses can be fabricated by milling or three dimensional (3D) printing.*

Even though a commercial dental laboratory fabricates most of the removable prostheses, the allied oral health practitioner needs to be familiar with the materials and their uses, care, and repair. She or he must understand the materials used in prosthetic dentistry to better care for the patient and to assist the dentist. Patients who wear removable prostheses will often ask the dental assistant or hygienist questions that relate to the fit or home care of their prosthesis. This chapter covers the uses of acrylics for fabrication of complete and partial dentures and for relining, tissue conditioning, and repairing these prostheses. It also covers the use of acrylic denture teeth, porcelain denture teeth, and acrylic repair techniques. The instructions to be given to the patient for the care of these prostheses are presented.

REVIEW OF POLYMER FORMATION

POLYMERS

Polymers are large, long-chain molecules formed by chemically joining together smaller molecules, called *monomers*. The polymer chains will vary in length as the monomer is being consumed and may contain from 10,000 to 100,000 monomer units. The chains will lengthen until no more monomer is available. Most of the polymers shrink as they form, and this creates undesirable features in the final product.

COPOLYMERS

When two or more different types of **monomers** join together, the polymer formed from them is called a *copolymer*. Copolymers are produced to enhance the physical and mechanical properties of the material. They are used in dentures to make them more resistant to fracture, in soft reline materials to make them soft and pliable, and in mouth guards to improve their shock-absorbing capacity.

POLYMERIZATION

The act of forming polymers is called **polymerization**. In general, less than 100% of the monomer is used up. The remaining unused monomer is called the *residual monomer*. The best clinical results occur when there is little residual monomer.

Polymerization (Curing) Methods

The materials that react by chemical means are called *chemical-curing, self-curing,* or *autopolymerizing*. Materials that use heat to initiate the reaction are called *heat-curing polymers*. Materials in which the reaction is activated by light are called *photo-* or *light-curing*. Whether initiated by chemical means, light, or heat, the polymerization process releases heat (i.e., it is an exothermic reaction). The heat must be controlled during the process. If the temperature becomes too great,

the monomer will vaporize and produce porosity in the material. Porosity weakens the material, causes it to discolor as stains are absorbed into the pores, and can lead to retention and growth of oral microorganisms and development of an unpleasant odor ("denture breath").

CROSS-LINKED POLYMERS

Polymer chains often have short chains of atoms attached to their sides. When the side chains of adjacent polymers bond together, the polymers are termed **cross-linked polymers** (see Fig. 6-4 in Chapter 6 Composites, Glass Ionomers, and Compomers). When side chains of adjacent polymers are joined by weak bonds, the polymers are easily manipulated, bent, or stretched. When adjacent polymers are joined by highly charged side chains, the bond is stronger, and the cross-linked polymers are stronger and stiffer. They also are more wear resistant and, consequently, can be used in denture teeth. They polish more easily and are less affected by solvents such as alcohol.

POLYMERIZATION REACTIONS

There are two types of polymerization:
- Addition polymerization
- Condensation polymerization

The reactions are the same as for the impression polymers, addition silicones, and condensation silicones (see Chapter 15 Impression Materials).

Addition Polymerization

Addition polymerization is the most common form of polymerization for dental materials. It occurs in three stages:

Stage 1: Initiation (or induction)
Stage 2: Propagation
Stage 3: Termination

Unlike condensation polymerization, the reaction does not produce any by-products. Monomers have a core unit of two carbon atoms joined by a double bond. One carbon atom has two hydrogen atoms attached, and the other carbon atom has attached to it one hydrogen atom and one reactive group called a **free radical**. The free radical is made reactive by the chemical reaction of organic peroxide, such as benzoyl peroxide, with an activator or accelerator, such as a tertiary amine, or by heating.

Initiation. The free radical initiates the reaction by opening the bond between the two carbon atoms of the monomer. The broken carbon bond causes the monomer molecule to bond to another monomer. Each linkage leaves a free radical available for further reaction.

Propagation. The process of linking monomer units is termed *propagation*, and it continues until the monomer units are used up, or until a substance reacts with the free radical to tie it up.

Termination. When the free radical is tied up or destroyed, the process is terminated.

Condensation Polymerization

Materials formed by a condensation reaction do not have many uses in dentistry. The condensation silicone impression materials are the most commonly known, and even they are not used much today. Typically, more than one type of monomer is used. The reaction itself produces by-products such as water, hydrogen gas, or alcohol that may compromise the physical properties or handling characteristics.

ACRYLIC RESINS (PLASTICS)

Synthetic polymers used in prosthetic dentistry are called *acrylic resins,* because they are derived from acrylic acid. Acrylic resin forms when a liquid monomer (commonly methyl methacrylate) is mixed with a powder of small polymer beads, and the mixture undergoes polymerization. The polymerized resin is **poly(methyl methacrylate) (PMMA).** It is composed of numerous methyl methacrylate (MMA) monomer units linked together to form a long-chain polymer.

USES OF ACRYLICS

The resins are used for denture bases, denture teeth, relining and repair of prostheses, provisional acrylic partial dentures (flippers or stayplates), tissue conditioners, and custom impression trays. They also have uses as orthodontic retainers and removable tooth movement devices (Fig. 17.1), bruxism mouth guards and provisional restorations (see Chapter 18 Provisional Restorations). Specialized acrylic resins are used in esthetic tissue replacement for severe gingival recession and for facial reconstruction due to trauma, surgery, or birth defects. Acrylic resins are especially useful because they can be shaped to any contour and custom-colored to match the shade of the teeth, gingiva, or skin.

MODIFIERS

Acrylic resins used in dentistry are often modified by the addition of plasticizers, rubbers, and fillers to change their physical and mechanical properties. **Plasticizers** are liquids added to soften the acrylic plastics and make them more pliable. Oily liquids called *aromatic esters* are often used as plasticizers. Rubbers may be added to increase the impact fracture resistance of the acrylic resin. Fillers are added to strengthen the resin or change its optical properties. Chemical coupling agents may be used to bond the filler to the acrylic resin. This coupling prevents the filler particles from being plucked out of the resin by abrasion, the result of chewing on food, and makes the resin more wear resistant (similar to the use of silane to couple fillers in composite resins). These bonded fillers can be found in light-cured denture repair or impression tray materials.

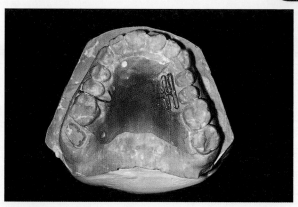

FIG. 17.1 Removable acrylic orthodontic tooth movement device.

PROPERTIES

Polymerization Shrinkage

Polymers undergo shrinkage as a result of the polymerization process. Heat-cured acrylic resins shrink about 6% by volume and about 0.2% to 0.5% linearly (from one point on the denture to another).

Dimensional Change

Sources of dimensional change in addition to polymerization shrinkage include water sorption and thermal expansion. A denture base will increase slightly in its overall size when it absorbs water. This expansion may help offset some of the shrinkage that occurs during polymerization. The coefficient of thermal expansion is more than twice that of composite resins.

Strength

The strength of the acrylic resins is fairly low, with a compressive strength of approximately 11,000 pounds per square inch (psi; or 75.8 megapascals [MPa]) and a tensile strength of 8000 psi (55.2 MPa). By comparison, amalgam has a compressive strength of about 60,000 psi (413.7 MPa). Acrylics are not very hard materials (Knoop hardness number, 16 to 18) and as a consequence are not very wear resistant. Although they have fairly good resistance to fatigue failure (can be flexed repeatedly before they break), they will break if dropped on the floor or in an empty sink during cleaning. To combat the brittleness and breakage problem, some manufacturers add butadiene-styrene rubber to the MMA to create a high-impact acrylic resin. An example of a high-impact acrylic resin is Lucitone 199 (Dentsply International), which comes in four gingival shades.

Thermal Conductivity

Denture bases do not conduct temperature well. Patients wearing dentures will notice a marked difference when they eat foods such as ice cream or drink hot beverages. Because the denture partially insulates against the temperature of the food or beverage, patients may burn themselves when they attempt to swallow foods that are too hot.

Table 17.1	Properties of Heat-Cured Acrylic Resins (PMMA)	
PROPERTY	**VALUE**
Polymerization shrinkage (by volume)	6%
Polymerization shrinkage (linear)	0.2%-0.5%
Coefficient of thermal expansion	More than twice that of composite
Compressive strength	75.8 MPa (11,000 psi)
Tensile strength	55.2 MPa (8000 psi)
Hardness (Knoop)	15-18 kg/mm^2
Biocompatibility	Good
Thermal conductivity	Poor
Wear resistance	Fair
Fatigue resistance (to flexing)	Good
Impact resistance (to breakage when dropped)	Poor

PMMA, poly(methyl methacrylate).

Chemical-Cured versus Heat-Cured Acrylics

The type of processing has some effect on the properties. Polymerization is never 100% complete, and varying amounts of free monomer may be present in the polymerized material. In general, chemical-cured acrylic resins are weaker, softer, more porous, and less color stable than the heat-cured acrylic resins. After polymerization, there is more residual monomer in the chemical-cured acrylic (up to 5%), and it initially adversely affects many of the physical and mechanical properties until the monomer leaches out in minute amounts over several days or weeks. Some dimensional change can occur during the first 24 hours in chemical-cured acrylic. For this reason, custom acrylic trays should not be used immediately, but should sit for 12 to 24 hours to allow most of the dimensional change to occur, so the impression will not be distorted. Heat-cured acrylics are harder, stronger, and less porous and have less than 1% residual monomer that leaches out of the surface relatively quickly. Properties of heat-cured acrylic resins are summarized in Table 17.1.

Porosity

Porosity in polymerized acrylic resin is characterized by the presence of many small or microscopic voids or pores. Porosity in the acrylic weakens it and makes it prone to collect debris and microorganisms. Denture odor and stains develop more readily. Porosity is a result of loss of monomer or inadequate pressure during processing. The monomer is highly volatile and can evaporate rapidly at room temperature during handling of the mixed powder and liquid. Monomer can vaporize during heat-curing of the resin if the temperature rises too much. Curing under pressure helps keep

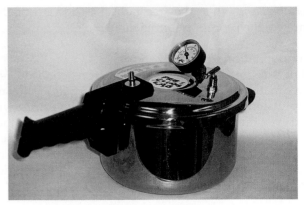

FIG. 17.2 Pressure pot used to provide a denser chemical-cured acrylic.

the monomer from evaporating during polymerization and creates a denser acrylic. When chemical-cured acrylic is cured in room temperature water and 15 to 20 pounds of air pressure in a pressure pot (Fig. 17.2), the resulting acrylic is stronger and has less porosity and shrinkage. A pressure pot is a laboratory device that resembles a pressure cooker. It is a thick-sided metal pot that seals well and can be pressurized by the addition of air through a one-way valve in its lid. Porosity can also occur by the entrapment of air during mixing of the powder and liquid acrylic resin components.

Caution

When using a pressure pot, it is not necessary to pressurize it with air to more than 20 psi. Although the pressure pot is constructed of heavy materials and can usually withstand high pressure and has a pressure release valve, excessive pressure—more than 30 psi—increases the risk of a mishap should the release valve malfunction.

ALLERGIC REACTION

Sensitive patients can react to the components of the denture materials. If excessive free monomer is present in the denture base, some people's tissues may be irritated and inflamed by the methacrylate monomer. Other components such as hydroquinone, benzoyl peroxide, and pigments can also cause irritation. Dental personnel who work with the materials can develop contact dermatitis through repeated exposure of unprotected skin to the materials. Personal protective equipment (PPE) should be used when handling these materials. Dental resins are not known to cause systemic toxic reactions.

Caution

To prevent contact dermatitis, avoid contact with methyl methacrylate even with gloved hands. Most resin monomers easily pass through gloves. Remove gloves and wash hands thoroughly if contact occurs.

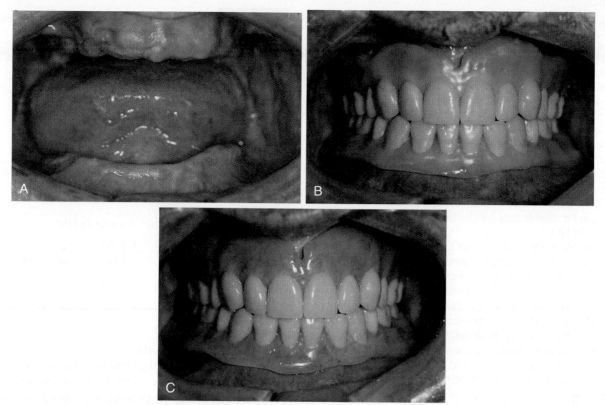

FIG. 17.3 Complete dentures. **A,** Edentulous ridges. **B,** Denture teeth set in wax for try-in. **C,** Dentures processed in acrylic, polished, and delivered to patient.

ACRYLIC RESINS FOR DENTURE BASES

The functions of the acrylic resin denture base are to
- Retain the artificial teeth in the **prosthesis**
- Adapt to the supporting structures for stability
- Distribute forces of mastication over a wide area to reduce pressure on the ridges that might contribute to resorption of the underlying bone
- Replace missing tissues or rebuild the contours of tissues lost when the underlying bone resorbs
- Establish a seal along the periphery of a complete denture that aids in retention (Fig. 17.3)

POLYMERIZATION REACTION

Acrylic resins polymerize by an addition reaction. Acrylic resins are supplied as a powder and a liquid. The powder is composed mostly of small beads of PMMA and benzoyl peroxide (the initiator). Inorganic pigments are added to give the acrylic resin colors resembling those of the oral mucosa, and titanium dioxide is added to keep the acrylic from being too transparent. Small, colored fibers may be added to simulate small blood vessels. Several shades of acrylic are available, so that the clinician can attempt to match the variations of racial pigmentation that can occur in the gingiva and mucosa of patients (Fig. 17.4). The liquid contains MMA, hydroquinone as an inhibitor or preservative to prevent polymerization of the MMA during storage, and glycol

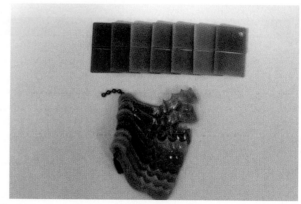

FIG. 17.4 Acrylic shade guides for matching the color of the gingiva. (Courtesy of Mark Dellinges, School of Dentistry, University of California, San Francisco [San Francisco, CA].)

dimethacrylate as a cross-linking agent. Cross-linking of the acrylic polymer chains helps prevent surface cracks, and it improves resistance to structural fatigue that can lead to fracture. The liquid is supplied in dark brown bottles to prevent ultraviolet light from initiating polymerization during storage. When the powder and the liquid are mixed, chemical- and heat-cured materials go through a similar reaction, except that chemical-cured materials have a tertiary amine in the liquid as an activator, whereas heat-cured materials do not (Table 17.2).

Steps in Complete Denture Fabrication

1. Make preliminary alginate impressions of edentulous ridges (by dental assistant/hygienist).
2. Pour impressions into stone for preliminary casts (by dental assistant/hygienist).
3. Fabricate custom impression trays from preliminary casts (by dental assistant/hygienist or laboratory technician).
4. Border mold trays with compound (or other thermoplastic material) and make final impressions with elastomer (by dentist or extended-function dental assistant/hygienist).
5. Box impressions with utility wax and pour into die stone for master cast (by dental assistant/hygienist or sent to lab).
6. Fabricate record bases (used to capture relations between upper and lower jaws; also called wax rims) (by dental assistant/hygienist or laboratory technician).
7. With record bases, record jaw relations, midline and lip line. Make facebow transfer—not used by all dentists (by dentist or extended functions dental assistant/hygienist).
8. Select shade and mold of teeth (by dentist with help from assistant/hygienist and patient).
9. Mount casts on articulator and set teeth in wax of record bases (by dentist or laboratory technician).
10. Try teeth in wax in the patient's mouth to check appearance and occlusion (by dentist).
11. Return wax try-in to laboratory for final processing in acrylic resin.

⚠ Caution

Liquid monomer should be considered a hazardous material. It is flammable and vaporizes easily when the lid is off of the container. Use in a well-ventilated area, ideally under a vapor hood. Avoid prolonged direct breathing of the vapor. Because all of its potential hazards have not been defined, it is advisable for pregnant workers and patients to avoid breathing the fumes. It can irritate eyes, nose, skin, and lungs and may affect the nervous system.

Physical Stages of Polymerization

Sandy stage. The first stage seen when the powder (polymer) and the liquid (monomer) are mixed is called the *sandy stage,* because the mixture looks grainy, similar to sand and water, and has a runny consistency.

Stringy stage. The second stage occurs when the powder particles absorb the liquid into their surface. It is called the *stringy stage,* because the mixture is stringy when handled and is thicker in consistency.

Dough stage. In the next stage, called the *dough stage,* more of the powder goes into solution and the mixture changes from stringy to doughy and is more easily manipulated.

Rubber stage. In the final stage, called the *rubber stage,* the mixture has a rubbery consistency that can no longer be manipulated for forming the denture base.

Table 17.2	Ingredients of Acrylic Resin and Their Function
COMPONENT	**FUNCTION**
Liquid	
Methyl methacrylate	Monomer
Hydroquinone	Inhibitor to prevent polymerization of monomer during storage
Glycol dimethacrylate	Cross-linking agent
Tertiary amine	Activator for chemical-cured resin
Powder	
Poly(methyl methacrylate)	Polymer beads
Benzoyl peroxide	Initiator
Titanium dioxide	Reduces translucency
Pigments	Simulate tissue colors
Colored fibers	Simulate small blood vessels

Chemical-Cured Resins

Polymerization of chemical-cured acrylic resins is set into action when the tertiary amine in the liquid activates the benzoyl peroxide in the powder to produce free radicals. The hydroquinone initially inhibits the reaction from progressing by destroying free radicals. This inhibition increases the working time so that the materials can be manipulated for a reasonable period of time, usually while the material progresses from the stringy stage to the dough stage. As the hydroquinone is depleted, the reaction proceeds more rapidly and advances from the dough stage to the rubber stage. The reaction is exothermic (releases heat) and ultimately becomes quite hot. When the reaction is complete, the material is hard and stiff.

Pour technique. Some chemical-cured materials can be mixed to a thin, fluid consistency and poured into a mold and cured under pressure.

Heat-Cured Resins

The most common method for processing denture bases uses heat and pressure during polymerization of the acrylic resin. Heat-cured acrylic resins go through initial stages of polymerization that are similar to those of chemical-cured resins.

Processing the Complete Denture

After the dentist has tried in the denture teeth set in wax and the patient approves the appearance, the denture is returned to the laboratory, where the technician places the cast of the edentulous arch, along with the denture setup (teeth mounted in wax on a record base), in a specially designed processing flask. The flask separates in the middle into two sections. The denture setup mounted on the cast is invested in a plaster investing material in the flask in such a manner that the flask can be opened in the middle to allow removal of the wax and record base after heating in a water bath. The teeth are held in place by the plaster. All remnants of the wax are removed. A liquid, called a *separating medium,* is placed and air-dried on the plaster and the cast to prevent the acrylic resin from sticking to or absorbing moisture from the gypsum materials. Mixed acrylic resin in the dough stage is placed in the space created by removal of the wax and record base. (It has a longer dough stage than chemical-cured acrylic, because it does not have the tertiary amine activator.) This space is where the denture base will be formed. A sheet of polyethylene material is placed over the resin and the flask is reassembled and closed under pressure. The flask is reopened to remove excess material that exudes out of the sides of the flask. This process is repeated until no excess material appears and the polyethylene sheet is removed. The flask is put into a device called a *pneumatic press* that maintains pressure on it, and it is placed into a temperature-controlled water bath for at least 8 hours. Heat activates the benzoyl peroxide, causing the formation of free radicals and allowing polymerization to occur. Applying pressure and controlling the heat minimize porosity by preventing the monomer from vaporizing. More of the monomer is consumed during the polymerization, so less free monomer is present in the cured denture base with heat-processed dentures. Similar to the chemical-cured resins, the material is hard and stiff when the polymerization is complete. It also shrinks when it is polymerized. Shrinkage is seen most readily in the palatal area and can cause the acrylic to lift from the cast as much as 0.25 mm. If a room temperature processing technique is used, shrinkage is less, but the properties of the denture are poorer initially, because of the presence of much more free monomer. The properties improve as the free monomer leaches out.

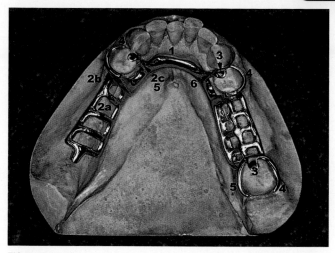

FIG. 17.5 Components of a removable partial denture framework. (From Carr AB, Brown DT: *McCracken's removable partial prosthodontics,* (ed 13). St Louis, 2016, Mosby.)

Components of a Complete Denture

- Denture Base—acrylic resin component that rests on the edentulous ridge and adjacent oral mucosa and contains the denture teeth. In the maxillary denture it also covers and rests on the hard palate.
- Flange—that portion of the denture that extends vertically from the base of the denture into the facial or lingual vestibule. In Fig. 17.3, panel B, it is the pink acrylic that extends on the facial from the base of the denture teeth to the depth of the vestibule.
- Peripheral seal—a seal created around the outer edge of the denture by its intimate contact with the oral soft tissues. It is needed to provide retention of the denture.
- Posterior Palatal Seal (also called Postdam)—a seal formed in the posterior extent of the maxillary denture base at the junction of the hard and soft palates. It is the part of the peripheral seal of the denture that resists tipping of the denture when biting with the anterior teeth.
- Denture Teeth—acrylic, composite resin or porcelain teeth used to replace missing natural teeth

Processing of a Removable Partial Denture (RPD)

A similar process is performed for applying a denture base to a removable partial denture, except that the partial denture will have a metal framework (see Fig. 17.5 for framework components) invested in the mold, as well as the teeth set in wax. Because the acrylic resin does not adhere well to the metal, a retentive mesh or lattice is made as part of the partial denture framework to lock the acrylic in place (Fig. 17.6).

Components of a Removable Partial Denture (RPD) Framework

The framework is the structure that supports the denture base and the teeth and provides stability and retention of the prosthesis. Its components include:
- Major Connector—joins the components of the framework on one side of the arch to the other side. In Fig. 17.4 it is the lingual bar. A maxillary RPD would have a palatal connector. The major connector provides cross-arch stability and aids in resisting displacement of the RPD by functional forces.
- Minor connectors—join the major connector to the other components of the framework such as the retentive clasp assembly, occlusal or cingulum rests and indirect retainers
- Direct retainer—the clasp assembly that has a retentive clasp arm (that engage undercuts on the crown of the support tooth), a reciprocal arm opposite the retentive arm (that braces against lateral stresses) and rests (metal stops on the occlusal of posterior teeth or cingulum of anterior teeth that prevent the partial denture from seating too far and putting too much pressure on the gingiva and bony ridge and directs occlusal forces along the long axis of the support teeth)
- Indirect Retainer—when an RPD has no support teeth at the distal extent of the arch on one or both sides, the indirect retainer aids the direct retainer in preventing displacement of the distal extension denture base. In Fig. 17.6 the upper right quadrant has a distal extension denture base replacing teeth #2 to #5.
- Retentive meshwork—a metal grid overlying the edentulous ridge into which the denture acrylic will be forced during processing for retention of the denture base
- Denture Base—acrylic resin component that rests on the edentulous ridge and adjacent oral mucosa and contains the denture teeth
- Denture Teeth—acrylic, composite resin or porcelain teeth used to replace missing natural teeth

Microwave Processing

The same denture resins used for the heat processing technique can be used for processing in a microwave oven. If a special monomer liquid is used in place of regular monomer, less porosity is found. Processing time is greatly speeded up, and processing is completed in about 5 minutes instead of the several hours needed for heat processing.

Injection Molding

Some vinyl acrylic resins can be processed by injecting the material into a mold when it is in a doughy form. With some materials, shrinkage and porosity are reduced by injection molding. Some laboratories use this technique because it is faster than the traditional heat processing.

Light-Cured Resins

In addition to heat- and chemical-curing, dental resins can be light-cured. The light-polymerized resins have photoinitiators such as camphorquinone and amine activators. These react to form free radicals when exposed to blue light and initiate the polymerization reaction (see Chapter 6). One of the commercially available light-cured materials (Triad VLC; Dentsply International) contains urethane dimethacrylate resin and silica fillers for thickening the material and reinforcing it. It comes in flat sheets or ropes depending on the application. Each sheet is individually packaged in a thick black plastic bag to prevent room light from reaching it and causing premature polymerization. The light-cured materials are fast and easy to use but require the purchase of an expensive light-curing unit (see Fig. 17.33 in Procedure 17.2). The material is available in limited acrylic colors. It is used for denture bases, record bases (see Procedure 17.2), custom trays, and denture repairs. It also has applications for removable orthodontic appliances.

DIGITAL DENTURES

The use of CAD/CAM technology in dentistry has expanded beyond crown and bridge applications to many other clinical facets of dentistry including removable partial and complete dentures. In Chapter 15 digital scanners were discussed and they can scan the edentulous ridges for complete dentures. However, the scanners are not able to determine with accuracy where the flange of the denture should end in the vestibule. Therefore, they cannot be used for complete denture final impressions since the peripheral seal needed for retention cannot be established from the scan. A mix of traditional denture construction techniques and CAD/CAM techniques are needed.

The clinician that wants to provide digital dentures has two options in order to participate. First, the clinician can use traditional denture methods up to the point of processing the denture and then can have the records entered into a CAD/CAM system for design

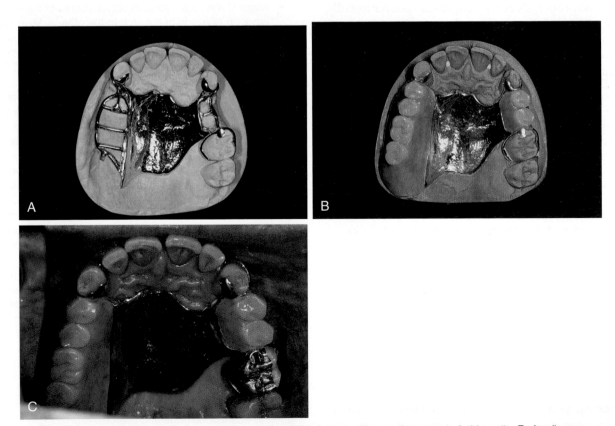

FIG. 17.6 A, Metal frameworks for upper removable partial denture with retentive areas to hold acrylic. **B,** Acrylic processed over retentive structure with denture teeth added. **C,** Maxillary partial denture in the mouth.

and fabrication by milling or 3-D printing. The second option is to use methods and devices developed by companies for digital denture systems. These systems allow final impressions and records of the bite and other jaw relations, occlusal plane orientation, tooth shade and mold and maxillary anterior tooth position all to be gathered in the first appointment and sent to the company to be scanned and entered into their CAD/CAM software. Then, denture can be designed and processed.

There are two main systems presently: AvaDent Digital Denture Solutions (Global Dental Science) and Pala Digital Dentures (Heraeus Kulzer). The two systems differ in their records collections methods, design software and method of fabricating the dentures. The two systems use trays that can be customized to take final impressions at the first visit and use their own devices for capturing jaw records and the other features (mentioned above) needed to design the denture. The impression and other records are sent to the company. A technician scans the records into the software and designs the denture based upon the records (Fig. 17.7). The dentist can receive this image and view it with the patient in the dental office and make adjustments on the arrangement, size and shade of the teeth before the denture is processed. If desired, a try-in denture can be made and sent to the dentist for the patient to evaluate.

The AvaDent system mills the denture base from large, thick preformed disks of acrylic that has been polymerized under heat and much more pressure than conventionally processed denture bases (Fig. 17.8). As a consequence, when the denture base is milled there will be no polymerization shrinkage because it occurred when the disk was made and porosity will be greatly reduced. The acrylic disk is highly cross-linked producing a stronger acrylic. The AvaDent system bonds artificial teeth to the denture base (Fig. 17.9).

The Pala Digital Denture system also designs the denture and allows the clinician to review it with the patient. Processing of the denture is by 3-D printing. The denture base and teeth are printed as one unit. It produces a denture with similar improvements in physical properties.

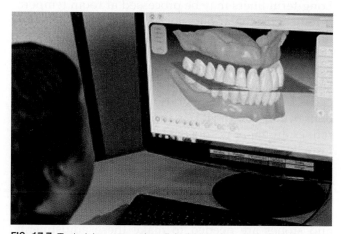

FIG. 17.7 Technician scans the clinical records and designs the denture. (Courtesy of AvaDent.)

Advantages of Digital Dentures

- Reduced number of appointments—usually 2 instead of 5 for conventional denture techniques
- Time savings for dentist and patient
- Dentures can be ready in a matter of days rather than weeks with conventional dentures
- Better fit of the denture because polymerization shrinkage is eliminated
- Porosity is reduced or eliminated reducing staining and development of odor
- Records can be stored for futures needs
- Duplicate or replacement dentures can be made without additional appointments

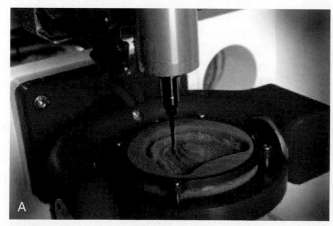
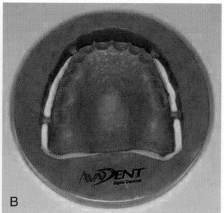

FIG. 17.8 Denture base is being milled from a preformed, thick acrylic disk. **A,** Milling of the denture base. **B,** Completed denture base with spaces created for the denture teeth. (**A,** courtesy Loma Linda University Dentistry Summer/Autumn 2012, CAD/CAM technology: application to complete dentures by Mathew Kattadiyil, DDS, MSD and Charles J. Goodacre, DDS, MSD. **B,** Courtesy of AvaDent.)

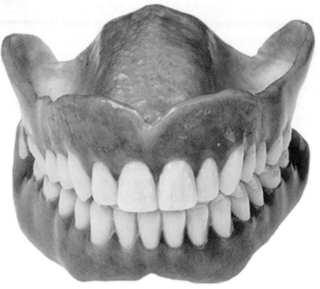

FIG. 17.9 Completed dentures after teeth have been bonded to the denture base. (Courtesy of AvaDent.)

DENTURE RELINE MATERIALS (LINERS)

Relining a denture is done for several reasons. A reline will fix looseness that occurs as the bony ridges resorb and the gums shrink. An upper denture will occasionally crack lengthwise through the palatal area as the ridges resorb. The reline readapts the denture to the ridges and repairs the fracture. A soft temporary reline material may act as a tissue conditioner to improve the health of the tissues before a hard reline is done. Some soft temporary reline materials will flow gradually to adapt to the tissues when worn for a day or two and will serve as a functional impression for a hard reline. A reline may serve to prolong the life of the denture as an alternative to making a new one.

Long-term denture relines can be made with either a hard setting material or a soft, flexible one. Both types of materials can be applied to the denture at chairside or may be sent to the dental laboratory for processing. In general, the laboratory processed reline gives a better result and will last longer. The chairside relines are more porous, more likely to break down sooner, and will stain more readily. The laboratory processed reline requires that the patient leave the denture out for 12 to 24 hours to allow the tissues to return to an uncompressed state before taking the impression for the reline: Pressure from wearing and eating with the denture will compress the tissues.

SOFT RELINING MATERIALS

Complete and partial dentures sometimes have a soft lining material placed on the tissue-bearing surface of the denture base. Soft liners may be used as short-term treatment for a few days up to a few weeks to allow tissues to heal after surgery, or when denture sores have formed. Soft liners may also be used for long-term treatment for patients who have chronic soreness with hard denture bases because of sharp bony spicules or thin mucosa over the ridges. Patients feel more comfortable with a lining that has a cushioning effect, especially if the denture is opposing natural teeth. Long-term soft liners are also used for patients with bony tissue undercuts that cannot be surgically corrected. A hard denture base rubs the mucosa in the area of the undercut, whereas a soft liner cushions the tissues and will flex in and out of the undercut when the denture is placed and removed. Soft liners are used with palatal defects such as cleft palate or tissue loss from cancer surgery or trauma. On average, long-term soft liner materials last about 1 to 3 years.

Long-Term Soft Liners

Long-term soft liners are made from silicone rubber or acrylics such as ethyl or methyl methacrylate that have been made pliable by the addition of plasticizers such as aromatic esters and alcohol (Fig. 17.10). Long-term liners may be processed at room temperature or with the application of heat. Although some long-term silicone and acrylic liners can be placed at chairside, others are placed at the commercial laboratory. Heat-cured silicone liners are processed in the laboratory, because they release acetic acid that can cause tissue burns. Laboratory-processed relines are denser and last longer (1 to 3 years). Chairside soft relines are more porous and stain more easily. Long-term liners composed of acrylic will harden over time as the plasticizers leach out and will need replacement. The silicone liners are more stable over the long term, because they do not have softeners to leach out. However, they can be difficult to adjust. Special burs and stones are needed to make these adjustments. Another problem with long-term soft liners is that they often do not form a good bond to old acrylic. Therefore, they may separate from the denture base at the edges and leak between the liner and the denture base.

Silicone liners support the growth of yeasts such as *Candida albicans* and may cause tissue irritation that requires antifungal therapy. Cleaning soft liners on a daily basis in benzalkonium chloride will reduce the growth of yeasts.

Short-term soft liners (tissue conditioners). **Short-term soft liners** are referred to as *tissue conditioners* or *treatment liners* and are usually placed at chairside. They are supplied as a powder composed of poly(ethyl methacrylate) and softeners or plasticizers of aromatic oils and ethanol (Fig. 17.11).

Application of short-term liner. The powder and liquid are mixed thoroughly according to the manufacturer's directions and are flowed onto the tissue-bearing surface of the denture, which was previously cleaned with

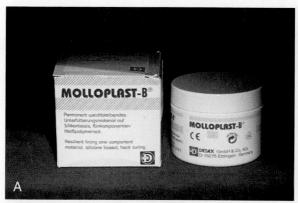

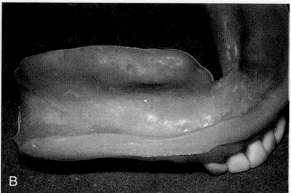

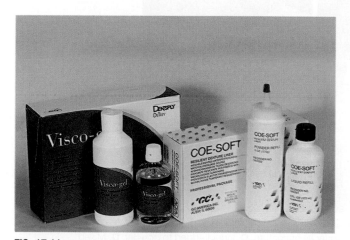

FIG. 17.10 Long-term soft liners. **A,** Heat-cured, silicone-based soft lining material. **B,** Soft liner processed in lower denture. **C,** Chairside, chemical-cured, silicone-based soft liner in cartridges dispensed with a mixing gun and tip. (Courtesy of Mark Dellinges, School of Dentistry, University of California, San Francisco [San Francisco, CA].)

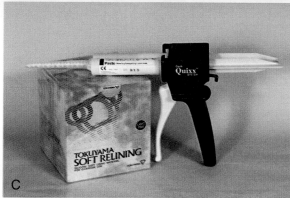

FIG. 17.11 Two tissue conditioners (short-term soft liners) (Visco-gel, Courtesy of Dentsply International, York, PA; Coe-Soft, Courtesy of GC America, Alsip, IL). They come with two components—powder and liquid.)

soap and water. The denture is reseated in the patient's mouth, and the patient is instructed to gently close into normal occlusion until the material cures (see sequence in Fig. 17.12). These liners are capable of readapting to the patient's tissues as they heal, because they have a high degree of flow. Because this flow property is greatest the first day, hard foods should be avoided to prevent distortion of the material. As the plasticizers leach out, the resin becomes stiffer. The plasticizers leach out more quickly in the short-term liners than in the long-

term liners and therefore need frequent replacement. Some short-term liners last for only 1 week; others last for 2 to 4 weeks.

Use of appropriate denture soaks can prolong the useful life of soft liners, and therefore the manufacturer's recommendations are important. The dental assistant and hygienist must be familiar with materials and procedures for the placement of liners at chairside and for the home care of both chairside and laboratory-processed liners.

DETECTION AND MANAGEMENT OF DENTURE SORES

Denture sores are common with new dentures as the tissues adapt to the new prosthesis. Older dentures may also produce sore spots as the bony ridges slowly resorb and the denture becomes loose. Sore spots can also occur after a denture reline since a whole new tissue-bearing surface has been created.

Signs and Symptoms

Typically, the patient first senses some mild soreness under the denture when eating or placing and removing the denture. After a few days mild soreness may become outright pain. Initially, the affected area may be slightly red as inflammation begins, and then can become a larger, bright red area in a couple days (Fig. 17.13). If not treated right away, the tissue can ulcerate leaving a painful raw area that will take longer to heal.

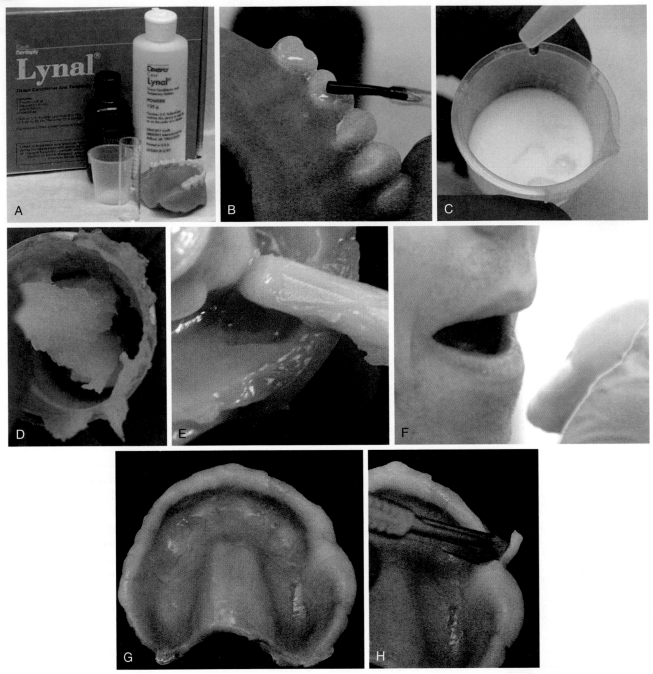

FIG. 17.12 Application of a tissue conditioner. It flows and adapts to the tissues as they heal. **A,** Tissue conditioner. **B,** Separating material to keep conditioner from sticking to outer surfaces of denture. **C,** Liquid added to powder. **D,** Mixed conditioner material. **E,** Conditioner added to tissue-bearing surfaces. **F,** Denture inserted into patient's mouth, seated evenly, and left until it gels. **G,** Excess material around denture border. **H,** Scalpel blade used to trim excess from border. (From Powers JM, Wataha JC: *Dental Materials: Properties and Manipulation* (ed 10). St. Louis, 2013, Elsevier. Courtesy of Richard Lee, Sr., and Bradley Jones, University of Washington Department of Restorative Dentistry, Seattle, WA.)

Causes of Denture Sores

Elastomeric impression materials used for complete dentures by their rubbery nature are flexible when set and will flex out of tissue undercuts and return to their original shape (elastic recovery). The cast made from these impressions will exhibit the undercuts the way they were in the mouth. When the denture is processed on these casts, the acrylic resin will flow into the undercuts and harden as it sets. When the patient is fit with the dentures some of the resin that went into the undercut is removed, but often not all of it. The soft tissues under the denture will compress to a limited degree allowing the denture to seat even with mild undercuts. When the patient wears the dentures for a few days and takes them in and out of the mouth, the acrylic will rub the soft tissues and create a sore spot. Another way a sore spot develops is when the occlusion is too heavy in one area and puts excessive

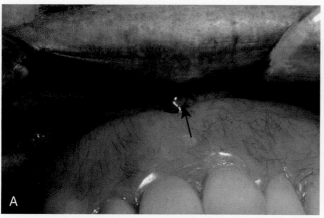
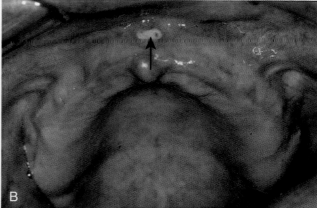

FIG. 17.13 Denture sore. **A,** Denture flange impinged upon maxillary frenum. **B,** Denture sore resulted. (Courtesy of Dr. Mark Dellinges.)

pressure on the ridge. A denture sore can develop when the borders are overextended. Still another way is when the denture presses on sharp edges of bone that were part of the sockets left when teeth were removed. The tissues overlying the sharp bone become irritated (These sharp bony edges may take months to remodel and become rounded. Sometimes they need to be surgically corrected). Dentures that have become loose and slide around under function can also cause sore spots.

Common Causes of Denture Sores

- Bony or soft tissue undercuts
- Sharp bony edges to sockets of extracted teeth
- Overextended denture borders
- Loose dentures
- Uneven occlusion on the denture causing pressure areas

Treatment

The denture requires some adjustment to eliminate the source of the irritation. The source needs to be detected. Sometimes there is an obvious projection on the inside of the denture that can readily be removed with rotary instruments such as an acrylic bur (a metal bur made for grinding acrylic) or abrasive stone. Other times it is necessary to discover precisely where the offending acrylic is located. There are two common methods for finding the acrylic that rubs the tissues:

- use of a paste painted inside the denture that shows the area of pressure
- colored dye that is applied to the denture sore and transferred to the inside of the denture

Use of Pressure Indicating Paste (PIP). Paste used to show pressure areas inside the denture (Pressure Indicating Paste (PIP) | Keystone Industries) is an opaque white silicone paste (Fig. 17.14) that is painted inside the denture with a brush. A thin layer of the paste should be evenly distributed across the entire tissue-bearing surface of the denture if there are

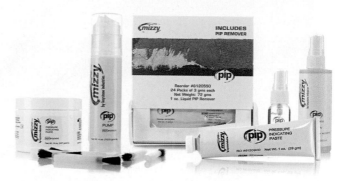

FIG. 17.14 Pressure Indicator Paste (Pressure Indicator Paste [PIP], Keystone Industries) Available in bulk jar, pump, tube or single-use packets with brush. Spray bottles of PIP removal agent and wetting agent (to keep PIP from sticking to the tissues).

multiple sore areas or limited to one area if there is only one sore. The brush supplied with the paste (PIP) will produce fine lines in the paste. Try to make the lines all go in the same direction. When the denture is seated, the operator or the patient can apply mild pressure to the denture by pressing evenly on the first molar/second premolar region with the thumbs (upper denture) or index and middle fingers (lower denture). An alternative to holding the denture with the fingers is to place cotton rolls over the occlusal surfaces of the posterior teeth and have the patient close with mild pressure. Carefully remove the denture after about 20 seconds. Ideally, there should be even contact throughout the denture surface. A thin layer of the paste will be evenly spread out where the denture contacted the tissues (Fig. 17.15). Lines in the paste from the brush will still be present in areas where the denture failed to touch the soft tissues. The PIP will be displaced in areas of excessive pressure exposing the denture base. This is the area to be adjusted (see sequence of figures below).

Use of Dye Transfer Method A small wooden applicator with dry purple dye on one end (Dr. Thompson's Sanitary Color Transfer Applicators, Great Plains Dental Products) is used to mark the denture

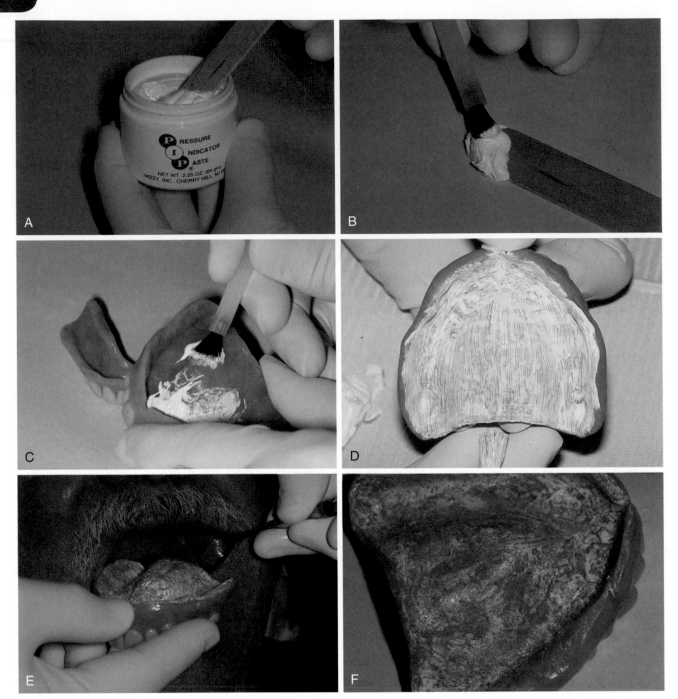

FIG. 17.15 Use of Pressure Indicating Paste (PIP) at delivery of a new denture or after a hard reline. **A,** A tongue blade is used to remove enough PIP to coat the denture a couple times. **B,** PIP is picked up on a disposable brush. **C,** PIP is spread on the tissue-bearing portion of the denture. **D,** PIP is spread in a even coating leaving brush marks that all course in the same direction. This pattern helps in reading tissue contact with the denture. **E,** Denture with PIP is seated in the mouth with light pressure for about 20 seconds. **F,** When the denture is removed, the brush marks are gone and an even distribution of PIP has occurred. No pressure spots are evident. Pressure spots would show as areas where PIP was displaced and the denture base exposed. Areas where the denture did not have contact with the tissues would show as PIP with remaining brush marks. (Courtesy of Dr. Mark Dellinges, University of California, SF.)

sore (Fig. 17.16). Excess moisture is wiped away from the denture sore with gauze. Next, the tip of the applicator with dye is wet with a drop of water and touched to the sore depositing the dye (Fig. 17.17). The inside of the denture should be dry. The denture is seated over the ridge and gently held in place for 10 to 20 seconds. The denture is removed and the purple dye

will have been picked up by the denture in the area of the sore. This marks the spot to be adjusted (Fig. 17.18).

Occasionally, the mouth is so sore that the patient cannot eat with the dentures. In this case, a tissue conditioner (temporary, soft denture liner) may be placed for a few days to a few weeks depending on the severity of the mouth soreness. An alternative is to have the

HARD RELINING MATERIALS

Immediate dentures are those placed immediately after extraction of the teeth. They become loose rapidly (usually within 6 to 12 months) as the extraction sites heal and the bone resorbs. These loose dentures can often be made to fit well again by placement of a **hard liner** to fill in the spaces. Conventionally placed dentures will loosen as well but over a longer period of time. The most common material used for this purpose is an acrylic resin similar to the original denture base material. This hard liner is placed directly into the patient's mouth at chairside or indirectly in the dental laboratory.

When to Use a Reline Material

- Inadequate seal of denture borders
- Lack of retention of the denture
- Looseness and poor denture stability
- Over-closed bite (loss of vertical dimension of occlusion)

Chairside Reline

With the chairside technique, a chemical-cured acrylic resin [poly(methyl methacrylate)] supplied as polymer powder and liquid monomer is commonly used. First, an acrylic bur is used to remove a thin layer of the tissue-bearing surface of the denture base, so that a fresh, clean surface is available for chemical bonding of the lining material to the denture. A lubricant such as petroleum jelly is applied to the denture teeth and to non–tissue-bearing surfaces to which the liner should not adhere. The freshened surface is primed with some of the liquid (methyl methacrylate monomer) to make it ready for the liner. The monomer is a good solvent and will slightly soften the surface, allowing the liner to bond better. The powder and the liquid are mixed thoroughly and applied to the primed denture base. The patient should be advised that the material has a strong smell and bad taste. The denture is reseated in the patient's mouth. The lips, cheeks, and tongue are moved through appropriate motions to reestablish the peripheral borders (a process called *border molding*). In essence, the reline material makes an impression of the tissues. The patient is asked to close into the normal occlusion. This position is held until the material just begins to harden. It should be removed from the mouth before polymerization is complete, because the chemical reaction is exothermic and the heat generated could burn the tissues. Also, the hardened material could lock into tissue undercuts, making it difficult and painful to remove. Gross excess material extending over the borders is removed with sharp iris scissors or a scalpel blade. The denture is placed into a plastic bag and sprayed with an appropriate disinfectant before taking it to the laboratory. The denture is placed into warm water (not hot) in a pressure pot in the office laboratory at 20 psi of pressure for about 15 to 20 minutes while the final set

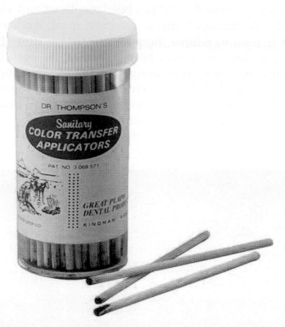

FIG. 17.16 Color Transfer Applicators. (Dr. Thompson's Sanitary Color Transfer Applicators, Great Plains Dental Products).

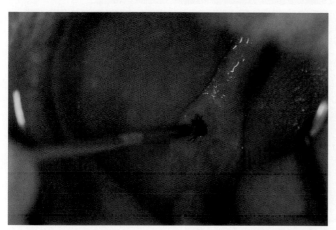

FIG. 17.17 Color transfer applicator used to mark denture sore and transfer the location to the denture. (Courtesy of Dr. Mark Dellinges, University of California, SF.)

patient leave the dentures out for a few days. However, most patients do not want to be seen without teeth and do not select this option.

HOME CARE

Warm salt water rinses can be useful to reduce inflammation and speed healing when used 3 to 4 times a day. Going to a soft diet will also reduce the pressure produced with eating. When possible, leaving the dentures out for a few hours a day will also help with healing. Good oral hygiene is necessary to reduce oral debris and bacteria. Over-the-counter numbing pastes, gels and rinses can be helpful in reducing symptoms and help to reduce pain while eating. Acidic and spicy foods may irritate the ulcerated tissue, so they should be avoided.

occurs. The pressure will reduce porosity that may contribute to staining and odor formation. Once completely hardened, the excess material is trimmed away and the denture borders are carefully polished.

The denture is disinfected before returning it to chairside. Pressure-indicating paste (PIP) is evenly coated on the internal aspect of the denture with an application brush. The denture is seated evenly in the mouth with gentle pressure. The denture is removed

and areas where the PIP has been displaced and acrylic shows through indicate pressure spots. An acrylic bur is used to relieve the pressure spots. After all of the pressure spots have been removed, the occlusion is checked with articulating paper and adjustments made as needed. The patient is advised that the interior of the denture is now entirely new and may cause sore spots much like a new denture. One or more visits may be necessary to complete the adjustments.

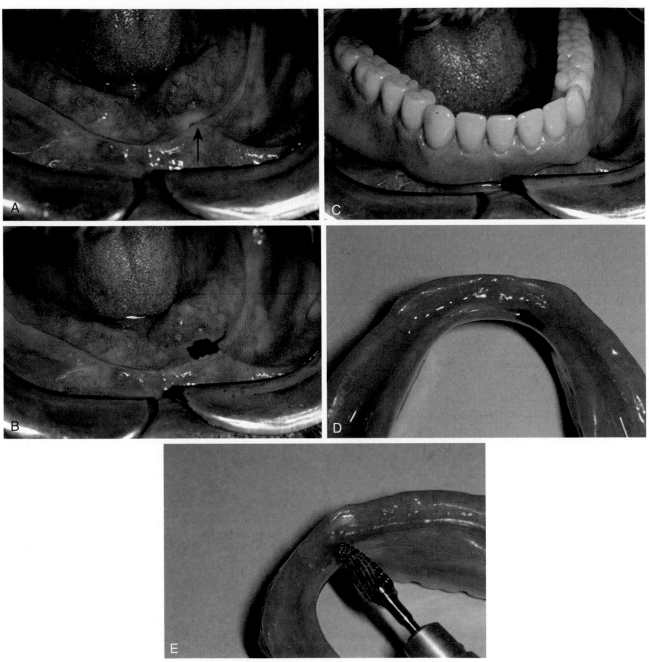

FIG. 17.18 A, Ulcer in soft tissue lingual to mandibular edentulous ridge caused by the lower denture. **B,** Denture sore marked with dye from Color Transfer Applicator. **C,** Denture dried and reseated. **D,** The dye is transferred to the denture indicating the location of the offending pressure area. **E,** An acrylic bur in a low speed handpiece is used to relieve the pressure area. **F,** Now that the location of the irritating denture part has been located, pressure indicating paste (PIP) is used to detect any remaining pressure spots. **G,** The denture is reseated and the interior inspected. Areas where pressure from the denture is evenly distributed will show a thin layer of PIP. PIP will be wiped away in areas of heavy pressure. **H,** Readjust areas of heavy pressure. **I,** Final check with PIP shows no pressure spots. (Courtesy of Dr. Mark Dellinges, University of California, SF.)

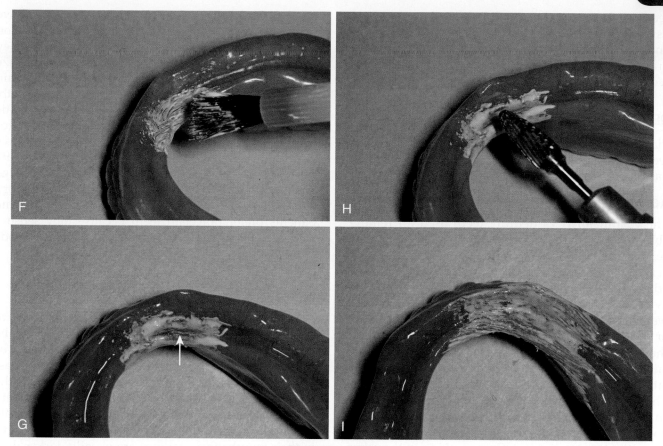

FIG. 17.18—cont'd

An alternative hard reline material (Ufi Gel hard; VOCO) is free of methyl methacrylate. It uses polymer beads and dimethacrylate as the monomer. It is hand mixed or is available in a cartridge for direct application to the denture. The self-mixing cartridge makes it easy to use and provides a homogeneous, bubble-free mix. The liner does not generate heat as it polymerizes, so it can be left in the patient's mouth until it fully cures, improving the accuracy of the fit. It is more pleasant for the patient because it is odorless and tasteless.

Problems Associated with Chairside Reline with Poly(Methyl Methacrylate)

- Porosity from mixing or applying, causing staining and odor
- Bad taste and smell
- Potential soft tissue irritation from free monomer
- Poor bonding with the denture base
- Heat generation with potential tissue burn if not removed soon enough

---

⚠ Caution

When doing a chairside hard reline with poly(methyl methacrylate), be sure to remove the denture before the reline material completely hardens. The heat released can burn the tissues and the material could lock into undercuts, making it difficult and painful to remove.

LABORATORY RELINE

The laboratory reline uses an indirect technique in which an impression of the tissues is made inside the existing denture and a cast is made from this impression. The technician uses an indexing instrument called a *reline jig* or device to establish the relationship between the cast and the denture. The impression material is removed, along with a thin layer of the tissue-bearing denture base surface, as with the chairside technique. The lining material is placed and the denture is returned to the reline jig, and then the lining material is heat- and pressure-processed to the denture base. This process produces a denser, longer lasting reline that is less prone to staining than a chairside reline. However, the negative part of the laboratory reline is that the patient will be without the denture for a period of time. On occasion, the heat from processing can warp the denture base and the occlusion can be changed.

OVER-THE-COUNTER LINERS

Some patients are "do-it-yourselfers" who purchase reline materials in the drugstore and apply them at home. They do not receive professional advice on the use and care of these liners and often use the liners far beyond their useful life. These materials can stiffen with time and can cause damage to the tissues, particularly if the occlusion is not properly reestablished with the new lining in place. They are usually porous and promote the growth of fungi, and patients can end up with fungal infection of the oral tissues. These over-the-counter products are not recommended.

DENTURE TEETH

Plastic (acrylic resin), composite resin, and porcelain teeth are used for complete and partial dentures. Each has certain advantages and disadvantages.

ACRYLIC RESIN TEETH

The vast majority of denture teeth used for removable dental prostheses are made from acrylic resin. Acrylic teeth are tough and chemically bond to the acrylic base of the denture. They are easy to grind to adjust the occlusion or to reshape a tooth to fit the available space and easy to repolish. They do not wear down the opposing natural or artificial teeth or restorations. Their main disadvantage is that they are softer and wear more readily than porcelain teeth. Plastic teeth are made in layers to simulate the colors and translucencies of natural teeth. The gingival portion of the teeth is manufactured so that the acrylic has minimal cross-linking. The bond of the acrylic tooth to the denture base is better without cross-linking. Cross-linking in the other portions of denture teeth makes them tougher and better able to hold up under function. Plastic teeth are used more often than porcelain teeth, because they are somewhat resilient and are thought not to stress the underlying ridges as much as porcelain teeth.

COMPOSITE RESIN TEETH

Nanohybrid composite material is used to make denture teeth that have improved properties compared with the simple acrylic resin teeth. Various filler particles have been used. Highly cross-linked macrofillers have been used to increase the strength and color stability. High-density microfillers are used to improve the wear resistance, and silanized silica-based nanofillers are used to improve optical properties such as light reflection. (See Chapter 6 for discussion of composite resin filler particles.) Composite resin teeth have a more natural appearance and translucency. The teeth made from hybrid composite resin and nanofillers can be made by two techniques: (1) pressing the materials together into a mold or (2) injecting the materials into a mold. Teeth made by the injection technique have better esthetics.

PORCELAIN TEETH

Porcelain teeth are brittle, hard, and very resistant to wear. Because of their brittleness, they are prone to fracture if the denture is dropped or is overstressed by hard foods or accidental biting on a fork. They do not

bond to the acrylic of the denture base and must have mechanical retention such as metal pins or retention holes to keep them in the acrylic denture base. They have a good esthetic appearance until the surface glaze is lost through wear or abrasive polishing. Porcelain teeth cannot be easily repolished, as can plastic teeth. They are highly stain resistant, whereas some plastic teeth will stain over time. They are not indicated for use against the natural dentition or most restorative materials, because they are very abrasive (Fig. 17.19). They also transmit heavier occlusal forces to the ridge and therefore may be a factor in patient discomfort, denture sores, and accelerated ridge resorption. Some patients prefer porcelain teeth because they sense a better ability to chew harder or more fibrous foods (Fig. 17.20).

CHARACTERIZATION OF DENTURES

Dentures can be given individual characteristics to make them seem more lifelike. Denture teeth can be arranged in the standard "ideal" arch alignment, or teeth can be arranged to recreate spaces (diastemas) (Fig. 17.21) or overlapping or crooked teeth that the patient had with the natural teeth. The denture teeth can be all one shade or can be selected to simulate the lighter and darker teeth that most people have in their mouths (e.g., canines are usually darker than incisors). Some patients request that restorations be placed in the denture teeth to simulate restorations they had in their natural teeth. The denture base acrylic itself is made in several shades, and these can be selected to replicate the color of the patient's mucosa and gingiva (see Fig. 17.4). The dental technician can do custom-shading with pigmented resins to simulate racial pigmentation in the denture base, because racial pigmentation is not always uniformly distributed in the tissues.

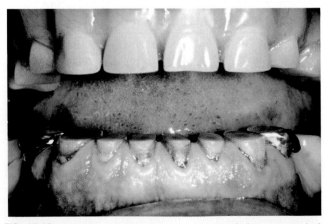

FIG. 17.19 Maxillary dentures with porcelain teeth have excessively worn opposing natural teeth. (Courtesy of Steve Eakle, University of California School of Dentistry, San Francisco, CA.)

PLASTICS FOR MAXILLOFACIAL PROSTHESES

A specialized aspect of a prosthodontic practice may include the fabrication of maxillofacial prostheses to replace facial tissues lost as the result of trauma, disease, surgery, or birth defect. These prostheses must have specialized characteristics so that they can be colored to match the surrounding skin, tear resistant in thin layers, resistant to staining, very flexible, and able to be attached to the surrounding skin with adhesives (Fig. 17.22). Materials that have been used are synthetic latex, plasticized vinyl resins, and silicone rubbers. Of these materials, the best for maxillofacial prostheses is silicone rubber.

DENTURE REPAIR

Acrylic complete and partial dentures can be repaired rather easily when they are broken. The repair of a partial denture with a metal framework is more complex, depending on the location of the break. If the break occurs through the framework or the clasp, it can sometimes be repaired by welding in the dental laboratory. However, many times such a break means that a new partial denture must be made. With the acrylic denture base lost or broken, teeth can be chemically bonded in place with repair acrylic. Likewise, broken denture bases can be repaired if the fragments can be reassembled.

CHEMICAL-CURED ACRYLIC REPAIR MATERIAL

The broken prosthesis should be disinfected at chairside before it is transported to the laboratory. For repair of an all-acrylic denture or partial denture, the broken parts are pieced together and are held with sticky wax. Plaster or stone is poured into the prosthesis to create a cast on which the parts can be stabilized while they are being repaired. Sometimes an impression of the patient's mouth must be taken to assemble the broken pieces. After the plaster has set, the fracture line is cut with an acrylic bur to create room for a sufficient bulk of repair material, and the adjacent surfaces several millimeters around the fracture line are ground to expose fresh surfaces for bonding. Often mechanical locks or dovetails are cut into the acrylic fragments to ensure a good, strong union between fragments. A coating of the liquid monomer is placed on the roughened surfaces to wet and prime them, as with the chairside reline procedure. Often the repair material is the same as the chairside reline material. The repair material is applied to the fracture in bulk or by the "salt and pepper" technique. With the salt and pepper technique, a small quantity of powder is sprinkled onto the wet fracture site and is wet with more liquid. This process of alternately adding powder and liquid continues until the fracture site is slightly overfilled. The prosthesis on the cast is then placed into a pressure pot with warm (not hot) water and about 20 pounds of pressure until cured (at least 20 minutes). Once the repair acrylic has cured, the prosthesis is removed, and excess material is cut back and polished. The prosthesis is disinfected and returned to chairside to try in the patient's mouth to confirm the fit and comfort.

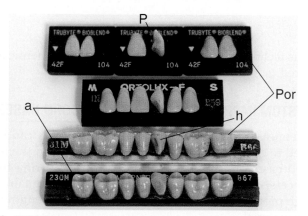

FIG. 17.20 Plastic and porcelain denture teeth. Porcelain teeth (*Por*) do not chemically bond to the denture base, as do plastic teeth (*a*); therefore, they have metal pins (*P*) or retention holes (*h*) to lock into the acrylic.

> **!** **Caution**
>
> Liquid monomer repair material is highly flammable; do not use it around an open flame such as a Bunsen burner.

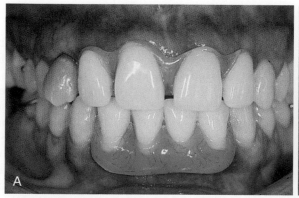
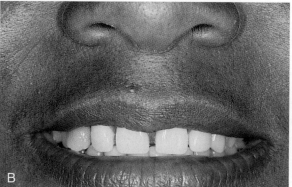

FIG. 17.21 Characterized temporary partial denture (stayplate) to create a lifelike appearance. Patient had naturally occurring diastemas between her maxillary incisors and wanted to have diastemas in the prosthesis. **A,** Stayplate with diastemas between the incisors. **B,** Natural-looking smile. (Courtesy of Arun Sharma, School of Dentistry, University of California, San Francisco [San Frncisco, CA].)

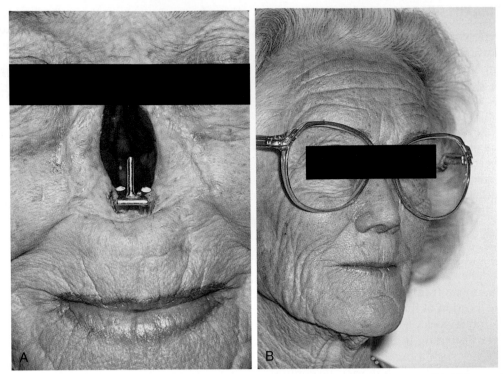

FIG. 17.22 Flexible acrylic prosthesis for nose lost to cancer. **A,** Metal implant at site of lost nose will hold the prosthesis in place. **B,** Lifelike prosthesis made of silicone rubber replaces the nose. (Courtesy of Arun Sharma, School of Dentistry, University of California, San Francisco [San Francisco, CA].)

LIGHT-CURED REPAIR MATERIAL

See Procedure 17.2 for more details.

Light-cured dimethacrylates have a number of useful applications, including repair of broken acrylic prostheses and fabrication of custom trays and record bases (e.g., Triad VLC; Dentsply International). Dimethacrylate is an acrylic resin that contains a chemical activated by light in the blue wavelength range, as well as an accelerator, inorganic fillers, and pigments to simulate tissue colors. These materials are cross-linked to improve their stiffness and strength.

Repair Technique

When used for denture repair, the prosthesis is prepared in the same manner as for chemical-cured material, except that a different liquid is painted on the fractured pieces before the repair material is applied. The repair material is removed from its light-proof package and is placed into the prepared fracture site. The repair material is coated with a liquid to prevent the development of an oxygen-inhibited layer of uncured material on the surface (see "Resin-to-Resin Bonding" in Chapter 6). Uncured material at the surface makes it more difficult to polish. The prosthesis on the cast is placed into a chamber with intense blue light (Triad 2000 VLC Unit [Dentsply International]; see Fig. 17.33 in Procedure 17.2) for about 10 minutes, and it is rotated on a turntable while the light polymerizes the repair material. After curing, it is shaped and polished and delivered to the patient.

This technique is somewhat faster than the chemical-cured method.

CUSTOM IMPRESSION TRAYS AND RECORD BASES

Chemical-cured and light-cured acrylic resins can be used to construct custom impression trays and the record bases on which wax rims are placed during the process of making dentures. The acrylics contain a high proportion of filler particles to impart strength to the material.

CHEMICAL-CURED TRAY AND RECORD BASE MATERIAL

See Procedure 17.1 for details.

Custom Tray Fabrication

Similar to the other chemical-cured acrylics, the tray materials are supplied as a powder and a liquid. Before the acrylic is mixed, the cast is prepared so that the acrylic does not stick to it. It is handled in one of three ways: (1) soaking in cold water, (2) coating with a separating material, or (3) lightly coating with petroleum jelly. Next, a spacer made from one layer of baseplate wax is applied to the cast. Some clinicians place three or four holes about 2 mm in diameter in the wax in the anterior and posterior ridge regions. The acrylic powder and liquid are mixed, and when the mixture reaches the dough stage, the material is adapted over the tissue portion of the cast and pressed into the holes in the wax so that some of the acrylic contacts the ridge in the anterior and posterior regions. This leaves acrylic elevations inside the tray after the wax is removed. These elevations create stops against the tissues when the impression is taken. The space left after removal of the wax creates a uniform thickness for impression material, and tissue stops keep the tray from being seated too heavily and compressing large areas of tissue during impression making. After the tray material is adapted to the cast and is still in the dough stage, excess material is cut away with a knife and is used to make a handle for the tray. The polymerization reaction is exothermic and the material becomes quite hot. After the acrylic has cooled, the tray should be carefully pried off the cast and the wax spacer removed. The tray is trimmed to the appropriate length with acrylic burs or abrasive bands on a lathe.

Record Bases

Record bases are rigid bases that correspond roughly to the denture base. They are used in the construction stage of the denture and have wax rims added to them over the ridge areas. They are used initially to establish the proper dimension between upper and lower arches, as well as the position of the centric occlusion. Marks can be made in the wax to denote the location of the border of the upper lip, the "smile" line, and the midline of the face as guides for placement of the denture teeth. Later, the denture teeth are set in the wax rims, and the record bases serve to stabilize the wax rims during the try-in appointment.

Record Base Fabrication

Record bases are also constructed from the same materials as the trays. The difference in their construction is that wax spacers, tissue stops, and handles are not used. If significant tissue undercuts are present on the cast, they are blocked out with wax before the record bases are constructed.

LIGHT-CURED TRAY AND RECORD BASE MATERIAL

Light-cured dimethacrylates can be used for construction of custom trays and record bases (Procedure 17.2). They are similar to light-cured repair materials but come in one color and do not have fibers to simulate blood vessels.

The technique for making custom trays and record bases is the same as for the chemical-cured materials, except that instead of mixing powder and liquid, a sheet of the preformed material is removed from its lightproof package and adapted over the cast or wax spacer. After excess material is trimmed (and a handle is formed if a tray), the tray or record base on the cast is placed in the light-curing unit as described previously for light-cured repair materials. The light-cured material generates very little heat during polymerization and is much easier to use because no mixing is required. It eliminates the concerns about inhaling and handling the monomer

associated with the chemical-cured material. These materials have largely replaced the chemical-cured materials in many offices and laboratories.

INFECTION CONTROL PROCEDURES

Contaminated dentures, custom trays, record bases, laboratory relines and other materials that are transported back and forth between the dental office and the dental laboratory should be treated following proper infection control procedures. The dental office is responsible for disinfecting these items that have been in the patient's mouth before they are sent to the laboratory. Likewise, the laboratory should disinfect the items before delivering them to the dental office. However, the dental office is ultimately responsible for assuring that items have been disinfected (or sterilized when possible) before placing them in the patient's mouth (see the box "Disinfecting Prostheses").

Disinfecting Prostheses

- Properly disinfect all prostheses before trying in the patient's mouth.
- Disinfect at chairside all prostheses going from the patient to the commercial or office laboratory, and package properly for transport.
- Iodophors and synthetic phenols are suitable disinfectants for most prostheses.
- Immerse prostheses for 15 minutes in one of these disinfectants in a denture cup or a plastic bag.

INSTRUCTIONS FOR NEW DENTURE WEARERS

Approximately 44 million people in the United States wear dentures. Losing one's teeth can have a physical and psychological effect on some people. Trying to adjust to acrylic prostheses can become a frustrating experience if patients do not know what to expect from their new dentures. It is vitally important to the acceptance of the dentures that hygienists and dental assistants as part of the dental team be able to instruct patients on what to expect, how to manage use of their new dentures, and how to care for them. The following is information you can provide to the new denture wearer.

WHAT TO EXPECT

Speaking

Dentures may create a feeling of fullness to the mouth as you adapt to the additional thickness of the dentures. Some people may feel a gagging sensation as they swallow. The tissues and muscles will adapt with time.

Most people will have some difficulty pronouncing some words, especially those with "f" and "s" sounds. Try reading the newspaper out loud and practice words that are difficult to pronounce. The lower denture will move when you talk or eat, because the tongue and cheeks move. Avoid the tendency to tongue thrust because it will dislodge your dentures.

Eating

The biting force with your dentures is about 20% of that with your natural teeth. The dentures sit on top of tissues that are compressible, so there will be some movement of the dentures while eating. Start with soft foods that are easy to chew. Biting into food with the front teeth will tend to dislodge the dentures. People with dentures tend not to chew the food long enough to grind it into small pieces, because it takes longer than with natural teeth. This can put you at risk for choking. Chew the food well before swallowing. Cut the food into smaller pieces than you usually do.

To help balance the dentures, chew with food on both sides of your mouth at the same time. Your dentures cover many of your oral tissues, so you may not be aware of foods or beverages that are very hot. Take care not to burn yourself.

Excess Saliva

Saliva is important to help you swallow your food, lubricate your mouth tissues, and help form a seal with your dentures. However, your mouth will react to the presence of the new dentures by producing more saliva than usual. Your mouth will usually adapt and return to its normal salivary flow in a week or two.

Fit

Your upper denture rests on the bony ridges and the hard palate. The borders of the denture help create a seal with the tissues and saliva fills in the gaps between the denture and the tissues, so suction is created to hold the denture in place. Your lower denture will feel looser, because it does not have the large surface area of the palate for support and the tongue is continually moving and lifting the lower denture. You will need to learn how to position your tongue to help keep the lower denture seated. Avoid using denture adhesive if possible while you learn to adapt to the new dentures.

Soreness

Like a new pair of shoes, your dentures may rub the tissues and create sore spots. Biting your cheeks is not unusual in the first few weeks. Do not attempt to adjust the dentures yourself. Call the office and we will get you in quickly to relieve the soreness. It might take several visits to eliminate all of the pressure spots.

Looseness

If you had teeth extracted just before placement of the dentures, some looseness will occur as the extraction sites heal and the gum shrinks. Your dentist will discuss with you when it is time to put a lining material inside the dentures to adapt them to the new position of the gums.

Regular Dental Checkups

Even though you no longer have your natural teeth, you will need to visit the dentist periodically to have your mouth checked for cancer or other mouth disorders. In addition, your dentist will check the fit of your dentures and professionally clean them. The dentist will advise you as to how often you should come in.

You should come in sooner than your regular checkups if you notice soreness, exceptional looseness, chipped teeth or acrylic, or if you have dropped and broken your dentures. Do not attempt to repair them yourself, as you could cause damage that may make a repair more difficult or impossible.

CARE OF ACRYLIC RESIN DENTURES

Cleaning the dentures is important in maintaining the health of the oral tissues. Improper or inadequate home care can lead to fungal infections of the tissues or damage to the dentures. The most commonly used home cleaning aids for dentures are denture brushes and denture soaks or cleaners. Denture brushes, when used with water or mild soaps, are not abrasive to the acrylic surface. Household cleaners can be very abrasive to the acrylic and should not be used. Denture cleaners can be found as tablets (Efferdent [Prestige Brands] and Polident [GlaxoSmithKline]) or powders. They may contain detergents, sodium perborate, alkaline compounds, and flavoring agents. When sodium perborate is placed in water it releases oxygen and effervesces, loosening debris. Diluted household bleach (hypochlorite) will remove some stains and will have an antimicrobial effect. However, it will remove the tissue color from the denture base over time. Bleach should not be used with prostheses containing metal such as partial denture frameworks or removable orthodontic appliances, because it will attack the metal and corrode it.

The patient needs to be instructed on how to care for new dentures. The following are home care instructions you can provide.

HOME CARE

Clean the dentures every day, twice if possible, to remove plaque and debris. Hold them over a towel or put water in the sink, so if you drop them they will not break. Clean the tissue surfaces and the teeth and outer surfaces of the denture with a denture brush. Many denture brushes have medium or hard bristles. The stiffness of the bristles is not as critical to the abrasion of the acrylic as the cleaner used on the brush. Use liquid soap, mild hand soap, or a nonabrasive denture cleaning paste to remove surface debris.

Expect some food to get under the denture when you eat. Remove and rinse the dentures after each meal if you cannot brush them, but do not use hot water as it may warp the dentures. Rinse your mouth as well to remove food particles.

At bedtime, clean the tissues that the dentures sit on and those surrounding the dentures. Use a soft tooth-brush and water to gently clean your gums, palate, tongue, and lining of your cheeks.

Remove the dentures overnight or at least for 4 hours during the day to give the gums a rest. You can prepare a denture soak with commercial denture cleaning tablets (such as Efferdent or Polident). Cal-culus that accumulates on the denture can be soft-ened and more easily removed by soaking the den-ture in a solution of white vinegar diluted 1:1 with water. Dentures are soaked overnight in commercial or homemade soaks. Be sure to rinse them thor-oughly before putting them back into your mouth, because the soaks may contain chemicals that can irritate the tissues. Bleach is an effective organic sol-vent and eliminates yeasts. It should be diluted: 1 part bleach to 10 parts water. Undiluted household bleach should not be used as an overnight soak for complete or partial dentures. It will fade the color from the acrylic and attack the metal framework and clasps of a partial denture, causing them to darken and corrode. Partial dentures with metal compo-nents should be soaked in commercial products that do not contain bleach.

Store your denture in water when you are not wear-ing it to keep it from drying and distorting.

Clasps on partial dentures can be cleaned with the pointed brush on the end of the denture brush if the two-headed variety is used. Use care to keep from damaging or distorting the clasps. Gently clean the tis-sue-bearing surfaces of dentures with soft liners, using a soft toothbrush. Liquid soap can also be used (Fig. 17.23).

Long- and short-term soft liners may be adversely affected by some of the effervescent commercial soaks (Efferdent or Polident). Do not soak them in mouth-wash containing alcohol, because it dries out the material. Use only cleaners recommended by the man-ufacturer. Clean soft temporary liners with damp cot-ton balls or cotton-tipped applicators for a few days. After about a week it will harden enough to clean with a soft bristle toothbrush.

Wearing a partial denture increases your risk of get-ting tooth decay. Be sure to brush your remaining teeth at least twice a day with a fluoride toothpaste, and floss at least once a day. Avoid starchy or sugary snacks.

IN-OFFICE CARE

Patients will accumulate calculus on the denture around the surfaces of the maxillary molars and the mandibular anterior teeth, just as they did with their natural dentition. The dental hygienist can provide a service by removing the calculus before returning the denture to the patient. Calculus can be removed by placing the prosthesis in a denture cleaning solution inside a zippered bag placed into an ultrasonic cleaner. It can also be carefully scaled off with hand instru-ments and the area polished with flour of pumice, then tin oxide or acrylic polishing compounds (Fig. 17.24). Care must be taken not to wear down the teeth and acrylic base during the polishing process. In addition, tissue-bearing surfaces of the complete denture or par-tial denture should not be polished.

STORAGE OF DENTURES

Acrylic resin prostheses absorb water and also are sen-sitive to water loss. The patient should be instructed to keep the prosthesis wet during periods of storage. This will prevent dimensional changes and distortion that can affect the fit. The prosthesis should be kept wet during the dental appointment. It can be stored in a denture cup to which water and a little mouthwash have been added to freshen it. Prostheses with soft liners should not be placed in mouthwash containing alcohol, because the alcohol may adversely affect the properties of the soft liner. Instructions for care of com-plete and partial dentures should be given to nursing home staff and to caregivers for homebound or inca-pacitated individuals.

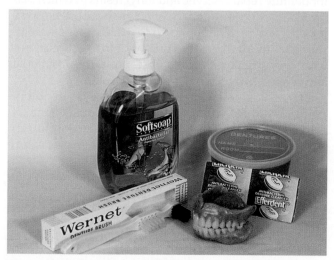

FIG. 17.23 Home care products for cleaning dentures: Brush, liquid soap, denture cleaner tablets, denture cup.

Precautions for Patients with Partial or Complete Dentures

- Store dentures in water to prevent warping from loss of moisture.
- Do not clean dentures in hot water, because they may warp.
- Avoid soaking dentures in undiluted chlorine bleach, because it will remove color from the resin and will at-tack metal components of partial dentures.
- Clean dentures over a sink partially filled with water or a towel to avoid breaking the denture if dropped.
- Avoid abrasive toothpastes or household cleaners, because they will scratch or wear the plastic.

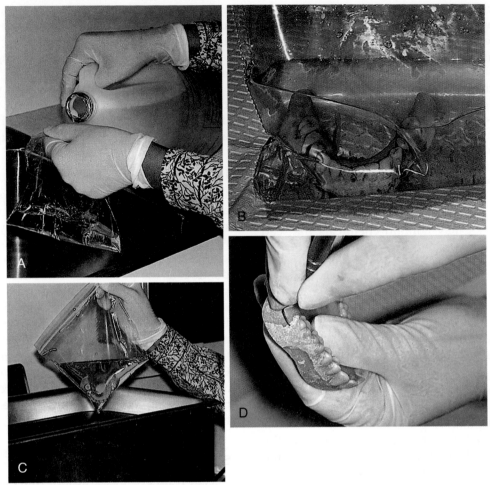

FIG. 17.24 Cleaning a denture in an ultrasonic cleaner. **A,** Cleaning solution (to remove stain and calculus) placed in plastic zippered bag. **B,** Denture placed in bag and sealed. **C,** Bag placed in ultrasonic cleaner for 10 to 14 minutes. D, Dentures with large calculus deposits need initial scaling with hand instruments before placing in ultrasonic cleaner. (From Darby ML, Walsh MM: *Dental Hygiene: Theory and Practice* (ed 4). St. Louis, 2015, Elsevier. Courtesy of Bertha Chan.)

SUMMARY

Acrylic resins are vitally important to the success of prosthetic dentistry. They are versatile materials that can be used to replace missing oral structures. The ability of these resins to chemically bond to one another is important when plastic teeth are linked to the denture base or when they are relined or repaired. When properly handled, they are strong and durable. They can readily be relined to improve the fit as the alveolar bone resorbs over time. Lining materials can be similar to the denture base material or can be modified with plasticizers to create soft liners for tissue conditioning or long-term cushioning for patients who cannot tolerate hard liners. Many relining procedures can be accomplished in the office at chairside, so that the patient does not have to be without the prosthesis for any length of time. Simple fractures of the resin also can be repaired readily in the dental office. The acrylic resins can be colored with pigments to simulate racial pigmentation, so the denture can be customized to match the tissue coloration of the patient.

Other resins chemically similar to the methyl methacrylate resins are also used in prosthetic dentistry. The addition of photoinitiators and amine activators produces light-cured materials that are easy to use, require no mixing, and eliminate the volatile monomer that is potentially hazardous. The light-cured resins have application for fabrication of custom trays and record bases and for denture repair. Acrylic and vinyl resins to which plasticizers have been added to soften them are often used in maxillofacial prosthodontics for replacement of facial tissues after trauma or cancer surgery. Noses, cheeks, ears, and other structures can be made from these materials and colored to match the surrounding skin.

The allied oral health provider plays an important role in delivering care to individuals who require prostheses. She or he may be called on to mix, place, remove, or repair any number of these materials. Therefore an intimate knowledge of the properties and handling characteristics of these materials is very important. In addition, patients need instructions in proper home care of the prostheses to maintain them and to prevent injury to the oral tissues. Knowledge of proper cleaning agents and methods is also necessary.

INSTRUCTIONAL VIDEOS

See the Evolve Resources site for a variety of educational videos that reinforce the material covered in this chapter.

Procedure 17.1 Fabrication of Custom Acrylic Impression Trays

See Evolve site for Competency Sheet

Consider the following with this procedure: safety glasses are recommended for the patient, PPE is required for the operator, and ensure appropriate safety protocols are followed.

NOTE: Figs. 17.25 through 17.32, Courtesy of Mark Dellinges, School of Dentistry, University of California, San Francisco (San Francisco, CA).

EQUIPMENT/SUPPLIES (FIG. 17.25)

- Maxillary or mandibular edentulous cast
- Sheet of baseplate wax, Bunsen burner, laboratory knife
- Tray powder and liquid, tongue blade or cement spatula, waxed paper cup
- Laboratory handpiece and acrylic bur, sandpaper drum (arbor band), and dental lathe
- Cast-separating medium, disposable brush, petroleum jelly

PROCEDURE STEPS

1. Using the disposable brush, coat the cast with separating medium and allow it to dry.

NOTE: The separating medium keeps the tray material and the wax from sticking to the cast.

2. Warm a sheet of baseplate wax over the Bunsen burner and place it on the cast. Adapt it to the cast over the edentulous ridges and into the vestibular folds. Use the laboratory knife to trim excess wax away until it is about 2 mm from the depth of the folds.

NOTE: The wax will be removed after the tray is fabricated and will create an even space within the tray for the impression material.

3. Cut three 2 × 2-mm square holes in the wax over the ridges for the maxillary and mandibular casts: two in the molar area, and one in the incisor area.

NOTE: As tray material is adapted into these holes, resin squares will appear inside the tray. When the impression is taken, these squares will contact the tissues over the ridges and act as stops. The stops will create an even thickness of impression material within the tray (except for the very small area of the square) and will prevent an uneven seating of the tray (Fig. 17.26). Some clinicians do not use these stops.

4. Mix the powder and liquid components of the tray material in the wax cup, in proportions recommended by the manufacturer. Stir with a tongue blade or cement spatula until thoroughly mixed (Fig. 17.27).

NOTE: The mix will be too wet to handle at this stage. Use only in a well ventilated area.

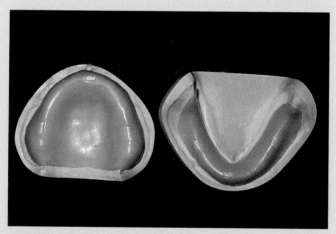

FIG. 17.26

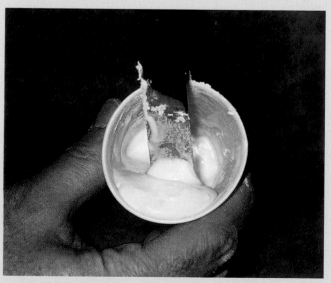

FIG. 17.27

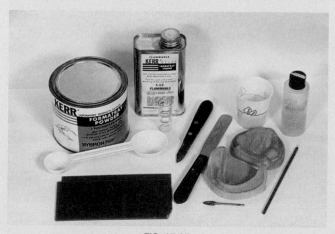

FIG. 17.25

Continued

Procedure 17.1 Fabrication of Custom Acrylic Impression Trays—cont'd

5. Apply petroleum jelly to the gloved hands. When the mixture is doughy, form it into a thick, wide rope that is long enough to fit around the entire ridge (Fig. 17.28).

   NOTE: Petroleum jelly keeps the tray material from sticking to the gloves.

6. Adapt the resin over the wax, into the holes in the wax, and into the depth of the vestibular folds. The tray should be 1 to 2 mm thick (Fig. 17.29).

   NOTE: If the tray is too thin, it might be too flexible to keep the impression from distorting.

7. Cut away excess tray material with the laboratory knife and quickly adapt it into the shape of a handle. Wet the tray end of the handle with monomer and place it on the tray. Smooth it into place with the fingers. The handle should be positioned so that it will not be in the way of the lips when seated in the patient's mouth.

   NOTE: Wetting the end of the tray with monomer (liquid) dissolves some material at the surface and allows it to stick to the polymerizing tray material.

8. Readapt the tray material to the cast continually as polymerization takes place.

   NOTE: The tray material shrinks as it polymerizes and tends to pull away from the cast.

9. Remove the tray from the cast once the heat of the reaction has cooled. Remove wax from inside the tray. If difficult to remove, heat the wax in warm (not hot) water (Fig. 17.30).

   NOTE: Residual wax must be removed, or it might prevent the impression material from adhering to the tray.

10. Trim the tray with an acrylic bur or arbor band to remove excess material (Fig. 17.31), and smooth the rough edges. The completed tray should extend 2 mm short of the vestibular folds. Confirm the fit of the tray on the cast (Fig. 17.32).

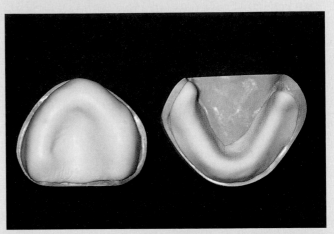

FIG. 17.29

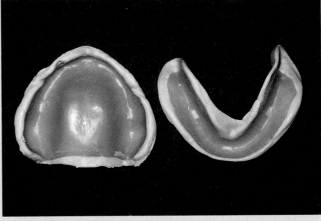

FIG. 17.30

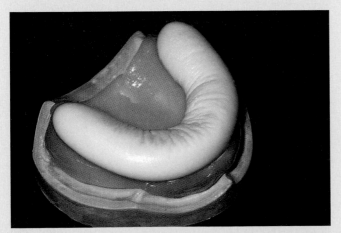

FIG. 17.28

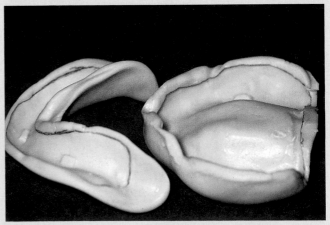

FIG. 17.31

Procedure 17.1   Fabrication of Custom Acrylic Impression Trays—cont'd

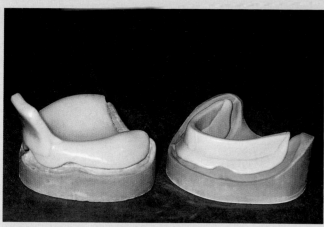

FIG. 17.32

NOTE: The tray must be smooth to the touch, or it will be uncomfortable in the patient's mouth. The tray is left short of the depth of the folds to allow room for stick compound to be added for border molding. Border molding uses softened compound to shape the location for the borders of the denture as the patient's cheeks and tongue are manipulated through simulated functional movements.

NOTE: Some dentists use addition silicone putty or special thermoplastic materials for border molding.

11. Disinfect the tray by immersion in appropriate disinfectant and store in a sealed bag labeled with the patient's name until ready for use.

Procedure 17.2   Fabrication of Record Bases with Light-Cured Acrylic Resin

See Evolve site for Competency Sheet

Consider the following with this procedure: safety glasses are recommended for the patient, PPE is required for the operator, and ensure appropriate safety protocols are followed.

NOTE: Figs. 17.33 through 17.39, Courtesy of Dr. Mark Dellinges, School of Dentistry, University of California, San Francisco (San Francisco, CA).

EQUIPMENT/SUPPLIES (FIG. 17.33)

- Edentulous casts (maxillary, mandibular, or both)
- Light-cured record base material (Triad VLC; Dentsply International)
- Model-releasing agent
- Light-curing unit (Triad 2000 VLC Unit)
- Disposable scalpel blade and handle
- 2 × 2 gauze soaked with alcohol
- Low-speed handpiece with acrylic bur
- Laboratory lathe with sandpaper drum (arbor band), rag wheel, and pumice

PROCEDURE STEPS

1. Apply a thin layer of model-releasing agent to the surface of the edentulous casts with a disposable brush, and let it dry (Fig. 17.34).
2. Remove a sheet of the Triad VLC material from the protective packaging, and place it over the cast.

NOTE: The packaging prevents light from polymerizing the material.

3. Press the material gently onto the cast, being careful not to trap air between the cast and the material (Fig. 17.35).

4. Press the material into the vestibule areas of the cast, using the blunt end of the disposable scalpel.

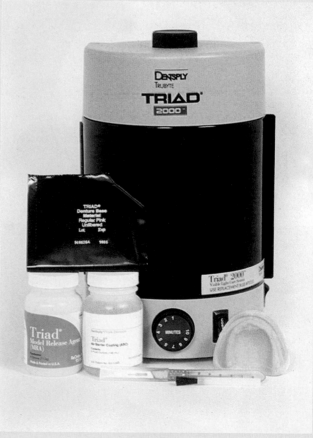

FIG. 17.33

Continued

Procedure 17.2 **Fabrication of Custom Acrylic Impression Trays—cont'd**

5. Trim away the excess material that extends beyond the depth of the vestibule with the scalpel blade. Smooth the edges with the fingers.

6. (Optional) Cut a 2-cm-long slit in the back of the palate of the maxillary record base material to allow for curing shrinkage.

NOTE: Resins shrink when polymerized. Because there is a large volume of material, the shrinkage will be greater. Too much shrinkage will cause the record base to fit poorly. The slit allows shrinkage to occur without lifting material away from the palate (Fig. 17.36).

7. Place the cast and record base into the light-curing unit on the turntable according to manufacturer's directions. Activate the turntable and cure for 2 to 4 minutes (Fig. 17.37).

8. (Optional) Place a small amount of the excess uncured base over the slit, and press with your fingers. Cure again.

NOTE: This step seals the slit; most of the polymerization shrinkage has already occurred.

9. Remove the record base from the cast, invert the record base, and cure again.

NOTE: The record base is inverted to cure the internal surface and ensure complete polymerization. The material is opaque, and light does not penetrate enough to cure entirely through it from the outside.

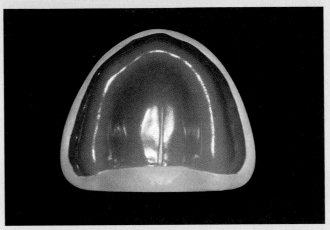

Fig. 17.36

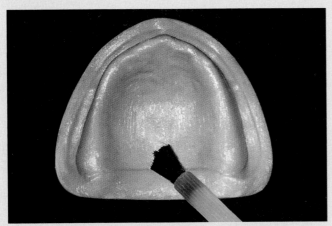

FIG. 17.34

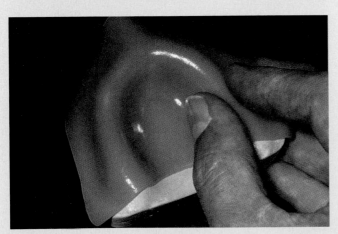

FIG. 17.35

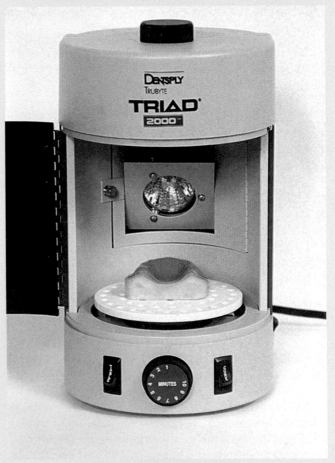

FIG. 17.37

Procedure 17.2 Fabrication of Custom Acrylic Impression Trays—cont'd

10. Wipe the record base after curing with the alcohol-soaked 2 × 2 gauze to remove the slippery film on the surface.

    NOTE: Resins will have a thin layer of unpolymerized resin on surfaces in contact with air. Oxygen inhibits the polymerization of resin at the surface. This same phenomenon is seen on the surfaces of composites and sealants.

11. Mark with a pencil the excess acrylic that extends beyond the border of the vestibule. Grind the excess with an acrylic bur or a sandpaper drum on a lathe in the laboratory to the correct thickness and length, as directed by the dentist (Fig. 17.38).

12. Thin the area over the ridges with the sandpaper drum or acrylic bur. Leave it approximately 0.5 mm thick.

    NOTE: If the material is too thick over the ridges, it will interfere with placement of denture teeth when they are set for the wax try-in appointment.

13. Smooth the periphery with pumice on a rag wheel.

    NOTE: This is for the patient's comfort.

14. Confirm the fit on the cast. The record base is now ready for the application of wax rims (Fig. 17.39).

15. Apply sticky wax to the ridge of the record base (Fig. 17.40).

16. Cut off one third from a sheet of baseplate wax (Fig. 17.41).

17. Use the remaining two thirds of the sheet. Warm it and roll it into a tight cylinder (Fig. 17.42).

18. Bend the rolled wax into a U-shape. Adapt it to the ridge crest of the record base (Fig. 17.43).

19. Smooth the facial and occlusal surfaces of the wax with a hot metal plate (Figs. 17.44 and 17.45).

20. Use the hot plate to shape the wax rim until it is approximately 17 mm high from the apical end of the record base to the anterior top edge of the wax and 10 mm wide (Fig. 17.46).

21. The wax rim can be used to mark the midline of the patient's smile and the location of the facial surfaces and incisal edges of the anterior teeth. It can also be used to determine the proper vertical dimension of occlusion, so the patient's bite is

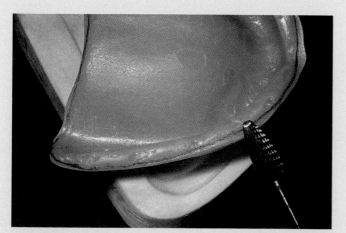

FIG. 17.38

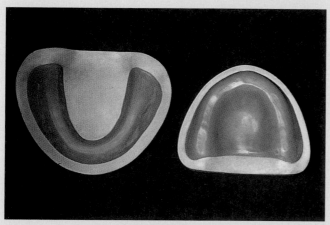

FIG. 17.39

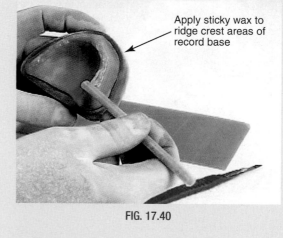

Apply sticky wax to ridge crest areas of record base

FIG. 17.40

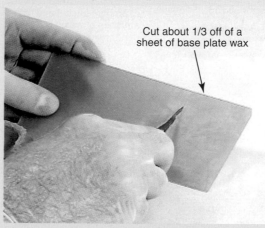

Cut about 1/3 off of a sheet of base plate wax

FIG. 17.41

Continued

Procedure 17.2 Fabrication of Custom Acrylic Impression Trays—cont'd

not propped open or overclosed. If the patient is totally edentulous, a lower record base will be used with the upper to record the location of the centric

occlusion. Indices are cut into the wax rims and a softer wax (e.g., Aluwax; Aluwax Dental Products) will be warmed and placed in the indices. The patient will close into the centric occlusion position and the wax will be cooled to lock in the position of the upper and lower record bases (Fig. 17.47).

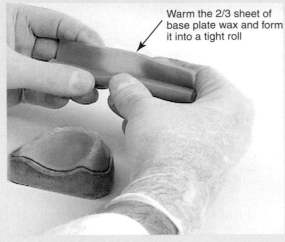

Warm the 2/3 sheet of base plate wax and form it into a tight roll

FIG. 17.42

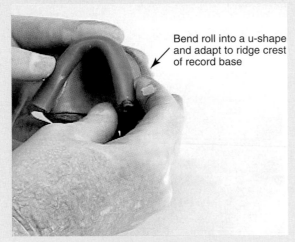

Bend roll into a u-shape and adapt to ridge crest of record base

FIG. 17.43

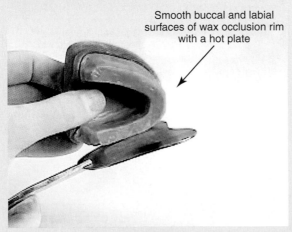

Smooth buccal and labial surfaces of wax occlusion rim with a hot plate

FIG. 17.44

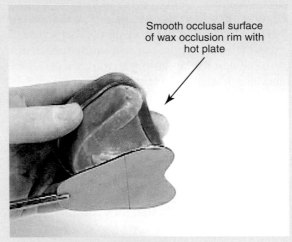

Smooth occlusal surface of wax occlusion rim with hot plate

FIG. 17.45

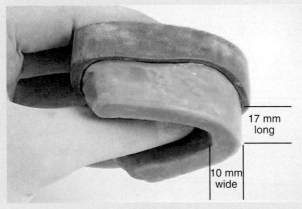

17 mm long

10 mm wide

FIG. 17.46

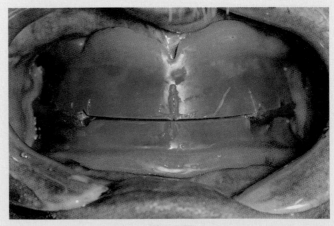

FIG. 17.47

Get Ready for Exams!

Review Questions

Select the one correct response for each of the following multiple-choice questions.

1. A polymer is formed by
   a. Breaking down chains of complex, high molecular weight molecules by heating them
   b. Mixing polysulfide and polyether
   c. Joining monomer molecules together in a long chain through carbon bonds
   d. Fusing acrylic powder beads together at high temperature

2. Cross-linking of polymers
   a. Is used to improve the physical and mechanical properties of the final resin product
   b. Occurs when long-chain polymers are mixed together and the chains physically wrap around each other
   c. Usually results in a weaker material as the degree of cross-linking increases
   d. Occurs when long chains link end-to-end

3. Addition polymerization
   a. Results in porosity in the final material
   b. Is the least common method of polymerization used in dentistry
   c. Produces numerous by-products such as alcohol and acetone
   d. Is initiated by a free radical

4. The physical stages of the addition polymerization reaction are
   a. Sandy, stringy, dough, and rubber
   b. Wet, flexible, and stiff
   c. Sol, gel, and solid
   d. Initial, thermal, and terminal

5. A heat-processed denture differs from a chemical-cured denture. Which one of the following is NOT true for the heat-processed denture?
   a. It is stronger.
   b. It is more porous.
   c. It is harder.
   d. It has less dimensional change during the first 24 hours after curing.

6. High-impact resins are created by
   a. Removal of free monomer
   b. Addition of plasticizers
   c. Heat-treating the resin after it has polymerized
   d. Addition of rubber particles to the acrylic

7. Which stage of polymerization of acrylic resins is longer for heat-cured resins during denture processing to allow adequate time to pack the acrylic resin into the denture flask?
   a. Sandy
   b. Stringy
   c. Dough
   d. Exothermic

8. What is the effect on a denture if it is left on the night-stand overnight?
   a. It will lose water and shrink.
   b. It will expand.
   c. It will crack.
   d. It will oxidize and lose color.

9. What is the effect on a partial denture framework if soaked in a chlorine-containing cleaner?
   a. Nothing will happen.
   b. The metal will clean rapidly and become shiny.
   c. The metal will dissolve and fracture.
   d. The metal will darken and corrode.

10. The effect that porosity has on an acrylic denture can be seen as all of the following EXCEPT one. Which one?
    a. It contributes to staining.
    b. It contributes to growth of microorganisms.
    c. It weakens the acrylic.
    d. It decreases the thermal conductivity of the acrylic.

11. The purpose of the use of a pressure pot during polymerization of a chemical-cured acrylic resin is
    a. To increase the strength of the acrylic
    b. To decrease the porosity
    c. To decrease the shrinkage
    d. All of the above

12. Which type of hard liner has the best physical properties?
    a. Chairside chemical-cured liner
    b. Laboratory chemical-cured liner
    c. Laboratory heat-cured liner
    d. None (they are all the same)

13. Methyl methacrylate is which one of the following?
    a. An inhibitor
    b. An accelerator
    c. Powder polymer
    d. Liquid monomer

14. Long-term soft liners are indicated for all of the following reasons EXCEPT one. Which one?
    a. Chronic soreness with hard acrylic denture bases
    b. Severe soft tissue undercuts
    c. Sharp, knife-edge ridges
    d. Soft tissues with chronic fungal infection

15. Acrylic resins can be made soft and pliable by the
    a. Use of less monomer in the mix
    b. Use of less powder in the mix
    c. Addition of plasticizers
    d. Addition of filler particles

16. All of the following statements about short-term soft liners are true EXCEPT one. Which one?
    a. They are also called *tissue conditioners.*
    b. They can readapt to the tissues as healing takes place, because they have a high degree of flow.
    c. They do not need frequent replacement because they absorb water and get softer over time.
    d. They are adversely affected by some commercial denture soaks.

Continued

Get Ready for Exams!

17. Over-the-counter denture liners have which of the following shortcomings?
   a. May not reestablish proper occlusion
   b. Are generally porous
   c. Promote growth of yeasts
   d. All of the above

18. All of the following are advantages of acrylic denture teeth over porcelain teeth EXCEPT one. Which one?
   a. They are more wear resistant
   b. They chemically bond to the denture base
   c. They are kind to the opposing teeth or ridges
   d. They can easily be ground and shaped to fit the available space

19. When a denture is repaired with a chemical-cured acrylic resin, all of the following procedures are performed EXCEPT one. Which one?
   a. the pieces are reassembled and held with sticky wax while a cast is poured inside the denture
   b. a layer of the old resin surrounding the fracture site is removed
   c. the resin surrounding the fracture site is wet with monomer to enhance the chemical bond with the repair acrylic
   d. the repair acrylic is mixed, applied to the fracture site, and allowed to cure at room temperature on the laboratory bench for the best results

20. Which one of the following statements regarding construction of custom impression trays is FALSE?
   a. Tray material may be chemical-cured or light-cured.
   b. Tray material is adapted directly to the cast.
   c. During polymerization, the chemical-cured material gets very hot.
   d. Baseplate wax is adapted over the cast to develop space for the impression material.

21. Which one of the following statements is FALSE regarding the care of dentures by the patient?
   a. Dentures should be stored in water to prevent warping.
   b. Dentures should be cleaned over a sink filled with water or over a towel to prevent fracture if dropped.
   c. Abrasive pastes or cleaners should not be used, or they will scratch the acrylic.
   d. The denture should be cleaned in hot water periodically to kill microorganisms.

22. Which one of the following statements about liquid monomer is FALSE?
   a. Gives a pleasant taste to a hard reline done at chairside
   b. Is potentially harmful to breathe
   c. Can cause allergic reactions or skin irritation
   d. May be present in small quantities in a new denture
   e. Evaporates readily so do not leave the cap to the bottle off

23. All of the following can have an adverse effect on soft denture liners EXCEPT one. Which one?
   a. Some effervescent commercial denture soaks
   b. Liquid hand soap
   c. Mouthwash containing alcohol
   d. Hot water

For answers to Review Questions, see the Appendix.

Case-Based Discussion Topics

1. A thin, frail 76-year-old widow had complete dentures made about 3 years ago. She comes to the dental office with a chief complaint of "my lower denture hurts me when I eat." In the 3 years since her dentures were made, she has had the lower denture relined twice with hard acrylic. This has not improved her comfort. Her lower ridge is sharp and thin.
Can you suggest a process that might make her more comfortable? Is the procedure best done in the office or in a commercial dental laboratory? What kinds of materials are often used?

2. A 62-year-old retired janitor comes to the dental office to get his teeth cleaned. He wears an upper complete denture and a lower partial denture with a metal framework that replaces teeth #22 to #26. In addition to calculus on his teeth, he has calculus on his denture and partial denture.
Describe a method of removing the calculus without scratching the acrylic. What home care measures can you recommend for care of his prostheses? What type of cleaner should he avoid on his partial denture? What types of brushes should he use to clean his prostheses?

3. A 57-year-old truck driver comes to the dental office with a broken maxillary denture. It is broken in two pieces through the midline of the palatal portion of the denture base. The pieces fit together easily. He said he dropped it in the sink while cleaning it.
What steps should be taken to prepare the denture for repair in the office? What materials could be used for the repair? What is the function of the pressure pot? What advice can be given to the patient to avoid a similar mishap in the future?

4. A 71-year-old retired teacher had an upper denture made 6 months ago. She returns to the office complaining that the denture has stained heavily in the palatal portion of the denture base and has developed a foul odor.
When you inspect the denture, you confirm a dark stain in the mid-palate but also notice numerous small porosities in the acrylic. Cite causes of porosity during processing of the denture. Why has the denture stained and developed a foul odor? What effect does porosity have on the physical and mechanical properties of the acrylic?

5. A 43 year-old beautician lost her upper teeth last year due to rapidly progressing periodontal disease associated with her uncontrolled diabetes. She comes to the dental office complaining of soreness in her palate beneath her denture. It has been getting progressive worse over the past three weeks. She wears her denture to bed so her husband will not see her without teeth.
What is the likely cause of the soreness? What should the dentist prescribe to help her? What can you advise her to do regarding her home care? If the denture had been new and she had only worn it for a few days and was taking it out at night, what else could cause irritation of the palatal tissues?

BIBLIOGRAPHY

Anusavice KL, Shen C, Rawls HR: Prosthetic polymers and resins. In *Phillips' Science of Dental Materials* (ed 12). Philadelphia, 2013, Saunders.

Bird DL, Robinson DS: Removable prosthodontics. In *Modern Dental Assisting* (ed 12). St. Louis, 2018. Elsevier.

Darby ML, Walsh MM: (editors): Persons with fixed and removable prostheses. In Dental Hygiene Theory and Practice (ed 4). St. Louis, 2015. Elsevier/Saunders.

Ferracane JL: Polymers for prosthetics. In *Materials in Dentistry* (ed 2). Philadelphia, 2001, Lippincott Williams & Wilkins.

Leinfelder KF, Terry DA, Connelly ME: The art of denture relining. *Inside Dentistry*, 3(5), 2007.

Powers JM, Wataha JC: Polymers in prosthodontics. In *Dental Materials: Properties and Manipulation* (ed 10). St. Louis, 2013, Mosby.

Vaidyanathan J, Vaidyanathan TK: Dynamic mechanical analysis of heat, microwave and visible light cure denture base resins. *J Mater Sci Mater Med*, 6:670–674, 1995.

18 | Provisional Restorations

Chapter Objectives

Upon completion of this chapter, the student should be able to:

1. Explain the purpose of provisional coverage.
2. Describe examples of circumstances that may require provisional coverage.
3. Identify the criteria necessary for a high-quality provisional restoration.
4. Describe the properties of provisional materials.
5. Distinguish among properties that are important for coverage in the posterior, anterior, and both areas.
6. Differentiate between intracoronal and extracoronal restorations.
7. Summarize the advantages and disadvantages of preformed and custom crowns.
8. Differentiate among direct and indirect fabrication techniques.
9. Summarize the advantages and disadvantages of acrylic and composite resin provisional materials.
10. Describe the technique for fabrication of preformed metal and polycarbonate crowns, custom crowns, and intracoronal cement provisional restorations.
11. Summarize patient education and home care instructions.
12. Fabricate and cement metal, polycarbonate and custom provisional crowns.
13. Place an intracoronal cement provisional restoration.

Key Terms

Provisional Coverage a restoration that temporarily takes the place of a permanent restoration, typically for up to 2 to 4 weeks. In the case of implant, complex prosthodontic and periodontal treatments, provisional restorations may be required to last for extended periods of time and are called interim restorations

Finish Line the continuous edge that borders the preparation to which the restoration is fit or finished; it is also called the *margin*

Extracoronal Restoration a restoration that covers all or part of the external surface of the clinical crown of the tooth and may extend over the cusp tips on facial or lingual surfaces or may include the removal of cusps, such as onlays, three-quarter crowns, full crowns, and veneers

Indirect Fabrication provisional restorations made on a cast or milled in a computer-directed machine outside the patient's mouth before delivery

Intracoronal Restoration a restoration within the crown of the tooth, such as an inlay or amalgam

Direct Fabrication provisional restorations made directly on the prepared tooth/teeth inside the patient's mouth

---

The increased retention of natural teeth and advances in technology in restoring and replacing tooth structure have increased the need for high-quality fixed prosthodontic, pedodontic, and endodontic treatments. Fabricating provisional restorations, also referred to as temporary or interim restorations, is an important component of fixed prosthodontic treatment. While the definitive restorations are being fabricated, provisional restorations are critical for both the biological and biomechanical health of the tooth and periodontium as well as the comfort of the patient. Once the tooth has been prepared, the exposed dentin must be protected from the thermal, chemical, mechanical, and bacterial effects from the oral environment. Adjacent soft tissues must be protected, and the position of the tooth must be maintained. All of this must be accomplished with provisional restorations, with additional considerations of esthetics, function, and patient comfort.

The dental auxiliary may be called on to provide a variety of functions such as fabricate, repair, remove, or maintain the provisional restoration as well as give home care instructions. Good provisional coverage not only helps to ensure the success of the final restoration, it is also an important component in patient satisfaction. Patients who need to return to the dental office to have their provisional crowns recemented or replaced or do not like the esthetics of the restoration may lose confidence in the doctor's ability.

DENTAL PROCEDURES THAT MAY REQUIRE PROVISIONAL COVERAGE

Provisional coverage may be required in general, pedodontic, endodontic, and prosthodontic cases. Whenever a situation arises wherein a permanent restorative material cannot be placed at the time of preparation, a provisional (temporary) material will be chosen (Table 18.1).

The patient wears this provisional restoration to protect the tooth for a short period of time, generally 2 weeks to a month. In cases involving complex treatments such as implants and complex prosthodontic procedures, a longer time may be required, 6 to 18 months.

This short-term or interim period of time may be used to make a final diagnosis, develop a treatment plan, allow hard or soft tissue healing, and communicate with the laboratory for the optimal success of the final restoration. In some cases, the patient may be asked to evaluate the provisional restoration to make cosmetic decisions regarding the final restoration. For instance, the patient wishing to close a large diastema (space) between teeth #8 and #9 may find that the resultant size of the restorations necessary to close this space is less esthetically pleasing than the space they wished to close.

CRITERIA FOR PROVISIONAL COVERAGE

Criteria for a properly fabricated and cemented provisional restoration include the following:
- Maintenance of tooth function and position in the arch
- Protection of hard and soft oral structures including the pulp
- Establishment of esthetics and retention
- Provide patient comfort

If these criteria are not met, pulpal and periodontal irritation, tooth migration, and patient dissatisfaction may very likely occur. Keeping these criteria in mind, the clinician can choose the most appropriate material, technique, provisional cement, and postoperative instructions for the patient.

MAINTAIN PREPARED TOOTH POSITION RELATIVE TO ADJACENT AND OPPOSING TEETH

When a tooth has been prepared to receive a crown, sufficient tooth structure has been removed to create a space between the adjacent teeth and the opposing teeth. The provisional restoration must contact adjacent teeth on the mesial and distal sides as well as be in occlusion with the opposing teeth. Otherwise, the tooth's position can shift within a couple days. When shifting occurs the restoration, which was designed to fit the tooth in its original position, may now be too high because of occlusal/incisal migration or may not seat properly as a result of lateral migration of the prepared tooth. This shifting will likely require the patient to have additional chairtime for adjustments before final cementation or possibly result in the need to take a new impression and fabricate a new restoration. Provisional restorations should share the load from forces during normal function or bruxing. If the provisional restoration itself is too high, the results may be those associated with trauma from occlusion, which may cause the tooth be become sore and mobile.

PROTECT THE EXPOSED TOOTH SURFACES AND MARGINS

When the tooth is prepared, the dentinal tubules are exposed to potentially harmful thermal, chemical, mechanical, and bacterial insults. Provisional materials placed near the pulp must have no adverse chemical effect and must be sufficiently insulating to protect the pulp from thermal assaults. Some of the materials generate heat as they set and must be handled properly to avoid pulpal damage. Maintaining the comfort of the patient is paramount.

The **finish line (or margin)** of the preparation is particularly susceptible to fracture if not adequately protected. Well-adapted provisional restorations protect the finish line from fracture and from marginal leakage of oral fluids and bacteria. If the finish line is damaged, the permanent restoration will no longer fit precisely, leaving space for future leakage of oral fluids and bacteria. The process of caries may even begin during the time the provisional restoration is in place.

Table 18.1	Dental Procedures Requiring Provisional Coverage
PROCEDURE	**TYPE OF PROVISIONAL COVERAGE**
Endodontic access preparation	Closes endodontic access preparations between appointments
Vitality of the tooth is in question	Allows the pulp to respond to therapeutic agents or to recover from the trauma of preparation
Emergency care	Prevents additional damage and improves esthetics and function while awaiting a permanent solution
Awaiting permanent restoration	Allows time for laboratory fabrication of cast and ceramic restorations
Restoration of implants	For long-term provisional coverage while the implant site is allowed to heal
Restoration of primary teeth	Placed on primary teeth because of extensive caries, pulpotomies, or pulpectomies until permanent teeth erupt

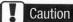 Caution

Because provisional luting agents are highly soluble and may wash out from under a provisional restoration, they cannot be expected to make up for marginal deficiencies in the restoration.

PROTECT THE GINGIVAL TISSUES

Many crown preparations extend 0.5 to 1 mm subgingivally, making the margins and the overall contour of the provisional restoration critical to periodontal health. Periodontal tissues are susceptible to irritation from overcontoured, overextended, or overhanging margins; trauma from food impaction; and buildup of plaque. Margins of the provisional must be flush with the preparation. If a margin is overextended, the resultant tissue irritation may lead to bleeding, inflammation and gingival recession, adversely affecting the cosmetic effect of the permanent restoration. If the margin is short of the finish line, the tooth may experience sensitivity.

All surfaces of the provisional restoration must be properly contoured, polished and maintain contact with adjacent teeth. If surfaces are undercontoured the process of chewing will excessively force food directly onto the gingiva rather than deflecting it facially and lingually. An overcontoured restoration may trap plaque by not allowing for any self-cleansing or gingival stimulation from the chewing process (Fig. 18.1).

Inadequate or open contacts likewise can lead to food impaction. Rough surfaces will act as plaque traps and may abrade the tongue or oral mucosa. These scenarios may also lead to irritation, inflammation, and recession.

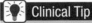 **Clinical Tip**

A properly contoured, polished and well-fitting provisional restoration is critical to maintaining periodontal health around the prepared tooth. Inflamed gingival tissue will bleed profusely at the delivery of the final restoration and potentially interfere with bonding or cementation.

PROVIDE FUNCTION

The provisional restoration should restore ideal occlusal/incisal contact with the opposing teeth and have functional contours and proximal contacts (Fig. 18.2). As previously mentioned, deficiencies in contour or contact of the provisional restoration may lead to problems that compromise or prevent the ideal placement of a permanent restoration. Patients must be able to chew normally and clean the provisional restoration as they would a permanent restoration. However, the provisional restoration is not intended to function exactly like the permanent restoration. Modifications in diet, including the avoidance of sticky and hard foods, may be necessary to prevent dislodging or fracturing of the provisional restoration.

ESTHETICS AND SPEECH

In addition, it is important to consider the esthetics along with concerns for function. Provisional restorations must have the appearance of natural tooth structure whenever esthetics is important.

For anterior esthetic restorations, provisional restorations may be used as a guide for color, contour, length, and positioning of the final restoration. This is an important component for patient satisfaction, as the patient now has an opportunity to give input concerning the esthetics of the restoration.

Speech is also influenced by the position of the teeth. Anterior provisionals that are too bulky, thin, long, short or do not occlude properly can change the patient's speech patterns causing lisps or whistling sounds when they speak. The provisional restoration must not interfere with normal speech patterns.

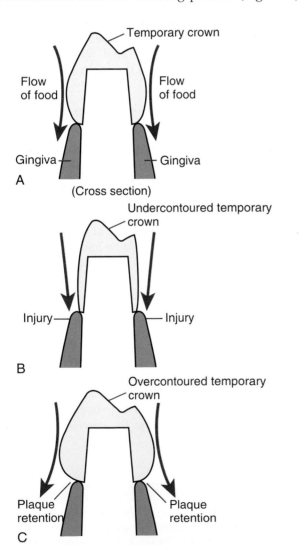

FIG. 18.1 A, Properly contoured provisional crown. **B,** Under-contoured provisional crown. **C,** Over-contoured provisional crown.

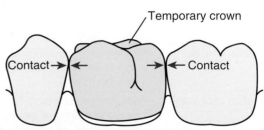

FIG. 18.2 Provisional crown duplicates natural tooth contour, contact, and occlusion.

Clinical Tip

Matching shades and customizing provisional materials to duplicate the natural teeth will greatly enhance patient acceptance and thus the success of the provisional restoration.

RETENTION

The cementation of the provisional restoration is accomplished with provisional cement which is not designed to be retentive for extended periods of time. Like a permanent restoration, the fit of the provisional crown is partly responsible for its retention. The design, height and taper of the crown preparation are also responsible for the retention of the provisional restoration. For many patients, a well-fabricated provisional restoration is a direct reflection on how the final restoration will turn out. The provisional restoration must be retentive enough to ensure patient confidence during the period in which the final restoration is being constructed.

Criteria for Provisional Coverage

Provisional coverage must:
- Reproduce proper proximal contacts and occlusal alignment
- Fit the tooth at the finish line (margins)
- Reproduce natural tooth contours
- Promote gingival health
- Provide pulpal protection
- Provide function, esthetics, and phonetics (speech)
- Remain stable and retentive
- Provide smooth surfaces

PROPERTIES OF PROVISIONAL MATERIALS

Materials used to fabricate provisional restorations must have properties that meet the specific requirement of the clinical treatment and the part of the mouth in which they are placed. Although most provisional restorations are in place typically for 2 to 4 weeks, provisional coverage on occasion may be required for extended periods of time. Strength and hardness are important for single and multi-unit **extracoronal restorations**. Biocompatibility with hard and soft tissues is also important. Provisional restorations located in the smile zone must be esthetic. In areas of the mouth with difficult access, the ability to manipulate the materials is also an important consideration.

STRENGTH

Materials must have sufficient compressive and tensile strength to resist the forces of mastication. Materials that are used for provisional bridges must also have sufficient flexural strength to resist deformation from flexing during mastication. Acrylics have more fracture toughness than brittle materials such as composite

resins that do not hold up well when used for long-span bridges or with patients who are bruxers. The material chosen must be able to resist the forces of chewing without breaking or coming off the tooth. In addition, the restoration should remain intact when removed so that it can be reused when necessary.

HARDNESS

Acrylic materials wear more readily than composite resin materials. Surface hardness must be sufficient to resist abrasion and wear for the period through which the provisional restoration is to be worn. The material should also be able to be polished to a smooth finish and should retain that smooth surface throughout its use. Smooth, polished surfaces will not irritate the tongue or oral mucosa, attract less plaque and make homecare easier resulting in healthier gingival tissues.

TISSUE COMPATIBILITY

Ideally, the material should not produce any additional irritation to pulpal or gingival tissues during or after setting reactions. Materials that generate heat when setting must be carefully selected depending on the clinical situation (i.e., deep preparation) and may be more appropriate for the **indirect fabrication** technique. In addition, for patient comfort, materials should not absorb or give off odors or taste.

ESTHETICS

Materials used in areas of esthetic concern must match adjacent teeth and must have good color stability and stain resistance. Shade selection is important in the management of patient expectations; many materials are not accurate in this area. Color stability is influenced by the surface quality and porosity of the material chosen as well as by the patient's oral hygiene and consumption of foods and beverages that tend to stain (e.g., berries, red wine, coffee, tea).

 Clinical Tip

It is advisable to pick a shade before a tooth is prepared; enamel dehydration from isolation during preparation procedures leaves the teeth lighter in color.

PROVISIONAL CROWN MATERIALS

The selection of provisional materials is typically based upon cost, ease of handling, esthetics, strength and accuracy of margins. Provisional materials include metals, polycarbonate, acrylics, composites, and cements. These materials may be used alone or in combination, such as an aluminum shell crown lined with acrylic. Provisional restorations may be preformed (e.g., stainless steel, tin-silver, aluminum, or polycarbonate crowns) or made specifically for individual procedures (e.g., custom acrylic or composite crowns and intracoronal restorations).

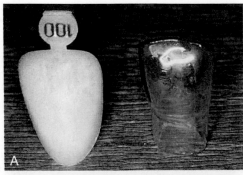

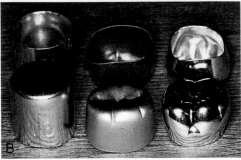

FIG. 18.3 **A.** Polycarbonate and celluloid crown forms. **B.** Aluminum shell, anodized aluminum and silver-tin crowns. (From Rosenstiel SF, Land MF, Fujimoto J: *Contemporary Fixed Prosthodontics*, (ed 5). St Louis, 2016, Elsevier.)

Provisional materials, whether they are cement, acrylic, or bis-acrylic composite, are mixed and placed in a plastic state and allowed to harden directly in/on the preparation or on a stone model. Cements are limited to intracoronal placement; provisional acrylic and composite resin can be used for extracoronal coverage as well.

Preformed crowns have the advantage of convenience, in that they are already premade in a variety of sizes and anatomic forms. This saves time because it eliminates the need for a crown template and is particularly useful in emergency situations and for badly broken-down teeth. Even though they come in different sizes, time must be spent in establishing contact, contour, occlusion, and marginal integrity.

Customized crowns are more versatile and more consistently meet the criteria for successful provisional restorations. They do, however, require the additional step of making a template or matrix for the final product. This template captures the external shape of the tooth structures as they exist before the preparation. This additional step can be further complicated if the original tooth is badly broken down or fractured.

PREFORMED CROWNS

The process of temporization using preformed crowns includes the use of metal (including stainless steel, aluminum or tin-silver), polycarbonate, and celluloid crown forms lined with acrylic, bis-acrylic composite or zinc oxide eugenol materials (Fig. 18.3). The preformed crown will become the outer surface of the provisional crown, and an acrylic or bis-acrylic composite material or thick, hard cement will occupy the inner portion of the crown. As previously mentioned, this

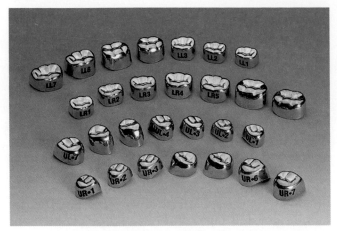

FIG. 18.4 A selection of pedatric stainless steel crowns. (Courtesy of Denovo Stainless Steel Crowns.)

method may be time saving, particularly in emergency situations when the patient has a fractured tooth, but does not consistently produce the most esthetic or well-fitting provisional crown.

Preformed crowns come in many sizes and tooth forms available in kits containing anterior or posterior crown forms or both. Because the prepared tooth is much smaller than this preformed shell, a reline of acrylic or bis-acrylic composite material is generally required for a close fit. Metal crowns are typically used only in posterior cases, while polycarbonate and celluloid forms are used on anterior teeth or premolars. Preformed crowns may only be used for single crowns and are not appropriate for temporary bridges.

Clinical Tip

If the kit of provisional crowns does not come with a measuring gauge, use a millimeter ruler to select the most appropriate crown size, measuring the width from mesial to distal contacts. All crowns that are tried in and not used must be sterilized before they are returned to the crown kit.

Stainless Steel Crowns

The stainless steel crown does not tarnish or corrode and is the most durable and abrasion-resistant of the preformed crowns, providing provisional coverage lasting months and even years (Fig. 18.4). The stainless steel crown has been used traditionally to restore primary teeth (Fig. 18.5). These durable and economical restorations are also used for adults, in cases where financial or health concerns would otherwise prohibit restoration of the tooth and result in the recommendation to extract. The primary advantage of these crowns is their malleability, which allows them to be bent and burnished to provide for good contacts, occlusion, and marginal integrity. The crown is cut with crown and bridge scissors and is crimped and contoured at the contact and margins with crimping and contouring pliers. Some manufacturers make their crowns pre-crimped at the cervical.

If the stainless steel crown is an alternate to a cast restoration for prolonged periods of time, minimal

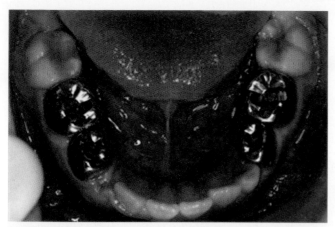

FIG. 18.5 Stainless steel crowns on mandibular primary molars. (Courtesy of DentalGama.)

reduction of the tooth is ideal to preserve natural tooth strength and provide protection for the pulp. With the marginal seal and occlusion intact, these crowns may be a solution to long-term provisional coverage of posterior teeth even though the adaptations of margins, the occlusion and overall contours are never as precise as those of cast restorations.

An alternative to stainless steel crowns is nickel-chromium crowns (e.g., Ni-Chro Crown, 3M ESPE) which have similar durability, handling characteristics and appearance.

Aluminum Shell and Tin-Silver Alloy Crowns

Aluminum, anodized aluminum shell crowns and tin-silver alloy crowns (e.g. Iso-Form, 3M ESPE) are used for provisional coverage of posterior teeth (see Fig. 18.3B). They are lined with acrylics, bis-acrylic composites or a thick mix of reinforced ZOE cement to support the soft metal. Without adequate support under functional forces the crown will distort and come off. For patients who brux their teeth a hard liner is preferred over ZOE. A well-fitted aluminum shell or tin-silver crown can last a few weeks. (Anodized aluminum shells go through an electrochemical process to create oxides on the surface of the aluminum to make it more durable and corrosion-resistant.)

Tin-silver crowns are the softest and most ductile of the preformed metal crowns and as a consequence, are easily burnished. They may be pre-crimped (constricted) at the cervical margins. For crown preparations with a thin finish line, these pre-crimped crowns when seated on the prepared tooth will stretch over the margins and be closely adapted to the tooth. For crowns with wider finish lines such as a shoulder margin, the crown may need to be expanded to allow it to fit over the margins. A plastic stretch block with a series of tapered stumps is supplied with the Iso-Form kit to expand the crown. The crown is pressed down on the tapered stumps that come in a variety of diameters (Fig. 18.6).

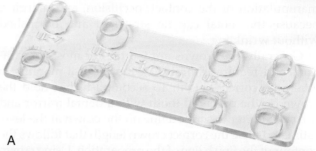

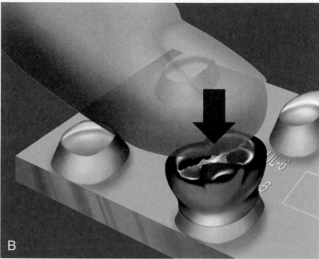

FIG. 18.6 Plastic stretch block for tin-silver alloy provisional crowns. **A,** Series of tapered stumps of various sizes for different size crowns. **B,** Preformed crown is pre-crimped at the cervical and needs to be stretched by pressing it down on the tapered stump. This will allow it to pass over the margins of the prepared tooth. (Courtesy of 3M ESPE.)

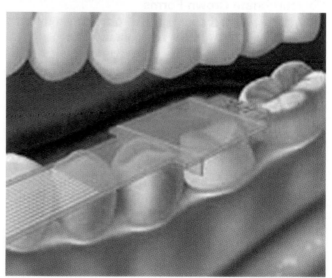

FIG. 18.7 Plastic measuring gauge used to determine the mesio-distal width for selecting a posterior provisional crown. (Courtesy of 3M ESPE.)

Fitting the crown. The mesial-distal width is measured for the most appropriate fit, and some crown kits provide a gauge for measuring the mesial-distal width (Fig. 18.7). To confirm the correct width of the selected provisional crown without trying it on the tooth, simply turn it upside down and see if the coronal portion fits the space. The softness of the metal allows for easy manipulation of the contact, occlusion, and margins, because the metal can be stretched and burnished without wrinkling.

Generally, the crowns are too tall for most preparations and require trimming at the cervical margins to attain the correct height. To accomplish this, hold the crown on the prepared tooth with a dental mirror and use an explorer to scribe a line on the crown at the level estimated to be the correct crown length that follows the contour of the finish line of the preparation. Using crown and bridge scissors begin trimming a little at a time to avoid overtrimming. If ragged edges are present after trimming, the margins should be smoothed with a finishing bur, sandpaper disk or a fine stone. Margins can be smoothed with a rubber wheel or polishing points. Contouring pliers are used to form the cervical contours and crimp the margins so they will closely adapt to the tooth. Prior to placing the supporting liner, the patient can bite on the crown a few times to begin forming the occlusal contacts. Because of their softness, these crowns wear easily, especially in patients who brux and must be checked for occlusal integrity if they will be worn for more than a few weeks (see Procedure 18.1).

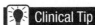 **Clinical Tip**

When selecting a preformed provisional crown, it is better to chose one that is slightly larger than the space rather than one that is smaller, because a larger one can be shaped and trimmed to fit. The smaller one cannot.

Polycarbonate Crown Forms

Preformed polycarbonate crown forms are composed of polycarbonate resin which contains microglass fibers which allow margins to be crimped with pliers and provide strength and durability. These crowns come in kits with several sizes and shapes for primary and permanent teeth and are available in tooth-colored shades, predominately in the A and B shades (see Fig. 18.3A). They are more rigid than the soft metal provisional crowns and may have to be adjusted with acrylic burs and disks or may be carefully cut with sharp crown scissors. The primary advantage is their esthetics for replacement of anterior and premolar teeth (some manufacturers even have molar forms) and their compatibility with acrylic resins to further customize the fit and margins. As an alternative to polycarbonate, tooth colored crown forms are also made from polymethylmethacrylate.

Fitting the crown. An appropriate size crown can be selected by measuring the mesial-to-distal space between the adjacent teeth to ensure adequate proximal contacts and confirming that it is long enough to cover the preparation. Most crowns are too long initially and must be trimmed at the cervical margin with scissors or an acrylic bur (see Procedure 18.2). After the crown has been adjusted for width and height, it is filled with acrylic resin or bis-acrylic composite,

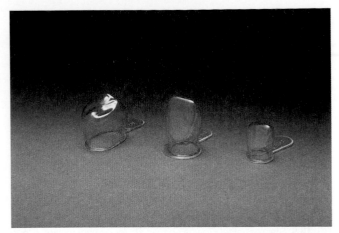

FIG. 18.8 Clear celluloid crown forms for permanent premolar and incisor and primary incisor. (Courtesy of 3M ESPE.)

which is matched to tooth shade, and then inserted onto the prepared tooth. The acrylic mix should reach the dough stage before seating the crown on the moistened preparation. Acrylic resins will chemically bond with the polycarbonate crown and composites will bond if the interior of the crown is first primed with methyl methacrylate liquid. Otherwise, retention can be obtained with the composite lining material by roughening the interior of the crown.

 Clinical Tip

Keep the tab of the polycarbonate crown form in place during fitting; it makes for a convenient handle for trying in and removing the crown.

Celluloid Crown Forms

Celluloid crown forms are thin, transparent shells made of cellulose acetate (Fig. 18.8). They are available in both primary and permanent anterior tooth shapes and sizes and primary posterior teeth.

Fiting the crown form. In order to select the appropriate form size, a measurement is made of the incisal width of the preparation space between the two adjacent teeth. The size of the celluloid crown form can be enlarged by warming the round end of an instrument such as a ball burnisher and pressing it into the form at the desired location. The size can also be reduced by slitting the crown form vertically on the lingual surface, lapping the cut edges to fit the crown preparation and then fusing the edges with a couple drops of acetone or a hot instrument (use caution). Preformed celluloid crown forms, like polycarbonate crown forms, are filled with acrylic or composite resin provisional material to create the tooth shape presented by the form. Usually one or two small holes are placed in the incisal corners of the crown form to allow excess resin or composite material to flow out when the crown form is seated. This prevents trapping air and the creation of voids in the material. After the fill material cures, the shell is slit with a scalpel and peeled off the tooth and adjustments to margins, contours or occlusion are done with an acrylic bur. Smoothing and polishing can be done with standard acrylic or composite polishers.

Advantages and Disadvantages. The advantage with the transparent form is that the shade selected to match the teeth is not affected by a predetermined color of the crown form allowing for a better color match. The disadvantage is that after the crown form is removed there is often a space left by the thickness of the crown form preventing contact with adjacent teeth and acrylic must be added to re-establish the interproximal contacts.

 Clinical Tip

If the margins are overextended when fitting preformed crowns, the gingival tissue will blanch when the patient bites on the crown or as the auxiliary seats the crown under finger pressure. This is a useful sign to know where to trim the excess, especially in areas where the margins cannot be viewed directly such as interproximal areas.

Modifying Preformed Crowns to Close Open Contacts

Metal crowns: Place the proximal surface on a paper pad and burnish the internal surface at the contact area with a ball burnisher. This stretches the metal outward to extend the contact area.

Polycarbonate crowns: Roughen the contact area and prime it with a drop of methyl methacrylate liquid. Add freshly mixed acrylic to the contact area. When it reaches the doughy stage, re-seat the crown on the prepared tooth to establish contact. Remove the crown and place in warm water to accelerate the set of the acrylic. Once set, remove excess acrylic and lightly polish the contact area.

An alternative material to use is flowable composite resin. Add the composite to the roughened and primed contact area, seat the crown on the prepared tooth, and then light cure the composite. Remove the crown and shape and polish the composite as with the acrylic material.

Celluloid crown forms: Use a warm ball burnisher to push out the contact area from the interior to extend the contact area. Try it on the prepared tooth and check the contact.

An alternative method is to make a hole where the contact area is located and allow the provisional crown material (acrylic or composite resin) to flow into contact with the adjacent tooth when the filled crown form is seated. Remove from the tooth before the acrylic sets fully so it does not get locked on the tooth. Remove excess material and reseat on the preparation a few times as it sets. With composite resin, use a 2 to 3 second tack cure and remove excess material from the margins and interproximal embrasure spaces before the final cure.

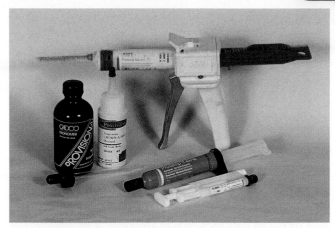

FIG. 18.9 Acrylic (liquid and powder) and composite provisional crown materials mixed by hand and automix.

CUSTOMIZED PROVISIONAL CROWNS

Custom provisional crowns more consistently meet the criteria for successful provisional restorations than preformed provisional crowns. A customized provisional allows for better function and fit. Superior esthetics improves patient acceptance and the ability to fabricate multi-unit provisional bridges makes these materials extremely popular.

Handling

Materials must be fast and easy to use, reliable, and inexpensive. The material should have sufficient working time and simplified technique to allow for fabrication of the provisional. For many customized provisional materials, the working time must also allow for removal from the mouth while still elastic for trimming before reinsertion. For these materials, tear strength, that is, the ability of the material to resist tearing or distortion on removal from the mouth or stone model, is a consideration. The setting time must be fast and must accommodate difficult-to-access areas when light-cured materials are used. Materials should be repairable to account for defects and to modify fit. Adding provisional material directly to the margins for repair will help provide good marginal integrity and relining the provisional crown with a new mix of material will ensure a good fit. Materials must be economical and efficient to use; provisional coverage must not be excessive in terms of cost of materials or time of fabrication.

MATERIALS FOR CUSTOM PROVISIONAL RESTORATIONS

Materials used for the fabrication of custom provisional restorations fall into two main categories: methacrylates and composite resins. (Fig. 18.9).

METHACRYLATE PROVISIONAL MATERIALS (ACRYLICS)

Acrylic materials in the form of methacrylates have been used for many years for custom provisionals.

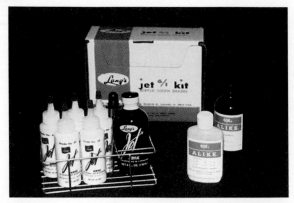

FIG. 18.10 Kit of methyl methacrylate (acrylic) materials: powders in a variety of shades and a bottle of liquid (monomer). (From Rosenstiel SF, Land MF, Fujimoto J: *Contemporary Fixed Prosthodontics*, (ed 4). St Louis, 2006, Elsevier.)

Their good esthetics, ease of manipulation, and low cost made them a popular choice over preformed crowns. However, these self-curing materials have high shrinkage and heat release during polymerization (exothermic reaction) and patients complain about the acrylic odor and bad taste. They have a low modulus of elasticity (relatively flexible), have adequate strength but wear easily. For the short time they will be in use, they are stain resistant and dimensionally stable.

The methacrylates can be placed into two subgroups: methyl methacrylate and ethyl methacrylate. These acrylics have several features in common: powder—liquid formulation, come in a variety of tooth colors, self-curing, shrink and release heat on setting, relatively strong, good polishability and material can be added to repair them. When the powder and liquid are mixed, the liquid partly dissolves the powder to produce a doughy mass that can be used to make provisional restorations.

Methyl Methacrylate

Methyl methacrylate (also called polymethyl methacrylate or PMMA) is the provisional material that has been used the longest. It consists of a powder – liquid formulation containing dibutyl or diethyl phthalate (polymer) powder and methyl methacrylate (monomer) liquid. It is available in a variety of tooth colors (Fig. 18.10). It has good strength for both single units and long-span bridges with good marginal fit. Of the two categories of methacrylates PMMA has the most shrinkage (3 - 8%) and heat generated on setting. The greater the volume of material, the more heat will be generated. The pontic area of bridges has the most volume and care must be taken so the patient does not receive a tissue burn from the heat. The monomer can be toxic to the pulp if in close proximity and any free monomer not reacted with the powder can cause irritation to the oral mucosa in sensitive individuals. Additionally, the taste

and odor is unpleasant. Examples of commercially available methyl methacrylate materials are *Duralay* (Reliance Dental Manufacturing) and *Jet* (Lang Dental Manufacturing Company). The setting time is approximately 5 to 6 minutes but fast set formulations are available with a 4-minute setting time, for example, Jet Set-4 (Lang Dental Manufacturing Company).

> **! Caution**
>
> Methyl methacrylate monomer is flammable, so keep it away from an open flame. It is not good to inhale the fumes or allow the material to contact the skin. Use in a well ventilated area.

Ethyl Methacrylate

Ethyl methacrylates (also called polyethyl methacrylates or PEMA) provide some improvements over methyl methacrylates. The powder – liquid formulation consists of polymer powder with coloring pigment and benzoyl peroxide which initiates the chemical reaction and ethyl methacrylate liquid. PEMA generates less heat and shrinkage when setting than methyl methacrylate and is better tolerated by the pulp and oral mucosa. However, they are not as strong as the methyl methacrylates and have less surface hardness. They are not suitable for long span provisional bridges or for use in patients who brux their teeth. Examples of these materials include Snap (Parkell) and Trim II (Keystone Industries).

> **! Caution**
>
> Heat generated during the polymerization of self-cured acrylic can potentially damage the pulp or burn soft tissues, especially when used in a large volume such as a bridge.

> **💡 Clinical Tip**
>
> Do not allow acrylic to set completely on a model or prepared tooth; this will cause the material to lock onto the preparation. Remove gross excess from the interproximal and "pump" the material on and off the tooth preparation until initial polymerization is complete.

COMPOSITE RESIN PROVISIONAL MATERIALS

Composite resin provisional materials were developed to overcome many of the undesirable features of the methacrylates. They are biocompatible and kinder to the pulp. These materials can be grouped into three categories: bis-acryl composite resin, bis-GMA composite resin and urethane dimethacrylate resin. They are a bit more expensive, but are easier to handle, with less odor, and bad taste and with better esthetics.

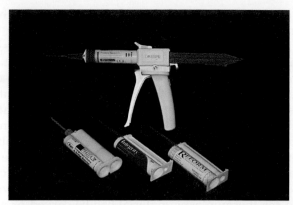

FIG. 18.11 Composite resin provisional materials in 2-paste cartridges with automixing delivery tips. (From Rosenstiel SF, Land MF, Fujimoto J: *Contemporary Fixed Prosthodontics*, (ed 4). St Louis, 2006, Elsevier.)

Table 18.2	Features of Acrylic and Composite Provisional Materials
ACRYLIC	**COMPOSITE**
High heat during polymerization	Low heat during curing
High shrinkage during polymerization	Low shrinkage during curing
Possible tissue irritation	Good tissue biocompatibility
Poor taste and smell	No unpleasant smell and mild taste
Difficult to repair	Easily repaired
Variety of color shades	Excellent esthetics.
Inexpensive	Expensive

Bis-acrylic Composite Resin Provisional Materials

Bis-acrylic composite provisional materials have a chemical structure between that of acrylic resins and dental composite materials. Low shrinkage and heat release during curing, imperceptible odor, good shade selection, and biocompatibility are distinct advantages over acrylic resins. The presence of micro- and nano-size glass fillers makes them more wear resistant than the acrylics, and they have good marginal fit. Early versions were self-curing but a newer variation is dual-cured. When they polymerize, they leave a thin layer of unset resin on the surface (oxygen inhibited layer) that should be removed. They are more brittle (higher modulus of elasticity) than the acrylics and therefore, must be limited in use to single units or short-span bridges that are not under significant occlusal loading. They are esthetically more pleasing in the anterior part of the mouth than the acrylics but more prone to stain. Examples of bis-acryl products include Integrity Temporary Crown and Bridge Material (self-curing) and Integrity MultiCure (both by Dentsply), Protemp Plus (3M ESPE) and Luxatemp Automix Plus (DMG America) (Fig. 18.11).

Bis-GMA Composite Resin Provisional Materials

Bis-GMA (bisphenol-A-glycidyl methacrylate) composite resins are an improvement over bis-acryl composites. They are stronger and less brittle, making them suitable for both single- and multiple-unit temporaries as well as long-term temporization. They have better esthetics, a wider shade selection and are less prone to staining. Polymerization shrinkage and exothermic heat are reduced, making them kind to the pulp. They also have good margins and polish well. The newest materials, made with nano-fillers, provide a smooth and lustrous surface with little finishing and polishing required. These smoother surfaces are more comfortable for the patient and are easier to keep clean, thereby promoting better periodontal health. Their chemistry is compatible with flowable composites which can be used for repairs and add-ons. If large repairs are to be made, it is advisable to apply a resin bonding agent to the surface first to ensure a good union between the provisional crown and the repair material. Examples of bis-GMA materials include TempSpan (Pentron Clinical Technologies) and Protemp Crown (3M ESPE).

Manipulation of Material. The two-paste material is typically mixed and dispensed from double-barrel cartridges placed into a mixing and dispensing gun. When the gun trigger is pressed the appropriate amounts of catalyst and base pastes are mixed and dispensed through automixing tips. Automixing helps to prevent operator error and unnecessary waste as well as ease of cleanup. Automix syringes also allow for direct delivery into a template without the incorporation of air voids.

Light-cured, self-cured, and dual-cured versions of these materials are available. Automixed self-cured materials are dispensed from syringes and may be used with any template. Light-cured materials require clear plastic templates and are difficult to cure in deep areas or those with limited access. Dual-cured materials require additional time to chemical-cure in areas the curing light can't reach, but they allow for removal from undercut areas while the materials are still flexible. Then they are trimmed and replaced for final curing (Table 18.2).

Urethane Dimethacrylate Resin Provisional Materials

Urethane dimethacrylate resins are the strongest of the custom provisional materials. Unlike the other composite resin materials, they are single component materials in a thick paste or putty form. They are light-cured with conventional curing lights or may require a special curing unit for the final cure.

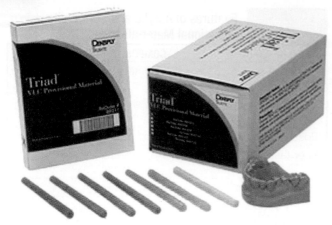

FIG. 18.12 Urethane dimethacrylate resin provisional material. (Triad VLC Provisional Material, Courtesy of Dentsply Prosthetic.)

Manipulation of Materials. Triad VLC Provisional Material (Dentsply) is a single component urethane dimethacrylate resin with a putty-like consistency that is available in seven shades including an enamel shade for creating incisal effects (Fig. 18.12). The shade (or shades if a layering technique is used) is selected, packed into a clear template made on a preoperative cast and pressed over the prepared teeth that have been lubricated with a water soluble lubricant such as KY jelly or glycerin. Partially lift and reseat the template several times to relieve undercuts and adapt the margins. A conventional curing light is used to harden the material. The template is removed with the provisional still in it. The material will not reach its maximum strength unless cured further in a Triad curing unit for two minutes. The provisional is removed from the template and reseated on the preparation to check the fit, margins and proximal and occlusal contacts. It is finished with an acrylic bur and then a coating of Triad Air Barrier Coating is placed to eliminate any unset air inhibited layer on the surface. It is returned to the Triad curing unit for eight minutes for its final cure. Remove any remaining air barrier coating with a soft brush or wheel.

Revotec LC (GC America) is also in a putty-like consistency. It is available in a single universal shade and lacks the esthetics of the bis-GMA composite resins. An appropriate size portion is cut from the tube-shaped material for the provisional being fabricated. It can be adapted directly to the prepared tooth and hand sculpted or could be placed in a template and adapted much the same way as the Triad material. If applied directly to the preparation, excess material is removed from the interproximal with a carver before completing the contours and margins. First, the provisional is light-cured for a total of 10 seconds from all angles with a halogen lamp to create a gel state so it can be removed without distortion. After the provisional is removed it is light-cured to its final cure outside the

mouth. Lastly, it is finished and polished as with other composite materials.

Radica (Dentsply Prosthetics) is a thermoplastic material in syringes that is heated in a special unit. A template made from impression putty is prepared on the preoperative cast. The teeth on the cast are lightly prepared to make room for a thin layer of the material. Warm material is expressed from the syringe into the template. Enamel and dentin shades are available if a layering technique will be used. The template is seated over the prepared teeth and allowed to cool and harden. The flexible putty template is removed and the thermoplastic material can be carved or additions made as needed. When the final shape has been achieved the material is cured in a special unit (Eclipse or Enterra unit, Dentsply Prosthetics). The thin provisional shell is lined with any of the methacrylates or composite resins and placed in the mouth on the fully prepared teeth using techniques as previously described.

Advantages of Composite Resin Provisional Materials

1. Easy to use
2. Set quickly
3. Flexible so easier to insert and remove
4. Minimal polymerization shrinkage and heat
5. Color stable and stain resistant
6. Minimal bad taste and odor
7. Easy to repair using flowable composite
8. Radiopaque

 Clinical Tip

When using automix dispenser guns, make sure there is compatibility with the cartridges and the dispenser gun. Different manufacturers' materials and dispenser guns are not always compatible.

METHODS OF FABRICATION OF CUSTOM PROVISIONALS

Custom provisional crowns can be made by direct fabrication (made directly on the prepared tooth) or by indirect fabrication (out of the mouth on a stone cast or by a combination of the two). Often a template is used as a carrier for the provisional material.

Types and Uses of Templates

A template (also called a mold or matrix) shapes the external contours and anatomy of the provisional, and the prepared tooth or stone cast creates the internal dimensions. Template materials include hard wax, impression materials (such as alginate, silicone, or polyvinyl siloxane), vacuum-formed plastic and thermoplastic resins (Fig. 18.13). A template can be made directly in the mouth prior to the preparation of the tooth or teeth or on a stone cast of the unprepared

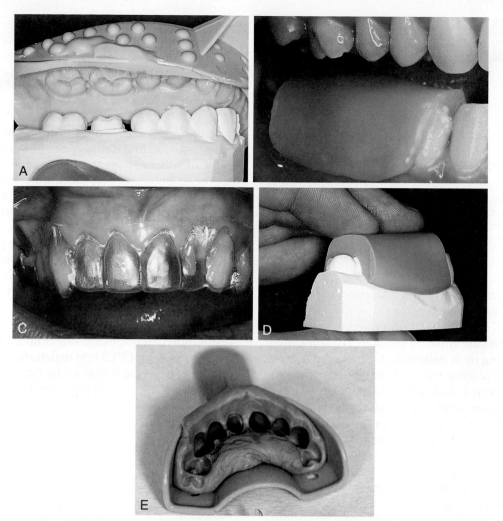

FIG. 18.13 Variety of templates used for fabrication of custom provisional restorations. **A,** Alginate impression **B,** Baseplate wax **C,** Clear vacuum-formed plastic **D,** Silicon putty E. Polyvinyl siloxane impression. (**A-D,** From Rosenstiel SF, Land MF, Fujimoto J: *Contemporary Fixed Prosthodontics*, (ed 5). St Louis, 2016, Elsevier.)

teeth. If the teeth are broken or require a change in shape for a more natural provisional, some repair or reshaping must be done in the mouth or on the stone cast.

Alginate and wax are the easiest to use and least expensive templates and are used extensively for single-unit, direct-technique provisionals. Polyvinyl siloxane (PVS) impression material is very popular and is often used in its putty form or regular body consistency in a tray. PVS, while more expensive, has an advantage over wax or alginate in that it can be reused later if the provisional should break.

Vacuum-formed plastic is the most common choice for multi-unit and indirect provisional techniques.

The vacuum-formed plastic template is made using a technique similar to that used to make whitening trays. A stone cast of the unprepared teeth is trimmed to remove borders that might entrap air. A thin sheet of the stiff plastic material (0.02 mm) is heated on a vacuum former until it sags 1 to 1.25 inches, and then the machine is activated to adapt the molten plastic to the cast. After the material cools it is removed from the cast and trimmed to include one or two teeth mesial and distal to the tooth/teeth to be prepared and approximately 3 to 4 mm below the gingival margin of the area of interest. The template is, then, ready for use with a direct or indirect fabrication technique.

Direct Technique *(See* Procedure 18.3*)*

Using the direct technique for provisional coverage, the provisional is fabricated directly on the prepared tooth using one of the provisional materials in a template. One popular technique uses a disposable triple tray impression with fast set material or bite registration material as the template. The impression used for the template is taken before the tooth is prepared. After the tooth is prepared, the impression is filled with a provisional material and seated on the prepared tooth.

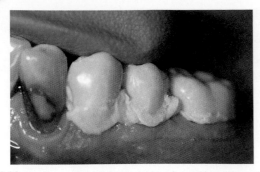

FIG. 18.14 Excess provisional material has flowed into the embrasure spaces and must be removed before it sets or the provisional restoration must be lifted and reseated several times before it sets to keep the restoration from being locked on the teeth. (From Rosenstiel SF, Land MF, Fujimoto J: *Contemporary Fixed Prosthodontics*, (ed 4). St Louis, 2006, Elsevier.)

If using an acrylic material for the provisional, powder and liquid must be mixed together to form a paste (see Fig. 18.30). It must be hand mixed to the proper consistency, and care must be taken to avoid trapping air during mixing or in delivering the material into the template. After placing the paste in the template, the template is inverted and seated over the moist prepared teeth. If gross voids are found on the occlusal or incisal, it may be necessary to place small holes in the occlusal or incisal corners of the template to alleviate hydrostatic pressure that has prevented the material from flowing into these areas.

Caution must be used when using this technique so that the provisional crown does not get locked on the prepared tooth. This happens when excess provisional material flows out of the template and hardens in the interproximal embrasure spaces locking under the contact areas of the adjacent teeth (Fig. 18.14). Not only is the crown very difficult to remove (and occasionally excess material must be cut from the undercuts with a bur), but heat generated during setting can burn tissues or damage the pulp. To avoid this mishap, the template with acrylic in place is "pumped" on and off the preparation when the material reaches a rubbery consistency. It can be removed just prior to its final set and the acrylic provisional crown can be removed from the template. Gross excess can be trimmed away with scissors. The provisional should, then, be placed in a cup of room temperature water to finish polymerization. (Hot water will accelerate the set but will cause more shrinkage and distortion.) If these materials are removed from the mouth too early and allowed to polymerize off the preparation, the amount of shrinkage may be sufficient to prevent them from seating back on the prepared tooth or the margins may be short. However, more material can be added to fill voids or correct deficient margins. The surface must be clean, and then some of the liquid (monomer) should be used to wet the surface so a new mix will bond to it. After it has set completely the rough provisional should be finished and polished for tissue health and patient comfort.

 Clinical Tip

Make sure the prepared tooth is slightly moist when seating the template containing acrylic. If the preparation is dry, the acrylic might stick to it and the provisional restoration may distort upon removal.

If using a composite resin paste-paste system with an automixing and delivery tip, be sure to keep the tip in the material as it is extruded to prevent the introduction of air bubbles. After placing the mixed material in the impression, reinsert it into the mouth. If using the triple tray, the patient is asked to bite into their normal occlusion while the material sets.

The impression is removed from the patient's mouth and the provisional crown is removed from the impression. If the triple tray is used, the occlusion should be very close to perfect. However, if the tray did not seat correctly, the occlusion could be quite high.

This technique is fast and provides a provisional restoration that duplicates the original tooth. Some clinicians use a clear PVS bite registration material so that they can speed the initial set by light-curing the material through the clear impression material.

 Clinical Tip

If bits of the provisional composite resin crown margins are going to come off, it is usually when the impression is removed from the prepared tooth. If the margins are thin, some the material may tear or stick to the prepared tooth. If the marginal defect is minor, seat the provisional crown back on the moistened preparation and add some flowable composite to repair the margin, then light-cure it. Be sure to lap the composite up onto the crown a couple millimeters so it has enough surface area to affect a good bond with the crown.

 Caution

Before using the direct technique, make sure there is adequate access to the preparation site, the template does not unduly impinge on the tissues, and tissues in the area are not inflamed and likely to bleed.

Indirect Technique

With the indirect technique the entire provisional is made outside of the mouth, then tried in and adjusted for fit. Any needed corrections to margins, contacts or voids can be made with the addition of new material either in the mouth or on the cast. Using the indirect technique, a pre-preparation impression of the area is made and poured into stone; the template is then made on this model. If it is necessary to account for missing tooth structure caused by caries or trauma, the defect can be corrected on the model with wax, acrylic, light-cured resin, or other materials. The template can be used indirectly with fabrication of the provisional on the model of the prepared teeth. The process of producing indirect provisional restorations is similar to the indirect composite procedure discussed in Chapter 6 Composites, Glass Ionomers, and Compomers.

The indirect technique has several advantages over the direct technique. The indirect technique allows for superior access to the preparations (stone replicas), saves chairtime and is more convenient for making multi-unit bridges or crowns in difficult-to-access areas. This technique is also desirable when the patient reports previous tissue irritation from methacrylate monomer or has difficulty maintaining an open mouth during the procedure. The indirect technique is also recommended when there is a concern for the health of the pulp due to deep caries or extensive prepping with the high-speed handpiece. By fabricating the crown indirectly, the tooth is not subjected to exothermic heat and chemical irritants of some provisional materials before they are set. The marginal fit is better when the material is allowed to set completely on the stone cast rather than with the direct technique where it is removed from the mouth before fully set.

> **Clinical Tip**
>
> Although the indirect technique requires additional time to fabricate a stone model or PVS die, this technique may well end up saving time in complicated cases and may be required if hard or soft tissue conditions would be further traumatized by direct fabrication. The indirect procedure can be delegated to the laboratory.

Indirect-Direct Technique

With the indirect-direct technique, a template is made on a pre-treatment cast. Next, the template is filled with a provisional material and seated on a lubricated stone cast where the teeth to be restored have been lightly prepared so that they are under-reduced compared to the actual tooth preparation. The result is a thin provisional shell that has the external form of the finished provisional but is too thin to serve as the functioning provisional restoration. At chairside, it is relined with freshly mixed provisional material and seated directly on the prepared tooth or teeth. So, half of the procedure is completed out of the mouth and half is completed directly on the teeth.

> **Clinical Tip**
>
> Coat the gypsum model with a separating medium to prevent the provisional material from sticking. If placing it in the patient's mouth, make sure the tooth is moist with saliva.

If using light-cured material, follow the manufacturer's directions for the required curing time. If using acrylic, remove the template while it is still doughy, trim away the excess with scissors, and then "pump" up and down on the preparation to prevent it from locking in the embrasures. When final set is achieved,

remove the provisional from the template and trim and polish.

> **Clinical Tip**
>
> If the custom provisional restoration is thin in areas, it is likely the result of one of two things:
> 1. the preparation has not been reduced enough to allow for adequate material
> 2. the template was pressed too hard onto the preparation causing it to compress toward the preparation

> Fabricating and cementing provisional restorations in many states are functions relegated to registered dental assistants and hygienists, while in other states they may be expanded functions. Check your state dental practice act for details.

ADVANCED TECHNIQUES

Many experienced dental auxiliary are equally capable of fabricating provisional coverage for complicated cases. At times, the dental laboratory technician may be called on to help in the fabrication of more difficult provisional coverage. Fabrication of provisional coverage over implants, for inlay and onlay preparations, and for long-term coverage will require specialized skills, knowledge of the requirements of the restorative procedure, and specialized alterations to provisional materials.

CAD/CAM Provisional (Temporary) Materials

Acrylate polymer (PMMA) blocks are available for use with CAD/CAM units to fabricate provisional restorations. These products provide many advantages over traditional provisional materials. Because they are processed with heat and pressure, there is no free monomer to irritate tissues and produce a bad taste. The polymers undergo more complete conversion and the materials have improved physical and mechanical properties, such as higher flexural strength, improved esthetics, and longer lasting color stability (due to decreased porosity). Polymerization shrinkage and exothermic heat are eliminated. CAD/CAM processing produces a superior fit and marginal integrity. They are durable and can be used for long-term provisionals (up to a year). They are indicated for single crowns, inlays, onlays and anterior and posterior bridges with up to two pontics. Some materials are available in up to six shades.

Examples of commercially available blocks include Telio CAD – Temp (Ivoclar Vivadent), VITA CAD – Temp in mono- and multi-color blocks (VITA North America), C-Temp (Kavo), artBlock – Temp (Merz Dental). Disks for multi-unit cases (such as PREMIOtemp CAD/CAM disks, Primotec USA) can also be used to fabricate provisional restoration in the office or in the laboratory using CAD/CAM technology and custom glazing and gingival effects (Fig. 18.15).

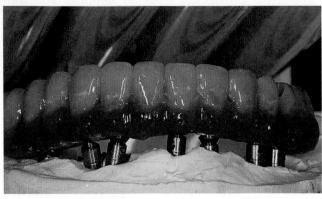

FIG. 18.15 Indirect multi-unit CAD/CAM acrylic provisional restorations customized by a skilled laboratory technician (Luke Kahng, CDT) with glaze and gingival colored composite resin. (From Kahng LS: Step-by-step: Fabricating temporaries with PMMA material. Dental Esthetics, May 2016.)

Provisional Materials for Inlays and Onlays

Any of the provisional materials discussed in this chapter could be used to make provisional restorations for inlay or onlay preparations for metal or ceramics using direct or indirect techniques. However, some of the materials, especially the acrylics, are much more difficult to handle in these complex cavity preparations with multiple walls and box forms.

Materials that are easier to use include:

Bis-acrylic and Bis-GMA Composite Resins – less shrinkage, low exothermic reaction

Urethane Dimethacrylate Resins – very strong, light – cured, putty consistency

Triad VLC Provisional Material

Revotec LC

Radica (thermoplastic material)

CAD/CAM materials – acrylate polymer blocks; eliminate exothermic reaction and polymerization shrinkage at the chair because they are already cured; increased strength and better fit. Drawback: requires in-office milling machine to deliver at the same appointment as the preparation.

Cements for Provisionals – use limited to entirely intracoronal preparations. Not for onlays.

ZOE and Reinforced ZOE

Zinc oxide/Calcium sulfate preparations (e.g., Cavit)

Polycarboxylate cement (paste-paste system)

HANDLING THE PROVISIONAL RESTORATION

CEMENTING THE PROVISIONAL RESTORATION

Provisional luting cements are used to cement provisional crowns. The choice of appropriate provisional luting cement is based on several factors:

- Properties of the provisional luting cement
- How long the provisional restoration will be in place
- How naturally retentive the preparation is
- What type of provisional restoration is being used

- What type of permanent restoration is being fabricated
- What type of permanent cement will be used

The cement must be retentive, have limited solubility to protect the tooth margins, not detract from the esthetics of the provisional restoration, be easily and completely removed, and not interfere with the bond of the permanent restoration.

A wide variety of provisional cements are available for the cementation of provisional restorations The most commonly used are zinc oxide eugenol (ZOE) or noneugenol formulations, polycarboxylate and resin cements. ZOE is self-curing, easy to handle, provides a sedative effect for sensitive teeth and has antibacterial properties. Polycarboxylate is also self-curing, is stronger than ZOE and is more retentive, because it sets harder and has weak bonds to tooth structure. Resin cements are the strongest, most esthetic and most versatile, since they can be self-cured, light-cured or dual-cured. If the provisional restoration is in an esthetic zone of the mouth and is thin, the stark, opaque white color of ZOE will show through. Resin cements are available in a variety of tooth colors and would be a better choice in this situation. However, because of their polymerization shrinkage, resin cements have more microleakage and discoloration at the margins. If the final restoration is to be cemented with permanent resin cement, a noneugenol provisional cement must be chosen, as eugenol in ZOE prevents resins from polymerizing. A detailed description of each type of provisional cement is discussed in Chapter 14 Dental Cement.

Before cementation of the provisional restoration, the preparation is dried and isolated with cotton rolls and the cement mixed according to the manufacturer's directions. The walls of the provisional crown are coated with the cement and then seated onto the tooth. Finger pressure is exerted, or the patient is asked to bite down firmly on a cotton roll placed on the provisional restoration. Excess cement is removed when appropriately set.

Removal of excess cement and the consequences of incomplete cement removal are covered extensively in Chapter 14 Dental Cements.

 Clinical Tip

If a light coating of a water-soluble lubricant or petroleum jelly is applied to the cervical half of the exterior of the provisional restoration before loading it with cement, clean up of the restoration after the cement sets will be much easier.

 Clinical Tip

Do not fill the entire interior of the crown with cement since the prepared tooth will displace most of it. Lightly coat the walls of the provisional crown with the cement.

All excess cement must be thoroughly removed, especially subgingivally, to prevent tissue irritation.

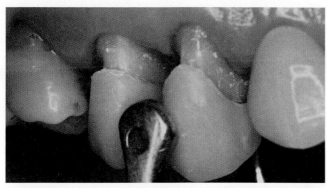

FIG. 18.16 To remove the provisional restoration, grasp it with removal forceps and gently rock it back and forth while applying mild force in an occlusal direction until the cement loosens. (From Rosenstiel SF, Land MF, Fujimoto J: *Contemporary Fixed Prosthodontics*, (ed 4). St Louis, 2006, Elsevier.)

REMOVING THE PROVISIONAL RESTORATION

The provisional restoration must be fabricated in a way that allows for easy removal without damage to the existing preparation. It is also desirable to preserve the provisional restoration in the event it may need to be used again.

Methods to remove the provisional restoration include the following:

- Using an instrument to engage the crown margin, pry the provisional off the preparation. Use caution not to damage the preparation margins.
- Using a chisel and mallet or crown and bridge removal instrument (also called a reverse hammer) to gently tap the restoration off the preparation. Keep the force directed along the long axis of the tooth to prevent damage to it.
- Using a pair of temporary removal forceps to grasp it, gently rock the provisional restoration back and forth and apply mild force in an occlusal direction until the cement loosens and then lift it from the preparation (Fig. 18.16).

If the provisional crown had a very snug fit when trying it on, only apply provisional cement to three or four millimeters of the crown walls around the margins. There will be less cement internally to hold the provisional crown making removal easier. Do not use this technique if the patient grinds his/her teeth. Another technique to make removal easier with a snug fitting crown is to add a small amount of petroleum jelly to the cement mix.

> **!** **Caution**
>
> All remnants of provisional cement must be completely removed and the tooth surface cleaned completely to prevent interference with bonding of the permanent restoration.

CLEAN-UP

After the provisional restoration has been removed there will be remnants of cement stuck to the tooth preparation. If the patient's tooth has been sensitive, a

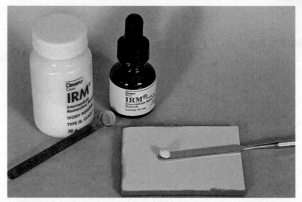

FIG. 18.17 Provisional cement used for intracoronal provisional coverage.

local anesthetic may be needed prior to removal of the provisional restoration. Carefully remove as much cement as possible with an instrument such as an explorer, interproximal carver or spoon excavator using light pressure so as not to damage the preparation. Usually very small fragments of cement will still remain. These must be removed to allow complete seating of the final restoration and prevent interference with bonding procedures. Use slurry of flour of pumice and water in a rubber prophy cup or a soft brush to complete the removal of these fine pieces of cement and rinse thoroughly. Do not discard the provisional restoration until the final restoration has been successfully cemented in case it is needed.

INTRACORONAL CEMENT PROVISIONAL RESTORATIONS

The main uses for intracoronal provisional cement restorations are for emergency treatments such as for deep caries or painful teeth, for protecting preparations for metal or ceramic inlays and to close endodontic access preparations. Cements used for inlay provisional restorations include: ZOE, reinforced ZOE (e.g., IRM, Dentsply), noneugenol zinc oxide, polycarboxylate, and zinc oxide/calcium sulfate materials. These cements can also be used to close endodontic access preparations and additional cements for this purpose include zinc phosphate cement and glass ionomer cement.

ZOE cement used for a provisional restoration has the added benefit of being soothing to inflamed pulp (Fig. 18.17). However, ZOE cements are highly soluble, have low strength, and have an unpleasant taste, limiting them to short-term and protected intracoronal placement. For these reasons, many clinicians use glass ionomer and resin-modified glass ionomer cements as an alternative. They are stronger, more durable, and provide an excellent seal to the tooth structure, preventing microleakage and the associated sensitivity. They are, however, more difficult to remove completely because of their bond to tooth structure and may not be the best choice when an inlay will be placed, because any remaining cement will prevent the inlay from seating.

Polycarboxylate cement (e.g., Ultra Temp, Ultradent Products) used for provisional restorations comes in a paste-paste, dual-barrel syringe delivery system. It is easy to remove when needed and is easy to clean up because it is water soluble until it sets.

Zinc oxide/calcium sulfate materials include Cavit-G (3M ESPE). Cavit is a premixed paste that sets in a moist environment. It expands on setting about twice that of ZOE from water sorption. It is relatively easy to remove from the preparation without having to use dental burs. Its drawbacks include low strength, softness, slow set and it breaks down with time. Its container should be re-capped soon after use because humidity will cause it to thicken.

 Clinical Tip

It should be noted that zinc oxide eugenol provisionals should not be used if a permanent restoration is to be cemented with a resin luting agent, because eugenol-containing cements inhibit polymerization of the resin cement.

Cements are placed directly into the cavity preparation with the aid of a matrix band and wedge when appropriate. The cement is carved and contoured, and then allowed to set. The final check of occlusion is done with articulating paper followed by additional carving as necessary (see Procedure 18.4).

PATIENT EDUCATION

Scheduled appointment times for fabricating provisional restorations must be adequate to instruct and demonstrate appropriate home care techniques, educate patients as to the limitations and expectations of the provisional restoration, and address patient concerns. Patients should understand that provisional restorations, although functional, are not as durable, well-fitting or esthetic as permanent restorations.

Because of limitations in the strength of provisional materials and the weak cements used to retain them, patients must be instructed that sticky foods may dislodge the provisional, hard foods may crack it and chewing gum may stick to it. Patients must be informed that there may be temperature sensitivity and an unpleasant taste associated with the provisional material. To avoid complications with treatment resulting from tooth movement or loss of tooth structure, patients must be told to immediately call the office if the provisional becomes dislodged, fractured or lost, even if the tooth is not sensitive. Teeth can shift in as little as 24 hours after loss of the provisional restoration. Strict adherence to appointment intervals is extremely important. Patients must return to the office at the appropriate time for placement of the permanent restoration due to the potential wear and breakdown of the provisional material or washing out of the provisional

cement. Limitations in esthetics of the provisional restoration may include imperfections in color matching, anatomic contour, and smoothness. Tobacco products and certain foods and beverages such as coffee, tea, red wine, berries and fruit juices may stain the provisional restoration. To avoid dissatisfaction, patients must be reminded that provisional restorations are not the same as permanent ones.

 Clinical Tip

If a provisional crown comes off during a time that the dental office is closed, the patient can be instructed to replace it after cleaning the interior of the crown and placing a small amount of denture adhesive into the crown. The patient should be instructed never to use any household cements.

HOME CARE INSTRUCTIONS

Home care instructions include brushing the restoration carefully along with the other teeth at least twice a day. Flossing should be done at least once a day and the floss should be pulled out to the side under the contact rather than back in an occlusal/incisal direction. Removing the floss back through the contact in an occlusal/incisal direction might dislodge the provisional restoration. If the provisional restoration includes a pontic, the additional use of floss threaders, Superfloss® (Oral B) or end-tufted brushes must be stressed for cleaning the tissue-contacting surface of the pontic and the proximal embrasures. Maintenance of healthy tissue during provisional coverage is crucial to the success of the permanent restoration. Inflamed gingival tissues can result in bleeding at the time of cementation of the permanent restoration that may compromise the cement seal.

SUMMARY

Provisional restorations protect teeth and periodontal structures in a variety of dental procedures. Regardless of the material and technique selected, a high-quality provisional restoration must be well adapted to the preparation, have proper contact, contour, and occlusion and must be functional and acceptable to the patient. If these criteria are not met, pulpal and periodontal irritation, tooth migration, and patient dissatisfaction will likely occur. There are many choices in the selection of provisional restorations and techniques for the fabrication of provisional restorations. The clinician must select materials and techniques on the basis of each patient's clinical needs and situation.

INSTRUCTIONAL VIDEOS

See the Evolve Resources site for a variety of educational videos that reinforce the material covered in this chapter.

Procedure 18.1 Metal Provisional Crown

See Evolve site for Competency Sheet.

Consider the following with this procedure: safety glasses are recommended for the patient, PPE is required for the operator, ensure appropriate safety protocols are followed, and check your local state guidelines before performing this procedure.

EQUIPMENT/SUPPLIES (Fig. 18.18)

- Mirror and explorer
- Selection of silver-tin alloy crowns
- Crown and bridge scissors
- Contouring pliers
- Ball burnisher
- Articulating paper
- Dental floss
- Isolation materials
- Cement and armamentarium
- Sandpaper disk and rubber wheel

PROCEDURE STEPS

1. Measure the mesiodistal width of the space between adjacent teeth.
2. Choose a crown that has a mesiodistal width equal to that of the original tooth.

   NOTE: If the crown does not fit, it may be sterilized and placed back in the kit.
3. Try in the crown, noting the occlusal relationship to adjacent and opposing dentition.

NOTE: The crown will be considerably higher than the adjacent teeth (Fig. 18.19).

4. Scribe a line on the facial and lingual crown surfaces to match the contour of the gingiva and approximate the amount of crown length that needs to be trimmed.

   NOTE: The crown is longer on the facial and lingual surfaces and shorter on the mesial and distal surfaces, forming a wavy line.
5. Trim to within 1 mm of the scribed line, using curved crown and bridge scissors.

   NOTE: Try to blend your cutting junctions to avoid producing burs of metal that will irritate the tissues (Fig. 18.20).
6. Contour the trimmed areas, using contouring pliers. Advance the pliers around the crown periphery as you continually squeeze the pliers with the ball portion of the pliers inside the crown and the curved beak on the outside of the crown.

   NOTE: This crimps the crown edge, adapting its circumference to the finish line (Fig. 18.21).
7. Retry the crown on the preparation to confirm fit. Adjust as needed.
8. Have patient tap the teeth together to adapt the soft metal to the occlusion

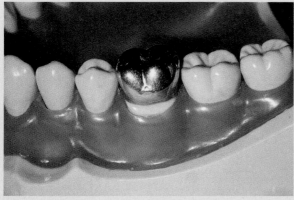

FIG. 18.18

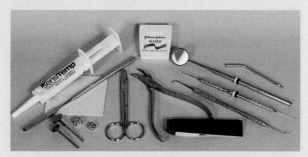

FIG. 18.19

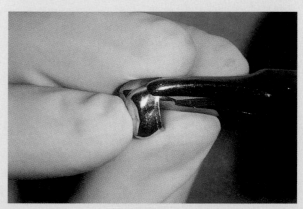

FIG. 18.20

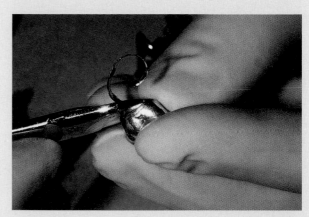

FIG. 18.21

Continued

Procedure 18.1   Metal Provisional Crown—cont'd

9. Check the bite with articulating paper; make sure the crown is occluding properly when the patient's teeth are fully together.

   NOTE: If the crown is interfering with occlusion, some reduction will be necessary. Only minor adjustments can be made on the occlusal surface before the surface is perforated (Fig. 18.22).

10. Check the contacts, using dental floss, to determine whether contacts are present and in the proper location.

    NOTE: If contact points need to be established, use the ball burnisher or contouring pliers with the ball portion inside and the curved beak outside, and gently squeeze to establish contact at the appropriate location.

11. Trim and polish the crown margins with disks and a rubber wheel to make the crown smooth and to prevent tissue irritation (Fig. 18.23).

12. Isolate the area and mix the cement according to the manufacturer's directions.

    NOTE: Because the metal is soft, the occlusal portion must be supported by a reinforced cement such as IRM. Plain ZOE cement such as TempBond is too weak for this purpose.

13. Seat the crown onto the preparation and have the patient bite on a cotton roll or a wooden stick in a mesiodistal direction to improve force distribution.

    NOTE: Make sure the patient is not biting only on the crown, but also on the adjacent teeth in the quadrant; biting only on the crown may force the crown too far in a gingival direction (Fig. 18.24).

14. When appropriate, remove excess facial and lingual cement. Remove interproximal cement by drawing a knotted piece of dental floss through the contact (Fig. 18.25) followed by an explorer.

Optional Steps

NOTE: The crown may be lined with an acrylic or bis-acrylic composite provisional material to further customize the internal fit and support the occlusal portion.

1. Mix the acrylic or composite provisional material according to the manufacturer's directions.

2. Place the material into the prepared crown, making sure to line the crown to avoid trapping air.

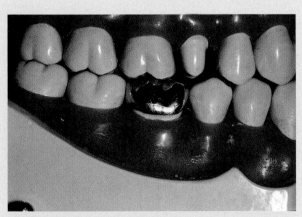

FIG. 18.22

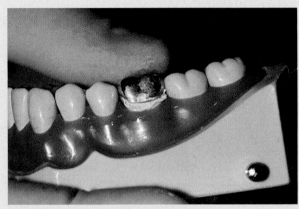

FIG. 18.24

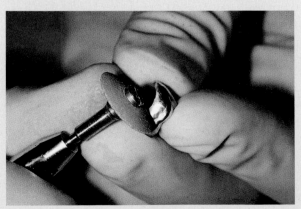

FIG. 18.23

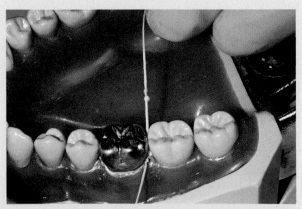

FIG. 18.25

Procedure 18.1   Metal Provisional Crown—cont'd

3. Place the crown back on the preparation, and have the patient bite in occlusion.
4. After the material has reached the desired consistency, remove the crown and remove the excess.
5. Because the acrylic supports the occlusal portion of the crown, it may be cemented with weaker

ZOE cement such as TempBond or a noneugenol version.

NOTE: Material should be removed while still elastic to avoid trapping the crown in undercuts.

6. Polish the crown and proceed with steps 12 through 14 above.

Procedure 18.2   Polycarbonate Provisional Crown

See Evolve site for Competency Sheet.

Consider the following with this procedure: safety glasses are recommended for the patient, PPE is required for the operator, ensure appropriate safety protocols are followed, and check your local state guidelines before performing this procedure.

EQUIPMENT/SUPPLIES (FIG. 18.26)

- Mirror and explorer
- Selection of polycarbonate crowns
- Articulating paper
- Dental floss
- Acrylic burs and sandpaper disks
- Pumice and rag wheel
- Isolation materials
- Cement and armamentarium

PROCEDURE STEPS

1. Measure the mesiodistal width of the space between adjacent teeth.
2. Choose a crown that has a mesiodistal width equal to that of the original tooth.

NOTE: Choose a crown that is slightly larger if an exact size cannot be found.

3. Try in the crown, noting the occlusal or incisal relationship to adjacent and opposing dentition.

NOTE: The crown will be considerably higher than the adjacent teeth. If the crown does not fit, it may be sterilized and placed back in the kit (Fig. 18.27).

NOTE: Keep the incisal identification tab in place to use as a handle for try in and removal.

4. Scribe a line on the facial and lingual crown surfaces to match the contour of the gingiva and approximate the amount of crown length that needs to be trimmed.

NOTE: The crown is longer on the facial and lingual surfaces and shorter on the mesial and distal surfaces, forming a wavy line.

5. Trim to within 1 mm of the scribed line with scissors or an acrylic bur on a slow-speed handpiece. Do not trim from the incisal/occlusal surface to adjust the length.

NOTE: Trim a small amount at a time while continuing to try and retry the crown until the desired amount is removed. If the crown was slightly larger than the space, it may be necessary to trim the proximal surfaces to establish a good seat (Fig. 18.28).

6. Check bite with articulating paper; make sure the crown is occluding properly when the patient's teeth are fully together.

NOTE: If the crown is interfering with occlusion, further reduction will be necessary. Only minor adjustments can be made on the incisal or occlusal surface before the surface is perforated. If the crown is fully seated and adjusting the occlusion has caused a perforation in the crown, it is possible that the preparation is under-reduced.

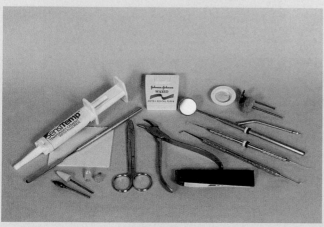

FIG. 18.26

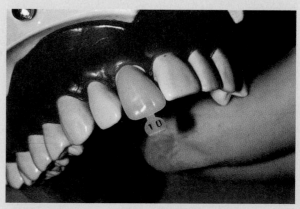

FIG. 18.27

Continued

Procedure 18.2 Polycarbonate Provisional Crown—cont'd

7. Check the contacts, using dental floss, to determine whether contacts are present and in the proper location.

   NOTE: If contact points are too tight or are not at appropriate locations, you will have to trim the proximal surface of the crown to establish correct location. If contact points are not present, you may have to add to the proximal surface with acrylic.

8. Trim and polish the crown margins with disks and pumice on a rag wheel to make the crown smooth and to prevent tissue irritation.

9. Isolate the area and cement the crown, following the manufacturer's directions for mixing the appropriate cement.

   NOTE: Completely coat the inside surfaces of the crown to avoid trapping air.

10. Seat the crown onto the preparation and have the patient bite on a cotton roll or a wooden stick in a mesiodistal direction to improve force distribution.

    NOTE: Make sure the patient is not biting only on the crown, but also on the adjacent teeth in the quadrant; biting only on the crown may force the crown too far in a gingival direction (Fig. 18.29).

11. When appropriate, remove excess facial and lingual cement. Remove interproximal cement by drawing a knotted piece of dental floss through the contact.

Optional Steps

NOTE: *If the crown is loosely fitting, it may be lined with an acrylic or bis-acrylic composite provisional material to further customize the internal fit.*

1. It may be necessary to place one or two small vent holes on the incisal corners or occlusal surface to prevent hydrostatic pressure from keeping the crown from fully seating.

2. Mix the provisional material according to the manufacturer's directions (Fig. 18.30).

3. Place the material into the prepared crown, making sure to line the crown to avoid trapping of air (Fig. 18.31).

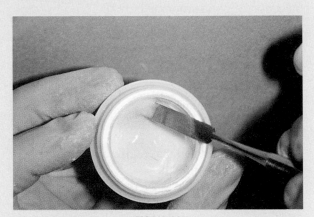

FIG. 18.30

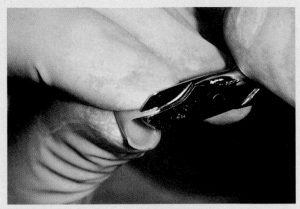

FIG. 18.28

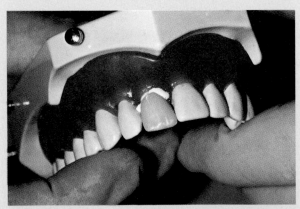

FIG. 18.29

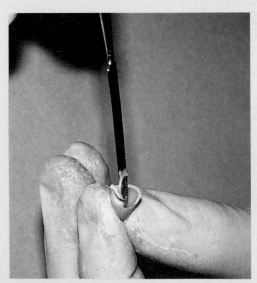

FIG. 18.31

Procedure 18.2   Polycarbonate Provisional Crown—cont'd

4. Place the crown back on the preparation, and have the patient bite in occlusion (Fig. 18.32).
5. After the material has reached the desired consistency, remove the crown, place it in room temperature water until set and then remove the excess.

NOTE: Crown should be pumped on and off the tooth while the lining material is still elastic to avoid trapping the crown in undercuts (Fig. 18.33).

6. Polish the crown, and proceed with steps 8 through 11 above (Figs. 18.34 and 18.35).

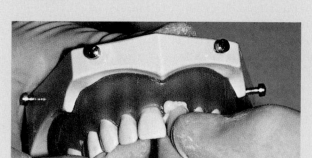

FIG. 18.32

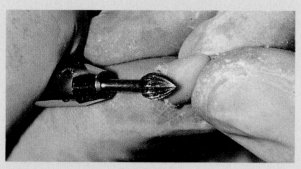

FIG. 18.34

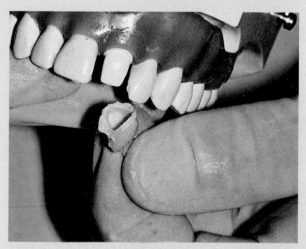

FIG. 18.33

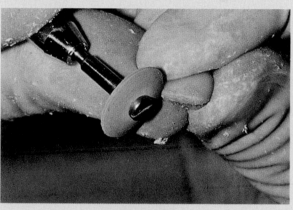

FIG. 18.35

Procedure 18.3 Custom Provisional Coverage: Direct Technique

See Evolve site for Competency Sheet.

Consider the following with this procedure: safety glasses are recommended for the patient, PPE is required for the operator, ensure appropriate safety protocols are followed, and check your local state guidelines before performing this procedure.

EQUIPMENT/SUPPLIES (FIG. 18.36)

- Mirror and explorer
- Template of the tooth before preparation
- Acrylic or composite provisional material
- Separating medium
- Dispensing syringe
- Acrylic stones and sandpaper disks
- Pumice and rag wheel
- Isolation materials
- Cement and armamentarium

PROCEDURE STEPS

Preparing the Template

1. Before preparing the tooth, make a template by taking an alginate or triple tray impression of it or by using a thermoplastic resin button or vacuum-formed plastic sheet on a stone cast of the unprepared tooth.

   NOTE: Alginate impressions should be kept moist until used.

2. Trim the template to remove undercuts or excess material.

Preparing the Provisional Coverage

Coat the prepared tooth with a water soluble lubricant such as KY Jelly or glycerin.

   NOTE: This will aid in separating the provisional material from the preparation while in a doughy stage (Fig. 18.37).

2. Remove excess moisture from the template.

3. Prepare the acrylic or composite resin provisional material according to the manufacturer's directions.

   NOTE: Custom shading must be considered at this time, with matching of adjacent teeth.

4. Dispense the provisional material directly into the template, making sure not to trap air.

   NOTE: An automixing tip on the syringe or cartridge that allows delivery of the mixed provisional material directly into the template is useful. Begin loading the template from the bottom and keep the tip buried in material until loading is complete to avoid introducing air into the mix. (Fig. 18.38).

5. Place the template back into the patient's mouth or onto the lubricated model, aligning it precisely on the prepared tooth.

   NOTE: A notch cut in the template at a visually accessible location in the mouth will facilitate replacement of the template to the correct position (Fig. 18.39).

6. Check the initial set of the material in the patient's mouth; initial set occurs within 1 to 3 minutes.

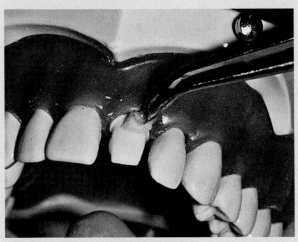

FIG. 18.37

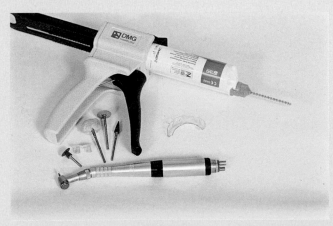

FIG. 18.36

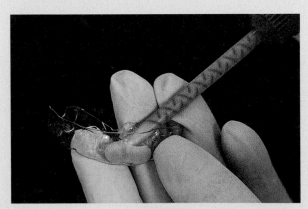

FIG. 18.38

NOTE: Check material in the patient's mouth, as heat and moisture will accelerate the set; use the material that has extruded from the location notch to test the set.

7. Remove the template with provisional material in place when a firm but still elastic consistency is reached.

NOTE: If the material is too soft, it will tear or stretch; if too hard, it may be difficult to remove it from undercut areas.

8. Remove the provisional material from the template and allow it to reach its final set.

NOTE: If acrylic materials are used, you must "pump" the provisional off and on the preparation when it reaches the doughy stage to avoid locking the material on the tooth or interproximal undercuts. Remove it from the mouth when it starts to get firm and warm.

If bis-acrylic composite resin materials are used, you should allow the material to reach its final set outside the mouth.

9. Trim excess material with acrylic burs and disks.

NOTE: If bis-acrylic composite material is used, you will first have to remove the greasy air-inhibited layer of unset resin with alcohol or it will tend to clog your disks and burs.

10. Reinsert the provisional and check margins, occlusion and contacts, adjusting as necessary.

NOTE: For acrylic: If slight air voids are present, they may be repaired with freshly mixed material (Figs. 18.40 and 18.41). For composite resin: fill voids or repair margins or contacts with flowable composite.

11. Finish polishing with flour of pumice or whiting polishing compound on a rag wheel.

12. Cement with an appropriate luting agent, and remove excess.

NOTE: The custom provisional may be completely fabricated on a stone model and then tried into the mouth and adjusted as necessary (indirect technique).

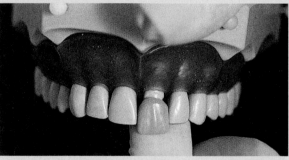

FIG. 18.40

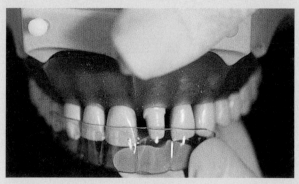

FIG. 18.39

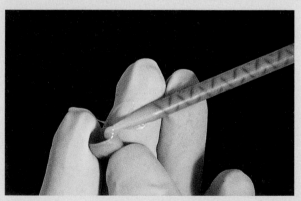

FIG. 18.41

Procedure 18.4 Intracoronal Cement Provisional Restoration

See Evolve site for Competency Sheet.

Consider the following with this procedure: safety glasses are recommended for the patient, PPE is required for the operator, ensure appropriate safety protocols are followed, and check your local state guidelines before performing this procedure.

EQUIPMENT/SUPPLIES (FIG. 18.42)

- Mouth mirror and explorer
- Isolation materials
- Matrix band and wedges
- Matrix retainer
- Cotton pliers
- Burnisher
- Temporary cement (powder/liquid)
- Paper mixing pad
- Cement spatula
- Plastic instrument
- Condenser
- Occlusal carver
- Interproximal carver
- Articulating paper
- Dental floss

PROCEDURE STEPS

1. Isolate the tooth, and note size and class of the cavity.

NOTE: This will determine the amount of cement necessary and the size of the matrix for placement.

2. Place the matrix and wedge.

NOTE: Be sure to obtain contact with adjacent teeth; insert the wedges firmly to create some separation of the teeth and use a burnisher to press the band to the adjacent tooth at the contact area.

3. Prepare a mix of the temporary cement to a putty-like consistency.

NOTE: The mix should be lightly coated in powder and should not stick to your gloved fingers (Fig. 18.43).

4. Roll the mix into a small ball, and place a portion into a proximal area.

NOTE: Begin by filling the proximal areas, then across the pulpal floor (Fig. 18.44).

5. Use the condenser to condense into the preparation, while packing the cement firmly to avoid trapping of air.

NOTE: Tap the end of the condenser into the remaining loose powder to prevent it from sticking to the cement.

6. Place and pack cement into the rest of the cavity with the condenser.

7. Do not overfill; pack cement only slightly higher than the cavosurface margin of the preparation.

8. Using the blade of the plastic instrument, wipe material toward the margin to ensure a good seal.

NOTE: Always wipe toward the margins; wiping away from the margins will pull material away from this important area (Fig. 18.45).

9. Remove excess material around the matrix in proximal areas and at occlusal margins.

NOTE: Remove excess carefully, as the material has not set. The material must be set enough so it is not pulled from the preparation margins.

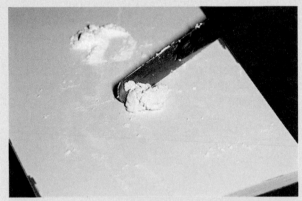

FIG. 18.43

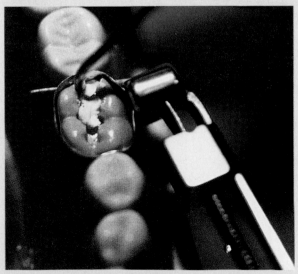

FIG. 18.44

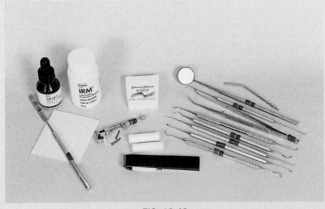

FIG. 18.42

Procedure 18.4 Intracoronal Cement Provisional Restoration—cont'd

10. Remove wedges, retainer, and matrix.

    NOTE: Be careful not to pull material away with the band.

11. Seal any open proximal margins by wiping still pliable cement toward them.

12. Remove proximal and gingival excess with an interproximal carver, and then from the marginal ridge.

    NOTE: The marginal ridge should be at the same height as that of the adjacent tooth.

13. Create embrasure.

14. Remove excess from the occlusal surface and carve the anatomic form with an occlusal carver.

    NOTE: The occlusal anatomy should approximate the original tooth form; it is not necessary to carve detailed anatomy (Fig. 18.46).

15. Carve from tooth to filling material, keeping half the instrument on the tooth and half on the filling.

    NOTE: This prevents breaking the material from the margins or ditching the margins of the material.

    NOTE: if you wish to accelerate the set of the material, pat a cotton pellet saturated in hot water on the surface of the material.

16. Check the occlusion with articulating paper, and adjust as necessary.

17. Check contacts with dental floss.

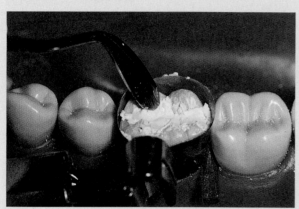

FIG. 18.45

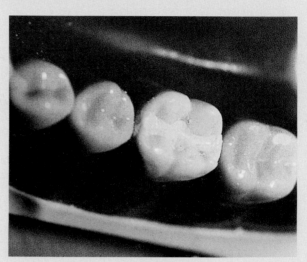

FIG. 18.46

Get Ready for Exams!

Review Questions

Select the one correct response for each of the following multiple-choice questions.

1. Intracoronal provisional Class II restorations must
   a. Contact adjacent teeth and be crimped with crimping pliers to fit snugly
   b. Contact adjacent teeth, be crimped with crimping pliers to fit snugly, and be sealed at the margins
   c. Contact adjacent teeth and be sealed at the margins
   d. Contact adjacent teeth, be crimped with crimping pliers to fit snugly, be sealed at the margins, and be made of metal for strength on posterior teeth

2. Polycarbonate crowns are used *primarily*
   a. On molars
   b. On anterior teeth and premolars
   c. For multiunit bridges
   d. For inlays

3. Which *one* of the following statements is most complete and correct? If the provisional restoration does not fit the tooth properly,
   a. Food impaction may occur and periodontal irritation may occur
   b. Periodontal irritation may occur and tooth migration may occur
   c. Food impaction may occur, periodontal irritation may occur, and hypersensitivity of the prepared tooth may occur
   d. Food impaction may occur, periodontal irritation may occur, hypersensitivity of the prepared tooth may occur, and tooth migration may occur

4. Important physical properties of provisional materials used for posterior teeth include the following
   a. Strength
   b. Tissue compatibility
   c. Ease of handling
   d. All of the above

5. Appropriate choices for extracoronal provisional restorations include
   a. Stainless steel crowns
   b. Acrylic and/or composite customized provisionals
   c. A and B
   d. None of the above

6. You will need to obtain a pre-preparation template of the tooth before fabricating
   a. Intracoronal provisional restorations
   b. Aluminum crown provisionals
   c. Polycarbonate crown provisionals
   d. Custom provisional restorations

7. The first step in fitting a stainless steel crown is
   a. Determining occlusal/incisal-to-gingival dimensions
   b. Determining mesial/distal dimensions
   c. Determining the contour of the finish line
   d. Determining occlusal height

8. Which of the following materials is NOT used to customize the internal fit of a preformed crown,
   a. Self-cured composite resin provisional material
   b. Acrylic provisional material
   c. Dual-cured composite resin provisional material
   d. Zinc phosphate cement

9. Provisional *custom* crowns placed on prepared teeth may be constructed of
   a. Celluloid
   b. Acrylic
   c. Stainless steel
   d. Polycarbonate

10. With intracoronal provisional restorations, place the cement and
    a. wipe the cement toward the margin
    b. wipe the cement away from the margin
    c. wipe the cement toward the matrix band
    d. allow the cement to harden before sealing the margins

11. Criteria for an intracoronal cement provisional restoration include all of the following *except*
    a. Marginal ridges at the same height as adjacent teeth
    b. Sufficient contact with adjacent teeth
    c. Detailed occlusal anatomy
    d. Reproduction of the gingival embrasure

12. Which *one* of the following statements regarding cementation of custom provisional crowns is true?
    a. The crown should be completely filled with cement to assure a good seal of the crown margins after seating it
    b. After cementation some excess cement can be left in the gingival sulcus to help with the retraction process for a separate impression appointment if bleeding has been a problem
    c. Placing a thin coat of lubricant around the cervical portion of the crown will make cleaning up the provisional crown easier after cementation
    d. A thick mix of the cement is preferred for luting for added strength

For answers to Review Questions, see the Appendix.

Case-Based Discussion Topics

1. How would each of the following situations be best handled?
   a. *A patient has a badly fractured central incisor. The preparation is close to the pulp. Which provisional material and technique would be most appropriate?*
   b. *A custom composite provisional crown is deficient at the gingival margin of the facial surface. How would you correct this problem?*
   c. *Your patient is concerned about the color match and smoothness of provisional crowns. Which provisional material and technique would be most appropriate?*
   d. *A patient is scheduled for a three-unit posterior bridge preparation. The patient has a limited opening because of temporomandibular joint pain. Which provisional material and technique would be most appropriate?*

BIBLIOGRAPHY

3M ESPE: Prefabricated Crowns – User Guide. Available at multimedia.3m.com/mws/media/68406O/prefabricated-crowns-user-guide.

Anglia L: Provisional restorations and patient satisfaction. *Gen Dent*, 46:197–199, 1998.

Berry T, Troendle K: Provisional restorations: Guidelines for proper selection, placement. *Dental Teamwork*, November/December:25–29, 1995. Available at: https://uthscsa.influuent.utsystem.edu/en/publications/provisional-restorations-guidelines-for-proper-selection-placemen

Berry T, Troendle K: Provisional restorations: Guidelines for custom fit, oral hygiene care. *Dental Teamwork*, January/February:23–27, 1996. Available at: https://uthscsa.influuent.utsystem.edu/en/publications/provisional-restorations-guidelines-for-a-custom-fit-oral-hygiene

Bird DL, Robinson DS (editors): *Provisional coverage. Modern Dental Assisting* , (ed 12), St. Louis, 2018, Elsevier.

Brinker SP: A modern guide to temporization materials and techniques. *Inside Dental Assisting*, 8(4), July/August 2012. Available at: https://www.aegisdentalnetwork.com/ida/2012/08/modern-guide-to-temporization-materials-and-techniques.

Comisi JC: Provisional materials: advances lead to extensive options for clinicians. *Compendium of Dental Education in Dentistry*, 36(1), January 2015. Available at https://www.aegisdentalnetwork.com/cced/2015/01/provisional-materials-advances-lead-to-extensive-options-for-clinicians.

Gegauff AG, Holloway JA: In Rosenstiel SF, Land MF, Fujimoto J, editors: *Interim Fixed Restorations in Contemporary Fixed Prosthodontics*, (ed 4). St Louis, 2006, Mosby.

Gottlieb M: Using an old technique with modern materials to fabricate esthetic temporary restorations. *J Am Dent Assoc*, 130:99–100, 1999.

Hester R: Fabricating high-quality provisional restorations for indirect inlays, onlays or crown preparations. *J Am Dent Assoc*, 130:1093–1094, 1997.

Kurtzman GM: Crown and bridge temporization part 1: provisional materials. *Inside Dentistry*, 14(8), September 2008. Available at https://www.aegisdentalnetwork.com/id/2008/09/crown-and-bridge-temporization-part-1-provisional-materials.

Kurtzman GM: Crown and bridge temporization part 2: provisional cements. *Inside Dentistry*, 14(9), October 2008. Available at https://www.aegisdentalnetwork.com/id/2008/10/crown-and-bridge-temporization-part-2-provisional-cements.

Leggat PA, Kedjarune U, Songkhla HY: Toxicity of methyl methacrylate in dentistry. *In Dent Journal*, 53(3):126–131, 2003.

Miller M (Ed.): *Provisional Crowns* (vol. 13). Houston, TX, 1999, REALITY Publishing, pp. 3–358 to 3–368

Schwedhelm ER: Direct technique for the fabrication of acrylic provisional restorations. *J Contemp Dent Pract*, 7:157–173, 2006.

Strassler HE: In-office provisional restorative materials for fixed prosthodontics part 1: polymeric resin provisional materials. *Inside Dentistry*, 5(4), April 2009. Available at https://www.aegisdentalnetwork.com/id/2009/04/in-office-provisional-restorative-materials-for-fixed-prosthodontics.

Strassler HE: In-office provisional restorative materials for fixed prosthodontics part 2: preformed crown forms. *Inside Dentistry*, 5(8), September 2009. Available at https://www.aegisdentalnetwork.com/id/2009/09/in-office-provisional-restorative-materials-for-fixed-prosthodontics-part-1-polymeric-resin-provisional-materials.

Strassler HE, Lowe RA: Chairside resin-based provisional restorative materials for fixed prosthodontics. *compendium of continuing education in dentistry*, November/December 2011. Available at: https://cced.cdeworld.com/courses/4552-Chairside_Resin-Based_Provisional_Restorative_Materials_for_Fixed_Prosthodontics.

Strassler HE, Morgan RJ: Provisional–temporary cements. *Inside Dental Assisting*, July/August 8(4), 2012. Available at:https://www.aegisdentalnetwork.com/ida/2012/08/provisional-temporary-cements.

Chapter Objectives

Upon completion of this chapter, the student should be able to:

1. Describe the uses of mouth guards.
2. List the materials for the fabrication of mouth guards.
3. Explain to a patient how to care for a mouth guard.
4. Fabricate a sports mouth guard.
5. Describe what obstructive sleep apnea is.
6. Describe the use of oral appliances to prevent snoring or obstructive sleep apnea.
7. Explain how preventive orthodontics prevent or eliminate the need for full-orthodontics.
8. Identify how interceptive orthodontics correct mal-alignments of the dentition.
9. Describe how thermoplastic orthodontic aligners work.
10. Identify how 3-D printing is being utilized in dentistry.

Key Terms

Mouth Guard an appliance made of hard or pliable material that protects teeth from trauma during sports activities or from grinding of the teeth

Custom-Fit made specifically to fit one individual

Obstructive Sleep Apnea a sleep disorder caused when the muscles that support the soft palate, uvula, and tongue relax and the airway narrows or closes

Space Maintainer a fixed or removable appliance used to prevent adjacent teeth from drifting into the space created when a tooth is lost

Thumb Sucking Device a fixed or removable appliance used to discourage tongue thrusting and thumb sucking

Palatal Expansion Device a fixed appliance used to expand the maxillary arch forcing the maxillary plates apart very slowly while the maxilla is still in development

Crossbite Corrector a fixed or removable appliance used to correct teeth in mal-alignment where the maxillary teeth are positioned lingual to the mandibular teeth

Orthodontic Tooth Aligners removable appliances that are designed to gently move teeth into predetermined positions

A number of oral appliances are available to the clinician to prevent damage to teeth, to keep teeth from shifting, to prevent sleep apnea and snoring, and to orthodontically move teeth. This chapter provides basic knowledge about these appliances. Most of these appliances can be fabricated in the dental office by trained staff or in a commercial dental laboratory. The dental auxiliary may be called on to fabricate these appliances or to instruct patients in their use and home care.

PREVENTIVE AND CORRECTIVE ORAL APPLIANCES

SPORTS MOUTH GUARDS

The purpose of sports guards is to protect the teeth and their supporting structures (gingival tissues and bone). The widespread use of **mouth guards** in school sports prevents thousands of injuries each year. According to the American Dental Association, more than 200,000 oral injuries are prevented on an annual basis by wearing mouthguards. The risk for oral/jaw injuries increases approximately 1.5 to 2 times when guards are not worn (Fig. 19.1, A). The National Youth Sports Foundation estimates that more than 5 million teeth will be knocked out in sporting activities this year alone. Dental injuries are the most common type of orofacial injury sustained during sports. The Centers for Disease Control and Prevention recommend and most states mandate that participants in school contact sports wear sports guards (also called *mouth protectors* or *mouth guards*) (Fig. 19.1, B).

Most professional and amateur adult athletes wear them too. The protective benefits of sports mouthguards have been well documented.

The three basic types of mouth guards for sports are:
- Stock guards
- Boil-and-bite guards
- Custom-fit guards

Stock Guards
(Fig. 19.2) Stock guard by Athletic Specialties

Stock guards can be purchased over the counter in sporting goods stores, in some retail stores or online. They usually cost less than $25 and come in sizes ranging from small, medium, and large. Along with being the least expensive, stock guards generally have the poorest fit, may be uncomfortable to wear, and provide the least amount of protection. In addition, they are not adapted to the patient's bite.

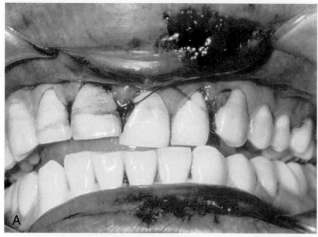

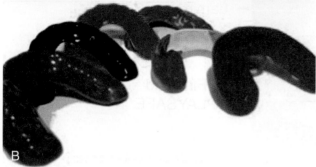

FIG. 19.1 Prevention of sports injuries. **A,** Injury to the lip and teeth that could be avoided with a sports guard. **B,** Multilayer sports guard. (Courtesy of Acacia Dental Group.)

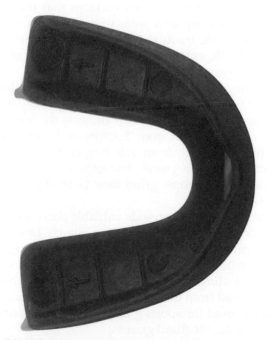

FIG. 19.2 Stock guard. (Courtesy of Athletic Specialties.)

Boil-and-Bite Guards
(Fig. 19.3) Boil and bite guard prior to and after fitting.

Similar to the stock guards, boil-and-bite guards can be found in sporting goods stores, retail stores and online costing less than $50. They are constructed of a horseshoe shaped, flexible thermoplastic material

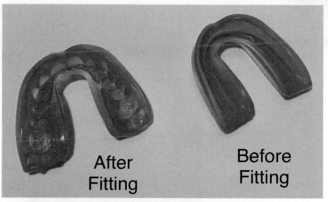

FIG. 19.3 Boil and bite guard prior to and after fitting.

that softens when heated. The material is softened in boiling water, placed in the mouth while still moldable, adapted to the teeth and arch by fingers, lips, and tongue, and then adapted to the bite by closing the teeth into the guard. Excess material is cut away with heavy-duty scissors. This type of guard is often difficult for inexperienced individuals to adapt properly and may have a poor fit interfering with breathing and speaking ability, but the fit is usually better than stock guards. Boil-and-bite guards can provide a false protection as they can become very thin when an athlete bites too far into them in a softened state.

Custom-Fit Guards
(Fig. 19.4) Custom-fit sports guards.

Professionally made guards are **custom-fit** to casts of the patient's mouth. Because of the added steps, materials, and time involved in their fabrication, custom guards may cost several times more than stock and boil-and-bite guards. Custom-fit guards can be made from a single layer of material or from pressure-laminated material in a commercial dental laboratory.

The single-layer guards can be fabricated in the dental office or a commercial laboratory. A sheet of thermoplastic material is heated in a vacuum-forming machine and vacuum adapted to the cast (Procedure 19.1). The material may be clear or a variety of colors (Fig. 19.1, B). A strap may be attached for sports such as football, where the athlete wears a helmet and wants to attach it to the facemask to make it readily accessible. Because the fit is excellent and the bite is comfortable, compliance with its use is much better than with the other types of guards.

Pressure-laminated sports guards fabricated in a commercial dental laboratory are highly recommended for contact sports such as hockey, basketball, and football. The thermoplastic material consists of two or three sheets that are heat-fused together. These guards are thicker than single-layer guards; provide more cushion, and durability.

Protection

Sports guards can absorb about 80% of the energy from a traumatic hit to the mouth. Sports guards

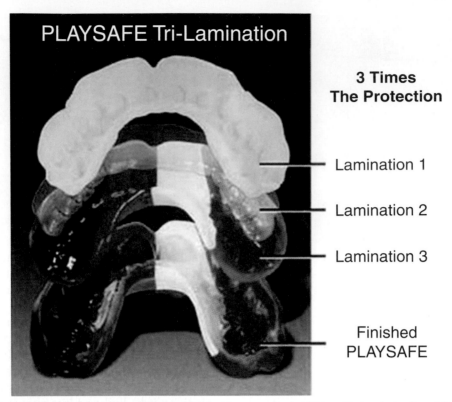

FIG. 19.4 Playsafe Tri-lamination custom-fit sportsguards. (Photo courtesy of Glidewell Laboratories Copyright © 2020.)

usually cover the upper teeth, gingiva, and bone. On occasion, they are made to cover both arches at the same time. They can protect the teeth and jaws from fracture by a direct blow or cushion the upper and lower teeth when an athlete's jaws are forced together by a blow to the lower jaw. Because these guards provide cushioning to the jaws during collision with another athlete or the ground, some concussions can be mitigated or prevented. The guard can prevent lacerations to lips for athletes with orthodontic braces or brackets and protect dental work such as bridges, anterior veneers, or crowns. Athletes should be directed to leave removable prostheses such as orthodontic retainers out when playing sports, because they could become dislodged and enter the throat.

Sports guards need a certain thickness and stiffness to maximize their protective qualities. The heavier the contact in the sport, the thicker the guard should be to provide maximal protection. For heavy-contact sports, where injuries are more likely, a thickness of about 5 mm is desirable. For less physical sports, 2 mm of thickness may suffice. Playsafe ™ was invented in 1982 and has become the leading custom fabricated sports mouthguard. Playsafe ™ mouthguards come in a variety of thicknesses depending on the age, dentition, and sports protection needed.

NIGHT GUARDS (BRUXISM MOUTH GUARDS)

Many patients who grind their teeth do so mostly at night while sleeping. They may not even be aware that they are grinding their teeth until the dental professional points out the wear evident on the teeth. Common signs of chronic bruxing include wear facets (flattened tooth surfaces that used to be convex), chipping and wear of incisal edges, stress cracks in teeth, fractured cusps, cracked teeth, mobility of teeth, enlarged masseters, and sore muscles of mastication.

Guards are recommended for patients who are bruxers (who grind their teeth). The guard does not stop the grinding habit, but it protects the teeth from wear, chipping, and even fracture of cusps. Guards to protect the teeth from grinding and clenching are also called *occlusal guards, bite splints,* or *night guards* (because many people grind their teeth at night when they are sleeping).

Dental offices can provide valuable preventive measures for their patients by offering guards. Dental auxiliaries can play an active role in recommending night guards, making impressions for their fabrication, and even fabricating them in the office laboratory. They can be fabricated from the same single-layer thermoplastic materials used for sports guards (soft guards) or from processed acrylic (hard guards).

Patients undergoing treatment for dysfunction of the temporomandibular joint (commonly called TMD) are often given devices (called TMJ splints) to wear that can serve three functions: (1) keeping the teeth separated, (2) taking stress off the joints, and (3) protecting the teeth. These splints can also be made from hard acrylic or soft thermoplastic material.

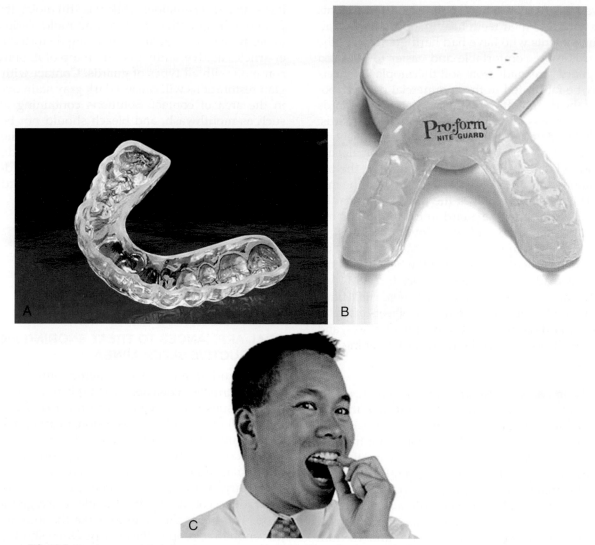

FIG. 19.5 Bruxism guard. **A,** Laboratory-processed hard acrylic occlusal guard. **B,** Soft guard made from thermoplastic material. **C,** Patient aligns the guard with the teeth and presses it in place. (**A,** Photo courtesy of Glidewell Laboratories Copyright © 2020. **B,** Courtesy Keystone Industries.)

Home Care Instructions for Soft Sports or Bruxism Guards

- Wash the guard with room temperature water and liquid soap on a toothbrush after each use.
- Do not soak a soft guard in a commercial denture cleaner or an alcohol-containing mouthwash, as these products will degrade the guard material over time.
- Allow the guard to air dry. Do not enclose it in an airtight container, because it will grow mold and bacteria. If storing it in a container, use one with perforations where air can circulate.
- Do not leave the guard in a closed automobile in the sun or expose it to hot water as this will cause warping.
- Do not chew on the guard when using it, as you may tear or distort it.
- Do not leave the guard where the family dog might reach it. They have been known to chew them up.
- Sports guards eventually wear out, so when it no longer fits well or has tears and holes in it, it is time to replace it.

Types of Materials

Three types of material are used in the making of night guards:

- *Hard:* Acrylic (methyl methacrylate resin and monomer)
- *Soft:* Thermoplastic sheets of poly(vinyl acetate)-polyethylene material
- *Hard and soft:* Laminates of hard and soft thermoplastic materials

Hard Acrylic Guard. Patients who grind their teeth heavily and frequently should have a hard acrylic guard, due to it being more durable than a soft guard. Hard acrylic guards are usually fabricated in the dental laboratory (Fig. 19.5).

They typically require more chair-time for adjustment, because the acrylic, like other resins, shrinks when it is cured. They also feel tight on the patient's teeth when first tried on.

Soft Guard. Soft guards are better suited for patients who do not grind their teeth heavily or regularly (daily). Some patients who have had hard guards find the soft guards more comfortable and easier to get used to. Soft guards are made from soft thermoplastic sheets and may be fabricated in the commercial dental laboratory or the dental office by the auxiliary. Soft guards require much less time to adjust than hard guards. Often chair-side adjustment can be made by heating the outside biting surface of the guard with an alcohol torch and, while it is still warm, placing it in the patient's mouth and having him or her bite into the materials. This process equalizes the bite. Care must be taken to avoid placing the guard in the mouth too hot and should be checked with the gloved hand first. A technique for using upper and lower casts mounted on a simple hinge articulator to adjust the bite at the time the guard is made is described in Procedure 19.1. Adjusting the bite on mounted casts will save chair-time. The poly(vinyl acetate)-polyethylene sheets used to make soft guards come in a variety of thicknesses, and the thinner sheets can also be used for whitening and fluoride trays.

Hard and Soft Laminate Guard. Patients who need the durability of a hard occlusal surface but like the feel of the soft material may prefer hard and soft laminate guards. Guards made from this material are hard on the biting surface and soft internally, allowing them to adapt readily to the teeth while being gentle on the soft tissues. The material comes in sheets that have a firm thermoplastic material laminated with a soft material. A sheet of the material is softened in a vacuum machine similar to the soft guard material and vacuum adapted to the cast.

Design of the Guard

Most night guards and TMD splints cover the maxillary teeth, but some dentists cover the mandibular teeth. Some guards or TMD treatment splints may only cover a few of the anterior teeth (e.g., NTI splints; NTI-Chairside Splints), but some experts contend that these may actually create a fulcrum that displaces the condyles from their ideal position in the joints. Some guards may cover both lingual and occlusal surfaces of the teeth and just lap over cusps of the posterior teeth and the incisal edges of the anterior teeth. Others cover all of the anterior and posterior teeth.

Maintenance

The auxiliary should instruct the patient in proper home care of the guard. First and foremost, the guard should be cleaned daily. When it is removed from the mouth, it should be rinsed thoroughly to remove saliva and then brushed with a toothbrush or denture brush and liquid soap. After the final rinsing, excess water should be shaken off and the guard stored in a rigid container that is left open so that it can air-dry. If it is sealed in a container while it is still moist, this may promote the growth of bacteria and mold. A rigid container prevents the guard from being distorted by other articles inadvertently placed on top of it. Staining is common with all types of guards. Contact with amalgam restorations will cause a dark gray stain over time in the area of contact. Solutions containing alcohol, such as mouthwash, and bleach should not be used, because they will degrade the material. Commercially available soaks for orthodontic retainers or dentures are useful to freshen the hard guards but can degrade the soft poly(vinyl acetate)-polyethylene guards over time.

 Caution

Patients should be advised not to immerse their sport guards or night guards in hot water, because it can cause distortion of the guard.

ORAL APPLIANCES TO TREAT SNORING AND OBSTRUCTIVE SLEEP APNEA

While snoring may be considered only an annoyance, **obstructive sleep apnea (OSA)** can lead to serious health issues if not treated. The most serious potential problems include hypertension, heart attack, heart failure, and stroke. Snoring and OSA are often caused by relaxation of the muscles that support the soft palate, uvula, and tongue, causing a narrowing or closing of the airway. Breathing becomes inadequate or stops for a few seconds, causing the blood oxygen level to drop. This alerts the brain to wake the individual up just enough to reopen the airway. Often short gasping breaths are taken until the oxygen level is restored. Someone with a serious problem may wake up 10 to 20 times an hour. They wake up in the morning feeling exhausted or, surprisingly, they may not notice the lack of sleep.

Risk Factors for OSA

Risk factors for OSA include a large neck, obesity, chronic nasal congestion, high blood pressure, diabetes, smoking, alcohol use, and a narrow airway. Men are twice as likely to have OSA as women. It is more common in people who are middle aged or older. To arrive at the proper diagnosis and plan of treatment, those afflicted may be sent to a sleep specialist at a sleep center for evaluation where sleep patterns may be monitored overnight.

Treatment of OSA

Treatment for mild OSA may include weight loss, exercise, reduced alcohol intake, smoking cessation, sleeping on one side, and use of nasal decongestants. Treatment for more severe OSA may involve the use of continuous positive airway pressure (CPAP). With CPAP a mask is worn on the face while sleeping and a device attached to it delivers a continuous positive flow of air to keep the airway open (Fig. 19.6).

Many people find the CPAP mask uncomfortable and have trouble adjusting to it. A more invasive approach to OSA is surgery to reduce the soft palate and uvula (uvulopalatopharyngoplasty) to open the airway. Many patients are willing to try oral appliances as a conservative alternative treatment.

Function of Appliances

Most appliances do one of three things: (1) lift the soft palate, (2) hold the tongue in a more forward position, or (3) reposition the mandible forward to bring the tongue away from the airway. There are at least 80 different designs for oral appliances. Oral appliances do not work for everyone and have the most success in those with mild to moderate OSA (Fig. 19.7).

PREVENTIVE ORTHODONTICS

Preventive orthodontics are intended to prevent or eliminate mal-positions and irregularities in the developing dentition and orofacial region. Preventive orthodontics eliminate the need for full orthodontics due

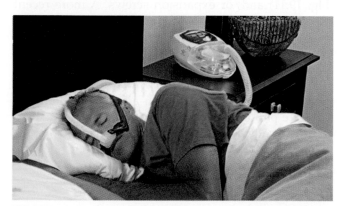

FIG. 19.6 Obstructive sleep apnea treatment device continuous positive airway pressure (CPAP) device for obstructive sleep apnea. (Courtesy of CPAP Global.)

to their application occurring while the dentition and face are still developing.

SPACE MAINTAINERS

Space maintainers are used most frequently in pediatric dentistry when a tooth is lost too soon. They prevent adjacent teeth from drifting and closing the space created by the lost tooth. The space is needed to allow the permanent tooth to erupt properly. Sometimes space maintainers are used in adults to hold the space from a lost tooth until an implant, bridge, or removable partial denture can be placed.

Types of Space Maintainers

Space maintainers can be removable or fixed. A removable space maintainer can be in the form of a stayplate or a retainer with a denture tooth or acrylic block attached. Fixed space maintainers are cemented in place and may have a wire loop attached to a stainless steel crown or an orthodontic band and extend from the crowned or banded tooth to contact the tooth on the opposite side of the space.

INTERCEPTIVE ORTHODONTICS

Interceptive orthodontics (corrective appliances) corrects problems in the orofacial region as they develop in an attempt to prevent the need for full orthodontics or, at a minimum, decrease the amount of time orthodontics are required. The appliance intervention is necessary to prevent a malocclusion.

THUMB SUCKING APPLIANCE

Thumb sucking and tongue thrusting are two main oral habits interceptive orthodontics or corrective appliances are utilized to treat. The **thumb sucking device** consists of metal protrusions, which resemble spikes or a rake. When the patient places the tongue or the thumb on the device, discomfort will occur. This discomfort is anticipated to break the tongue thrusting or thumb sucking habit (Fig. 19.8).

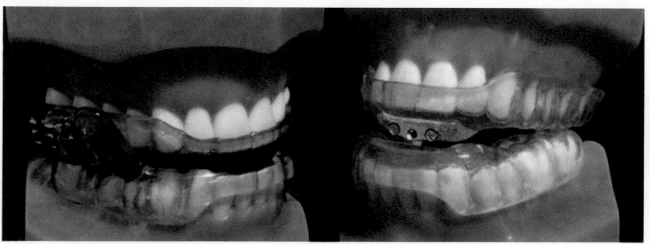

FIG. 19.7 Oral appliance for obstructive sleep apnea positions the lower jaw forward to prevent the tongue and soft tissues of the throat from obstructing the airway. (Courtesy of Dental Sleep Apnea Clinic.)

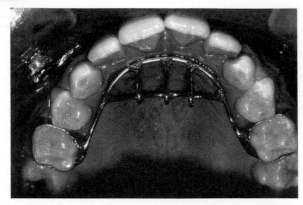

FIG. 19.8 Thumb sucking device. (Courtesy of Dr. Frank Hodges.)

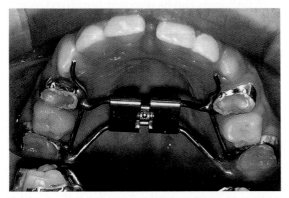

FIG. 19.9 Palatal expansion appliance. (Courtesy of Dr. Frank Hodges.)

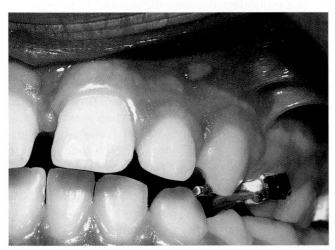

FIG. 19.10 Crossbite correcting device. (Courtesy of Dr. Frank Hodges.)

PALATAL EXPANSION APPLIANCES

Palatal expansion devices are utilized to expand the maxillary arch when it is too narrow and re-establish the balance between the width of the maxillary and mandibular jaws. Without expansion an abnormal relationship between dental arches would exist. The problems associated with a narrow palate could include the following: airway obstruction due to a narrow nasal cavity and crowding of the maxillary teeth (Fig. 19.9).

CROSSBITE CORRECTOR

A **crossbite corrector** corrects the area where the maxillary teeth are positioned lingual to the mandibular teeth. The crossbite is corrected by the use of a fixed or removable device. The device can be a band with an extension that guides the tooth into the appropriate place (Fig. 19.10).

ORTHODONTIC TOOTH ALIGNERS

Many types of minor tooth movement can be achieved with removable appliances that direct forces on the teeth to move them into proper alignment. Traditional removable appliances usually consist of an acrylic base with embedded stainless steel wires (see "Wrought Metal Alloys" in Chapter 11) bent into springs or bows (Fig. 19.11) and/or expansion screws. A more recent approach uses a series of clear thermoplastic aligners to gradually move the teeth into the desired position. Because these **orthodontic tooth aligners** are made from a clear thermoplastic material, their developer cleverly named the process *Invisalign* (Align Technology, Inc.). They are used more with adults than children. They are popular because they are more esthetic than conventional braces and brackets. However, complex malocclusions will require conventional orthodontic treatment with brackets and braces.

How Aligners Are Made

Design software creates a three-dimensional model from a digital scan of the teeth or a cast of the teeth. Next, technicians digitally move the individual teeth into the final desired position, using design software. Then, the software is used to simulate moving the teeth in gradual stages, and aligners (made of polyurethane) are fabricated for each stage of movement (Fig. 19.12).

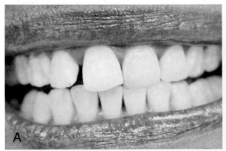
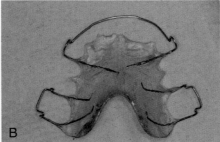
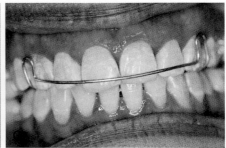

FIG. 19.11 Removable tooth movement appliance (Hawley appliance). **A,** Protruding right maxillary central incisor **B,** Hawley appliance with a labial bow that will be activated by tightening the loops. The pressure created on the incisor will move it lingually. The bow is reactivated as the tooth moves. **C,** Maxillary incisor has been repositioned with the Hawley appliance, and the appliance will now serve as a retainer. (Courtesy of Dr. Scott Rooker, Los Altos, CA.)

Treatment

The patient wears the aligners approximately 20 hours a day. Wearing the aligners for a shorter period of time each day will prolong the treatment. The aligners are removed only to eat, drink, or clean the teeth. Small nobs made of composite material (called *buttons* see Chapter 6) are bonded to the teeth (see Chapter 5) to help the aligners grip well and to facilitate tooth movement (Fig. 19.13).

Elastic may be needed to help rotate teeth or to intrude or extrude them.

A new aligner in the series is used every 2 to 4 weeks. This is repeated until the malocclusion or misalignment is corrected. The last and final step is to make a retainer that will keep the teeth from shifting. It is usually made from the same clear material as the aligners.

3-D Printing

The use of 3-D Printing is becoming increasingly popular in the field of dentistry. A common application of 3-D Printing is with the use of a desktop 3-D printer to fabricate (print) clear orthodontic aligners. The aligners can be utilized for the movement of teeth similar to the aligners shown in (see Fig. 19.12) or as a retainer to maintain the position of the dentition after orthodontic treatment has been concluded. The printer utilizes a resin type material to print the appliances.

3-D Printing is not new to the medical field; however, its use in dentistry is just now becoming more prevalent. It should be noted that 3-D Printing is not limited to orthodontic applications. Other applications for 3-D Printing include the following: prosthodontics, oral surgery, periodontics, and general dentistry.

SUMMARY

Sports guards prevent many oral injuries each year. The use of mouth guards not only helps those patients with TMJ disorders, but is effective in the prevention of excessive tooth wear and fracture. Space maintainers prevent loss of space by drifting of adjacent teeth when teeth are lost prematurely. Treatment of sleep apnea is a growing segment of the modern dental practice. More adults are requesting orthodontic treatment to correct misaligned teeth and they demand "invisible" braces when possible. So, dental auxiliary must be able to answer questions about the procedures and materials used. They must also be able to provide home care instructions for the appliances.

INSTRUCTIONAL VIDEOS

See the Evolve Resources site for a variety of educational videos that reinforce the material covered in this chapter.

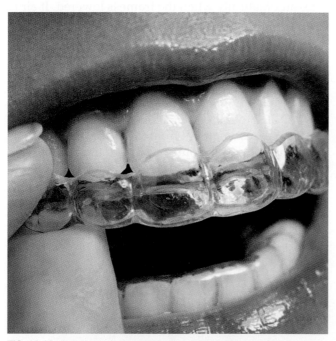

FIG. 19.12 Removable clear tooth aligner Invisalign. (Courtesy of Align Technology, San Jose, CA.)

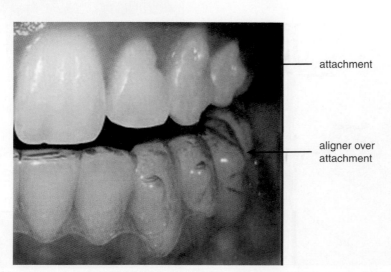

attachment

aligner over attachment

FIG. 19.13 Aligner buttons bonded to teeth. Spaces are created in an aligner over the facial surfaces of selected teeth. Composite resin is packed into these spaces. The teeth are prepared for bonding of the composite buttons. The aligner is positioned over the teeth and the composite buttons are bonded to the teeth. These buttons aid in tooth movement.

Procedure 19.1   Fabrication of a Sports Mouth Guard (Protector)

See Evolve site for Competency Sheet.

Consider the following with this procedure: safety glasses are recommended for the patient, PPE is required for the operator, ensure appropriate safety protocols are followed, and check your local state guidelines before performing this procedure.

EQUIPMENT/SUPPLIES (FIG. 19.14)

- Trimmed casts (study models)
- Mouth guard material: One sheet 6 × 6 inches, 0.15 inch thick
- Vacuum former unit
- Heavy-duty scissors
- Straight-line hinge articulator
- Petroleum jelly
- Alcohol torch
- Disinfectant spray and zippered plastic bag

PROCEDURE STEPS

1. Inspect casts (study models) and remove any blebs of dental stone on the teeth.

   NOTE: These blebs (bumps) of stone represent trapped air bubbles in the impression. Painting alginate on the occlusal surfaces of the teeth and in the palate just before inserting the loaded tray will help minimize trapped air in the impression.

2. Trim casts in a horseshoe shape so that the central portion representing the tongue and palate areas is mostly removed.

   NOTE: To save time trimming the casts, these areas can be blocked out with a piece of wet, crumpled paper towel once the impressions are poured.

3. Insert a sheet of mouth guard material in the frame of the vacuum former and clamp it in place. Lift the clamping frame up to a heating element and turn on the heat to soften the material.

NOTE: The guard material comes in sheets in a variety of colors that are appealing to young athletes, or they can be clear.

4. Place the maxillary cast on the platform and center it under the sheet of guard material.

5. Lower the frame when the sheet of material has softened and sags an inch or more. Turn on the vacuum when the molten guard material covers the cast. Leave the vacuum on for at least 30 seconds to allow the molten material to adapt to the cast (Fig. 19.15).

   NOTE: With some machines, the vacuum activates automatically when the frame is lowered. If air is trapped between the cast and the guard material, use a wet paper towel to quickly press the guard material against the cast while the vacuum is still on, to force the air out and closely adapt it to the cast.

6. Remove the guard material and the cast from the clamping frame and allow it to cool.

   NOTE: Hold it under cold water to cool it rapidly.

7. Trim excess material from the cast. Carefully remove the cast from the guard material.

   NOTE: Removing excess guard material at the sides of the cast will help free the cast more easily.

8. Place the maxillary and mandibular casts together in their proper bite relationship (centric occlusion) and mount them on the articulator, using fast-set plaster (Fig. 19.16).

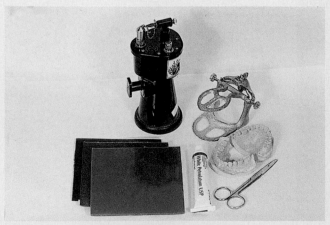

FIG. 19.14

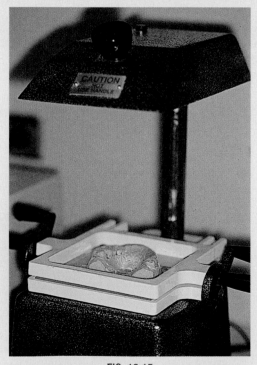

FIG. 19.15

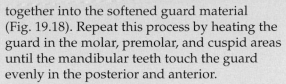

Procedure 19.1 Fabrication of a Sports Mouth Guard (Protector)—cont'd

NOTE: For patients whose bite relationship is not clear, a separate bite registration should be taken when the alginate impressions are made.

9. Trim excess guard material away, using heavy-duty scissors, until the guard extends about 3⁄8 inch onto the palatal and facial gingiva of the cast.

NOTE: The guard is extended over the gingiva to give added protection, but is kept short of the depth of the vestibule so that it will not irritate the tissues when the athlete bites on the guard.

10. Place the guard on the maxillary cast and check to see that the guard material is not too thick in the molar area (Fig. 19.17). The mandibular cast should close evenly onto the guard and not prop the bite open.

11. Correct the bite. If the guard hits the mandibular molars first, apply a thin coat of petroleum jelly to the occlusal surfaces of the mandibular cast, soften the guard in both right and left molar areas with an alcohol torch, and close the casts together into the softened guard material (Fig. 19.18). Repeat this process by heating the guard in the molar, premolar, and cuspid areas until the mandibular teeth touch the guard evenly in the posterior and anterior.

NOTE: A guard corrected in this manner will allow the athlete to close comfortably and not be in a strained jaw position.

12. Round out, using an acrylic bur in the laboratory handpiece, the indentations in the guard caused by the mandibular cast. Next, create smooth borders and an occlusal surface by flaming with an alcohol torch to soften the material, then lightly rubbing the surface of the guard with a gloved finger coated with petroleum jelly.

NOTE: Be careful not to overheat the guard. Just soften the surface by lightly flaming it. If it is too hot, it could cause a burn to the finger. Overheating the guard can also cause it to burn.

13. A commercially purchased strap can be added to the anterior part of the guard for those sports in which a face guard is used. The strap allows the athlete to remove the guard from the mouth while not in activity and have it attached to the face guard and ready to reinsert when needed. While still on the cast, heat the guard on the facial surface and heat the back surface of the strap attachment base with an alcohol torch and press the two soft surfaces together. Allow it to cool. Insert the face guard strap into the slot on the strap attachment base (Figs. 19.19 and 19.20)

14. Wash the guard with liquid soap and water. Rinse thoroughly and spray it with a disinfectant. Store it until the delivery appointment in a zippered plastic bag marked with the patient's name.

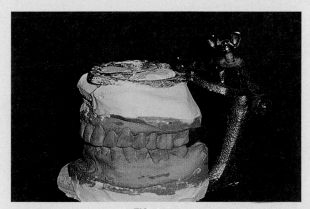

FIG. 19.16

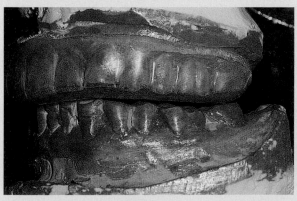

FIG. 19.17

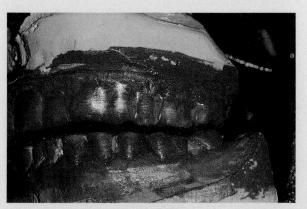

FIG. 19.18

Continued

Procedure 19.1   Fabrication of a Sports Mouth Guard (Protector)—cont'd

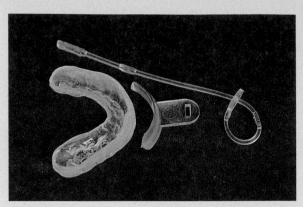

FIG. 19.19

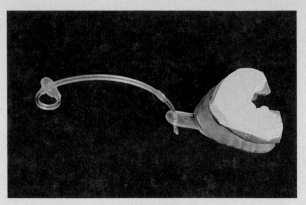

FIG. 19.20

Get Ready for Exams!

Review Questions

Select the one correct response for each of the following multiple-choice questions.

1. When a soft mouth guard is prescribed by the dentist, fabrication can be done by:
   a. The dental assistant
   b. The dental hygienist
   c. The laboratory technician
   d. All of the above

2. This appliance is utilized to correct a mal-occusion where the maxillary teeth are positioned lingual to the mandibular teeth:
   a. Thumb sucking device
   b. Palatal Expander
   c. Crossbite corrector
   d. Space maintainer

3. The main purpose of a sports mouth guard is:
   a. To help protect the teeth and supporting structures during contact sports
   b. To keep the airway open
   c. To keep the tongue out of the way
   d. To keep teeth in alignment after orthodontic treatment

4. Custom-made mouth guards and splints may be made of:
   a. A plastic material softened by boiling
   b. Thermoplastic resilient plastic or hard processed acrylic resin
   c. Composite resin
   d. Tray acrylic

5. A palatal expander is a fixed appliance used to expand the:
   a. Mandibular arch
   b. Maxillary arch
   c. Both maxillary and mandibular arches
   d. Neither maxillary nor mandibular arches

6. Obstructive sleep apnea can lead to:
   a. Chronic fatigue
   b. High blood pressure
   c. Heart problems
   d. All of the above

7. Oral appliances used for obstructive sleep apnea work by:
   a. Holding the tongue forward
   b. Holding the mandible forward
   c. Supporting the tissue of the soft palate
   d. Any one or more of the above

8. The treatment objectives of oral appliances for sleep apnea include all of the following *except* one. Which one?
   a. Lift the soft palate
   b. Hold the tongue in a more forward position
   c. Open the nasal passages
   d. Reposition the mandible forward to bring the tongue away from the airway

9. Which one of the following statements about space maintainers is *true*?
   a. They are always cemented into place.
   b. They are used only when primary teeth are lost.
   c. They prevent teeth adjacent to the space from drifting into the space.
   d. Denture teeth are never used in conjunction with space maintainers.

10. With Invisalign orthodontic treatment the removable aligners are changed about every:
    a. 2 to 4 weeks
    b. 5 to 8 weeks
    c. 9 to 12 weeks
    d. 13 to 15 weeks

Get Ready for Exams!—cont'd

11. Which one of the following statements about removable orthodontic aligners is *true?*
    a. All malocclusions can be treated with aligners.
    b. Aligners are made for each stage of tooth movement simulated by design software.
    c. Aligners are made from processed acrylic resin.
    d. Treatment with aligners takes much longer than conventional treatment because a series of aligners must be used.

12. Boil and Bite sports guards may appear to be protective but may not be. This is due to the material becoming very thin when athletes bite into them in a softened state.
    a. The first statement is true the second is false
    b. The first statement is false the second is true
    c. The first and second statement are true
    d. The first and second statement are false

For answers to Review Questions, see the Appendix.

Case-Based Discussion Topics

1. Upon examination, a 37-year-old truck driver is found to have chipped and worn incisal edges on the anterior teeth and flattened occlusal surfaces on the first and second molars. He has almost worn through the enamel. His teeth are not mobile, his periodontal health is good, and he has no caries. He suspects he clenches and grinds when he is driving in heavy traffic. His wife tells him he grinds his teeth in his sleep.

Is he a candidate for an occlusal guard? If so, what type of guard material would best be suited for his condition? Should he wear the guard at night, during the day, or both? Why?

2. A sixteen-year-old boy will be playing left tackle for his high school football team. He is 6 feet 2 inches, weighs 190 pounds, and is very strong.

Should he wear a sports guard? If so, is a single-layer guard appropriate? What types of injuries can a sports guard prevent?

BIBLIOGRAPHY

Academy for Sports Dentistry: Frequently asked questions. Available at: http://www.academyforsportsdentistry.org/faq-s.

American Academy of Dental Sleep Medicine: Oral appliances. Available at: http://www.aadsm.org/obstructive_sleep_apnea.php.

American Dental Association (ADA) Council on Access: Prevention and Interprofessional Relations; ADA Council on Scientific Affairs: Statement on Athletic Mouthguards 2009. Available at: http://www.ada.org/~/media/ADA/Science%20and%20Research/Files/SCI_Statement%20on%20Athletic%20Mouthguards_2016Oct24.pdf?la=en.

Bird DL, Robinson DS: Orthodontics. In *Modern Dental Assisting* (ed 12). Philadelphia, 2018, Elsevier/Saunders.

Darby ML, Walsh MM: Orthodontic care. In *Dental Hygiene: Theory and Practice*, St. Louis, 2015, Saunders/Elsevier.

Powers JM, Wataha JC: Mouth protectors. In *Dental Materials Properties and Manipulation*, St. Louis, 2013, Mosby.

Robinson DS, Bird DL: Orthodontics. In *Essentials of Dental Assisting*, St. Louis, 2017, Elsevier.

University of Washington: Classification of space maintainers. In: *Atlas of Pediatric Dentistry [web-based textbook]*. Atlas maintained by the Department of Pediatric Dentistry, University of Washington, Seattle, Washington. Available at: http://depts.washington.edu/peddent/AtlasDemo/space009.html.

Answers to Review Questions

Chapter 2
1. c
2. d
3. b
4. c
5. d
6. b
7. c
8. b
9. b
10. a
11. d
12. c
13. c
14. c
15. d
16. c
17. d

Chapter 3
1. a
2. b
3. c
4. c
5. d
6. b
7. a
8. b
9. c
10. b

Chapter 4
1. d
2. d
3. d
4. c
5. c
6. d
7. c

Chapter 5
1. d
2. a
3. d
4. c
5. b
6. a
7. b
8. e
9. a
10. b

11. c
12. a
13. b
14. c
15. b

Chapter 6
1. a
2. d
3. d
4. a
5. c
6. c
7. b
8. c
9. d
10. b
11. d
12. d
13. c
14. b
15. a
16. d
17. b
18. a
19. d
20. c
21. d
22. d
23. c

Chapter 7
1. b
2. b
3. c
4. c
5. d
6. c
7. b
8. a
9. c
10. b
11. d
12. b
13. b
14. a
15. d
16. d
17. a
18. a
19. a

20. c
21. a
22. c
23. c
24. b
25. a

Chapter 8
1. c
2. b
3. b
4. d
5. b
6. b
7. b
8. d
9. b
10. d

Chapter 9
1. a
2. c
3. a
4. a
5. d
6. d
7. d
8. b
9. d
10. c
11. b
12. d
13. c
14. b
15. c
16. c
17. b
18. a
19. d
20. b
21. c
22. c

Chapter 10
1. d
2. c
3. c
4. d
5. c
6. c
7. a

8. d
9. d
10. c
11. a
12. b
13. d
14. a
15. c
16. d
17. a
18. a

Chapter 11
1. b
2. a
3. a
4. a
5. d
6. b
7. a
8. d
9. c
10. c
11. d
12. a
13. d
14. d
15. d
16. a

Chapter 12
1. d
2. b
3. b
4. c
5. e
6. b
7. d
8. b
9. d
10. a
11. a
12. d
13. c
14. a
15. d
16. a
17. b
18. c
19. b

Chapter 13
1. d
2. c
3. d
4. d
5. b
6. c
7. c
8. b
9. a
10. a
11. b

Chapter 14
1. b
2. b
3. d
4. c
5. b
6. c
7. a
8. d
9. d
10. d
11. a
12. d
13. d
14. b
15. a
16. d
17. a
18. a

Chapter 15
1. b
2. a
3. c
4. d
5. c
6. d
7. d
8. a
9. b
10. a
11. c
12. d
13. b
14. c
15. a
16. b
17. b
18. d
19. d
20. b
21. b
22. a
23. d
24. a
25. d
26. c
27. b

Chapter 16
1. b
2. c
3. c
4. c
5. a
6. c
7. a
8. a
9. d
10. a
11. e
12. b
13. c
14. d
15. a
16. d
17. a

Chapter 17
1. c
2. a
3. d
4. a
5. b
6. d
7. c
8. a
9. d
10. d
11. d
12. c
13. d
14. d
15. c
16. c
17. d

18. a
19. d
20. b
21. d
22. a
23. b

Chapter 18
1. c
2. b
3. d
4. d
5. c
6. d
7. b
8. d
9. b
10. a
11. c
12. c

Chapter 19
1. d
2. c
3. a
4. b
5. b
6. d
7. d
8. c
9. c
10. a
11. b
12. c

Glossary

Abrasive: A material that comprises particles of sufficient hardness and sharpness to cut or scratch a softer material when drawn across its surface.

Addition Polymerization: common form of polymerization for dental materials; monomer molecules are added one to another sequentially as the reactive group on one molecule initiates bonding with an adjacent monomer molecule and frees another reactive group (free radical) to repeat the process

Addition silicone: A silicone rubber impression that also sets by linking of molecules in long chains but produces no by-product. The most commonly used addition silicones are the polyvinyl siloxanes.

Adhesion: The act of sticking two things together. In dentistry, it is used to describe the bonding or cementation process. Chemical adhesion occurs when atoms or molecules of dissimilar substances bond together and differs from cohesion in which attraction among atoms and molecules of like (similar) materials holds them together.

Adhesive: An intermediate material that causes two materials to stick together.

Agar: A powder derived from seaweed that is a major component of reversible hydrocolloid.

Air Polishing: the process of polishing or finishing using fine particles with air pressure to remove biofilm and stain for enamel surfaces and in pits and fissures; an alternative to prophy pastes. Air polishing uses soft particles (Mohs ranking of 3) and an air pressure of approximately 40 to 60 pounds per square inch (psi).

Air Abrasion or Microabrasion: like air polishing but using greater air pressure (40 to 160 psi) and harder particles (aluminum oxide; Mohs harness ranking of 9). Used to cleanse cast appliances before cementation, repair porcelain and composite restorations, prepare tooth surfaces before bonding, and cut tooth structure for restorative preparations.

Alginate: A versatile, irreversible hydrocolloid impression material that is used most often in the dental office; however, it lacks the accuracy and fine surface detail needed for impressions for crown and bridge procedures.

All-ceramic restoration: Ceramic restorations with no metal core.

Allograft: tissue taken from a donor (usually deceased) for grafting in another human

Alloplast: synthetic graft material

Alloy: A mixture of two or more metals.

Alloy, admixed: A mixture of lathe-cut and spherical alloys for amalgam.

Alloy, base metal: An alloy that comprises non-noble metals.

Alloy, high noble: An alloy that contains at least 60% noble metals, 40% of which must be gold.

Alloy, lathe-cut: Irregularly shaped particles formed by shaving fine particles from an alloy ingot for amalgam.

Alloy, noble: An alloy that comprises metals that do not corrode readily.

Alloy, porcelain bonding: Special casting alloy manufactured for its compatibility with porcelain that has been bonded to it at high temperature.

Alloy, spherical: Alloy particles produced as small spheres for amalgam.

Alloy, wrought metal: An alloy that has been mechanically changed into another form to improve its properties.

Amalgam, dental: Restorative material that comprises silver-based alloy mixed with mercury.

Amalgamation: A reaction that occurs when silver-based alloy is mixed with mercury.

Amalgam separator: a device that collects amalgam particles and mercury from evacuation systems that might otherwise escape into the wastewater and therefore enter the environment

Anneal: To modify physical properties of a metal by heating it.

Antibacterial mouth rinse: A liquid used to rinse the oral cavity to reduce or suppress bacteria associated with dental caries or periodontal disease.

Autograft: graft tissue harvested from the patient's own body

Barrier Membrane: protective membrane that prevents the in-growth of fibrous connective tissue into a graft site and also holds the graft material in place

Base: A thick layer of cement used in a cavity preparation to protect the pulp from chemical insult or to act as a thermal insulator and to support restorations in deep cavity preparations.

Base-Metal Alloy: alloy composed of non-noble metals which corrode more readily

Bioactive Dental Materials: materials that interact with living tissue and are used to remineralize and repair dentin.

Bio-aerosol: A cloud-like mist that contains droplets, tooth dust, materials dust, and bacteria of a particle size smaller than 5 μm in diameter.

Biocompatible: The property of a material that allows it not to impede or adversely affect living tissue.

Bite registration: An impression of the occlusal relationship of opposing teeth in centric occlusion (patient's normal bite).

Bleaching: A cosmetic process that uses chemicals to remove discolorations from teeth or to lighten them.

Bond or bonding: To connect or fasten; to bind (*Webster's New World Dictionary*). Basically, items are joined together at the surface in two ways: by mechanical adhesion (physical interlocking) and by chemical adhesion.

Bonding agent: A low-viscosity resin that penetrates porosities and irregularities in the surface of the tooth or restoration created by acid etching, for the purpose of facilitating bonding.

Brittleness: Hard and likely to break or crack.

Buildup: A restorative material such as amalgam, composite resin, or glass ionomer cement that is used to replace missing tooth structure in a badly broken-down tooth and to act as support for a restoration such as a crown.

CAD/CAM: Computer-assisted design/computer-assisted machining technology that uses a scanning device to capture an image of the preparation and integrates it with computer software to design and cut restorations from blocks of dental materials.

Calcium hydroxide: Used as a low-strength base and a direct pulp-capping material to stimulate secondary dentin formation.

Cariogenic: Substances or microorganisms that promote dental caries.

Casts: Hard replicas of hard and soft tissue of the patient's oral cavity made from gypsum products. They are also referred to as *models*.

Ceramics: Materials composed of inorganic metal oxide compounds, including porcelain and similar ceramic materials that require baking at high temperature to fuse small particles together to form the restoration, or a pre-formed ceramic block from which the restoration is milled using CAD/CAM techniques.

Chemical-set materials: Materials that set through a timed chemical reaction with the combination of a catalyst and base.

Chroma: The intensity or strength of a color (e.g., a bold yellow has more chroma than a pastel yellow).

Cleaning: The removal of soft deposits from the surface of restorations and tooth structure. Polishing and cleaning are done to remove surface stains and soft deposits from the clinical crowns and exposed root surfaces of teeth after all hard deposits are removed. Aside from abrasives, there are also chemical cleaning products that are used primarily for removable prostheses.

Coefficient of thermal expansion (CTE): The measurement of change of volume or length in relationship to change in temperature.

Colloid: Glue-like material composed of two or more substances in which one substance does not go into solution but is suspended within another substance. It has at least two phases: a liquid phase called a sol and a semisolid phase called a gel.

Compomer: A composite resin that has polyacid, fluoride-releasing groups added.

Composite, dual-cured: Composite that contains components of light-cured and self-cured composites. When the two parts are mixed together, it polymerizes by a chemical reaction that can be accelerated with blue light activation.

Composite, flowable: A light-cured, low-viscosity composite resin that contains fewer filler particles.

Composite, hybrid: Composite that contains both macrofiller and microfiller particles to obtain the strength of a macrofill and the polishability of a microfill.

Composite, light-cured: Composite that polymerizes when a chemical is activated by light in the blue wave range.

Composite, macrofilled: An early generation of composite that contained filler particles ranging from 10 to 100 μm.

Composite, microfilled: Composite that contains very small filler particles averaging 0.04 μm in diameter.

Composite, packable: A light-cured, highly viscous, heavily filled composite resin for dentists who use a placement technique with composite that is similar to that of amalgam.

Composite resin: Direct-placement tooth-colored material that comprises an organic resin matrix and inorganic filler particles.

Composite, self-cured: Composite that polymerizes by a chemical reaction when two resins are mixed together.

Compressive force: Force applied to compress an object.

Condensation silicone: A silicone rubber impression material that sets by linking of molecules in long chains but produces a liquid by-product through condensation.

Contamination: Contact with a substance that changes the chemical or mechanical properties (e.g., contamination of the etched surface of the tooth with saliva before bonding).

Coping: A thin covering like a thimble that serves as a substructure for a porcelain-bonded-to-metal crown.

Corrosion: Deterioration of a metal caused by a chemical attack or electrochemical reaction with dissimilar metals in the presence of a solution containing electrolytes (such as saliva).

Corrosive: Usually an acid or strong base that can cause damage to skin, clothing, metals, and equipment.

Creep: Gradual change in the shape of a restoration caused by compression from occlusion or adjacent teeth and can cause amalgam to bulge out of the cavity preparation.

Crossbite Corrector: a fixed or removable appliance used to correct teeth in mal-alignment where the maxillary teeth are positioned lingual to the mandibular teeth.

Cross-Linked Polymers: adjacent long-chain polymers joined by the bonding of short chains along their sides to enhance the properties of the polymer

Crown: an indirect restoration that covers all or part of the coronal tooth structure (extracoronal) and is composed of metal, ceramic or a combination of the two.

Cure or polymerization: A reaction that links low molecular weight resin molecules (monomers) together into high molecular weight chains (polymers) that harden or set. The reaction can be initiated by strictly a chemical reaction (self-cured), by light in the blue wave range (light-cured), by a combination of the two (dual-cured), or by heat.

Custom-made: Made specifically to fit one individual.

Delayed Expansion: expansion of amalgam containing zinc when it is contaminated with moisture (e.g., saliva) during condensation.

Demineralization: The action usually caused by acids that removes minerals from the tooth.

Density: The measure of the weight of a material compared with its volume.

Dental amalgam: Restorative material composed of silver-based alloy mixed with mercury.

Dental caries: A process whereby bacteria in plaque metabolize carbohydrates and produce acids that remove minerals from teeth and permit bacteria to invade.

Dental stone: A stronger, less porous form of gypsum product used in dentistry.

Depth of Cure: the depth to which light from a curing unit can penetrate and cure composite resin

Desensitizing agent: A chemical that seals open dentinal tubules to reduce tooth sensitivity to air, sweets, and temperature changes.

Diagnostic casts: casts generally made from dental plaster or stone and used for patient education, treatment planning, and tracking the progress of treatment, as with orthodontic models; these casts are also known as *study models*.

Dies: Replicas of the prepared teeth that are generally removable from the working cast.

Die stone: The densest form of gypsum product used in dentistry.

Digital Impression: detailed digital images of the preparation, surrounding and opposing teeth, and tissues taken by a digital scanner for the purpose of making a restoration

Dimensional change: A change in the size of matter. For dental materials, this usually manifests as expansion caused by heating and contraction caused by cooling.

Direct fabrication: Provisional restorations made directly inside the patient's mouth.

Direct restorative materials: Restorations placed directly into cavity preparations.

Dual set materials: Materials that polymerize by a chemical reaction that occurs when the material is mixed with a catalyst or that is initiated by exposure to blue light (or by a combination of chemical or light reaction).

Dual-cured composite: Composite that contains components of light-cured and self-cured composites. When the two parts are mixed together, it polymerizes by a chemical reaction that can be accelerated by blue light activation.

Ductility: The ability of an object to be pulled or stretched under tension without rupture.

Edge strength: The ability of a material to withstand fracture at a thin edge such as at the margins of a restoration.

Elastic deformation: deformation of a material that recovers its original shape and size when the force is removed

Elasticity: The ability of a material to recover its shape completely after deformation from an applied force.

Elastic Limit: the greatest stress a structure can withstand without permanent deformation

Elastic Modulus (also called Young's Modulus): a measure of the stiffness of a material; the higher the elastic modulus the stiffer the material

Elastomers: Highly accurate elastic impression materials that have qualities similar to rubber. They are used extensively in indirect restorative techniques, such as crown and bridge procedures.

Enamel Microabrasion: a process that uses hydrochloric acid and an abrasive such as pumice to remove shallow discolorations of the enamel.

Endosseous (endosteal) implant: Implant placed into the bone.

Erosion: The loss of tooth mineral caused by dietary or gastric acids, not by bacterial metabolism (caries process).

Esthetic materials, direct placement: Tooth-colored materials that can be placed directly into the cavity preparation without being constructed outside of the mouth first.

Esthetic materials, indirect placement: Tooth-colored materials that are used to construct restorations outside of the mouth on replicas of the prepared teeth in the dental laboratory or at chairside. Later, they are cemented to the teeth.

Etch-and-Rinse (also called Total-Etch) Technique: a clinical technique that includes etching of both enamel and dentin as a separate step from the application of bonding agents

Etching or conditioning: Terms used interchangeably to describe the process of preparing the surface of a tooth or a restoration for bonding. The most common etching material (etchant) used is phosphoric acid.

Excess residue: A wax film that remains on an object after the wax is removed.

Exothermic reaction: The production of heat resulting from the reactions of the components of some materials when they are mixed.

Extracoronal restoration: A restoration that covers all or part of the external surface of the tooth and may extend over the cusp tips on facial or lingual surfaces such as onlays, ¾ crown, full crowns, and veneers.

Extrinsic stains: Stains that occur on the tooth surface.

Fatigue failure: A fracture that results from repeated stresses that produce microscopic flaws that grow.

Film thickness: The minimum thickness obtainable by a layer of a material. It is particularly important to dental cements.

Final Impression: a detailed impression of oral structures used to make an accurate cast from which restorations or prostheses are made

Final set time: The time needed for the reaction that begins when the material is mixed to go to completion, and the material hardens to its permanent state .

Finish line: The continuous margin that borders the preparation to which the restoration is fit or finished.

Finishing: A procedure used to reduce excess restorative material to develop appropriate occlusion and contour. This usually is done with rotary instruments. Finishing removes surface blemishes and produces a smooth surface.

Firing: A process of heating porcelain at high temperature until it fuses.

Flash: Feather-like excess of material that extends beyond the cavity margins.

Flash point: The lowest temperature at which the vapor of a volatile substance will ignite with a flash. A low flash point means that a substance can catch fire very easily.

Flexural stress: Bending caused by a combination of tension and compression.

Flow: The movement of the wax as it approaches the melting range.

Flowable composite: A light-cured, low-viscosity composite resin that contains fewer filler particles.

Fluorapatite: A tooth mineral that results when fluoride is incorporated into hydroxyapatite.

Fluoride: A naturally occurring chemical that helps to protect tooth structure from dental caries.

Fluorosis: Enamel abnormality caused by consumption of excessive levels of fluoride.

Free radical: A reactive group on one end of a monomer that initiates the joining of adjacent monomer molecules to form a polymer.

Galvanism: An electrical current transmitted between two dissimilar metals.

Gamma-2 phase: A chemical reaction between tin in the silver-based alloy and mercury that causes corrosion in the amalgam.

Gauge: A measure of the thickness of a wire. For example, an 8-gauge wire is thicker than a 16-gauge wire.

Gel: A semisolid state in which colloidal particles form a framework that traps liquid (e.g., Jell-O).

Glass ionomer: A self-cured, tooth-colored, fluoride-releasing restorative material that bonds to tooth structure without an additional bonding agent.

Glass ionomer cement: One of the most versatile cements; used as a permanent luting agent and restorative material, and for low- and high-strength base and core buildups.

Glazing: Firing porcelain at high temperature to achieve a smooth, shiny surface.

Grit: The particle size of the abrasive, typically classified as coarse, medium, fine, and superfine.

Gypsum: A material found in nature and composed of the dihydrate of calcium sulfate; used to make dental casts and dies.

Hardness: The resistance of a solid to penetration.

Hazardous chemicals: a chemical that can cause burns to the skin, eyes, lungs, etc. poisonous or can cause fire.

Heat-pressing: Pressing molten ceramic material into a mold at high temperature and pressure

Hue: The color of the tooth or restoration. It may include a mixture of colors, such as yellow-brown.

Hybrid composite: Composite that contains both macrofill and microfill particles to obtain the strength of a macrofill and the polishability of a microfill.

Hybrid (resin-modified) glass ionomer: A glass ionomer to which resin has been added to improve its physical properties.

Hybrid layer: A resin/dentin layer formed by the penetration of the dentin bonding resin through collagen fibrils exposed by acid etching and into the etched dentin surface. It serves as an excellent resin-rich layer onto which the restorative material, such as composite resin, can be bonded.

Hydrocolloid: Glue-like material that comprises two or more substances in which one substance does not go into solution but is suspended within another substance. It has at least two phases: (1) a liquid phase called a sol and (2) a semisolid phase called a gel.

Hydrocolloid, irreversible: An impression material that is mixed to a sol state, and as it sets, it is converted to a gel by a chemical reaction that irreversibly changes its nature.

Hydrocolloid, reversible: An impression material that can be heated to change a gel into a fluid sol state that can flow around the teeth, then cooled to gel again to make an impression of the shapes of the oral structures.

Hydrodynamic theory of tooth sensitivity: Pain caused by movement of pulpal fluid in open (unsealed) dentinal tubules. Actions that cause a change in pressure on the fluid within the dentinal tubules stimulate nerve fibers in the processes of odontoblasts in the pulp to send out a pain response.

Hydrophilic: An attribute that allows a material to tolerate the presence of moisture.

Hydrophobic: An attribute that does not allow a material to tolerate or perform well in the presence of moisture.

Hysteresis: The property of a material to have two different temperatures for melting and solidifying, unlike water, which has one temperature for both.

Ignitable: A material or chemical that can erupt into fire easily.

Imbibition: The act of absorbing moisture.

Implant, endosseous (endosteal): Implant placed into the bone.

Implant, subperiosteal: Implant placed on top of the bone and under the periosteum.

Implant, transosteal: Implant that penetrates entirely through the bone.

Impression compound: An impression material that comprises resin and wax with fillers added to make it stronger and more stable than wax.

Impression plaster: An impression material that comprises a gypsum product similar to plaster of paris.

Incremental Placement: a technique for composites that places and cures small increments individually to reduce the overall polymerization shrinkage and shrinkage stress in the restoration and permit curing throughout the increment

Indirect fabrication: Construction of provisional or final restorations on a cast outside the patient's mouth.

Indirect restorative materials: Materials used to fabricate restorations outside the mouth that are subsequently placed into the mouth.

Indirect-placement esthetic materials: Tooth-colored materials that are used to construct restorations outside of the mouth in the dental laboratory or at chairside on replicas of the prepared teeth. They are later cemented to the teeth.

Initial set time: The time at which the material can no longer be manipulated within the mouth and coincides with the end of working time.

Inorganic filler particles: Fine particles of quartz, silica, or glass that give strength and wear resistance to the material.

Insulators: Materials that have low thermal conductivity.

Interface: The space between the walls of the preparation and the restoration.

Intermediate: Materials expected to last from a few weeks to a year.

Intracoronal restoration: A restoration within the crown of the tooth, such as an inlay.

Intraoral Scanner: a type of camera that takes digital images (typically in continuous video form) of oral structures for CAD/CAM procedures, such as crown preparations.

Intrinsic stains: Stains that are incorporated into the tooth structure, usually during the tooth's development.

Irreversible hydrocolloid: An alginate impression material that is mixed to a sol state and as it sets converts to a gel by a chemical reaction that irreversibly changes its nature.

Light-activated materials: Materials that require light in the blue wave range to initiate a reaction.

Light-cured composite: Composite that polymerizes when a chemical is activated by light in the blue wave range.

Liner: A thin layer of material used to protect the pulp from the chemical components of dental materials and microleakage, to stimulate reparative dentin, or to act as a pulp capping.

Lost wax casting technique: a technique for fabricating a metal restoration by encasing the wax pattern in stone then vaporizing the wax under high temperatures to leave an empty impression space (pattern) once occupied by the wax; Molten metal is then cast into the space and takes the shape of the pattern.

Luting: To cement two components together such as an indirect restoration cemented on or in a tooth (e.g., inlays, crowns, bridges, veneers, orthodontic bracket and bands, posts and pins).

Macrofilled composite: An early generation of composite that contained filler particles ranging from 10 to 100 μm.

Malleability: The ability to be compressed and formed into a thin sheet without rupture.

Margination: A procedure for removal of excessive restorative material from margins of restorations.

Safety Data Sheet (SDS): printed product report from the manufacturer that contains important information about the chemicals, hazards, cleanup, and special PPE related to a product.

Melting range: A range of melting points of the individual components of the wax.

Microfilled composite: Composite that contains very small filler particles averaging 0.04 μm in diameter.

Microleakage: Leakage of fluid and bacteria caused by microscopic gaps that occur at the interface of the tooth and the restoration margins.

Mixing time: The amount of time allotted to bring the components of a material together into a homogeneous mix.

Model plaster: The weakest, most porous form of gypsum product used in dentistry.

Monomer: small organic molecules that are joined in long chains to form polymers. As used in dentistry, monomers are usually liquids.

Mouth guard: A hard or pliable resin that protects teeth from trauma during sports activities or from teeth grinding.

Nitinol: An alloy of nickel and titanium often used for orthodontic wires.

Non-vital tooth: no longer has a living pulp and ceases to give response to electrical stimuli or temperature changes

Opaque: Optical property in which light is completely absorbed by an object.

Organic resin (polymer) matrix: Thick resin liquids made up of two or more organic molecules that form a matrix around filler particles.

Osseointegration: Bone growth in intimate contact with an implant.

Overhang: Excessive restorative material present at the cervical cavosurface margin.

Over-the-counter (OTC): Available in retail or drug stores without a doctor's prescription.

Packable composite: A light-cured, highly viscous, heavily filled composite resin for dentists who use a placement technique with a composite that is similar to that of amalgam.

Palatal Expander: a fixed appliance used to expand the maxillary arch forcing the maxillary plates apart very slowly while the maxilla is still in development.

Particulate matter: Very small particles (e.g., dust from dental plaster or stone).

Percolation: Movement of fluid within the microscopic gap of the restoration margin as a result of differences in the expansion and contraction rates of the tooth and the restoration with temperature changes associated with ingestion of cold or hot fluids or foods.

Peri-Implantitis: an infection around an implant that can cause gingival inflammation and loss of bone around the implant

Permanent: Lasting indefinitely.

Personal protective equipment (PPE): gloves, masks, gowns, eyewear, and other protective equipment for the employee.

Pigments: Coloring agents that give composites their color.

Plastic deformation: deformation of a material causing permanent changes in size or shape due to an applied force

Plasticizer: Liquid added to acrylic resin to soften it and make it more pliable.

Polishing: A procedure that produces a shiny, smooth surface by eliminating fine scratches, minor surface imperfections, and surface stains using mild abrasives frequently found in the form of pastes or compounds.

Poly (methyl methacrylate): A polymer that comprises numerous methyl methacrylate monomers linked together into a long chain.

Polyether: A rubber impression material with ether functional groups. It has high accuracy and is popular for crown and bridge procedures.

Polymer: A long-chain, high molecular weight molecule produced by the linking of many low molecular weight monomer molecules.

Polymerization: The act of forming polymers by joining monomers end-to-end.

Polymerization, addition: A common form of polymerization of dental materials. Monomer molecules are added to one another sequentially as the reactive group on one molecule initiates bonding with an adjacent monomer molecule and frees another reactive group to repeat the process.

Polymers, cross-linked: The joining of adjacent long-chain polymers by bonding of short chains along their sides.

Polysulfide: A rubber impression material that has sulfur-containing (mercaptan) functional groups.

Polyvinyl siloxane (also referred to as vinyl polysiloxane): Very accurate addition silicone elastomer impression material. It is used extensively for crown and bridge procedures because of its accuracy, dimensional stability, and ease of use.

Porcelain: A tooth-colored ceramic material that comprises crystals of feldspar, alumina, and silica that are fused together at high temperatures to form a hard, uniform, glass-like material.

Porcelain-metal restorations: Restorations that have a metal core over which porcelain is fused at high temperature.

Porosity: Numerous microscopic holes or voids within a material often caused during polymerization of resins when a monomer vaporizes and is lost.

Post: A metal or nonmetal dowel placed within the root canal to retain a core buildup.

Post, active: A post that engages the root canal surface like a screw.

Post, custom: A post cast to fit precisely within the root canal space; it usually has the core attached.

Post, passive: A post that sits within the prepared canal space but does not engage the root surface.

Post, pre-formed: A factory-made post supplied in several sizes.

Pouring: *pouring the cast* refers to the process of vibrating the flowable gypsum product into the impression; this process must produce a cast that is the exact replica of the structures captured in the impression.

Power whitening: in-office whitening procedure that uses strong whitening agents and may use a high-intensity light source to accelerate the whitening process.

Precious metal: The classification of metal based upon its high cost.

Preliminary Impression: an impression of the dentition or edentulous arch and surrounding tissues taken as a precursor to other treatment; often used to make casts (models) of oral structures for planning, and to construct custom trays or provisional restorations

Prevention/preventive aids: Chemicals, devices, or procedures that reduce or eliminate disease or tooth destruction in the oral cavity.

Primary bonds: The strongest bonds that hold atoms together because they involve the exchanging or sharing of electrons.

Primary consistency: Less-viscous mix of material that flows easily, can be drawn to a 1-inch string with a spatula when lifted from the center of its mass, and is suitable for luting.

Proportional limit: The greatest stress a structure can withstand without permanent deformation.

Prosthesis: A device used for the replacement of missing tissues. It can serve both cosmetic and functional roles.

Provisional coverage: A restoration that temporarily occupies the place of a permanent restoration, typically for up to 2 to 3 weeks. In the case of implant and complex prosthodontic and periodontally involved cases, provisional restorations may be used to last for extended periods of time. These restorations are also commonly referred to as temporaries.

Reactive: Ability of a substance to take part in a chemical reaction, resulting in a different end product.

Remineralization: process that replaces mineral lost from the tooth by an acid attack.

Resilience: The resistance of a material to permanent deformation.

Resin-based cement: Modified composite used to bond ceramic indirect restorations, conventional crowns and bridges, and orthodontic brackets.

Restorative agents: Materials used to reconstruct tooth structure.

Retention: A material's ability to maintain its position without displacement under stress.

Sealant: A protective coating usually composed of resin that is bonded to enamel to protect pits and fissures from dental caries.

Secondary bonds: The weaker bond that holds atoms together. Unlike with primary bonds, there is no transfer or sharing of electrons.

Secondary consistency: Thick, putty-like, condensable mix of material that can be rolled into a ball or rope and is suitable for use as an insulating base.

Sedative: To soothe or act in a sedative manner; to relieve pain.

Selective etching: technique where enamel is etched first with phosphoric acid prior to the application of self-etch acidic primers that lack sufficient acidity to produce a good etch of the enamel

Self-cured composite: Composite that polymerizes by a chemical reaction when two resins are mixed together.

Self-etch system: A bonding system that does not use a separate etching procedure with phosphoric acid. The acid is contained in the resin primer and no rinsing is needed.

Shearing force: Force applied when two surfaces slide against each other or in a twisting or rotating motion.

Shelf life: The useful life of a material before it deteriorates or changes in quality.

Silane coupling agent: A chemical that helps to bind the filler particles to the organic matrix.

Silicone, addition: A silicone rubber impression material that sets by linking of molecules in long chains but produces no by-product. It is commonly known as polyvinyl siloxane and is the most popular material for crown and bridge procedures because of its accuracy, dimensional stability, and ease of use.

Silicone, condensation: A silicone rubber impression material that sets by linking of molecules in long chains but produces a liquid by-product through condensation.

Sintering: Fusion of ceramic particles at their borders by heating them to the point that they just start to melt.

Slip-casting: Process whereby ceramic powder is mixed with a water-based liquid to form a mass or slip. The slip is pressed into a form and is baked at high temperature.

Smear layer: A tenacious layer of debris on the enamel or dentin surface resulting from cutting the tooth during cavity preparation. It comprises fine particles of cut tooth structure, bacteria, and salivary components.

Soft liner, long-term: A soft material that lines a denture for use in patients who have problems with hard-acrylic denture bases. It is expected to last 1 to 3 years.

Soft liner, short-term: A soft provisional material that lines a denture for a short period of time to improve tissue health. It is also called a tissue conditioner, and it typically lasts from a few days to a few weeks.

Sol: A liquid state in which colloidal particles are suspended. Through cooling or by chemical reaction, it can change into a gel.

Solder: An alloy used to join two metals together or to repair cast metal restorations.

Solubility: Susceptible to being dissolved.

Splatter: Small particles that may contain blood, saliva, oral particulate matter, water, and microbes.

Stiffness: A material's resistance to deformation.

Strain: Distortion or deformation that occurs when an object cannot resist a stress.

Stress: The internal force, which resists the applied force.

Subperiosteal implant: Implant placed on top of the bone and under the periosteum.

Substantivity: Property of a material to have a prolonged therapeutic effect after its initial use.

Surface energy: The electrical charge that attracts atoms to a surface.

Surfactant: A chemical that lowers the surface tension of a substance so it is more readily wetted. For example, oil beads on the surface of water, but soap acts as a surfactant to allow the oil to spread over the surface.

Sutures: natural or synthetic material with the appearance of thread used to hold tissues together or to reposition tissues after trauma or surgical procedures. They can be absorbable (sutures broken down naturally by the body's enzymes and absorbed) or non-absorbable (sutures made of materials that are not broken down by the body and require removal by a dental professional)

Syneresis: A characteristic of gels to contract and squeeze out some liquid, which then accumulates on the surface.

Tarnish: Discoloration that results from oxidation of a thin layer of metal at its surface. It is not as destructive as corrosion.

Temporary/Provisional: Materials expected to last from a few days to a few weeks.

Tensile force: Force applied in opposite directions to stretch an object.

Therapeutic agents: Materials used to treat disease.

Thermal conductivity: The rate at which heat flows through a material.

Thixotropic: a characteristic of some gels and liquids to flow more readily under mechanical force such as mixing, stirring or shaking.

Thumb Sucking Device: a fixed or removable appliance used to discourage tongue thrusting and thumb sucking

Total-etch (also called Etch and Rinse) system: A bonding system that includes etching of both enamel and dentin as a separate step from the application of bonding agents.

Toughness: The ability of a material to resist fracture.

Toxicity: The strength of a product or a of a chemical to cause damage to the body.

Translucency: Varying degrees of light passing through and being absorbed by an object.

Transosteal implant: Implant that penetrates entirely through the bone.

Transparent: Light passing directly through an object.

Trimming: The process of removing excess hardened gypsum from the cast for ease in working with the cast and for appearance in presentation.

Triturator (amalgamator): A mechanical device used to mix silver-based alloy particles with mercury to produce amalgam.

Ultimate strength: The maximum amount of stress a material can withstand without breaking.

Universal Bonding System: a bonding system capable of bonding to tooth structure as well as most restorative dental materials.

Value: How light or dark a color is. A low value is darker and a high value is brighter.

Varnish: A thin layer placed on the floor and walls of the cavity preparation to seal the dentinal tubules and minimize microleakage.

Veneer: Thin layer of ceramic or composite resin material that is bonded to the fronts of teeth to improve their appearance.

Viscosity: The ability of a liquid material to flow.

Vital tooth: has a living pulp, which produces response to temperature change or electrical stimuli.

Vitality: A life-like quality.

Walking bleach technique: whitening technique for non-vital teeth in which whitening materials are sealed inside the tooth crown for a few days and the patient "walks" around with the whitening material in place.

Water sorption: The ability to absorb moisture.

Wax pattern: A duplicate of the restoration carved in wax.

Wet dentin bonding: Bonding to dentin that is kept moist after acid etching to facilitate penetration of bonding resins into etched dentin.

Wetting: The ability of a liquid to wet or intimately contact a solid surface. Water beading on a waxed car is an example of poor wetting.

Working casts: Casts generally made from one of the dental stones and strong enough to resist the stresses of fabricating an indirect restoration or prosthesis; these casts are also known as *master casts or working models.*

Working time: The lapse of time from the start of mixing the material until it begins to harden and is no longer workable because it has reached its initial set

Xenograft: graft tissue taken from an animal (usually bovine) for use in a human

Yield strength: The amount of stress at which a substance deforms.

Yield stress: the stress at which plastic deformation begins; also called yield point on a stress-strain curve.

Young's Modulus or Elastic Modulus: measures the resistance of a material to being deformed or its stiffness.

Zinc oxide eugenol: A hard and brittle impression material used in complete denture procedures. A variation of this material is used as a provisional filling material.

Zinc oxide eugenol cement: A cement generally used as a provisional material or to temporarily cement provisional coverage.

Zinc phosphate cement: The oldest of the cements; used primarily for permanent luting.

Zinc polycarboxylate cement: The first cement developed with adhesive bonds; used primarily for permanent luting.

Index

Note: Page numbers by *f* indicate figures; *t,* indicate tables, and *b* indicate boxes.